Atlas of Deep Endometriosis

Alice Brandão • Claudio Peixoto Crispi
Marco Aurelio Pinho Oliveira

Atlas of Deep Endometriosis

MRI and Laparoscopic Correlations

Springer

Alice Brandão, MD
Fonte Imagem Clinic and Felippe Mattoso Clinic
Rio de Janeiro
Brazil

Claudio Peixoto Crispi, MD
São Vicente de Paulo Hospital
Rio de Janeiro
Brazil

Marco Aurelio Pinho Oliveira, MD, PhD
State University of Rio de Janeiro
Rio de Janeiro
Brazil

Original Portuguese edition published by Revinter, Rio de Janeiro, Brasil, 2014
ISBN 978-3-030-10095-7 ISBN 978-3-319-71697-8 (eBook)
https://doi.org/10.1007/978-3-319-71697-8

Printed on acid-free paper

This Springer imprint is published by Springer Nature
The registered company is Springer International Publishing AG
The registered company address is: Gewerbestrasse 11, 6330 Cham, Switzerland

Alice Brandão

As always, in all my books and in my life, I thank my parents and brothers, who have served as an example. To my husband, Rodrigo, and Matheus and Vinícius, my beloved sons, who support me in everything, and to Cida, a part of our family.

I would like to thank all my colleagues and patients for the confidence they have given to my work. Without them, I could not have done this book.

Cláudio Crispi

I would like to thank God for allowing me to participate in the development of minimally invasive surgeries. These techniques have contributed directly to the maintenance of health and to the treatment of our patients with much less trauma.

I would also like to thank my family for all their support and affection and, above all, for understanding the need for my absence in our daily lives.

I thank Dr. Alice Brandão for all her dedication to the study, understanding, and contribution to the diagnosis of endometriosis. Her ability to map the disease contributed greatly to reducing the number of incomplete surgeries.

Finally, I thank all my staff, for all personal and professional support, which allows me the time necessary for the development of surgical practice, research, and teaching of minimally invasive techniques.

Marco Aurelio Pinho de Oliveira

I would like to thank my parents, who, besides preparing me for life, also taught me the basis of gynecology.

To my family, for the happiness they give me and for the joy that I feel in having their understanding, help, and support.

I would also like to thank my patients, who trusted me for their treatment of deep endometriosis.

Foreword

The development of diagnostic imaging methods has brought a great revolution in the treatment of endometriosis, allowing the preoperative mapping of the disease sites and a precise planning of the surgical strategy, especially in cases of deep and intestinal endometriosis. It also allowed us to correctly handle cases in which we did not indicate surgery, as well as the postoperative follow-up of patients treated surgically.

This atlas was developed by highly competent professionals in the diagnosis and treatment of endometriosis, allowing the specialist to have an overview of the diagnosis and treatment of the disease, from the clinical aspects of the diagnosis through imaging and the correlation with surgical and histopathological findings, essential quadrilateral for those who want to deal comprehensively and completely with a disease as prevalent as endometriosis.

To preface this work is a great honor for me. I have known the authors for several years, and I have great respect for Alice, for Cláudio, and for Marco. During the 25 years that I have devoted my life to the research on endometriosis, I believe that this atlas is born in an era of important and growing awareness of the medical and non-medical society about the disease, when we observe a great dissemination of knowledge in this area. The atlas is published at a time when the recognition of Brazilian researchers in this area is increasing worldwide.

I hope you enjoy every detail of this book.

Mauricio S. Abrão, MD, PhD
Department of Obstetrics and Gynecology, Faculty of Medicine
University of São Paulo (USP), São Paulo, Brazil

Human Reproduction Center of the Sírio-Libanês
Hospital, São Paulo, Brazil

Contents

1 Introduction . . . 1
1.1 Location of Deep Endometriosis . . . 2
1.1.1 Pelvic Location . . . 2
1.1.2 Abdominal Location . . . 9
Reference . . . 11

2 Magnetic Resonance Imaging . . . 13
2.1 Technical Aspects . . . 13
2.1.1 Equipment . . . 13
2.2 Protocols . . . 13
2.2.1 Pelvic Endometriosis Protocol . . . 13
2.2.2 T1-Weighted Sequence . . . 14
2.2.3 T2-Weighted Sequence . . . 15
2.3 Endometriosis of the Abdominal Wall . . . 19
2.4 The Preparation of the Patient . . . 21
Reference . . . 23

3 MRI Aspects of Deep Endometriosis . . . 25
3.1 Features of Deep Endometriotic Lesions . . . 25
3.1.1 Morphology . . . 25
3.2 Signal Intensity . . . 35
3.2.1 Predominantly Fibrous Lesions . . . 35
3.2.2 Mixed Lesions (Fibrosis and Glandular Tissue) . . . 36
3.2.3 Lesions with a Prominent Glandular Component . . . 36
3.3 Additional Findings . . . 42
3.3.1 Enhancement Pattern . . . 42
3.3.2 Characterization of Adnexal Lesions . . . 42
3.3.3 Associated Inflammatory Process Identification . . . 45
3.3.4 Improved Identification of a Small Non-hemorrhagic Abdominal Wall Deep Endometriosis . . . 46
References . . . 57

4 Deep Endometriosis by Location . . . 59
4.1 Anterior Compartment . . . 65
4.1.1 Urinary Tract (Bladder and Distal Ureter) . . . 71
4.1.2 Round Ligament . . . 107
4.1.3 Myometrium . . . 122
4.2 Posterior Compartment . . . 134
4.2.1 Retrocervical Region . . . 137
4.2.2 Rectovaginal Space . . . 161
4.2.3 Uterosacral Ligaments . . . 175
4.2.4 Vagina (Posterior Vaginal Fornix) Anatomy . . . 195
4.2.5 Myometrium Anatomy: Posterior Compartment . . . 206

4.2.6 Rectum and Sigmoid . . . 219
4.3 Lateral Compartment . . . 239
4.3.1 Parametrium and Paracolpos Anatomy . . . 240
4.3.2 Ureter . . . 259
4.3.3 The Pelvic Autonomic Nerves: Hypogastric Nerve and Plexus . . . 259
4.3.4 Pelvic Floor . . . 275
4.3.5 Ovarian Fossa . . . 291
4.4 Abdominal Wall . . . 300
4.4.1 Cesarean Scar Line: Umbilicus . . . 300
4.4.2 Inguinal Region or Canal of Nuck . . . 308
4.5 Appendix, Cecum, and Terminal Ileum . . . 313
4.5.1 Anatomy . . . 313
4.5.2 Common Aspects of Endometriosis . . . 313
4.5.3 Clinical Condition . . . 318
4.5.4 MRI and Laparoscopic Findings . . . 318
4.5.5 Comments on Treatment . . . 322
4.5.6 Diaphragm . . . 322
References . . . 325

5 Stratification Risk and Monitoring of Patient by MRI . . . 327
5.1 Patient Risk Stratification . . . 327
References . . . 338

6 Postsurgical Findings in Deep Endometriosis . . . 339
6.1 Endometriosis Postsurgical Aspects . . . 339
6.2 Fibrocicatricial Tissue . . . 341
6.3 Foci of Signal Loss in Surgical Site . . . 343
6.4 Resection of Posterior Vaginal Fornix and Uterine Cervix . . . 345
6.5 Changes in the Parametrium . . . 347
6.6 Colorectal Anastomosis . . . 349
6.7 Complications . . . 351
6.8 Evacuatory Disturbance . . . 352
6.9 Bladder Dysfunction . . . 353
6.10 Rectovaginal Fistula . . . 354
6.11 Residual Lesions/Recurrence . . . 355
6.12 Ovary . . . 358
6.13 Infiltrative Endometriosis . . . 358
References . . . 358

Index . . . 359

Contributors

Brainner Campos Barbosa, MD Permanent Member of the Brazilian College of Radiology, Abdominal Imaging Observership—Hôpitaux Universitaires Paris Nord Val de Seine—Hôpital Beaujon, Beaujon, France

Fellowship in Internal Medicine—Rede D'Or Imaging Center, Rio de Janeiro, Brazil

Current Member and Director of Rio de Janeiro's Society of Radiology, Radiologist of the Fleury Group and of Rede D'Or Imaging Center, Rio de Janeiro, Brazil

Fábio Coelho Barros, MD Specialist in Radiology and Diagnostic Imaging at Pontifical Catholic University, Rio de Janeiro, Brazil

Specialist in Gynecology and Obstetrics—TEGO, Permanent Member of the Brazilian College of Radiology, Physician-Radiologist at Lumic—Santa Teresa Hospital—Petrópolis, Rio de Janeiro, Brazil

Physician-Radiologist at Bronstein Medicine, Rio de Janeiro, Brazil

Leon Cardeman, MD Fellow of the International Academy of Cytology, Member of the International Academy of Pathology, Adjunct Professor of Pathological Anatomy at the Rio de Janeiro Medicine and Surgery School, Rio de Janeiro, Brazil

Alice Brandão Costa Member of the Women Healthcare University Program, Medical Student in the Federal University of Piauí—UFPI, Picos, Piauí, Brazil

Camila da Motta Alves Barros, MD Specialist in Radiology and Diagnostic Imaging at Pontifical Catholic University, Rio de Janeiro, Brazil

Physician-Radiologist Specialist in Women's Imaging at Lumic—Santa Teresa Hospital—Petrópolis, Rio de Janeiro, Brazil

Physician-Radiologist at the IRM—Magnetic Resonance Imaging, Rio de Janeiro, Brazil

Physician-Radiologist at the Alcides Carneiro Hospital—Petrópolis, Rio de Janeiro, Brazil

Denise Campos da Paz Benevenuto, MD Professor of Pathological Anatomy at Gama Filho University, Rio de Janeiro, Brazil

Physician-Pathologist Doctor at the LabCardeman, Rio de Janeiro, Brazil

Fernanda Teixeira Azeredo de Andrade, MD Physician Graduated at Fluminense Federal University (UFF), Medical Residency in Radiology and Diagnostic Imaging at Marcílio Dias Naval Hospital, Rio de Janeiro, Brazil

Fellowship at the Felippe Mattoso Clinic, Rio de Janeiro, Brazil

Tania Maria Nery C. de Andrade, MD Pathologist at H.F.A., Pathologist at the LabCardeman, Course on Cytopathology and on Histology and Cytopathology Stages at Royal Surrey County Hospital and at Epsom District Hospital, Guildford, England

Renata Carneiro Leão Laranjeira, MSc Physician Graduated at Fluminense Federal University, Medical Residency in Radiology and Diagnostic Imaging at Federal University of Rio de Janeiro, Master's Degree in Radiology at Federal University of Rio de Janeiro, Rio de Janeiro, Brazil

Physician-Radiologist at Felippe Mattoso Clinic, Rio de Janeiro, Brazil

Physician-Radiologist at the Rio de Janeiro State Servers' Hospital, Rio de Janeiro, Brazil

Sheila Rochlin, MD Head of the Pathological Anatomy Sector at Fernando Magalhães Municipal Institute of Women, Pathologist at the LabCardeman, Rio de Janeiro, Brazil

1 Introduction

Endometriosis is characterized by the growth of endometrial tissue, containing both glands and stroma, in an ectopic location, outside the uterine limits. Deep endometriosis is a particular form of endometriosis defined when the endometrial tissue infiltrates more than 5 mm into the anatomical structure, either the peritoneal surface or the viscera.

The infiltrative process may have aggressive behavior, involving vital structures such as the bowel, ureter, and bladder, causing ureteral or intestinal stenosis, in addition to the involvement of the pelvic nerves.

Endometriosis is estimated to occur in 6–10% of women, and deep endometriosis is frequent, with 25–30% of patients having this form of presentation [1].

Persistent pelvic pain is frequently associated with this form of deep endometriosis. However, clinical manifestations may vary, and there may be little correlation with the extent of the disease.

Magnetic resonance imaging (MRI) is a noninvasive method with high spatial resolution, which can be used as part of the preoperative workup, allowing mapping of the exact location of deep retroperitoneal lesions, definition of surgical complexity, and appropriate therapeutic planning.

Its main advantage is that it can provide an overall assessment of the pelvis, identifying patients with multifocal disease and extra-pelvic involvement, as well as those with ureteral and intestinal stenosis, and nerve involvement. This MRI atlas provides information which facilitates the planning of one-step surgery. Furthermore, it is possible to characterize the lesion and diagnose associated pathologies such as benign myometrium disease and complex adnexal cysts.

This MRI and laparoscopic atlas was made to guide radiologists and gynecologists in the diagnosis of deep endometriosis, allow adequate preoperative evaluation, and, as a consequence, have a positive impact on treatment planning. It is based on the knowledge of a radiologist and two gynecologists, who each have 20 years' experience in this area and are dedicated to the diagnosis and treatment of endometriosis.

The atlas is divided into the following sections for teaching purposes:

1. Location of deep endometriosis
   This section describes the anatomic compartments: anterior, posterior, and lateral of the pelvis. It also includes aspects of morphology, signal intensity, and enhancement patterns of deep endometriosis in MRI.
2. Technical aspects
   This covers the ideal MRI protocols and the preparation of the patient for this exam.
3. Aspects of deep infiltrative endometriosis in MRI and laparoscopy
   This section is the heart of this atlas and covers the anatomy and common aspects of endometriosis of each site, as well as the clinical, laparoscopic, pathological, and MRI findings. It also includes a brief comment on treatment.
4. Use of MRI in risk stratification and patient monitoring
   The use of MRI can guide the therapy by selecting patients with higher surgical severity. Furthermore, we suggest a proposal for follow-up imaging in deep endometriosis.
5. Postsurgical findings
   With the increase in the surgical treatment of these patients, the radiologist must be prepared to characterize these findings and especially not interpret them as residual lesion.

We expect that the reader, at the end of this atlas, will share the passion that the authors have to work with the female pelvis, and especially with deep endometriosis, and thus positively affect the lives of these patients.

A. Brandão et al., *Atlas of Deep Endometriosis*, https://doi.org/10.1007/978-3-319-71697-8_1

1.1 Location of Deep Endometriosis

Deep endometriosis locations were divided into the pelvic and the abdominal.

1.1.1 Pelvic Location

1.1.1.1 Definition of Compartments

Deep pelvic endometriosis is distributed in three compartments: the anterior, posterior, and lateral (Fig. 1.1).

The central organ of the female pelvis, the uterus, delimits the compartments.

The anterior compartment is defined as the area anterior to the uterus, encompassing the bladder, the ureter, the ureteral ostia, the round ligaments, the anterior myometrium, and the vesicovaginal/vesicocervical space (Fig. 1.2).

The posterior compartment is defined as the area posterior to the uterus, which includes the myometrium, the retrocervical region, the rectovaginal septum, the vagina, the uterosacral ligaments, the rectum, and the sigmoid colon (Fig. 1.3).

The lateral compartment includes the ureters, the parametrium, the paracolpos, the broad ligaments, and the ovarian fossa (Figs. 1.4 and 1.5).

We include a special section on the pelvic floor and nerve involvement.

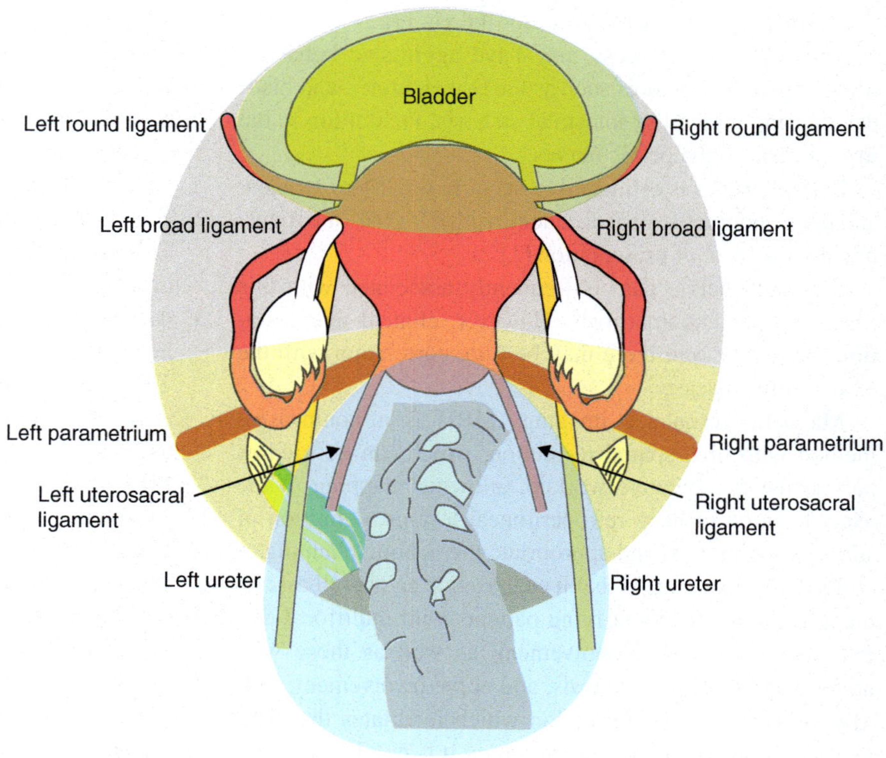

Fig. 1.1 Pelvic endometriosis compartments: anterior, posterior, and lateral, shown in different colors. Note that the left side is on the right, as in the laparoscopic view

Fig. 1.2 Anterior compartment. The area anterior to the uterus, encompassing the bladder, the ureteral ostia (red arrows in **a**), the round ligaments (blue arrows in **e**), the anterior myometrium, the vesicovaginal space (pink arrows in **c**), and the vesicouterine recess (red arrow in **c**). (**b**) Laparoscopic aspect (arrows indicate obliterated vesical umbilical arteries). (**d**) Laparoscopy of normal anterior compartment (arrow indicates round ligament). (**f**) Laparoscopy (arrows indicate round ligaments). (**a, c, e**) T2-weighted sequences. (**a, c**) Sagittal plane. (**e**) Short axis (coronal)

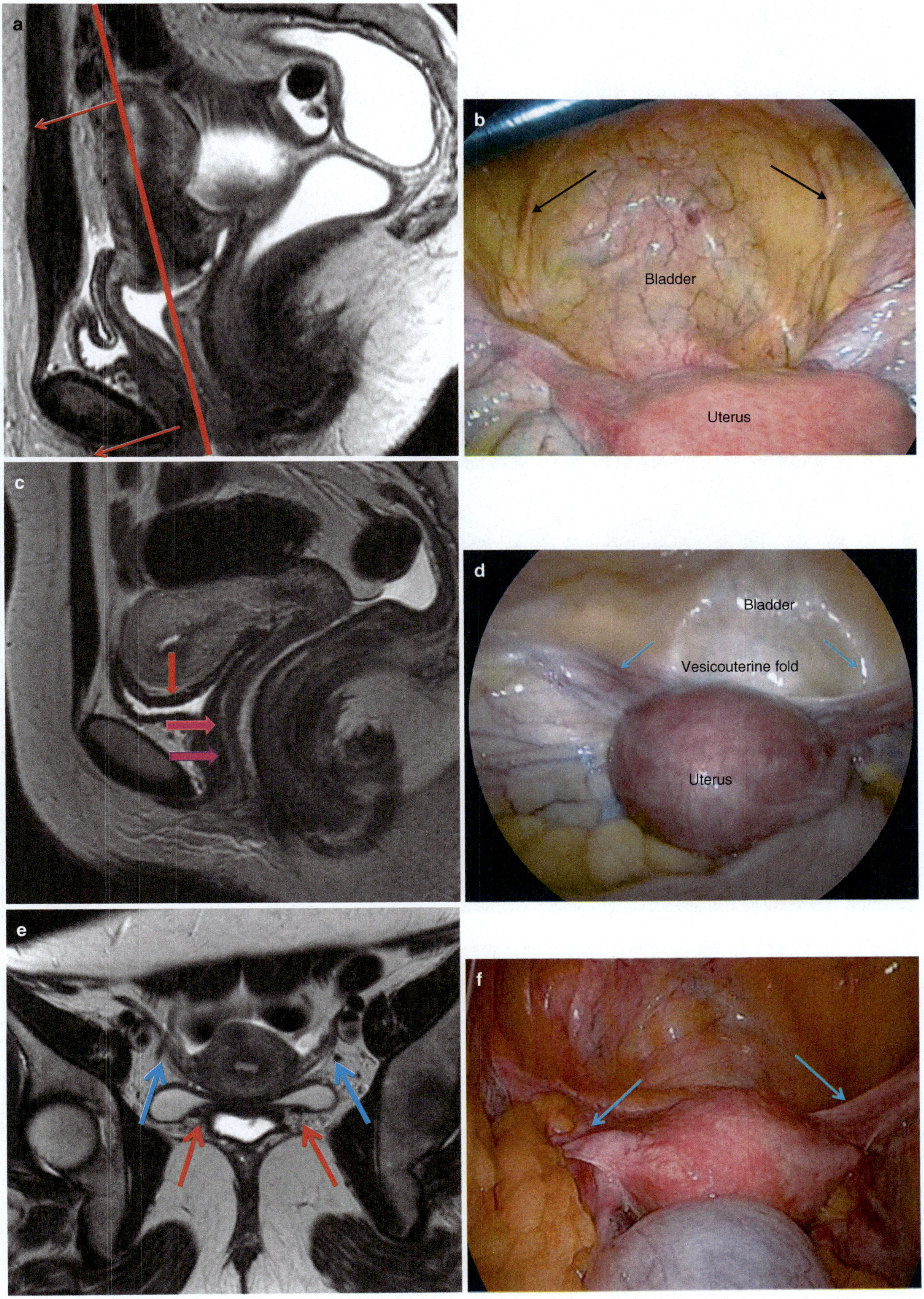
a
b
Bladder
Uterus
c
d
Bladder
Vesicouterine fold
Uterus
e
f

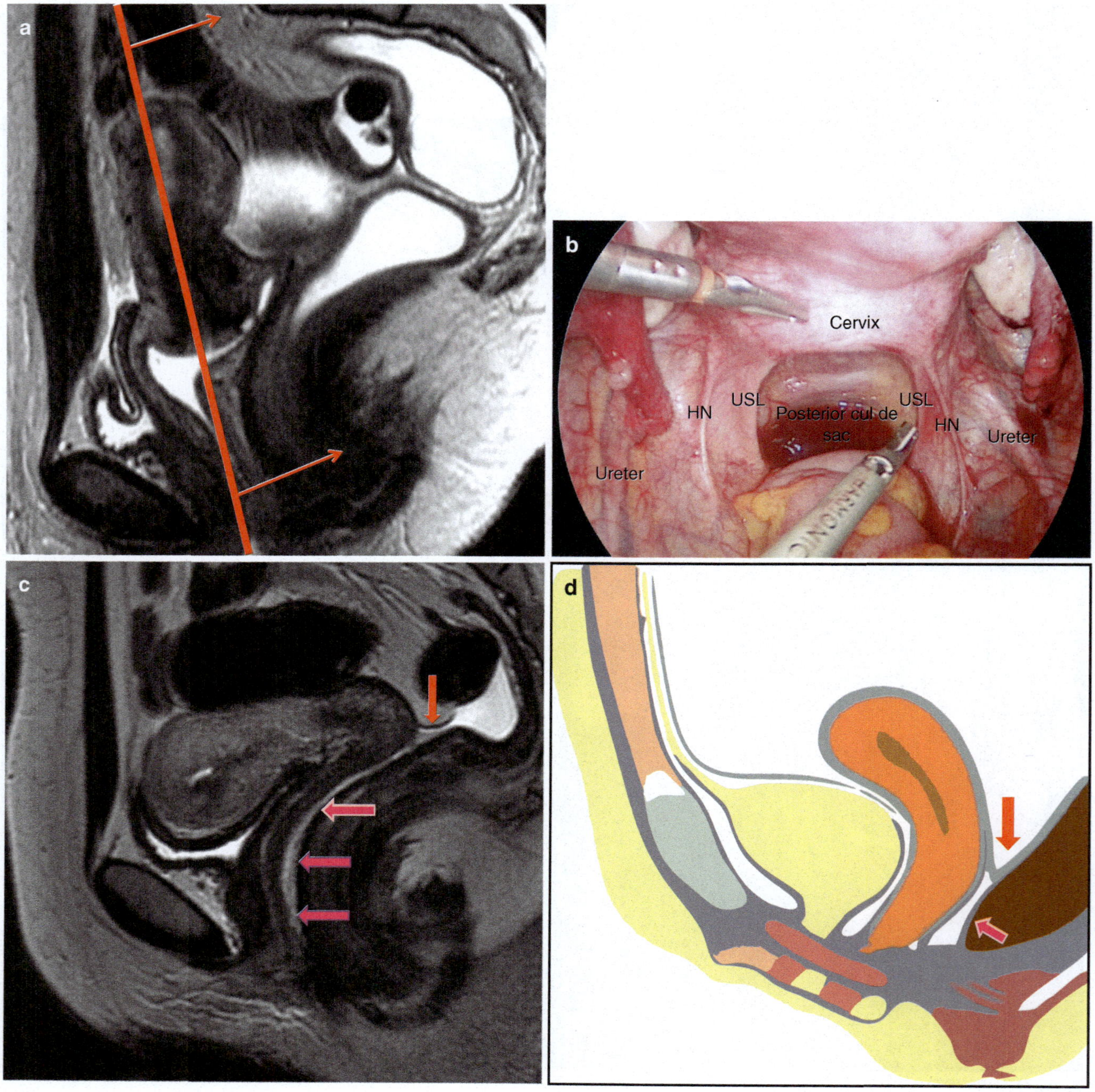

Fig. 1.3 Posterior compartment. The area posterior of the uterus, including the myometrium, retrocervical region, the rectovaginal septum (pink arrows in **c**, **d**), the vagina, the uterosacral ligaments (blue arrows in **e**), the posterior cul-de-sac (red arrow in **c**, **d**, **e**), the rectum (green arrow in **e**), and the distal sigmoid. (**a**, **c**, **e**, **g**, **h**) T2-weighted sequences. (**a**, **c**, **g**, **h**) Sagittal. (**e**) Axial. Note that the red line in the right paramedian axial plane (**g**) represents the plane of the uterosacral ligament in the sagittal plane (**h**). (**b**) Laparoscopy. *USL* uterosacral ligaments. *HN* hypogastric nerve. (**d**) Diagram. (**f**) Laparoscopy. View of the posterior compartment and its components

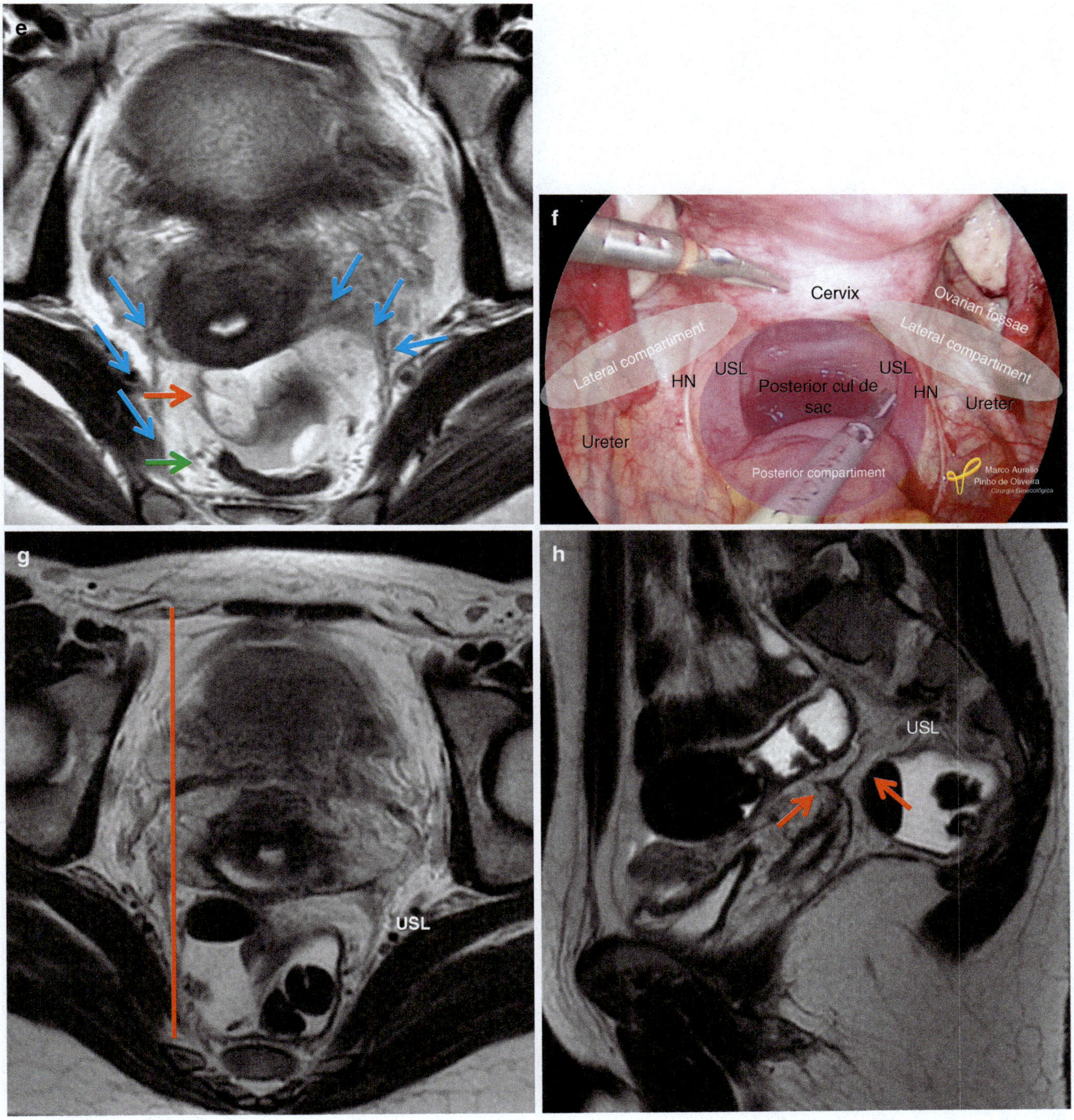

Fig. 1.3 (continued)

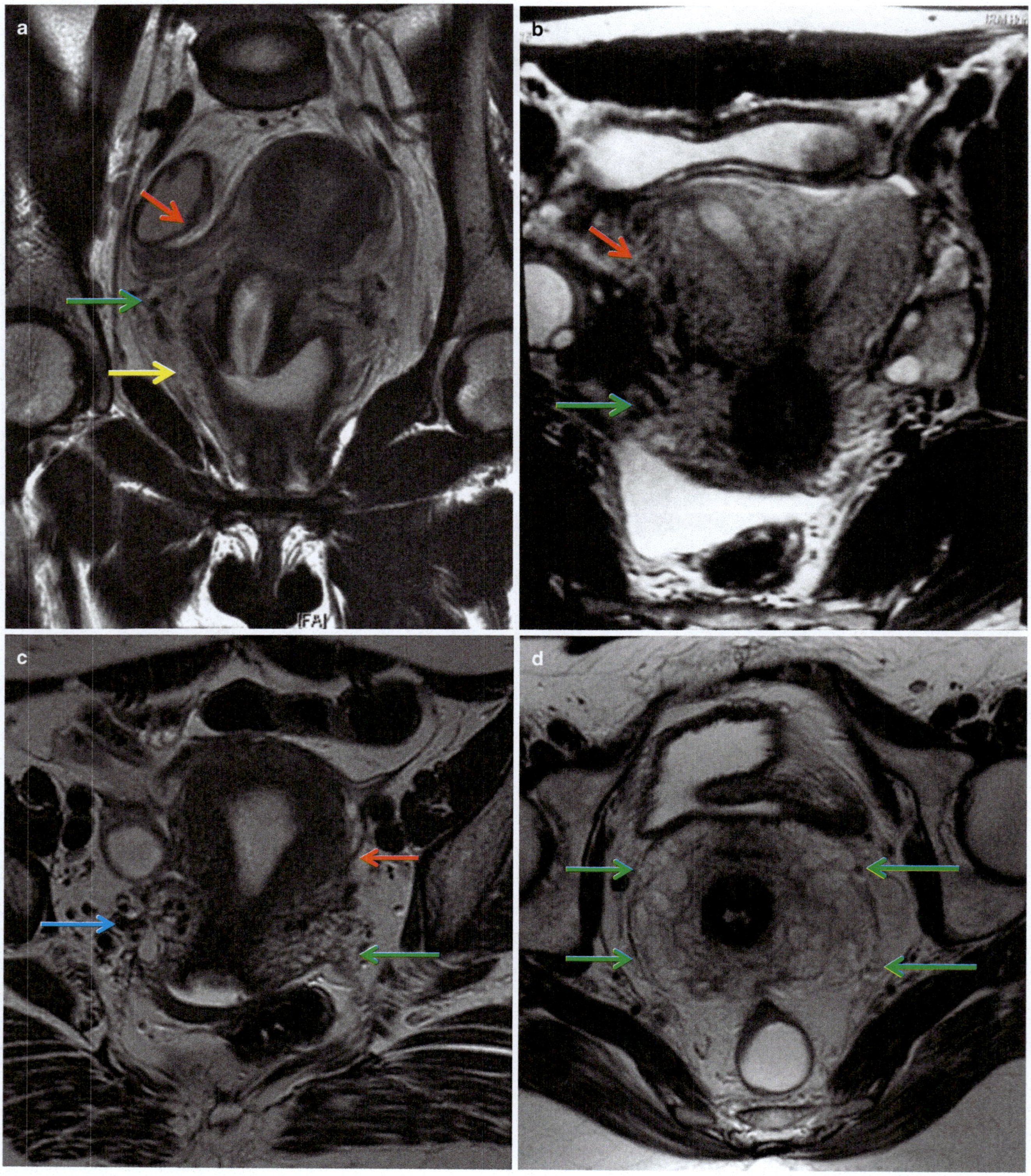

Fig. 1.4 Lateral compartment. Including ureters, parametrium (green arrow), uterine arteries (blue arrow), broad ligaments (red arrow), and paracolpos (yellow arrow). (**a–c**, **e**) T2-weighted sequences. (**a**) Coronal. (**b–d**) Axial. (**e**) Sagittal. (**e**, **g**) Laparoscopy. (**e**) USL = utero-sacral ligaments. *HN* hypogastric nerve. (**g**) Parametria topography (blue areas)

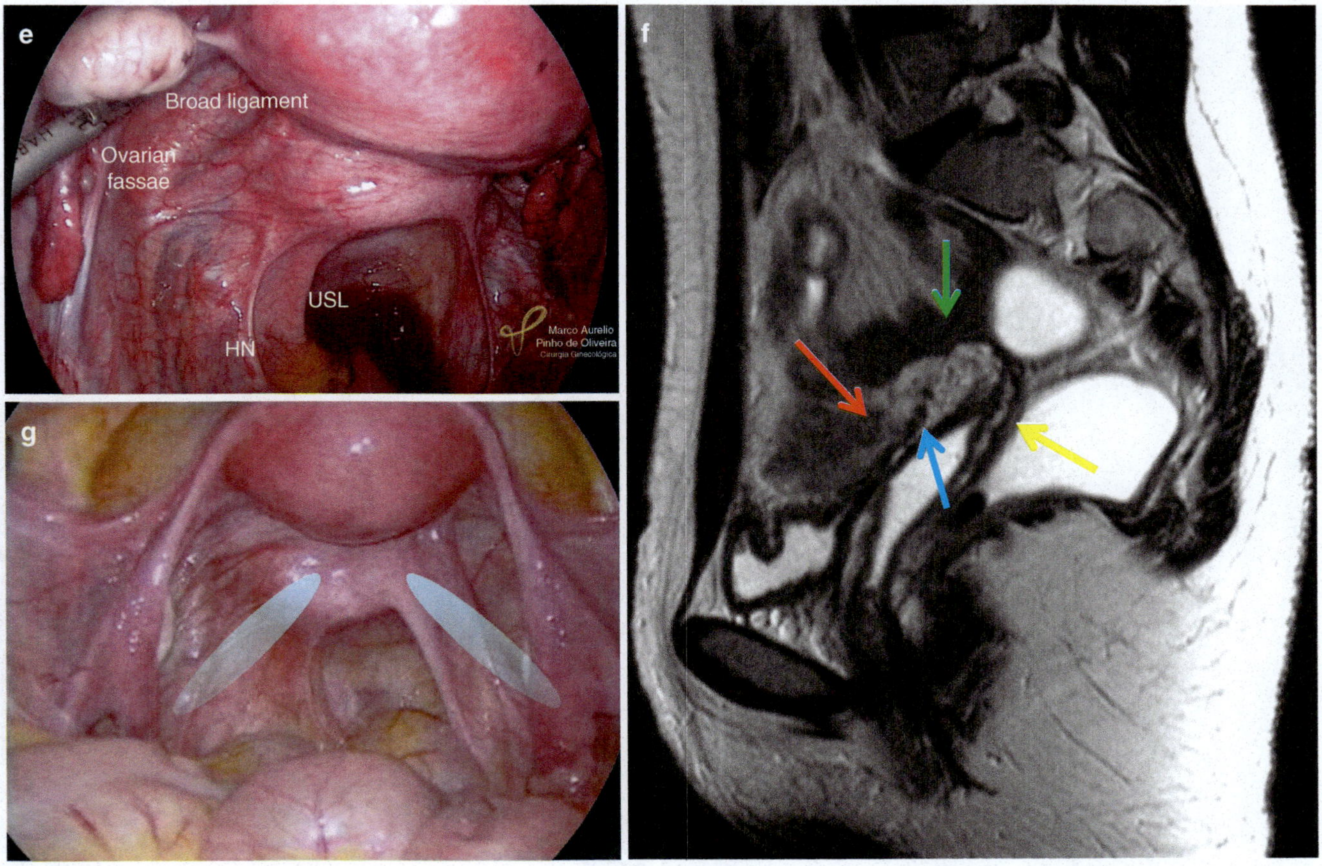

Fig. 1.4 (continued)

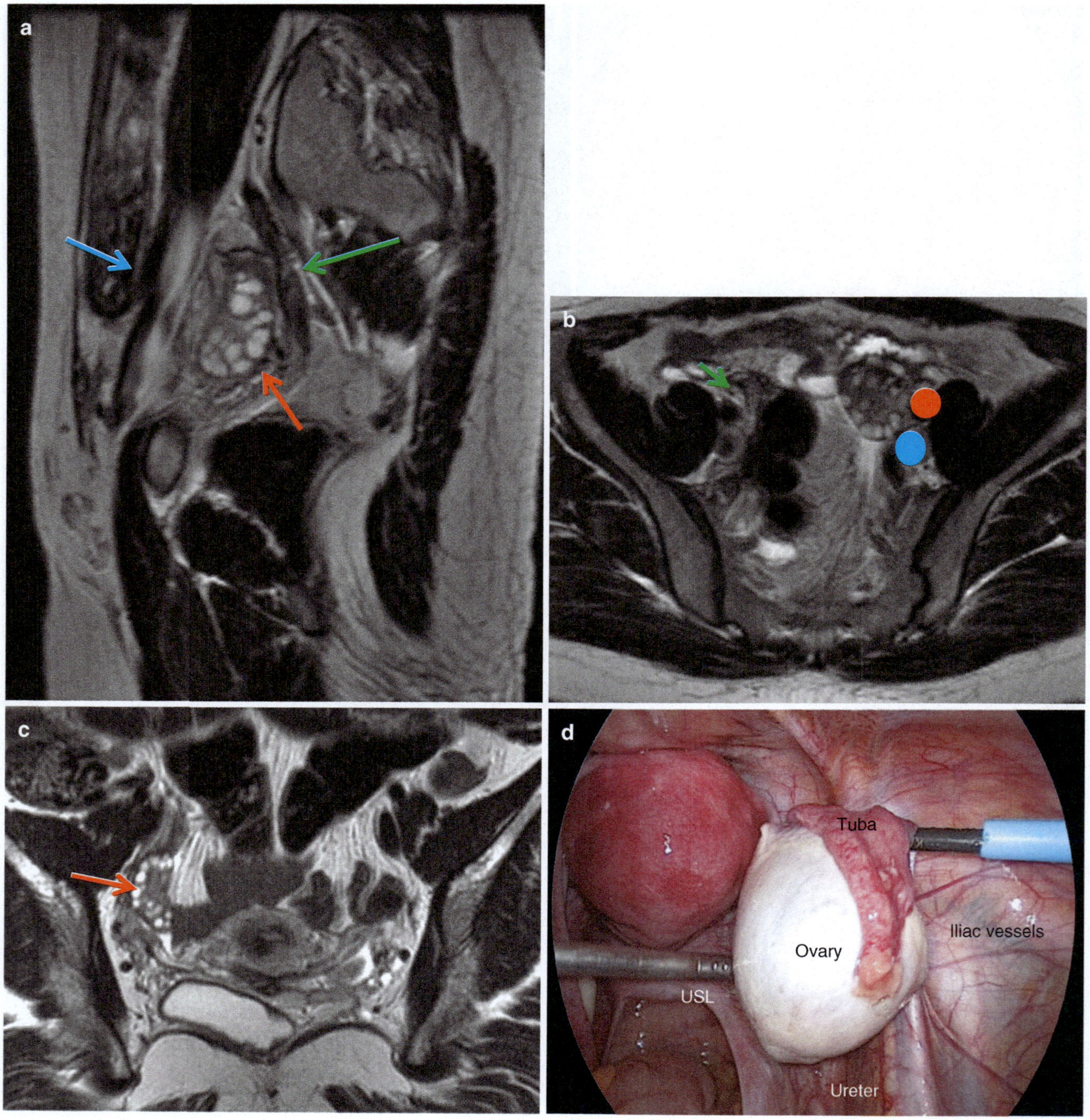

Fig. 1.5 Ovarian fossa. Including the external iliac vessels (blue arrow), the internal iliac vessels (green arrow in **a**, **b**, vein blue and artery red in **b**), the ovary (red arrow), and the ureter. (**ac**) T2-weighted sequences. (**a**) Sagittal. (**b**) Axial. (**c**) Coronal. (**d**) Laparoscopic view of the ovary and ovarian fossa

1.1.2 Abdominal Location

This location includes lesions that affect the abdominal wall (surgical scar, umbilical, and inguinal regions), the parieto-colic gutters, the small bowel, the appendix, the cecum, and ascending and descending colon, as well as the diaphragm (Fig. 1.6).

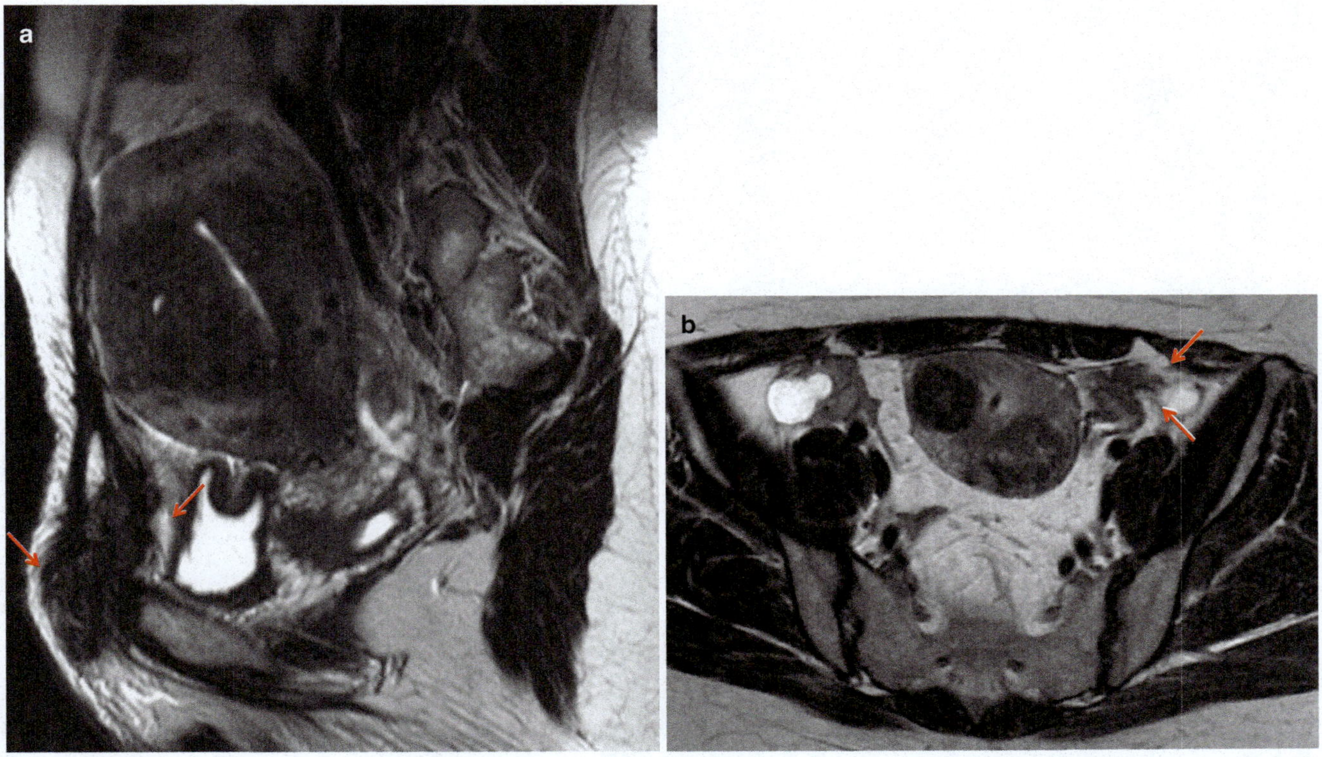

Fig. 1.6 Abdominal locations. (**a**) Abdominal wall. Large lesion on the cesarean scar (arrows). Note uterine adenomyosis. (**b, d**) Deep lesion in the left parieto-colic gutter, involving the sigmoid and round ligaments (arrows). (**c**) Cecum and small intestine. Lesion on the cecum involving the ileocecal valve (arrow) with mucocele of the appendix. (**e**) Diaphragmatic dome. Lesion in the right hemidiaphragm (arrow). Liver—lesion in right lobe (arrow). (**a–c, f**) T2-weighted sequences. (**e**) T1-weighted sequence with fat suppression. (**a**) Sagittal. (**b**) Axial. (**c–f**) Coronal

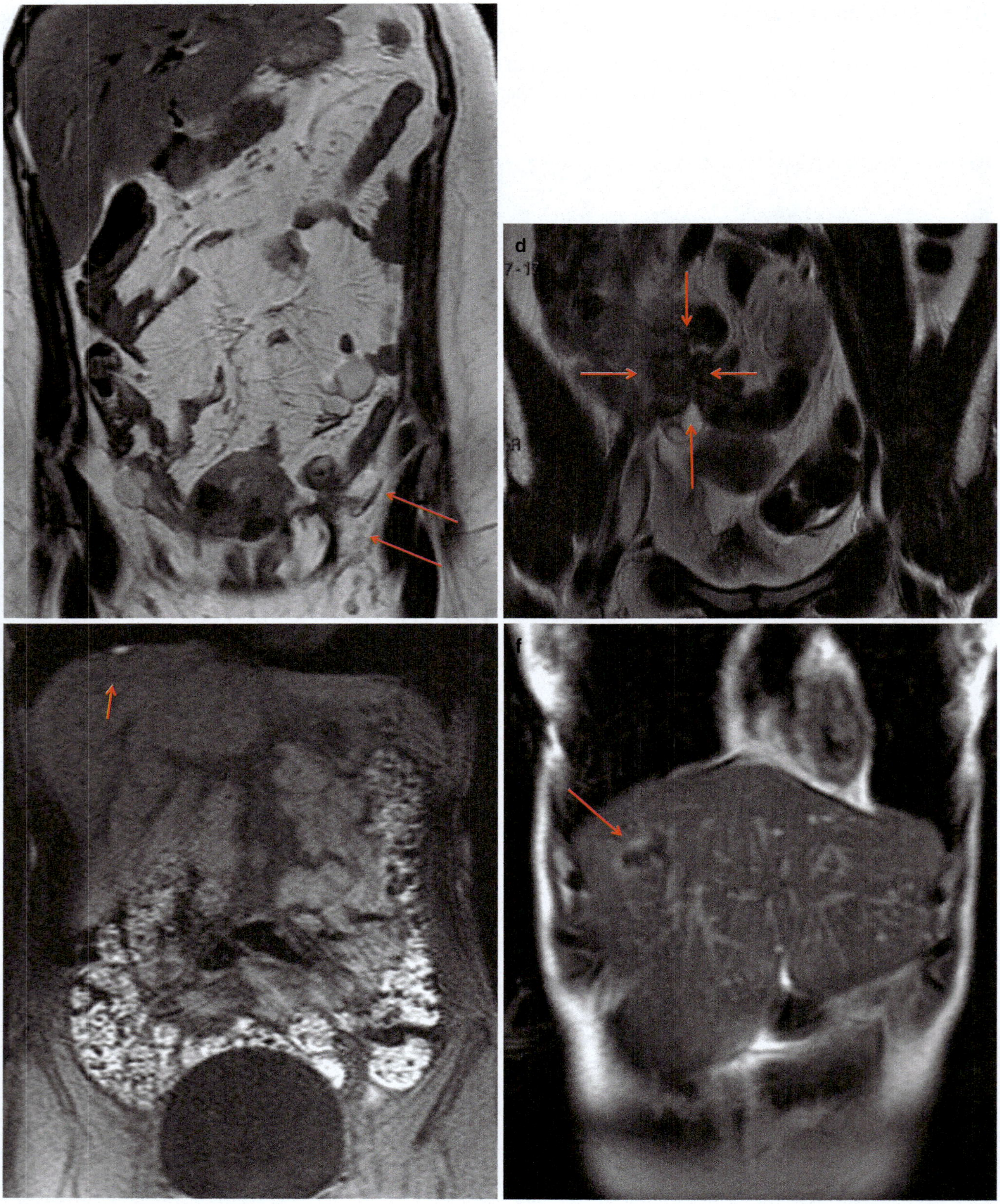

Fig. 1.6 (continued)

Reference

1. Crispi C. Tratado de Videoendoscopia e Cirurgia minimamente invasiva em Ginecologia. 5th ed. Rio de Janeiro: Revinter; 2011.

2 Magnetic Resonance Imaging

MRI is an imaging method with many applications in gynecology due to its high spatial resolution, multiplanar capability, and excellent tissue contrast, which provides high-quality images without exposing the patient to ionizing radiation.

2.1 Technical Aspects

2.1.1 Equipment

Ideally, for the study of the female pelvis, the examination should be performed using an MRI scanner with a high gradient and high field (1.5 T or greater), using surface coils in a phase arrangement, as described below (Fig. 2.1).

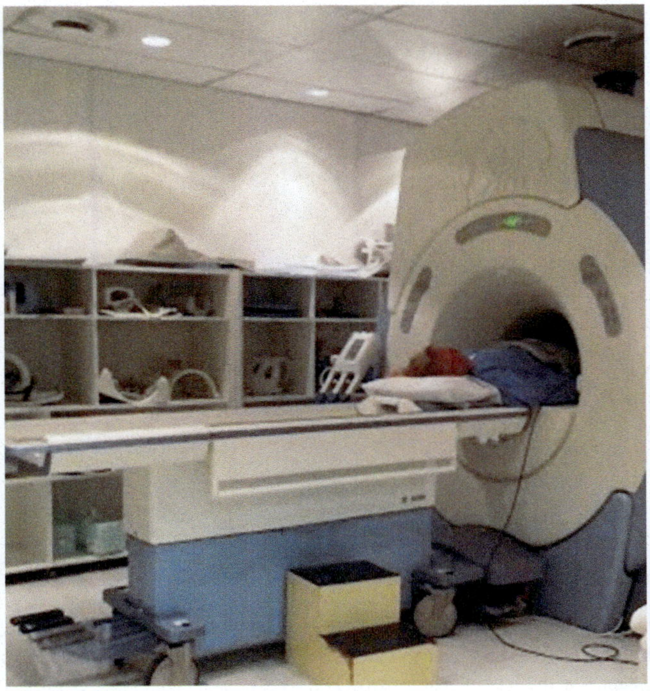

Fig. 2.1 Apparatus with high gradient and high field. Positioning of the patient to perform the exam

2.2 Protocols

The optimal strategy for abdominal and pelvic MRI investigation of endometriosis relies on standardization of a specific routine protocol.

2.2.1 Pelvic Endometriosis Protocol

The cornerstone of MRI is its ability to distinguish pathologic tissue from normal tissue, as well as to characterize soft tissues. The development of phase arrangement coils (phased-array) provided an improvement in the acquired images due to the increased signal to noise ratio, which is ideal for use in the study of the female pelvis. This type of MRI scanner allows the use of a smaller field of view (FOV) without loss of image quality. This relationship is directly related to the number of channels. Currently, surface coils are the ideal type of coils with at least eight channels (Fig. 2.2).

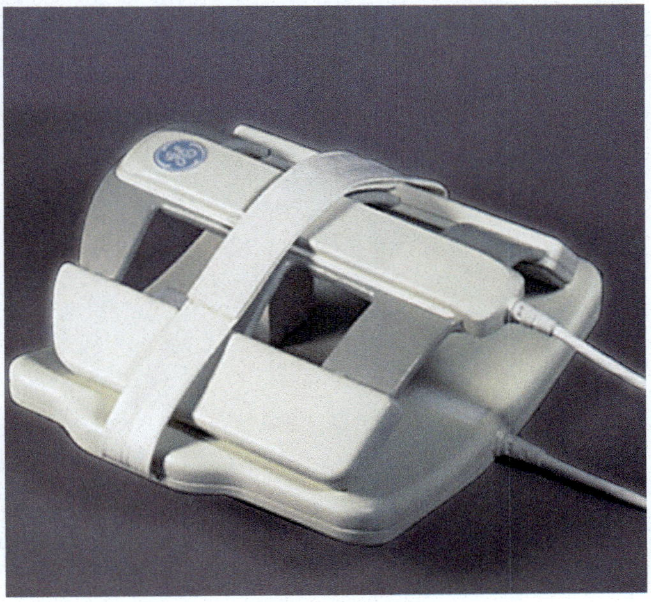

Fig. 2.2 Eight channel cardiac surface coil

A. Brandão et al., *Atlas of Deep Endometriosis*, https://doi.org/10.1007/978-3-319-71697-8_2

The MRI protocol for endometriosis in the female pelvis relies on the contrast between tissues obtained from the differences in T1 and T2 relaxation times and is divided into T1-weighted and T2-weighted sequences. The contrast study can include a T1-weighted sequence, obtained after gadolinium administration in the arterial, venous, and delayed phases, as well as functional examination (Table 2.1).

2.2.2 T1-Weighted Sequence

This sequence gives anatomical information and tissue characterization. The differences in tissue contrast between the fat, muscles, and pelvic organs can be better appreciated when the sequence is associated with a fat suppression pulse. Fluid content or fibrous tissue appears as low signal intensity, whereas fat, fluids with high protein concentrations, and blood will appear as high signal intensity. The addition of a fat suppression pulse enables the minimization of T1 signal from fat, such as those from adnexal teratoma, highlighting the blood. Thus, this sequence produces images with greater sensitivity for detection of bleeding spots (Fig. 2.3).

Gradient-recalled-echo (GRE) sequences are faster than the basic T1-weighted spin-echo sequence and minimize the artifacts related to breathing, vascular flow, and peristalsis. This sequence is acquired quickly, in 10–20 s, with breath holding (Table 2.1).

The ideal acquisition planes are the axial and sagittal.

Later in this section, there will be more detail about contrast-enhanced dynamic study.

Table 2.1 Pelvic examination protocol

Sequence	Plane	FOV	Thickness	Matrix	NEX	TR	TE	Slices
FSE T2-weighted	Axial	26	6.0/1.5	256 × 192	4	4400	90	30
FSE T2-weighted	Sagittal	26	4.0/0.2	384 × 224	4	4400	102	24
FSE T2-weighted	Coronal short axis	26	4.0/0.2	384 × 224	4	4200	101	24
FSE T2-weighted	Coronal long axis	26	4.0/0.2	384 × 224	4	4200	101	24
GRE T1-weighted	Axial	34	6.0/1.5	256 × 192	1		Minimum	24
GRE T1-weighted with fat suppression	Axial	34	6.0/1.5	256 × 192	1		Minimum	24

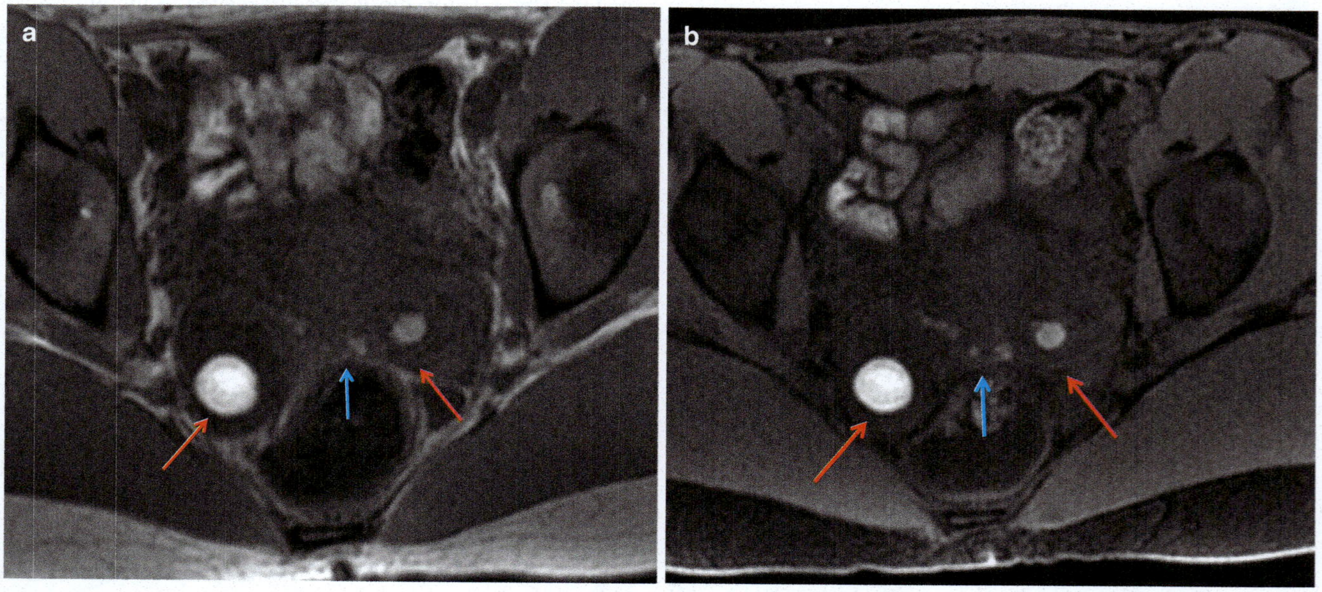

Fig. 2.3 T1-weighted sequences. (**a**–**c**) Axial plane. (**a**) Without the addition of a fat saturation pulse. (**b**) With fat saturation. (**c**) With fat saturation after administration of gadolinium. (**d**) Sagittal plane with fat saturation. (**e**) With fat saturation after administration of gadolinium. Note bilateral endometriomas (red arrows) and retrocervical endometriosis with bleeding (blue arrow)

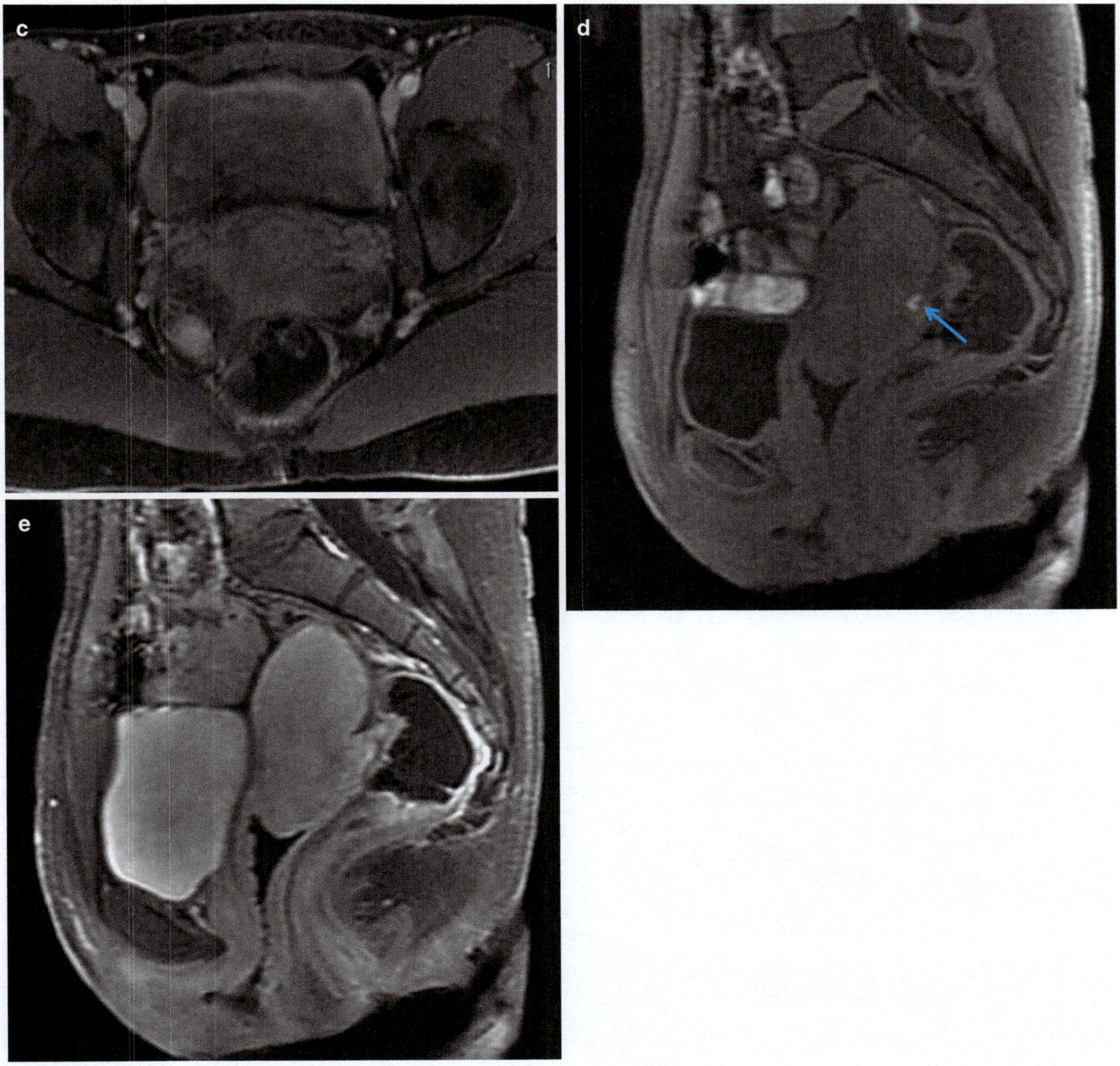

Fig. 2.3 (continued)

2.2.3 T2-Weighted Sequence

This sequence plays an important role in MRI of the female pelvis, providing high-resolution images, with high diagnostic performance and visibility of pathological lesions, such as deep infiltrative endometriosis.

The fast spin-echo (FSE) pulse sequence with a pelvic phased-array multicoil provides T2-weighted high-resolution images, which are very important for the deep pelvic endometriosis protocol, because they yield excellent soft-tissue contrast and allow assessment of the anatomy of the pelvic organs, peritoneal surface, ligaments, muscle, and fascia, as well as the ureters and parametrium.

Moreover, this particular form of endometriosis lesion is composed predominantly of fibrous tissue, with a small amount of bleeding, with plaque-like implants or nodules that are hard to see, commonly hypointense in all sequences. T2-weighted high-resolution imaging findings show an excellent correlation with surgical and histopathologic examination findings of deep endometriosis.

However, it requires a longer acquisition time compared to the T1-weighted sequence, taking between 2 and 4 min depending on the number of acquired slices, the gradient, the field, and the coil (Fig. 2.4).

Routinely, T2-weighted sequence is acquired in the four orthogonal planes (axial, sagittal, coronal short-axis, and long axis). A new imaging option is the 3D T2-weighted sequence..

In the axial plane, the entire true pelvis is studied, with good demonstration of the compartments, the peritoneal lining, and supporting structures, vessels, nerves, and the parametrium. The cecum and pericecal region can be evaluated when insinuated in the pelvis. If not, an upper abdominal MRI is needed in order to exclude lesion in the pericecal region (Fig. 2.5).

The T2-weighted axial plane slice position is similar to the T1-weighted axial sequence, acquired with 25-degree anterior and inferior direction, in order to follow the direction of the uterosacral ligaments, facilitating their identification. The thickness ranges between 3 and 6 mm and the interval 0–1 mm. The FOV varies according to the sequence, being around 30–36 cm for T1-weighted to maintain an appropriate signal to noise and 22–24 cm for the T2-weighted

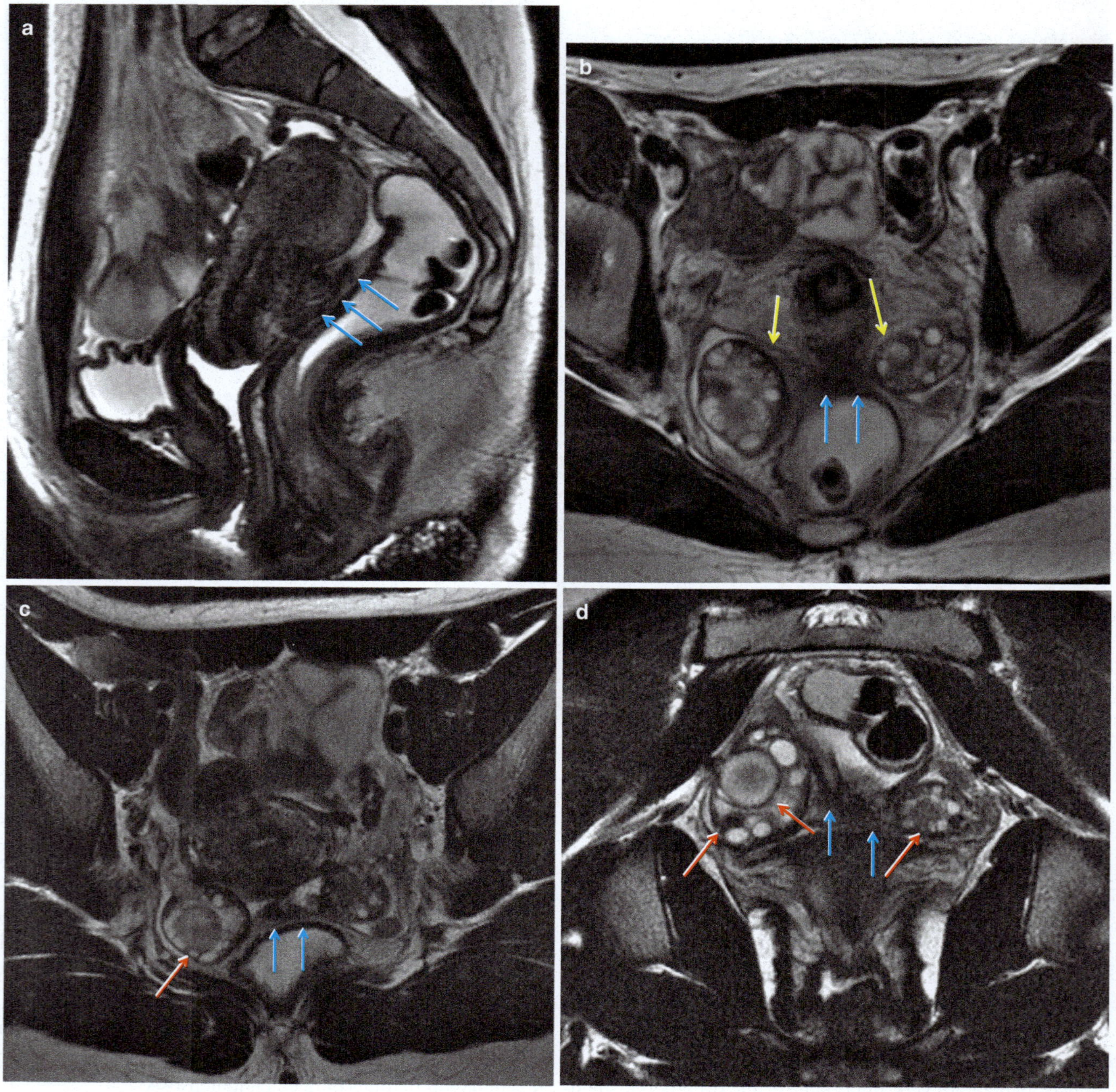

Fig. 2.4 T2-weighted sequence with high spatial resolution. As in Fig. 2.9. Notice retrocervical endometriosis (blue arrows), adherence with posterior and medial deviation of the appendages (**d**) (yellow arrows) and the endometriomas (red arrows). (**a**) Sagittal plane. (**b**) Axial. (**c**) Coronal with short axis. (**d**) Coronal with long axis. (**e**) Laparoscopy. Note the medial deviation of the adnexa, attached to the retrocervical lesion (black arrows)

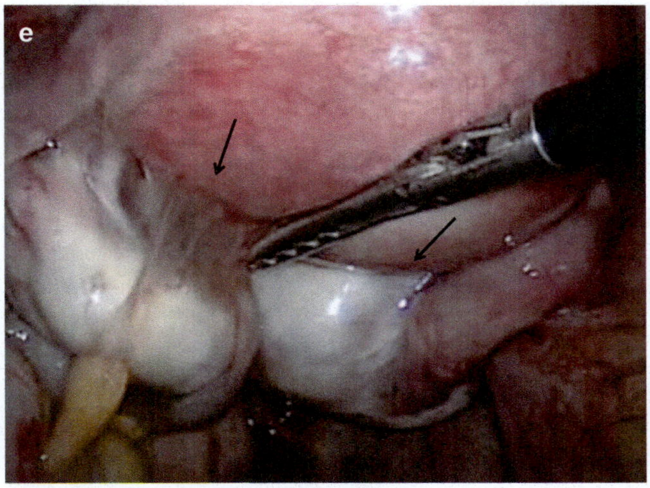

Fig. 2.4 (continued)

sequence. In other planes, the thickness is 4 mm, with a 10% range and a FOV around 22–26 cm.

The sagittal plane is programmed parallel to the uterine cavity in the axial plane in order to acquire anatomical images of the uterine zonal anatomy. The association of endometriosis with benign myometrial pathology is common. This plane adequately analyzes the support of the uterine ligaments, bladder, distal ureter, rectum, sigmoid, vagina, and anterior and posterior cul-de-sac, with good delineation of the anterior and posterior compartments (Fig. 2.6).

The coronal sections of the short axis are positioned perpendicularly to the uterine cavity, and the coronal long axis is parallel to the cavity, both of them in the sagittal plane. These two planes provide high-resolution images of the uterus (zonal anatomy), parametrium, ureters, broad ligaments, uterosacral and round ligaments, rectum, sigmoid, ovarian fossa, and pericecal region (Figs. 2.7 and 2.8) [1].

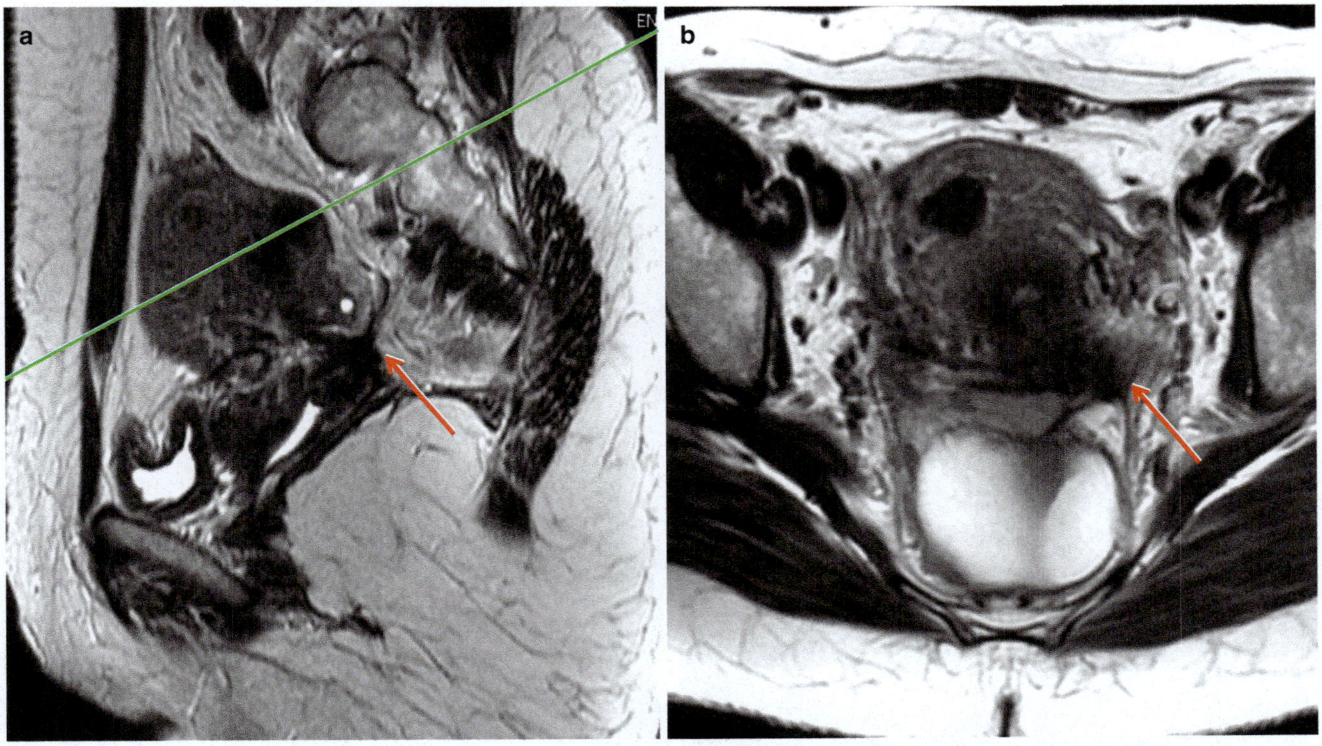

Fig. 2.5 Positioning of axial slices with 25% angulation, following the direction of the uterosacral ligament (arrow) in the sagittal plane. (**a**, **b**) T2-weighted sequences. (**a**) Sagittal. (**b**) Axial. Note endometriosis in the left uterosacral ligament (arrows in **a**, **b**)

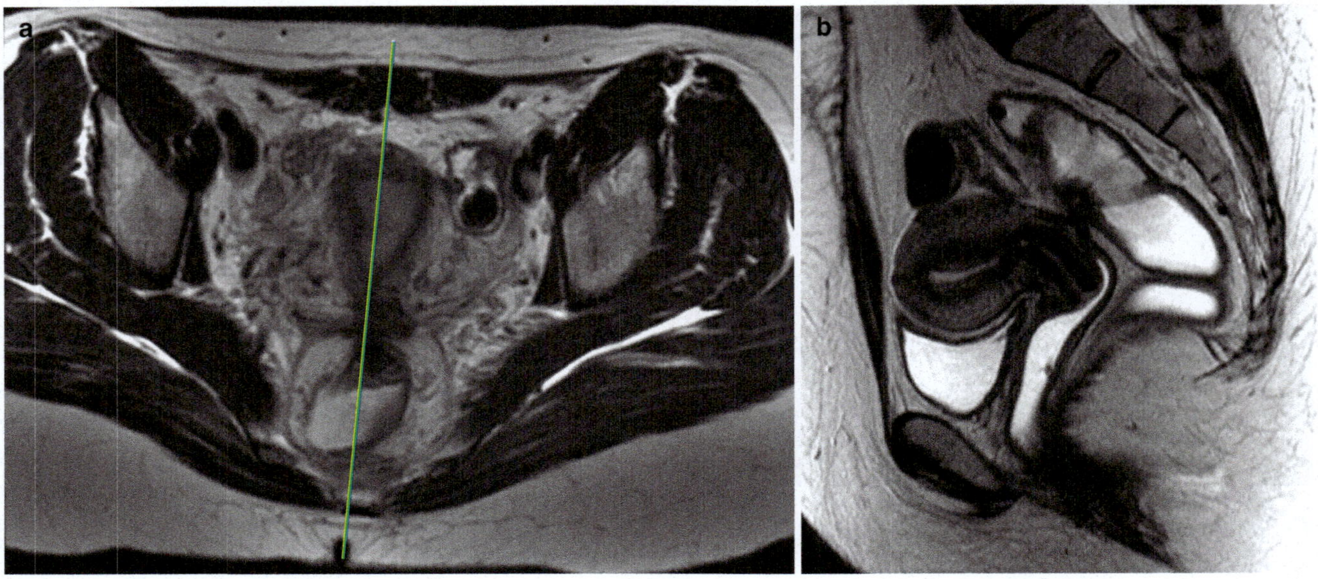

Fig. 2.6 Marking the sagittal plane, according to the angulation of the uterine cavity shown in the axial plane. (**ab**) T2-weighted sequences. (**a**) Axial. (**b**) Sagittal. Note retrocervical lesion with rectal nodule

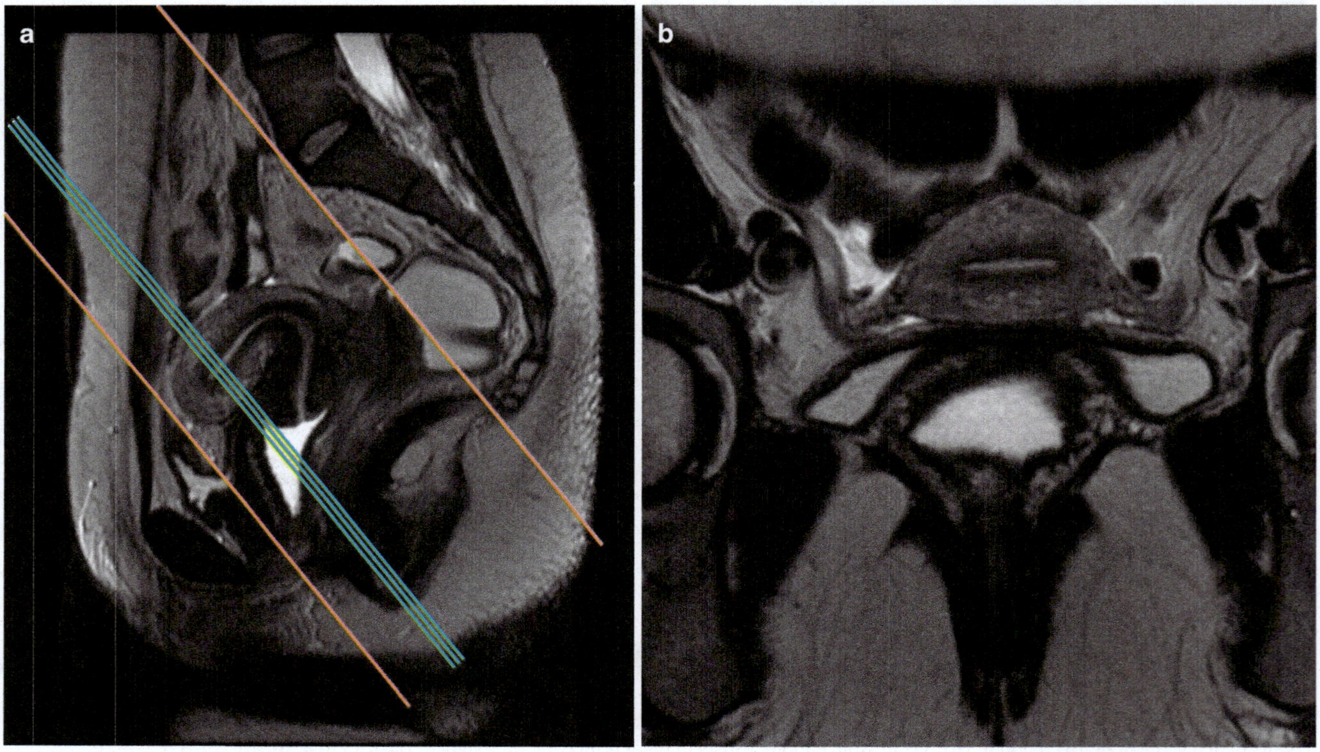

Fig. 2.7 Marking the sagittal plane, according to the angulation of the uterine cavity shown in the axial plane. (**ab**) T2-weighted sequences. (**a**) Axial. (**b**) Sagittal. Note retrocervical lesion with rectal nodule

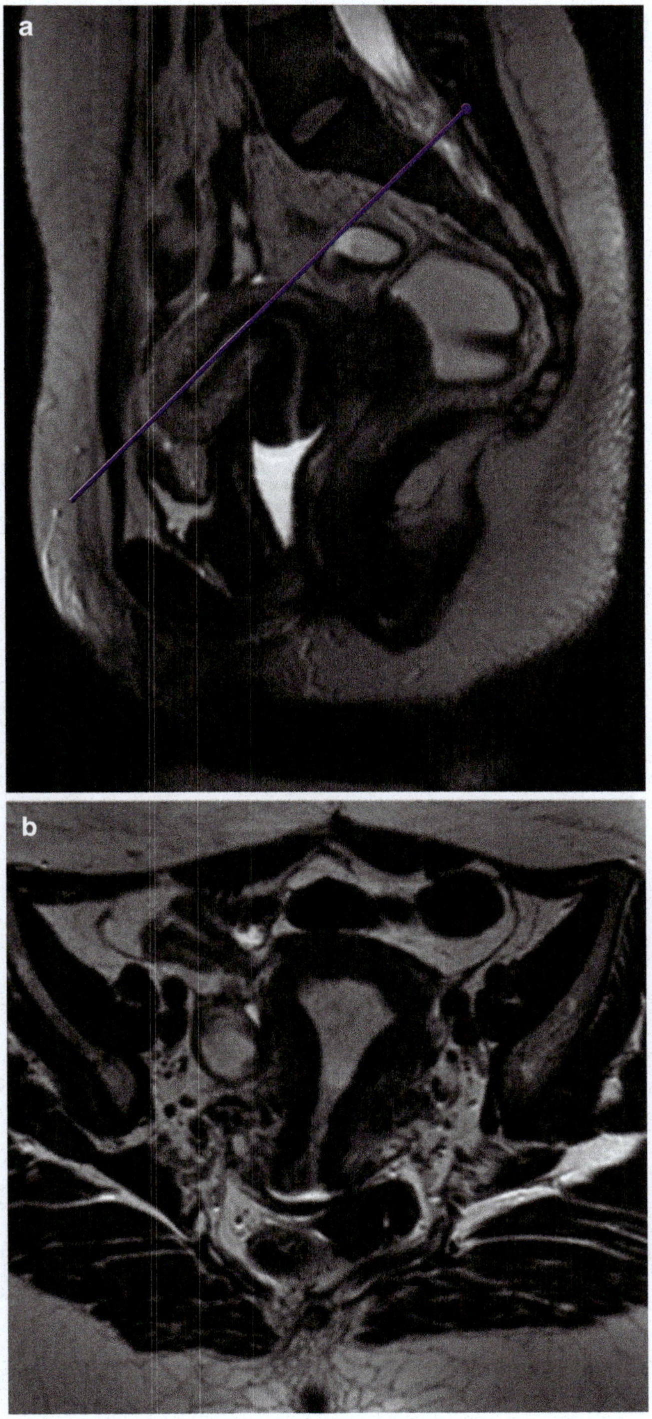

Fig. 2.8 Planning the coronal plane in the long axis, positioned in the sagittal plane, parallel to the uterine cavity. (**a**, **b**) T2-weighted sequences. (**a**) Sagittal. (**b**) Coronal long axis

2.3 Endometriosis of the Abdominal Wall

The protocol should be focused on the anterior abdominal wall, using a coil with a larger field of view. A skin marker should be positioned on the clinically suspected area, on the umbilical, inguinal, or scar endometriosis (Fig. 2.9).

The sequences may be different from those used in endometriosis of the pelvis. The FSE T2-weighted axial plane must include the umbilical and the inguinal region. The T2-weighted sagittal and coronal planes can be performed additionally with the patient in apnea, because breathing artifacts could harm the identification and analysis of the extent of the injury in this location, with and without fat suppression. A tip to acquire high-quality images during apnea is to increase the field of view (FOV), thinner thickness and no interval, with a suitable matrix.

The intravenous contrast medium can be important in small abdominal wall endometriosis. These lesions may have a predominance of fibrosis and no bleeding and, consequently, a signal similar to the muscle, which could go unnoticed. Increased contrast can enhance the lesion and improve its conspicuity (Fig. 2.10).

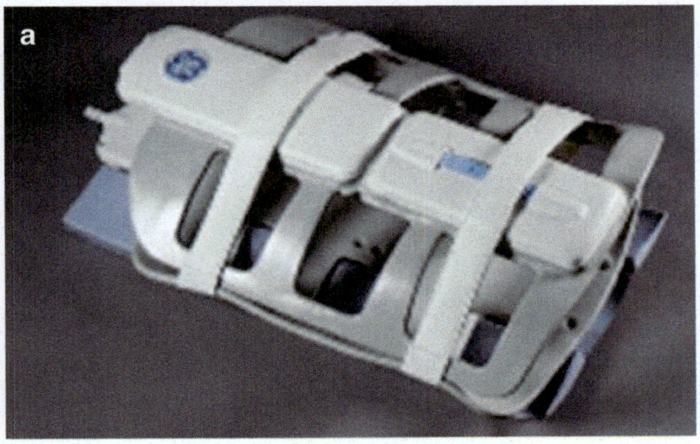

Fig. 2.9 Protocol for anterior abdominal wall endometriosis. (**a**) Coil with larger field of view. (**b**) Place the skin marker on the lesion (in the example, umbilical—arrow). T2-weighted sequence. Sagittal

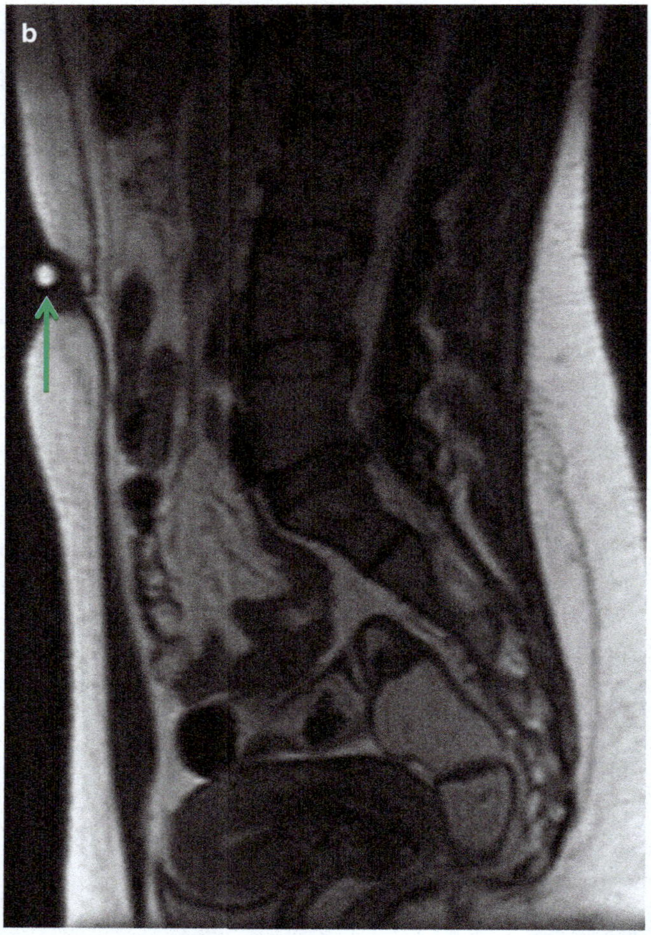

Fig. 2.9 (continued)

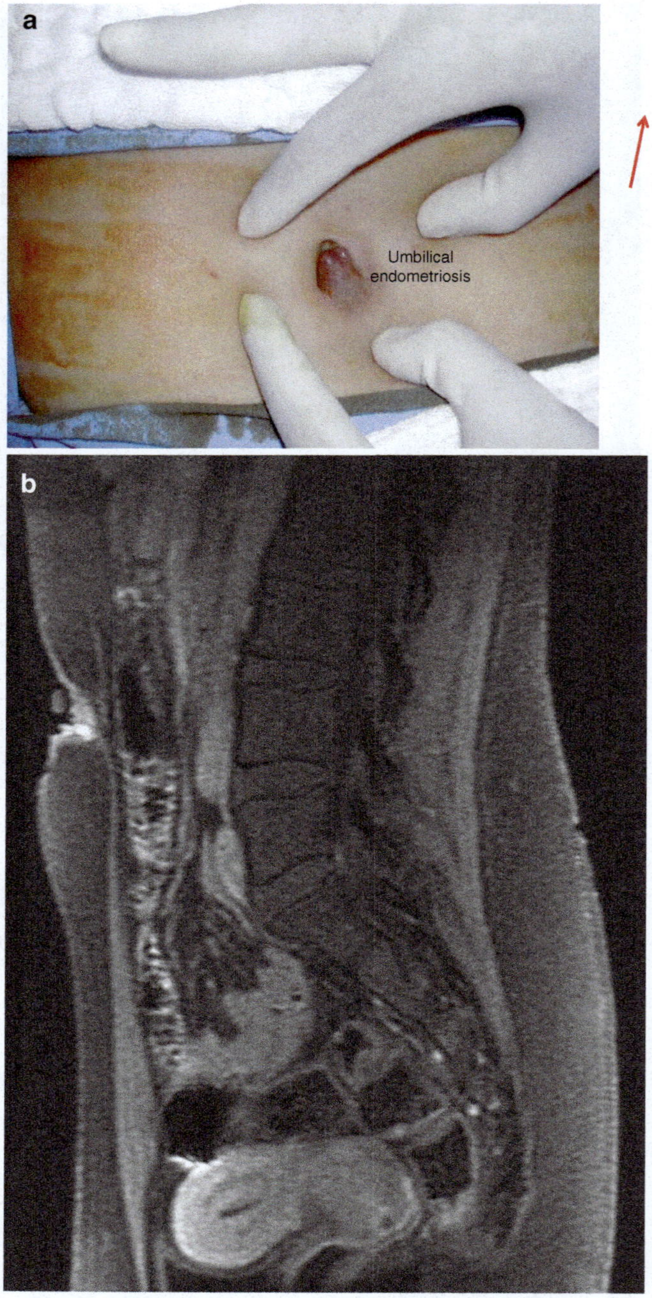

Fig. 2.10 Umbilical lesion (as in Fig. 2.9) enhanced by gadolinium. T1-weighted sequence with fat suppression and use of gadolinium. Sagittal

2.4 The Preparation of the Patient

The proper preparation of the patient is essential for the MRI exam. It is highly important to identify bowel lesions, especially small ones (Table 2.2).

Preparation is divided into two parts, preparation at home and at the radiology department. At home, we request the patient go on a 24-h low-fiber diet, ending with 4 h of fasting apart from a glycerin *suppository*. This can be administered during a period of 2–8 h before the exam, in order to facilitate the preparation (Fig. 2.11).

At the radiology department, before the exam, the patient is requested to empty their bladder. This will make the patient more comfortable and will also help to improve imaging quality, since there will be less artifacts related to the bladder distention, making it easier to identify small lesions. Moreover, the uterus will be in the anteversion position, reducing the artifacts from the small bowel (Fig. 2.12). The high-resolution T2-weighted sequences are more susceptible to peristalsis artifacts from the bowel, myometrium, and bladder.

Table 2.2 MRI protocol, with bowel preparation

At home	At the radiology site
Low fiber diet 24 h	120 ml of rectum saline solution
Fasting 4 h	10 mL of intravaginal ultrasound gel
Glycerin suppository	10 mg of butylescopolamine was injected intravenously

An intravenous antispasmodic agent should be administered in order to reduce peristalsis (10 mg butylscopolamine, Buscopan; Boehringer Ingelheim, Ingelheim, Germany). It is important that it is administered slowly with the patient lying down, to avoid tachycardia, a side effect from the medication.

In order to acquire a better evaluation of the vaginal fornix and paracervical region, 20 ml of gel is administered by the patient into the vagina, using a vaginal cream applicator (Fig. 2.13).

In addition, an intestinal preparation of 120 ml of saline solution is administered into the rectum, so as to detect smaller rectum lesions and identify and quantify stenosis (Fig. 2.13).

Before the MRI, the patient is positioned in the supine position, with their arms beside their body.

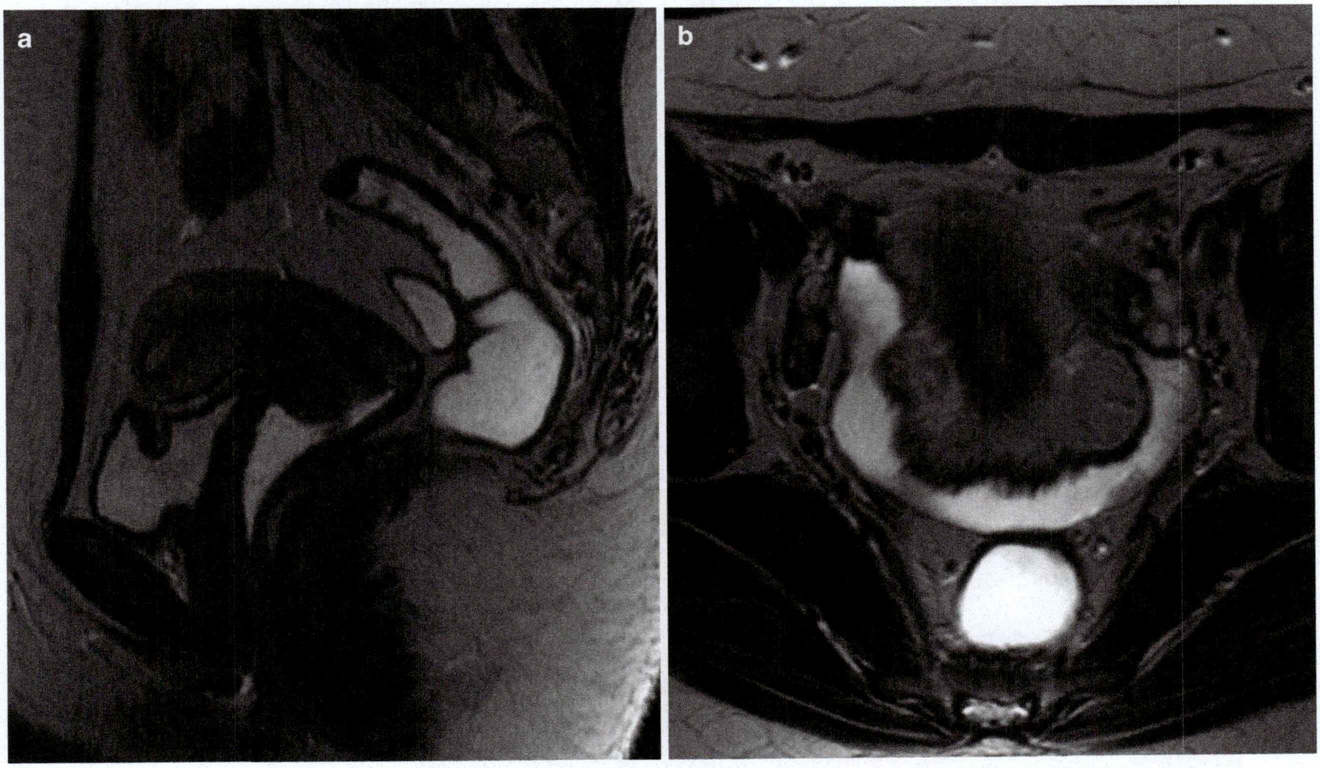

Fig. 2.11 Importance of preparation with an oral diet (without residue from the previous day and day of the exam), fasting (4 h), and use of Buscopan intravenously. Reduction of movement artifacts and better evaluation of intestinal loops. (**a, b**) Redundant rectum and sigmoid. (**c**) Ileal loops. (**a–c**) T2-weighted sequences. (**a**) Sagittal. (**b, c**) Axial

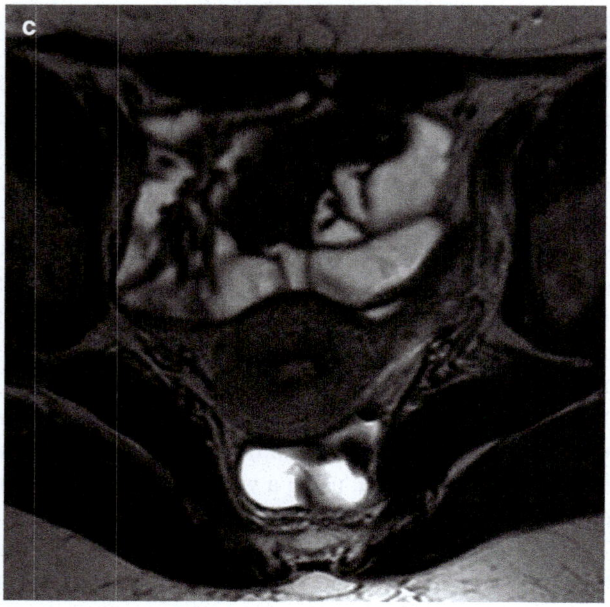

Fig. 2.11 (continued)

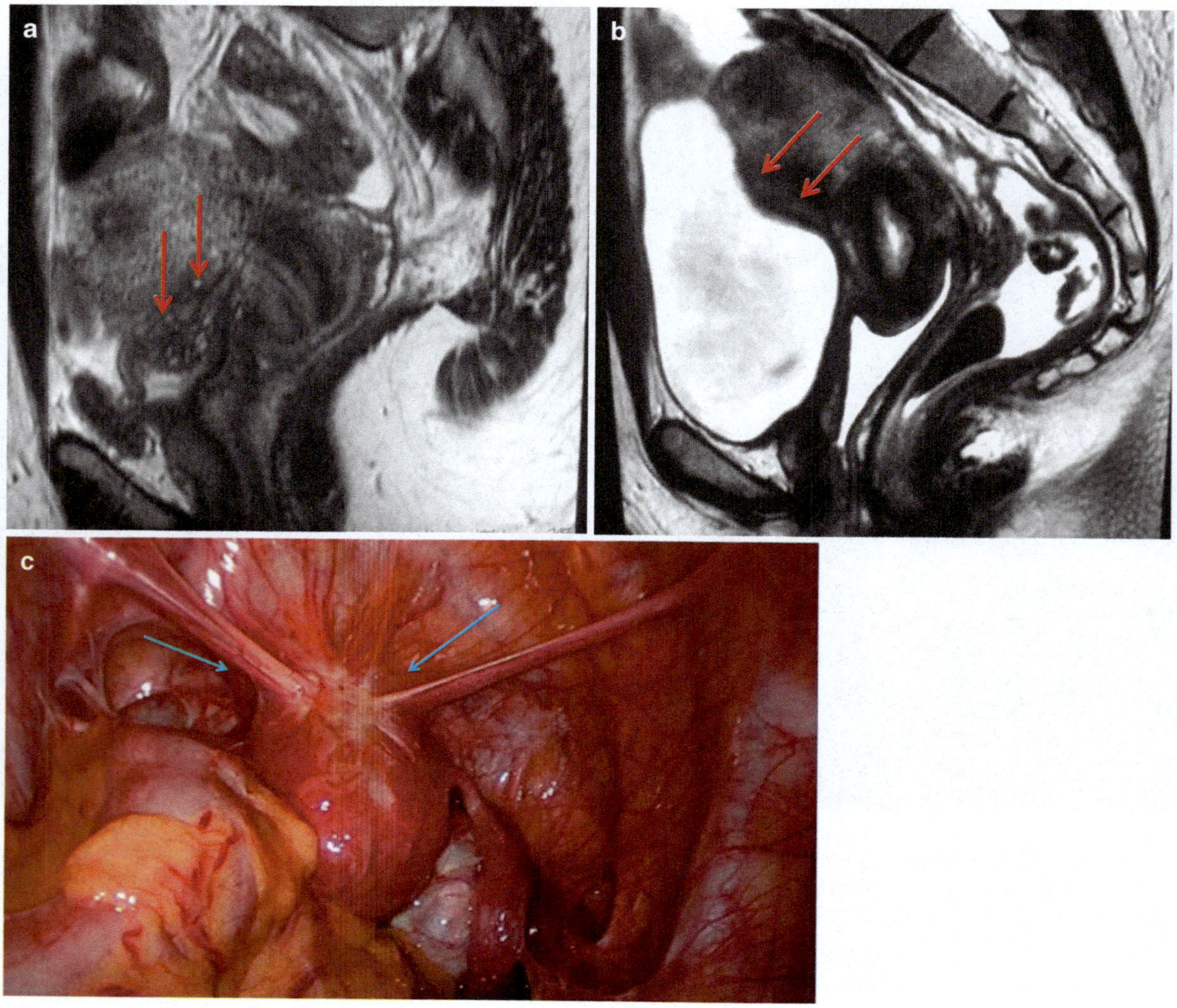

Fig. 2.12 Importance of bladder emptying. (**a**) Better identification of lesion in the anterior compartment, reduction of artifacts, and the uterus assuming anteversion position, avoiding artifacts in the image caused by intestinal loops. (**b**) Compare patient with full bladder. (**a**, **b**) T2-weighted sequences. Sagittal. (**c**) Laparoscopy of lesion in the anterior compartment (arrows)

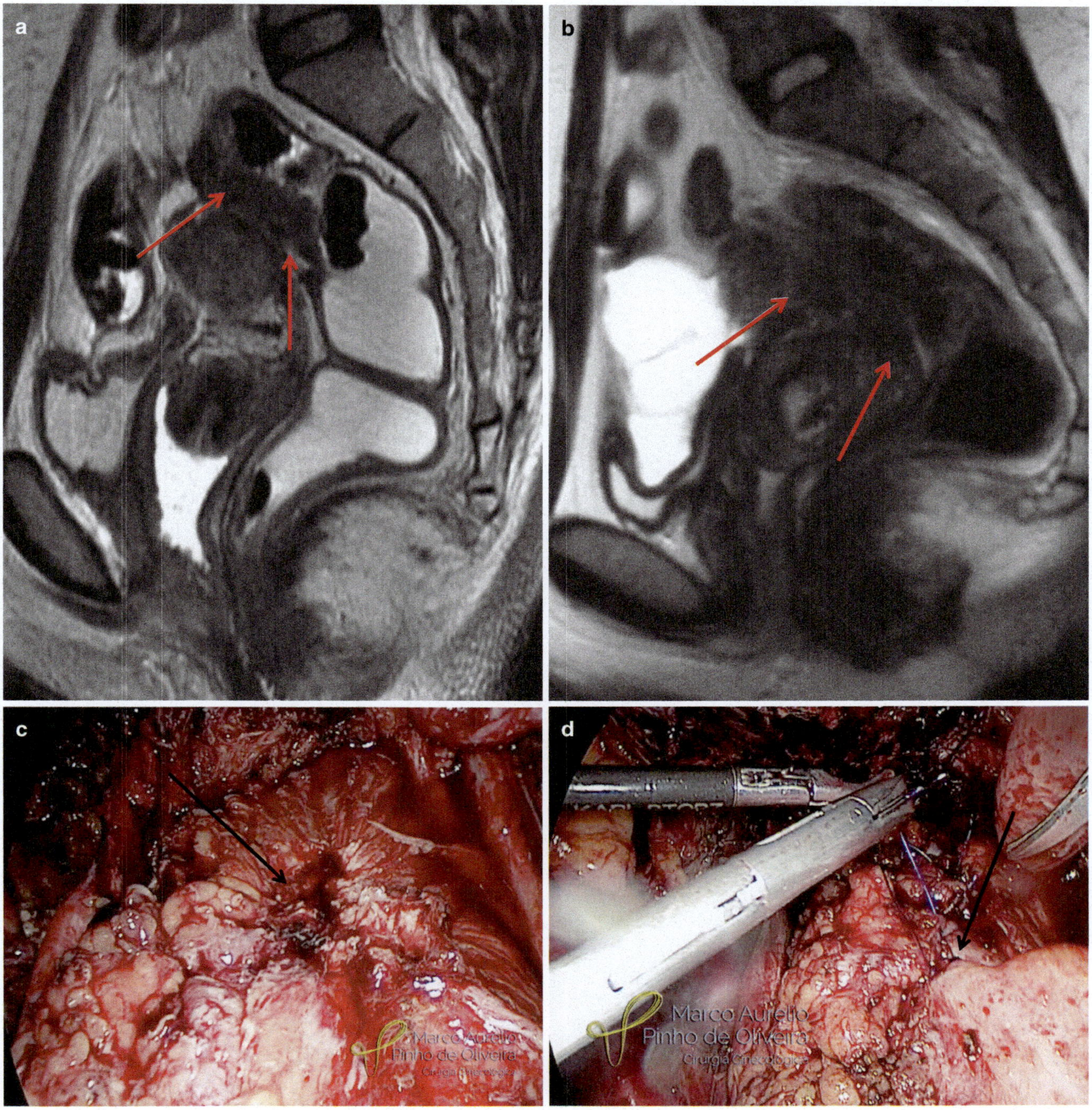

Fig. 2.13 Intestinal lesion (arrows). Improvement of evaluation of lesion with vaginal gel, intestinal preparation, and saline solution rectally. Compare the examination done with the appropriate preparation in (**a**) and without preparation in (**b**). (**c**, **d**) Laparoscopy of intestinal lesion in **c** (arrows) and start of discoid resection in (**d**). (**a**, **b**) T2-weighted sequences. Sagittal

Reference

1. Novellas S, Chassang M, Bouaziz J, Delotte J, Toullalan O, Chevallier E. Anterior pelvic endometriosis: MRI features. Abdom Imaging. 2010;35:742–9.

3 MRI Aspects of Deep Endometriosis

Deep endometriosis is defined as endometrial tissue (hemosiderin laden macrophages, endometrial glands and/or stroma) outside the uterine cavity infiltrating deeper than 5 mm into the peritoneum or an extraperitoneal organ. Although it is considered a benign disorder, it has an infiltrative behavior, causing inflammation and fibrosis, sometimes extensive, as well as adhesions. The deep disease has little hormonal response but may suffer hemorrhage.

The disease may have a complex and unpredictable clinical behavior among patients, including multifocal and multicentric lesions, and non-gynecological organ, lymphatic, and neural involvement.

The goal of the MRI evaluation, which should observe the epicenter of the lesion, is to detect its length and behavior and establish the most suitable treatment for each patient.

In this section, we discuss the aspects of deep endometriosis in the context of MRI. For didactic purposes, we have divided the features of deep endometriotic lesions by morphology, signal intensity, and enhancement pattern. In addition, we have devoted a section to analyzing the adnexal suspicious lesion and the signs of pelvic and abdominal adhesions using MRI.

3.1 Features of Deep Endometriotic Lesions

3.1.1 Morphology

The gross appearance of deep endometriotic lesions may vary and can present as ligamentous thickening, subperitoneal nodules, and poorly defined lesions with an aspect of a plaque, covering organ surfaces and promoting adhesions (Fig. 3.1).

3.1.1.1 Ligament Thickening

Abnormal ligament thickness is characterized by the authors as a thickness greater than 5 mm, based on the accepted criteria of deep endometriosis and also on Dzung's work on the anatomy of the uterosacral ligament. Thickening is usually associated with contour irregularity, ligamentous retraction, and adhesion (Fig. 3.2) [1].

When it affects the uterosacral ligament, adherence promotes posterior and medial displacement of the ovary and/or tube, as well as lateral and posterior positioning of the uterus, in addition to rectal and sigmoid retraction. The injury may involve the hypogastric nerve and extend to the parametrium involving the ureter and uterine artery (Fig. 3.3).

3.1.1.2 Subperitoneal Nodule

The subperitoneal nodule is a nodular lesion, of varying size, which exceeds the peritoneum limit or has extraperitoneal location. It can penetrate organs such as the sigmoid colon and bladder, with parietal involvement from the outer to the inner layer, sometimes even to the mucosa. As the mucosa is not usually involved, endoscopic study will be usual in most of these cases (Fig. 3.4).

The nodule morphology may vary from regular to irregular or spiculated, with its size being larger than 5 mm. It may cause associated retraction and infiltration in the surrounding structures and also involve important pelvic structures, such as the ureter, pelvic nerves, and vessels, and may affect bladder, rectal, and sexual functions (Fig. 3.5).

Bowel endometriosis may induce marked muscle hypertrophy, identical to that observed in cases of adenomyosis, leading to extramucosal parietal nodules that may cause stenosis [2].

A. Brandão et al., *Atlas of Deep Endometriosis*, https://doi.org/10.1007/978-3-319-71697-8_3

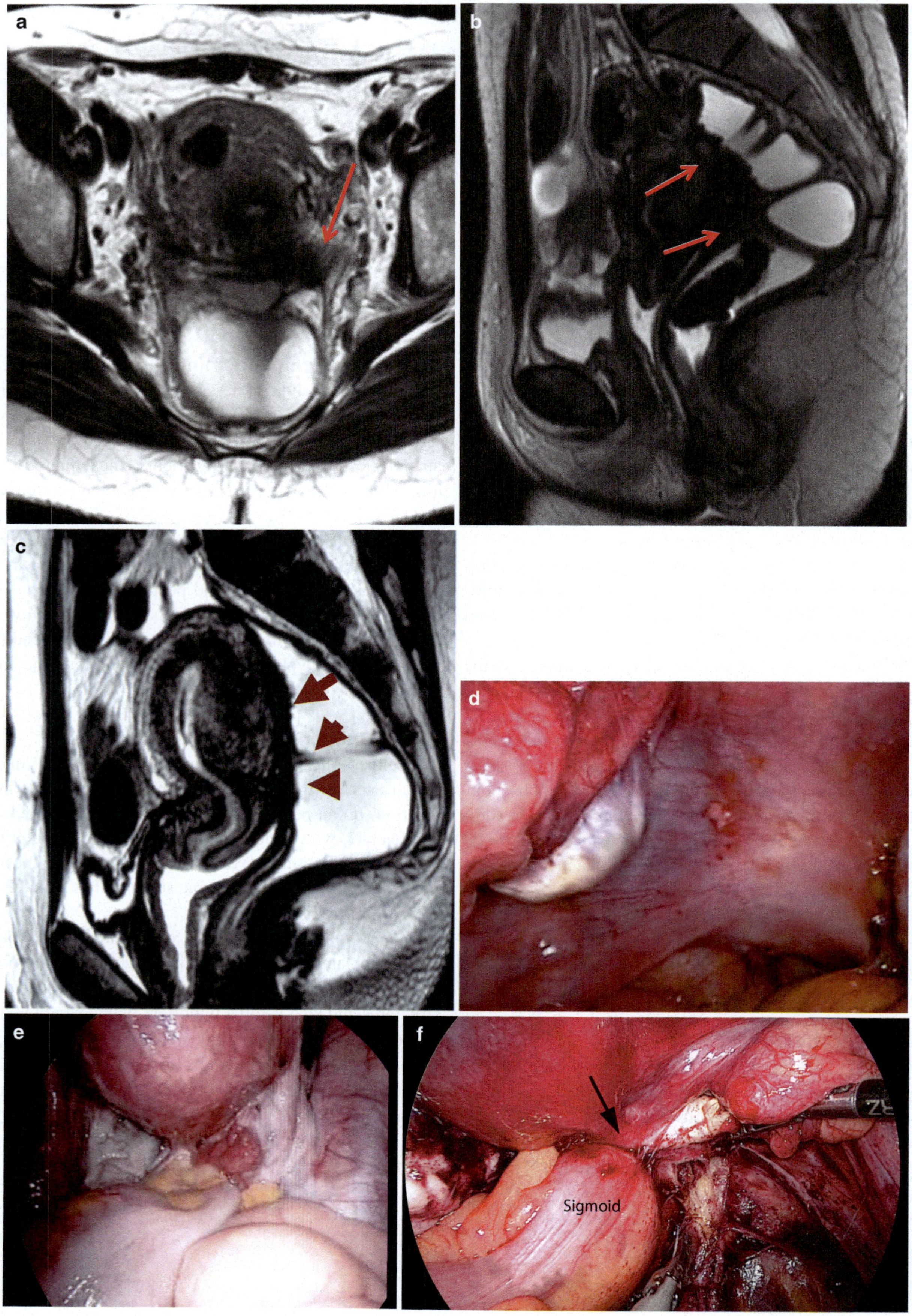

Fig. 3.1 Morphology of deep endometriosis. (**a**) Ligamentous thickening of the left uterus. (**b**) Retrocorporal and retrocervical nodule. (**c**) Mantle lesion covering the posterior uterine surface, promoting adhesions between organs. T2-weighted sequences. (**a**) Axial. (**b**, **c**) Sagittal. (**d**–**f**) Laparoscopies. (**d**) Uterosacral lesion (correlated with **a**). (**e**) Sigmoid lesion (correlated with **b**). (**f**) Retrouterine lesion with extensive adherence (correlated with **c**)

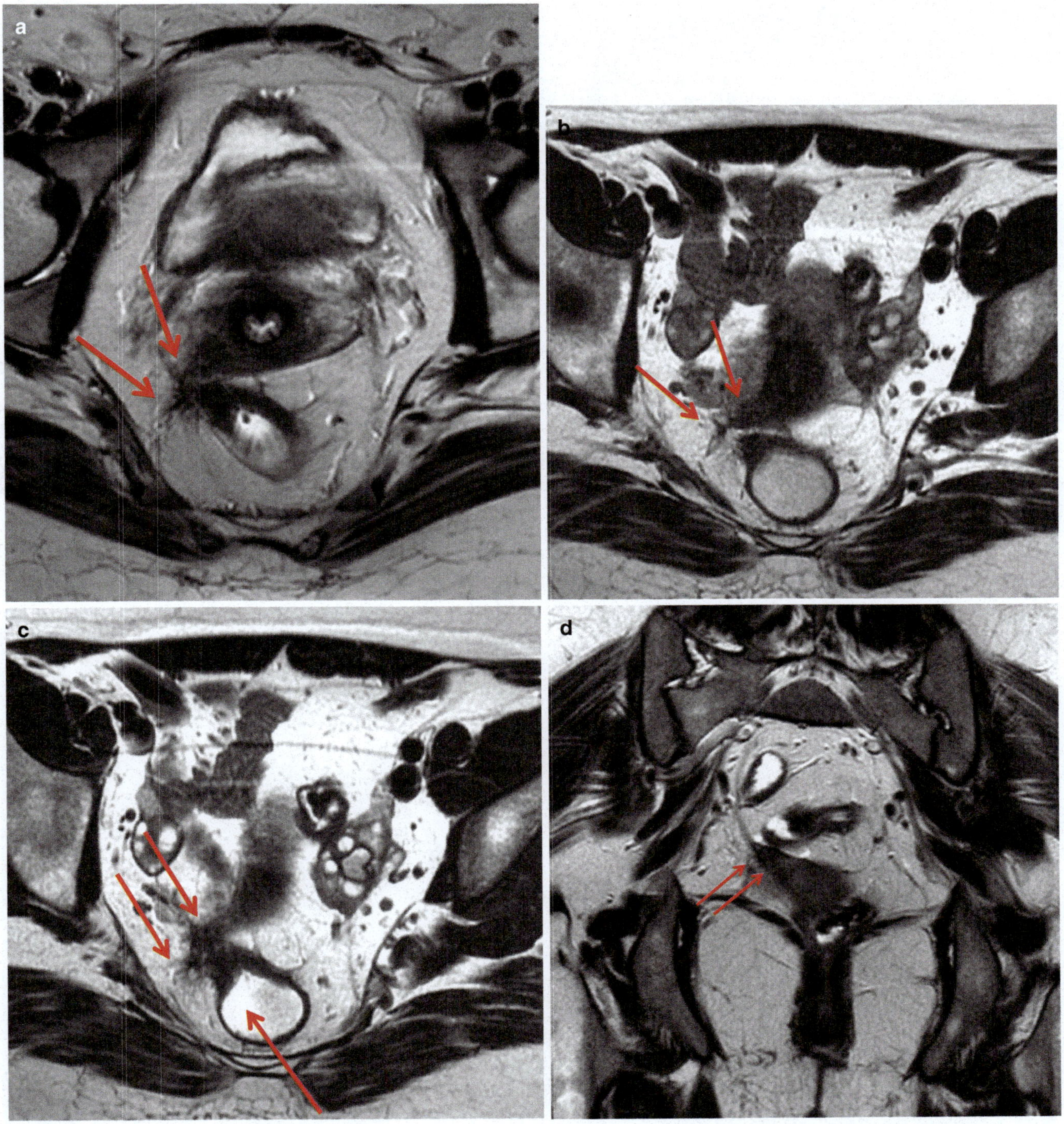

Fig. 3.2 Thickening, irregularities, and retraction of the right uterosacral ligament right. Adherence to the anterior wall of the rectum, with deep intestinal involvement. (**ae**) T2-weighted sequences. (**a–c**). (**d**) Short coronal axis. (**e**) Sagittal. (**f**) Laparoscopy

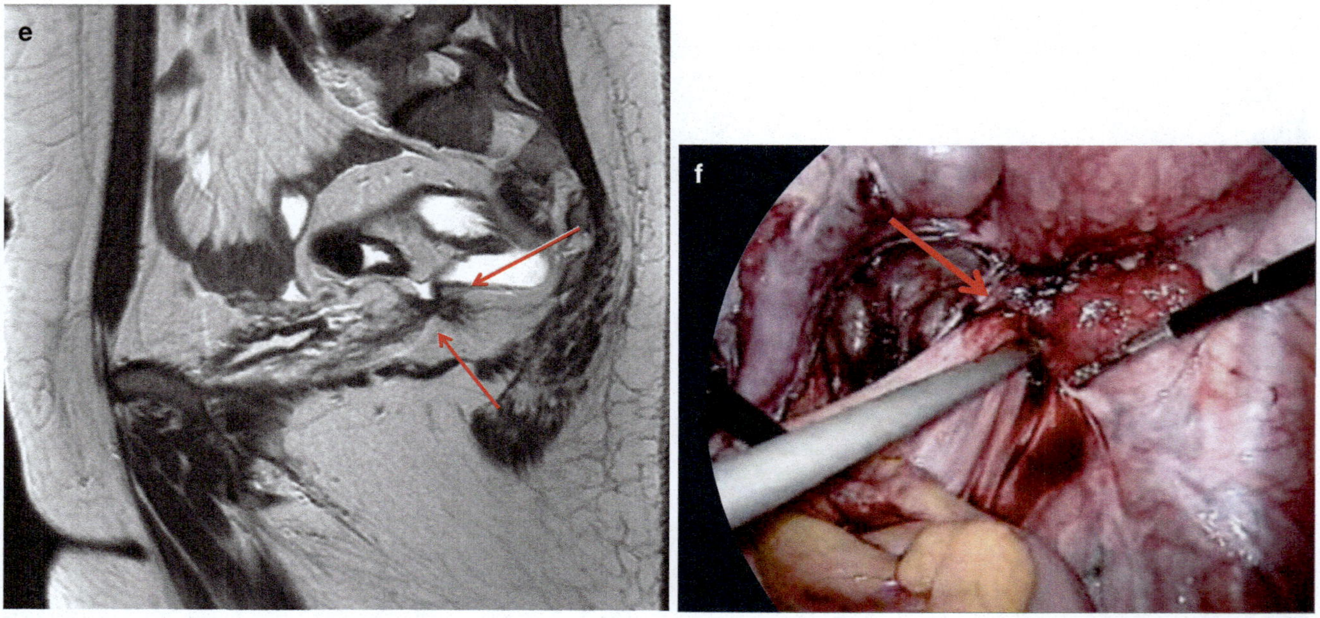

Fig. 3.2 (continued)

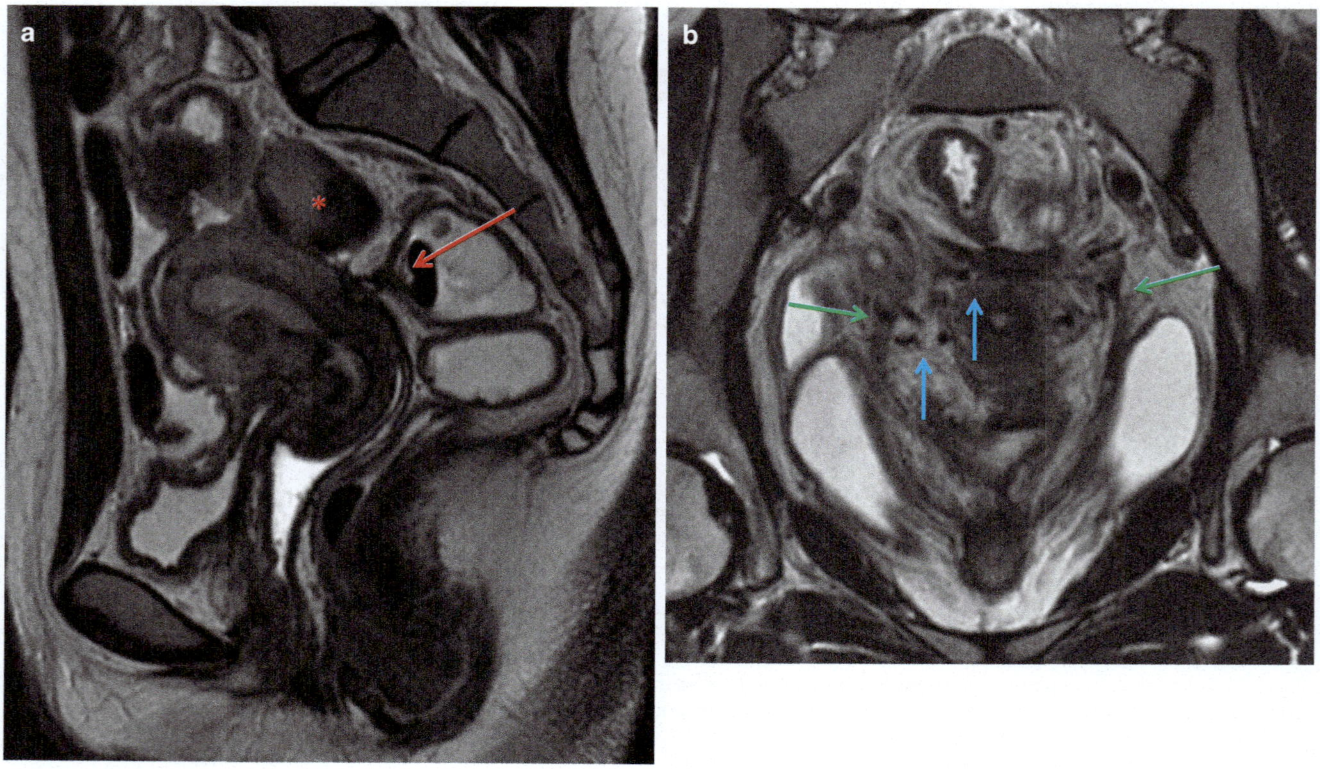

Fig. 3.3 Compromise of the bilateral uterosacral ligament, cervical insertion (yellow arrow), determining posterior and medial displacement of the annex (*), retrouterine, and anterior retraction of the upper rectal segment (red arrow). Note the proximity of the lesion to the ureters (green arrow) and uterine arteries (blue arrows). T2-weighted sequences. (**a**) Sagittal. (**b**) Short coronal axis. (**c**, **d**) Oblique axis

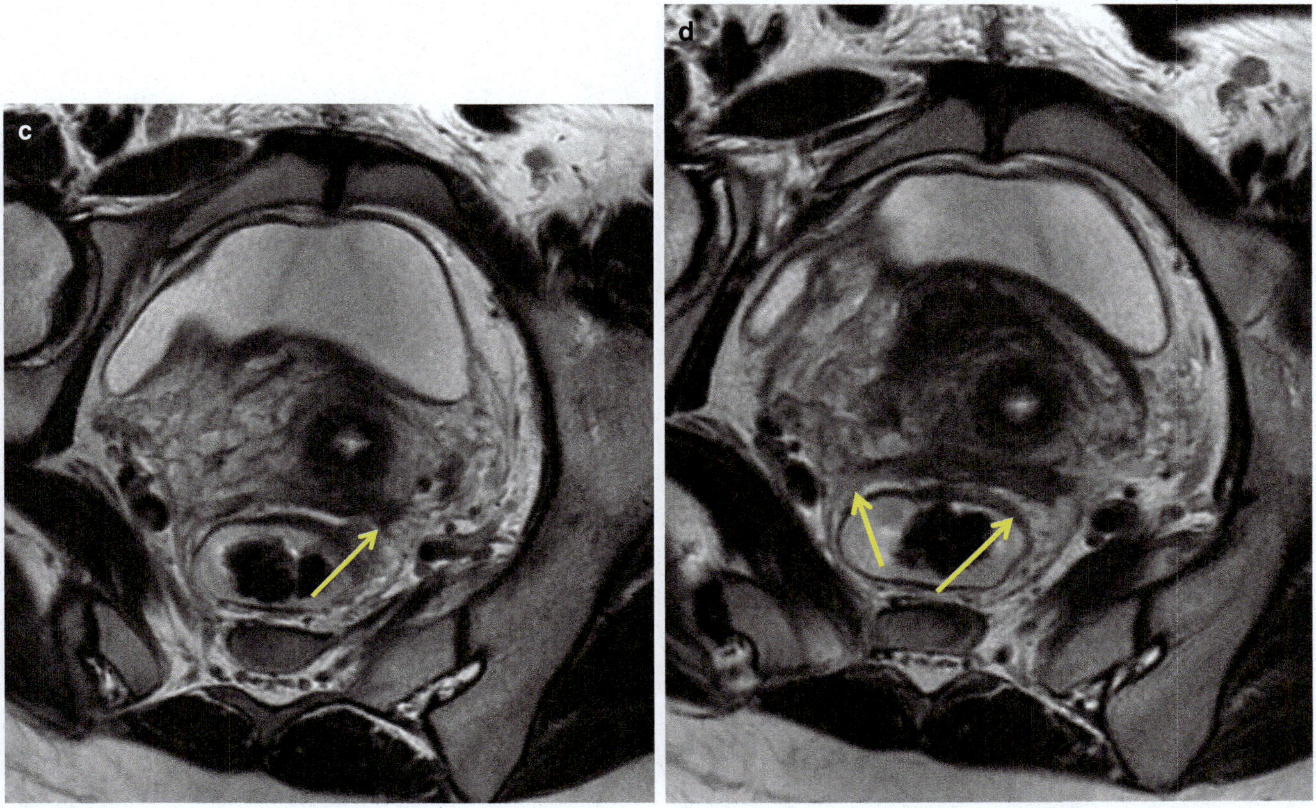

Fig. 3.3 (continued)

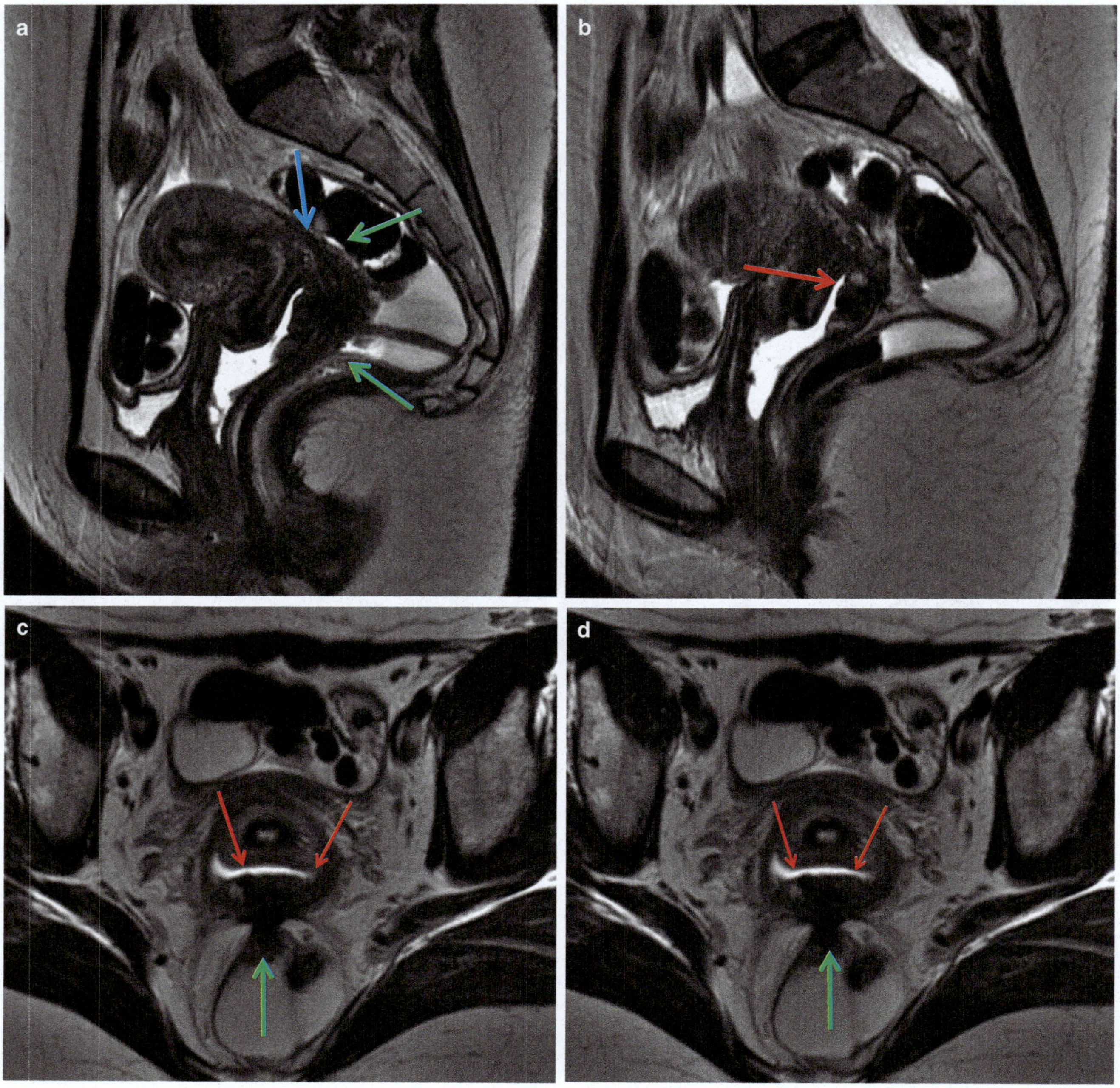

Fig. 3.4 (**a–f**) Nodule in the rectovaginal septum, irregular, with penetration in the rectal segments (green) to the mucosa, and posterior vagina obliterating the vaginal fornix (red) and posterior (blue) extending to paracolpos (**b**). (**g**, **h**) Control after hormone therapy with reduction of volume and signal intensity and important decrease of rectal extension. (**a–e**, **g**, **h**) T1-weighted sequence (hypointense lesion with hypersignal foci). (**f**) T1-weighted sequence (bleeding foci). (**a**, **b**, **g**) Sagittal plane. (**c–f**, **h**) Axial plane. (**i**) Laparoscopy showing a rectum nodule attached to the retrocervical region with extension to the rectovaginal septum

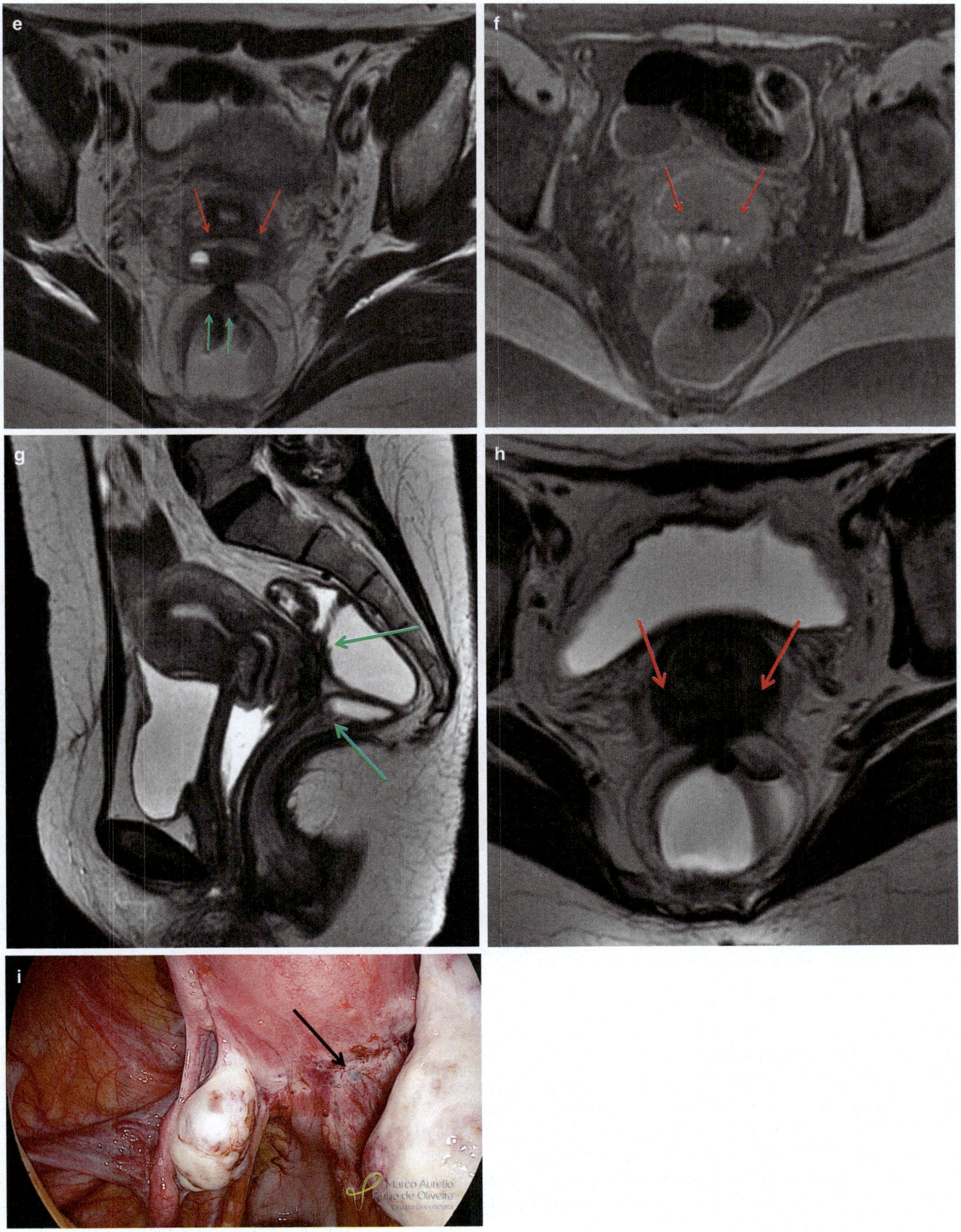

Fig. 3.4 (continued)

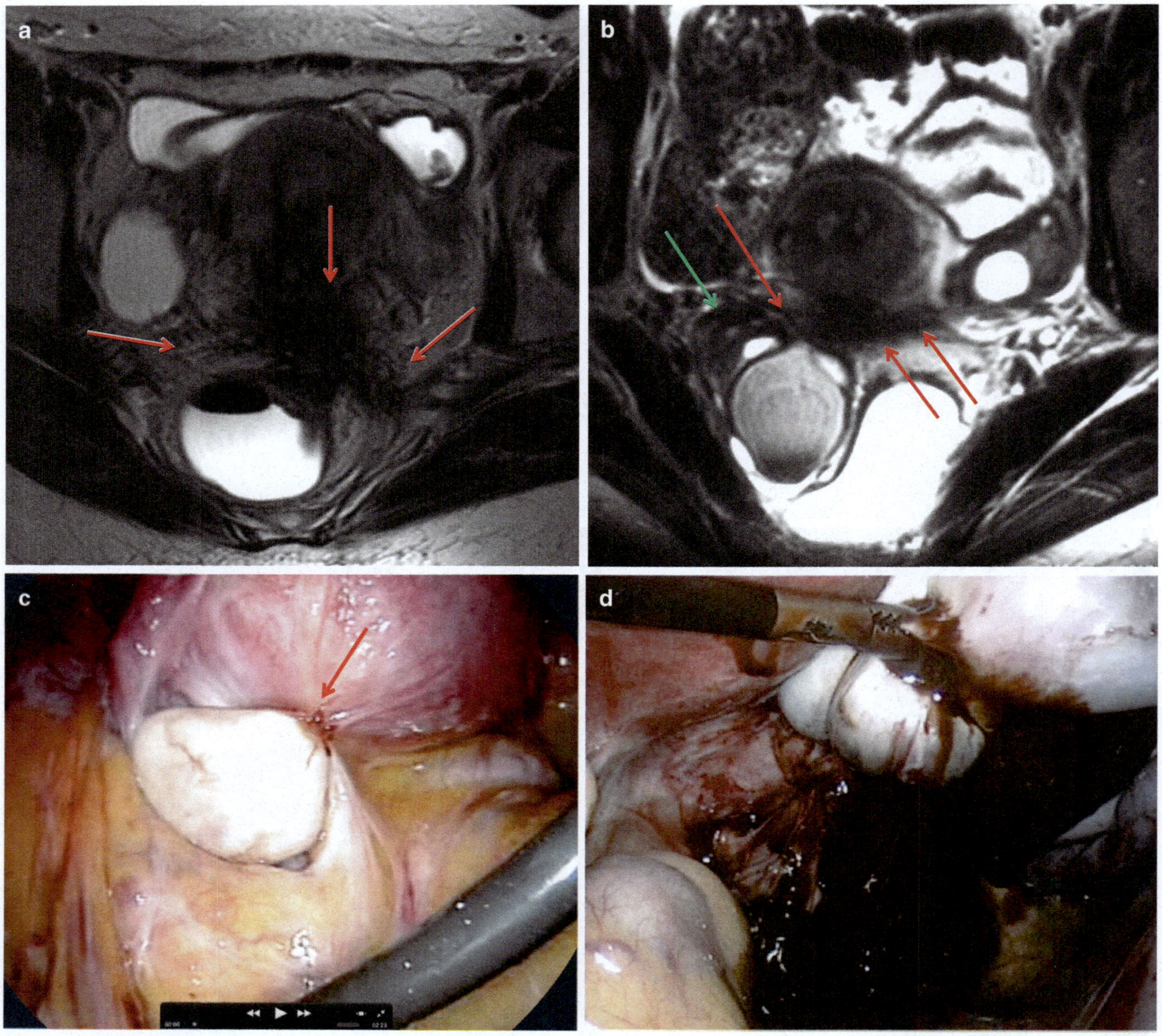

Fig. 3.5 Case 1: (**a**) Rectovaginal septum node, irregular, with penetration of the uterosacral ligaments, mostly to the left, causing adhesion between the vagina, rectum, and the ligament, in addition to retraction of the uterus and anterior rectal wall (arrows). Case 2: (**b**) Another lesion in the rectum and ligamentous septum (red arrows), later diverting the appendages, especially the right (green arrow), which intersects between the uterus and rectum. (**a**, **b**) T2-weighted sequences. (**a**) Axial. (**b**) Coronal with short axis. (**c**, **d**) Laparoscopy identifying the lesion (arrow)

3.1.1.3 Plaque-Like Lesions

These lesions have a plaque-like infiltrative morphology, with ill-defined margins, and cover the neighboring organs, such as the surface of the uterus, causing adhesions between pelvic or abdominal structures. Usually the adhesion process is prominent, promoting obliteration of the posterior and anterior cul-de-sac, as well as uterine, bladder, and bowel retractions (Fig. 3.6).

Usually, the plaque-like lesion has a longitudinal growth pattern, with a small anteroposterior diameter and fibrosis dominant signal intensity, promoting a hypointense signal in T2-weighted images. Thus, the diagnosis of this type of lesion by MRI may be difficult for less experienced professionals (Fig. 3.7).

On the other hand, the subperitoneal extension of the plaque-like lesion may be underestimated by physical exam, and laparoscopy and MRI may be required to provide a comprehensive survey of the extension of the lesion and its complications.

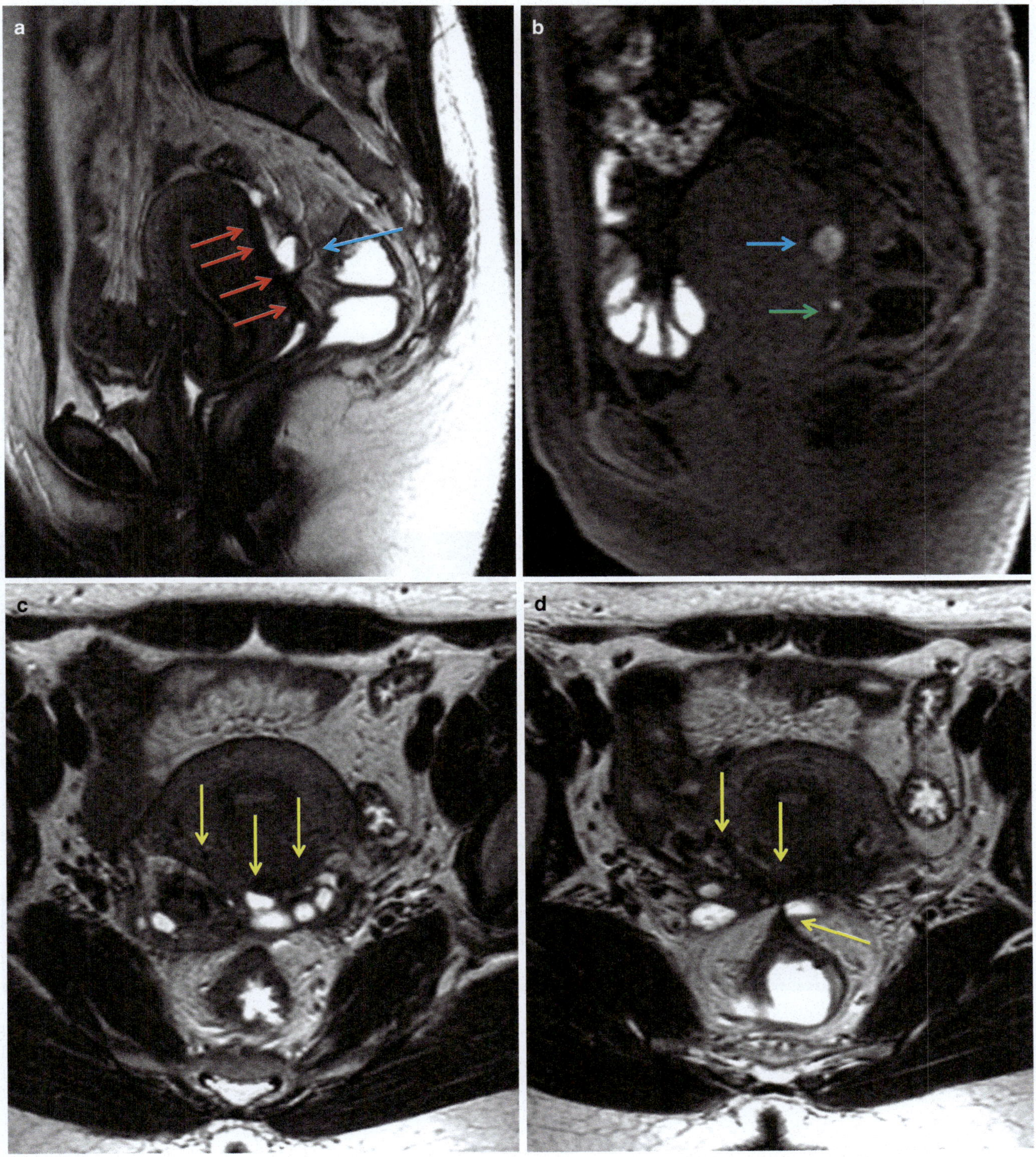

Fig. 3.6 Lesion in the mantle covering the posterior uterine surface (red arrows), from the fundus to the cervix, promoting adhesions with the uterus, rectum, and appendages (yellow arrows) and partial obliteration of the posterior fornix. The lesion is poorly delimited, hypointense in T2 (red arrow) with a bleeding focus in the vaginal fornix (green arrow). Note peritoneal endometriosis associated with fluid with containing blood (blue arrow). (**a**, **c**, **d**) T2-weighted sequences. (**b**) T1-weighted sequence with fat saturation. (**a**, **b**) Sagittal. (**c**, **d**) Axial. (**e**) Laparoscopy showing rectum lesion, sacral obliteration, and posterior adhesion with medial deviation of the appendages

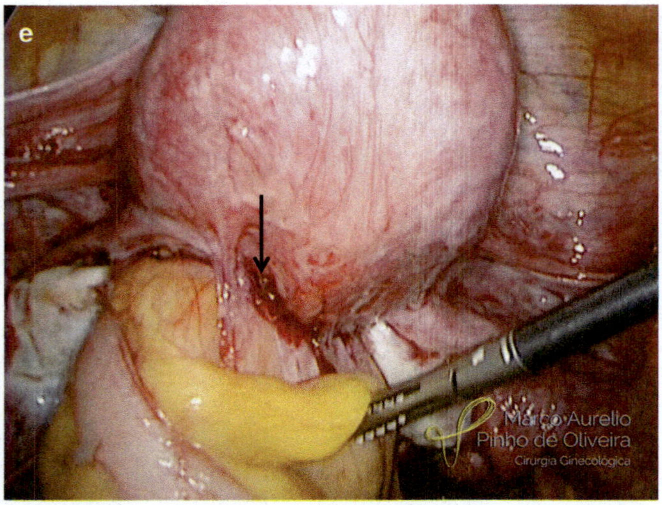

Fig. 3.6 (continued)

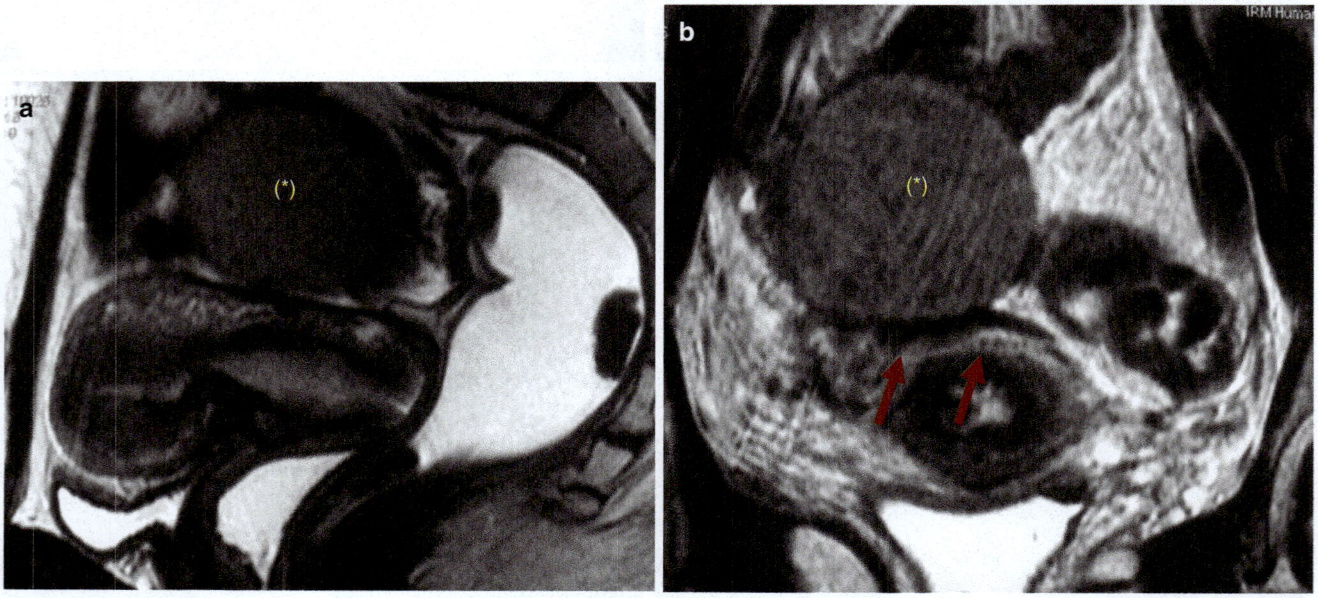

Fig. 3.7 Mantle lesion. Note the difficulty of identifying the lesion in the sagittal plane, due to the longitudinal growth pattern and the small anteroposterior diameter, in addition to the predominance of fibrosis with a hypointense signal in T2, without bleeding. Posterior and medial deviations of the right retrouterine ovary (*). (**a**, **b**) T2-weighted sequences. (**a**) Sagittal. (**b**) Coronal short axis

3.2 Signal Intensity

The signal intensity characteristics of deep endometriosis lesions may vary as well and are affected by the proportion of glands, stroma, and fibrosis. Deep endometriosis lesions have a higher fibrous component.

The presence of hemorrhage and the extent of the associated inflammatory reaction may also impact on signal intensity. Furthermore, the signal intensity of the lesion may be influenced by hormonal treatment and pregnancy. In the latter, a stromal decidual reaction may be observed and may present peritoneal nodules.

3.2.1 Predominantly Fibrous Lesions

Predominantly fibrous lesions present with lower glandular tissue and a predominance of stromal and interstitial fibrosis. In some cases, many histological sections may be necessary to identify the glandular component of endometriosis [3].

In MRI, this lesion presents low signal intensity in the T2-weighted sequence, an intermediate signal in the T1-weighted sequence, which may be enhanced after intravenous administration of gadolinium. The enhancement intensity is usually mild in these cases (Fig. 3.8).

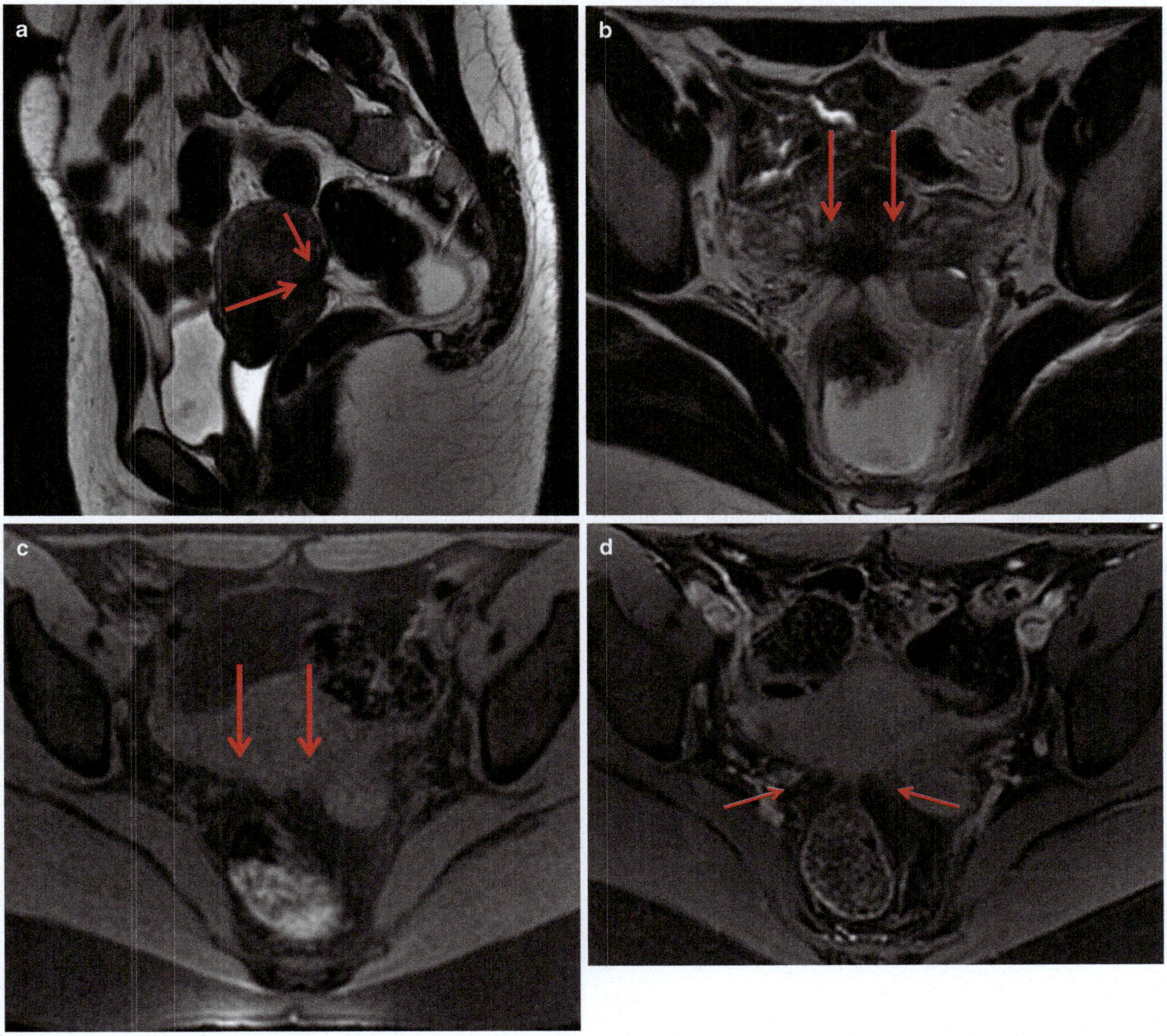

Fig. 3.8 Retrocervical lesion with a predominance of fibrosis (arrows) characterized by a hypointense signal in T2-weighted sequence (**a**, **b**), an intermediate signal in T1 (**c**) and discrete enhancement with gadolinium (**d**). (**a**) Sagittal. (**b–d**) Axial. (**e**) Histopathology. Note the lack of glandular tissue and predominance of stroma and interstitial fibrosis (thanks to Dr. Leon Cardeman). (**f**) Laparoscopy demonstrating involvement of the rectum adhered to the lesion, in addition to medial deviation of the ovaries

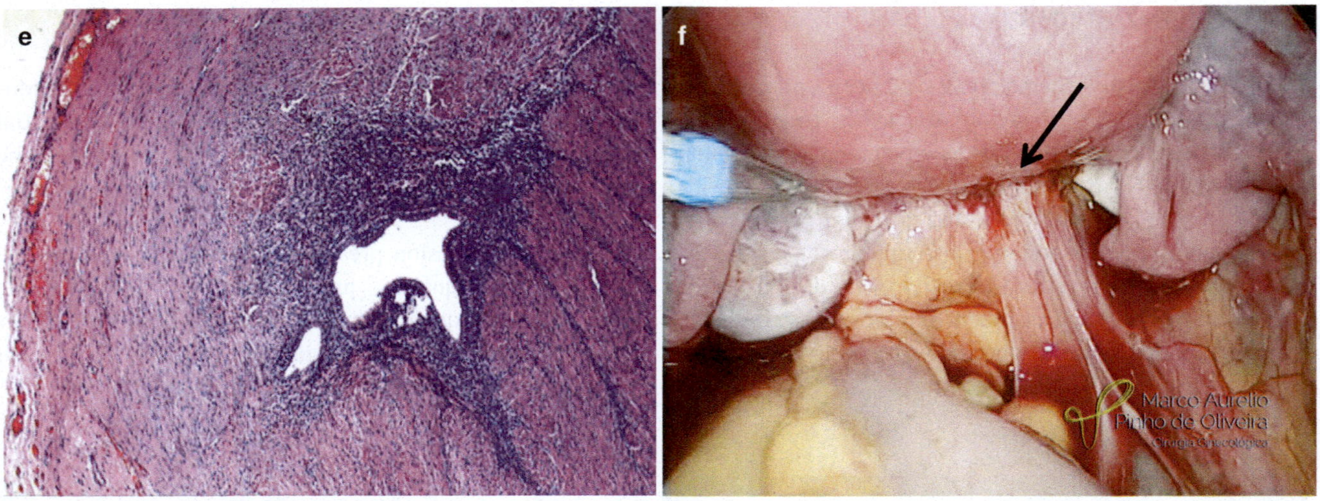

Fig. 3.8 (continued)

Endometriosis in places with smooth muscle component, such as the bowel, may induce marked muscle hypertrophy and be associated with fibrosis, contributing to wall thickening. Muscle reaction and interstitial fibrosis result in a nodule with an intermediate signal in the T1 and hypointense in the T2-weighted sequence (Fig. 3.9).

3.2.2 Mixed Lesions (Fibrosis and Glandular Tissue)

The heterotopic endometrial tissue permeates the fibrous component of the deep lesion and is characterized by islands of endometrial glands, cystic dilation of endometrial glands, or bleeding spots. Cysts represent the complete reabsorption of the gland wall by fibrotic process (Fig. 3.10).

Although endometriosis is a hormone-dependent disease, ectopic endometrial glands are sometimes resistant to hormonal stimulation and rarely undergo cyclical bleeding, which is, if present, restricted to a small area of the lesion. In these cases, it can be observed in the MRI, with a hyperintense foci in the T2-weighted sequence interposed with the fibrotic component of the lesion. When there is bleeding, hemorrhagic focus presents as a hyperintense signal in the T1-weighted sequence and, rarely, at a hematic level (Fig. 3.11).

3.2.3 Lesions with a Prominent Glandular Component

Lesions with a strong prominent glandular component are uncommon and present with a hyperintense signal in T1- and T2-weighted sequences (Fig. 3.12).

This signal can be related to pregnancy or hormone therapy with progesterone, as well as to taking tamoxifen for breast carcinoma, which promotes a decidual response. The lesion will present as a polypoid mass projecting from serosal surfaces, referred to as polypoid endometriosis. The mass is isointense to the myometrium in the T1-weighted sequence and hyperintense in the T2-weighted sequence, similar to the decidualized endometrium, with contrast enhancement and hyperintense focus in the T1-weighted images corresponding to hemorrhage.

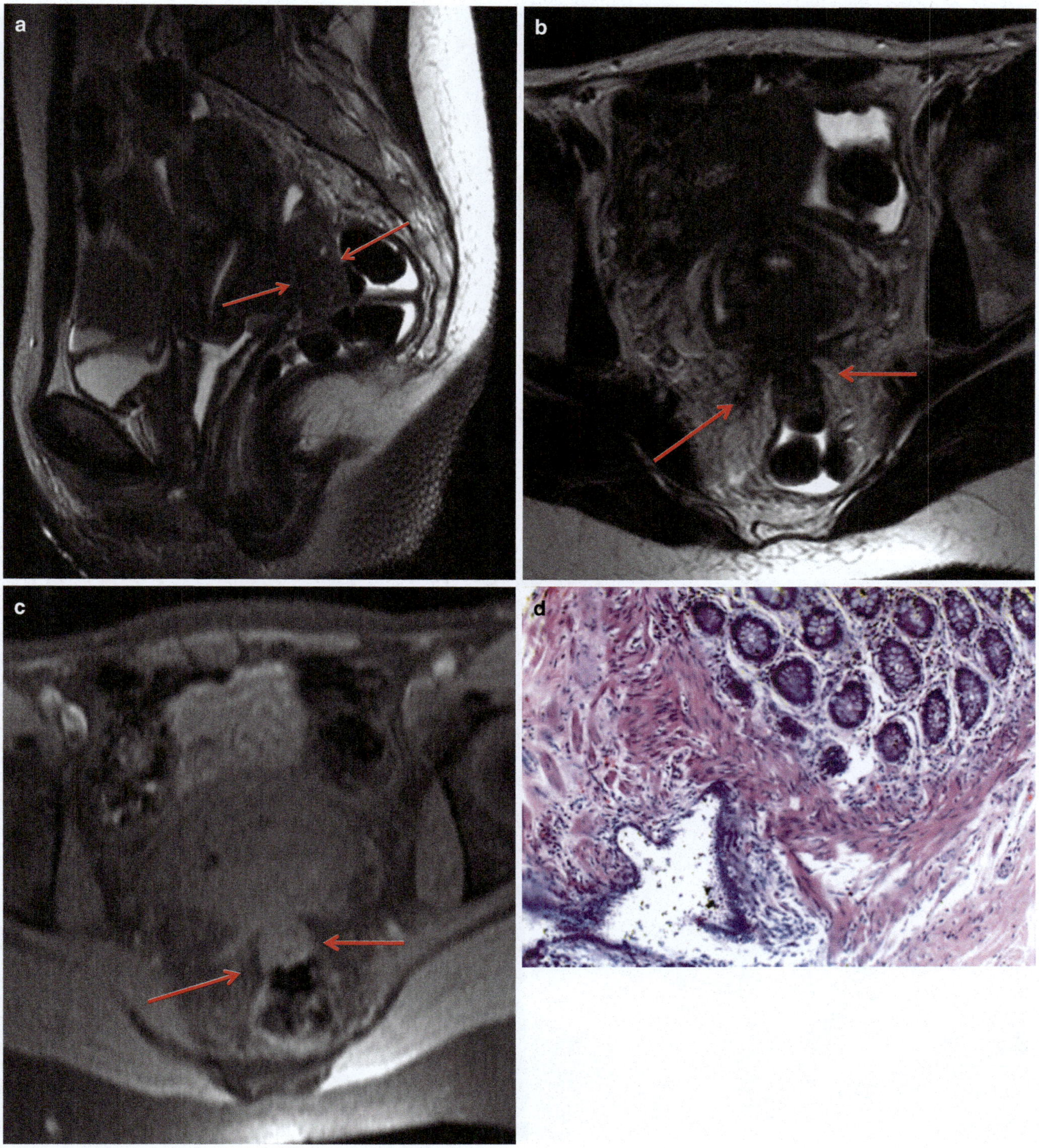

Fig. 3.9 Intestinal rectal endometriosis. Hypointense lesion in T2-weighted sequences (**a**, **b**) and with an intermediate signal in T1-weighted sequence (**c**), with anterior parietal thickening. (**a**) Sagittal. (**b**, **c**) Axial. (**d**) Histopathology demonstrates lack of glandular tissue, fibrosis, and muscular hyperplasia. Note endometriotic wedge near the intestinal glands

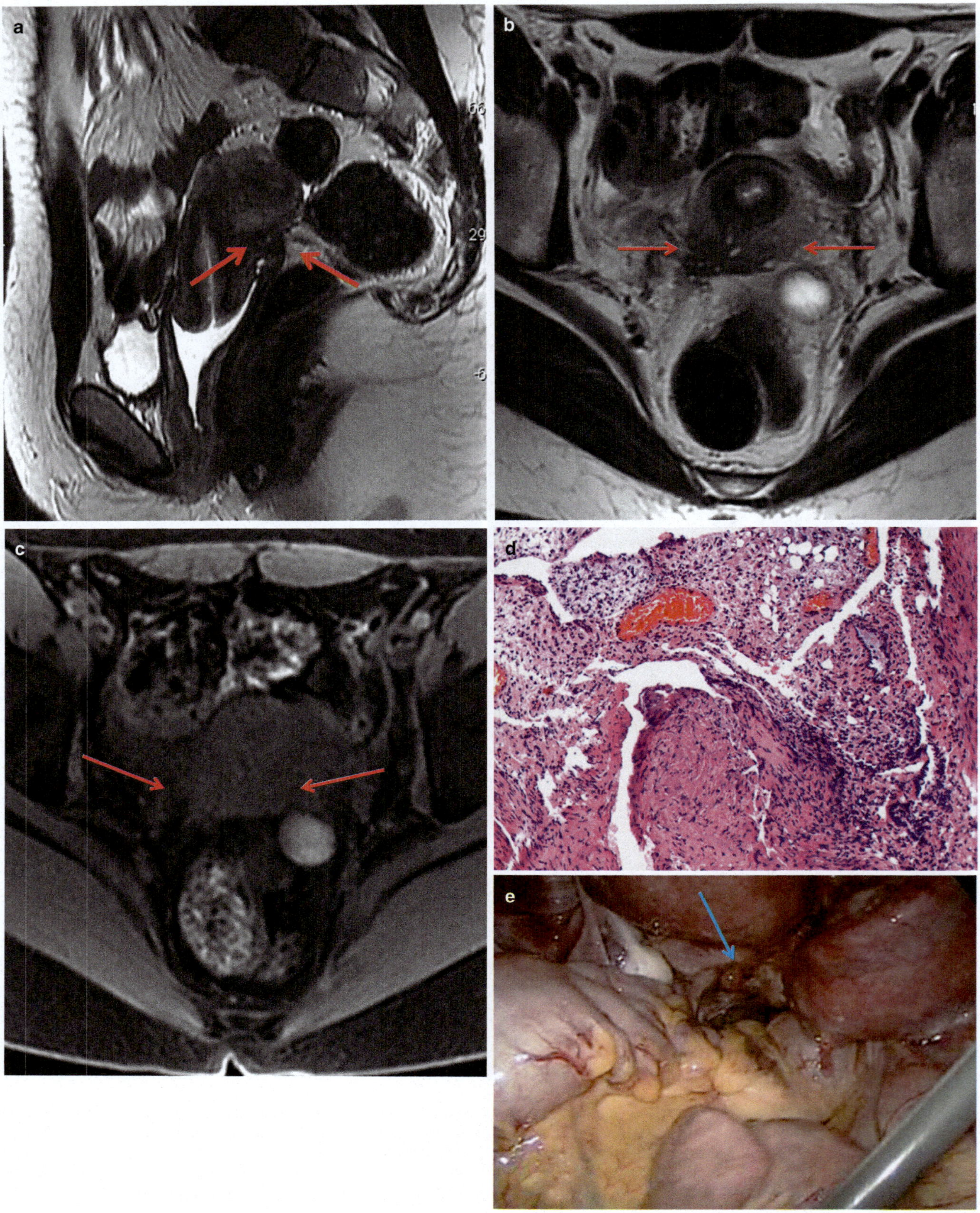

Fig. 3.10 Retrocervical lesion with heterotopic endometrial tissue permeating the fibrous component, islets of endometrial glands, cystic dilatation of the endometrial glands, and bleeding spots. (**a**, **b**) T2-weighted sequences. (**a**) Sagittal. (**b**) Axial. (**c**) T1-weighted sequence with fat saturation. (**d**) Histopathology demonstrates endometriosis, presenting little glandular component (400!) (thanks to Dr. Leon Cardeman). (**e**) Laparoscopy showing retrocervical nodule with vesicle (arrow)

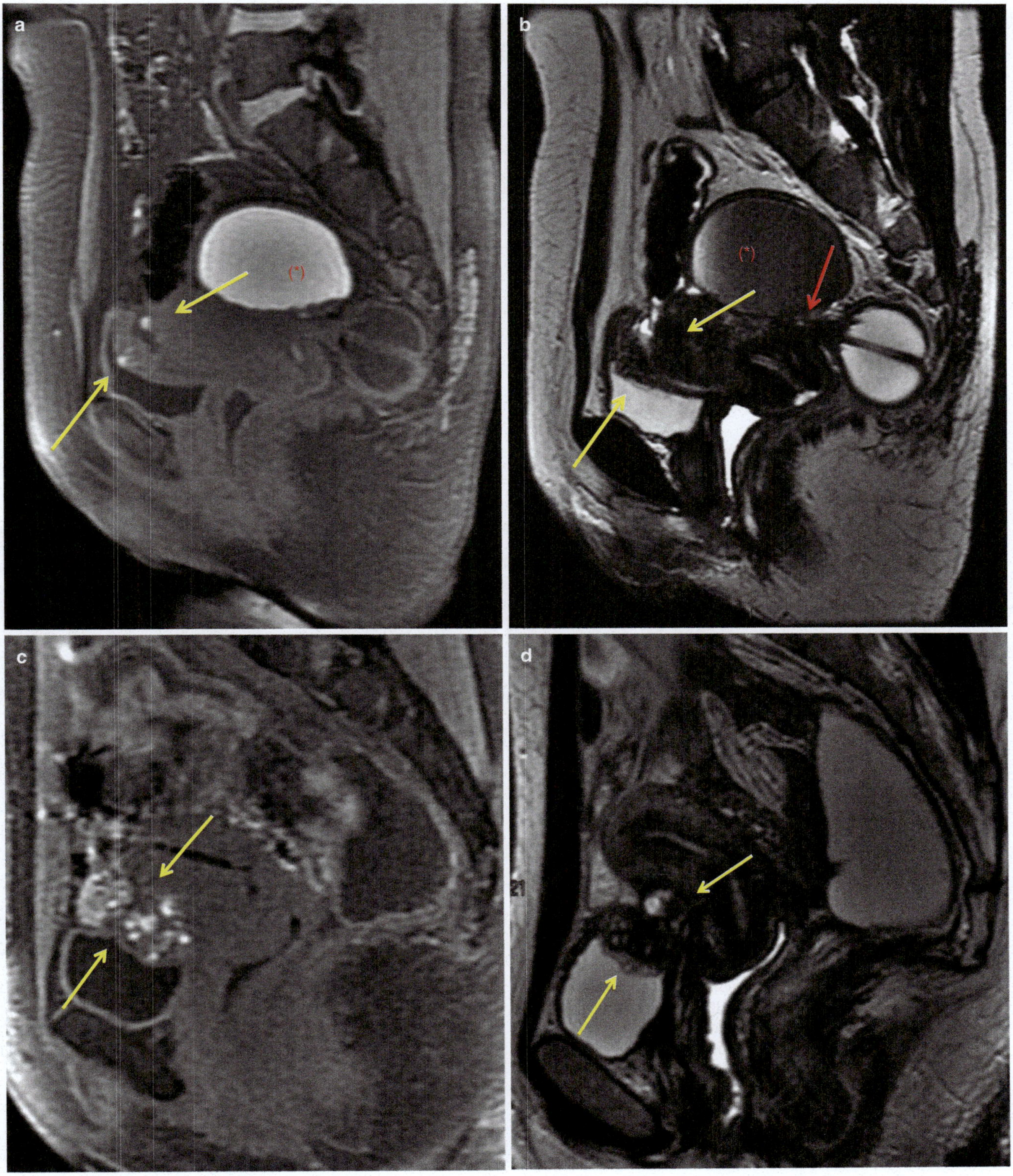

Fig. 3.11 Case 1 (**a**, **b**) and Case 2 (**c**, **d**). Anterior compartment lesions with fibrotic component and hyperintense foci in T2-weighted sequences (**b**, **d**) and T1 with fat suppression (**a**, **c**) due to bleeding (yellow arrows). Case 1: (**a**, **b**) Note additional retrocervical lesion (red arrow) and endometrioma (*). (**e**) Correlation with pathology (vesicouterine fold lesion with large endometriotic cyst). (**f**) Laparoscopy showing lesion in anterior compartment with bladder and right round ligament involvement with bleeding

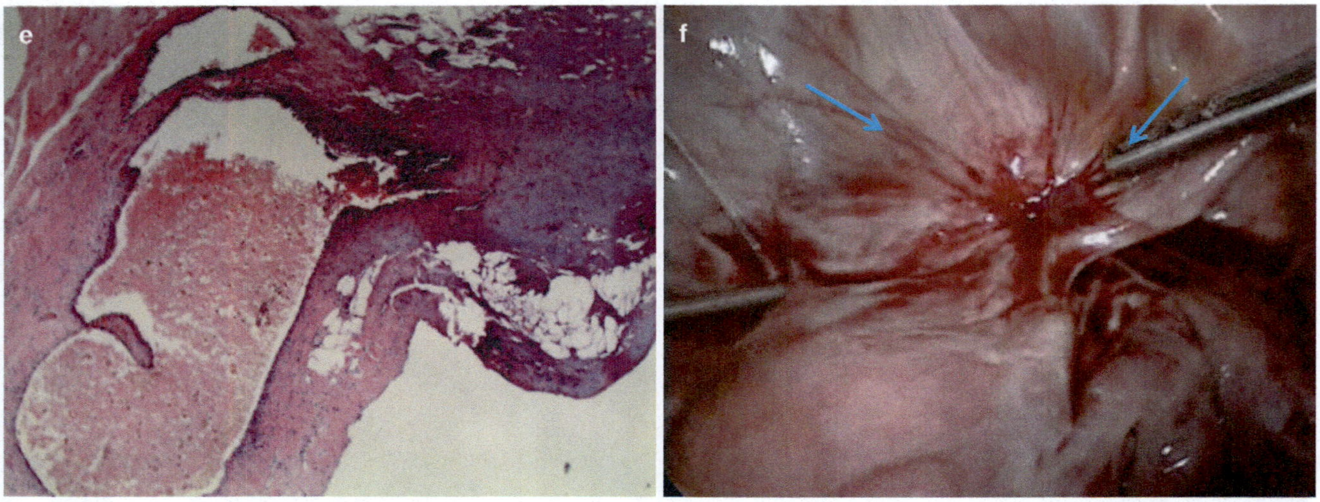

Fig. 3.11 (continued)

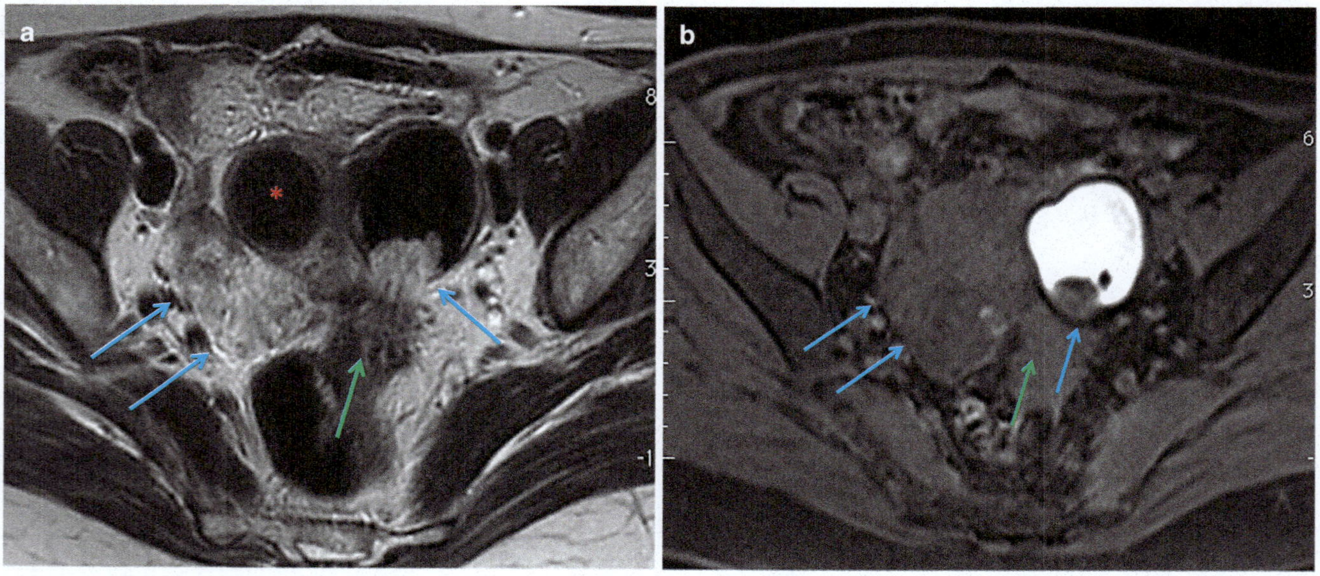

Fig. 3.12 Retrouterinal lesion, causing adhesion between the uterus, sigmoid, and left appendage, with a strong glandular component. Note hypersignal in T2-weighted sequences (green arrow) and enhancement by gadolinium. In addition, there is prominent peritoneal endometriosis with a hypersignal in T2, intense enhancement, without restricted diffusion (**d**), which also extends to the left endometrioma (blue). Patient on hormonal therapy (observe infarction of leiomyoma—*). (**a**) T2-weighted sequence. (**b**) T1-weighted sequence with fat saturation. (**c**) T1-weighted sequence with fat saturation and gadolinium. (**d**) ADC map, axial plane. (**e**) Laparoscopy demonstrating the adhesion and extensive decidual peritoneal component

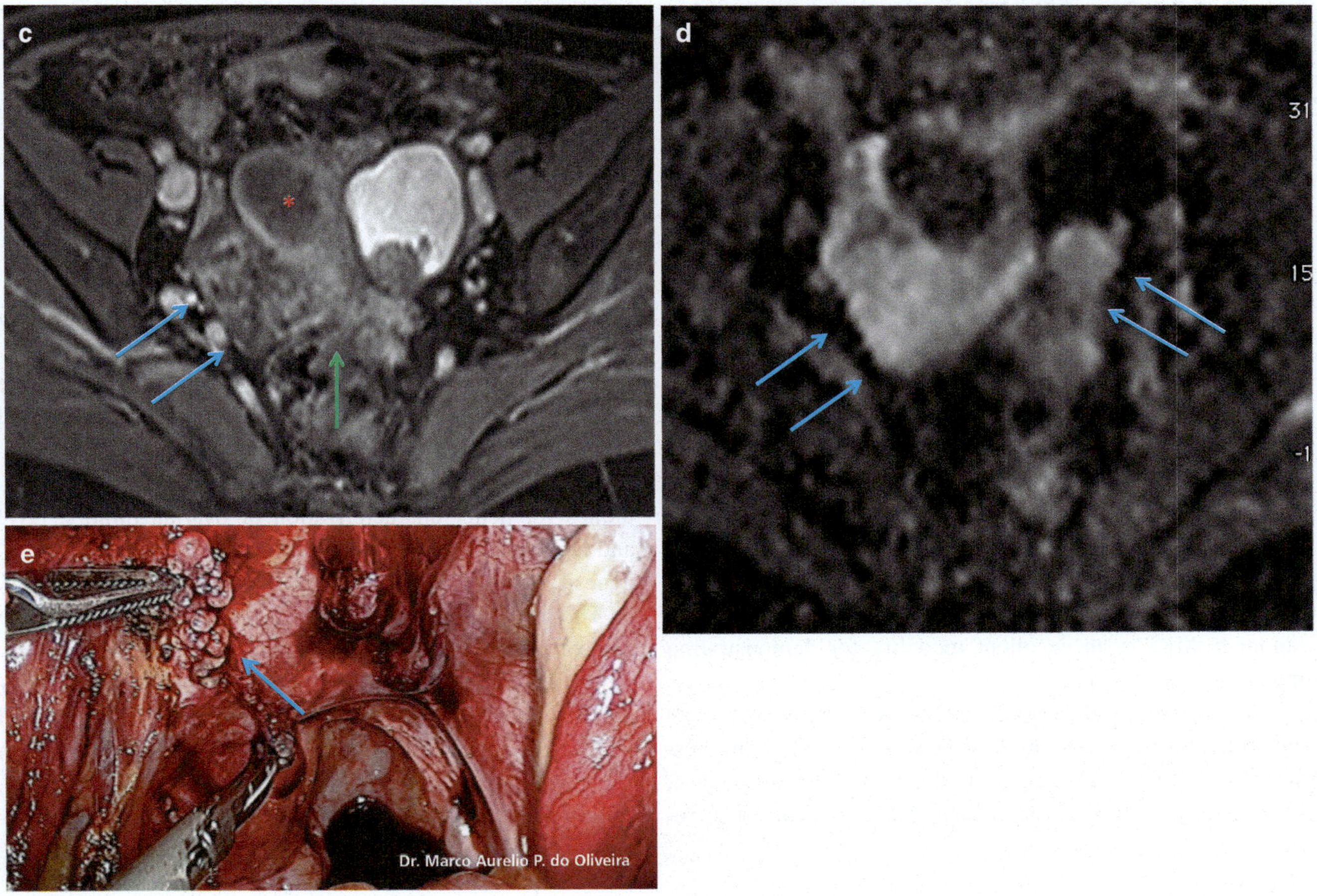

Fig. 3.12 (continued)

3.3 Additional Findings

3.3.1 Enhancement Pattern

The pattern of enhancement of deep endometriosis is variable, and, in general, the contrast does not contribute to the identification and characterization of deep endometriosis in the MRI. However, there are situations where it is important, such as in adnexal lesion characterization and improved identification of small, nonhemorrhagic abdominal wall deep endometriosis.

3.3.2 Characterization of Adnexal Lesions

Endometriosis has an increased risk of secondary carcinoma. The incidence of malignant ovarian endometriomas is estimated to be about 1%. Endometrioid and clear-cell carcinomas are the most common histologic subtypes of carcinomas. MRI is an excellent modality for demonstrating malignant transformation.

The imaging characteristics that suggest malignancy in an endometrioid ovary cyst are large lesion size, with a progressive loss of hypointense signal in the T2-weighted sequence, promoted by dilution of hemorrhagic fluid by the tumor secretion, as well as the solid component presented as a mural nodule.

The malignant mural nodule presents a low signal intensity in the T1-weighted sequence, a variable signal in the T2-weighted sequence, and increases its signal intensity with the contrast-enhanced sequence.

However, a mural nodule in an endometrioma is not pathognomonic of ovarian cancer. It can be related to a clot, decidual change, mucinous metaplasia, or polypoid changes. Polypoid endometriosis can mimic a malignant tumor (Fig. 3.13 and Table 3.1) [1, 4].

Furthermore, multiparametric MRI can evaluate the lesion's aggressiveness, using the diffusion-weighted sequence (DWI) and tumor permeability (DCE-MR imaging). Functional sequences are promising emerging techniques for better characterization of ovarian tumors. DWI and DCE-MR imaging evaluate tumor cellularity and angiogenesis, respectively [5].

Thomassin-Naggara et al. studied 41 patients with known adnexal lesions and showed that early enhancement characteristics, using an intensity curve vs. time, help to differentiate benign, borderline, and invasive tumors. A gradual increase in enhancement in the early phase of the perfusion study was defined as type 1 curve; a moderate initial increase, similar to the myometrium, followed by a plateau was classi-

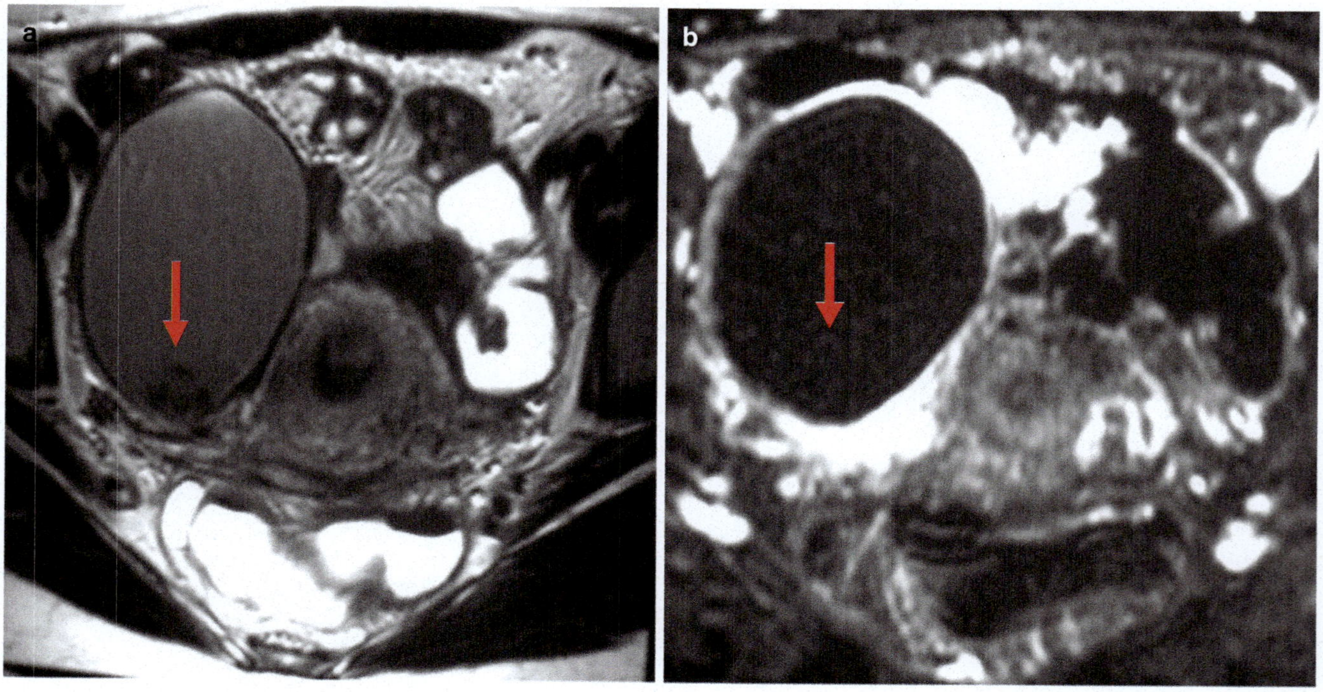

Fig. 3.13 Difference between endometrioma (Case 1) and endometrioid cystadenocarcinoma (Case 2). Case 1: (**a**, **b**) The endometrioma clot (arrows) is not enhanced by gadolinium (**b**). Case 2: (**c**–**e**) The mural nodule (arrows) enhances with the study contrast (E). (**a**, **c**, **d**) T2-weighted sequences. (**b**, **e**) T1-weighted with gadolinium, being (**b**) subtraction imaging. (**a**–**c**) Axial. (**d**, **e**) Sagittal

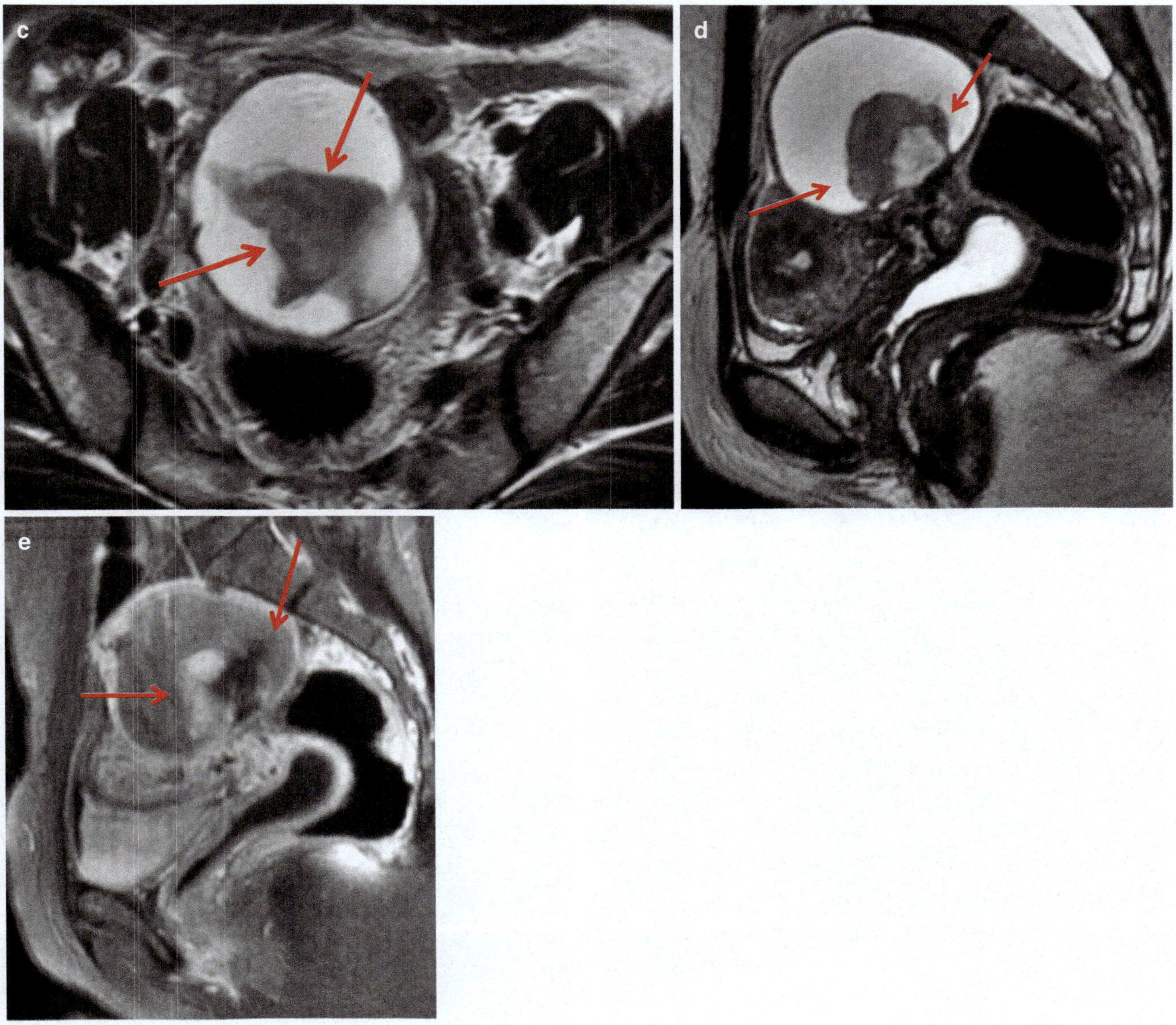

Fig. 3.13 (continued

Table 3.1 Mural nodule in an endometrioid cyst. Differential diagnosis

	T1	T2	Contrast-enhanced
Carcinoma	Hypointense	Variable	Enhancement
Clot	Hyperintense	Hypointense	No enhancement
Decidual change	Variable	Hyperintense	Minimum enhancement
Mucinous metaplasia	Variable	Hyperintense	No enhancement
Polypoid endometriosis	Hypointense	Intermediate	Enhancement

fied as type 2 curve; a rapid initial increase, more intense than the myometrium, was reported as type 3 curve. The type 3 curve is considered the most suspicious (Fig. 3.14) [5–7].

Moreover, a mural nodule displaying both low signal intensity on the T2-weighted sequence and nonrestricted diffusion has a 100% benign predictive value [5].

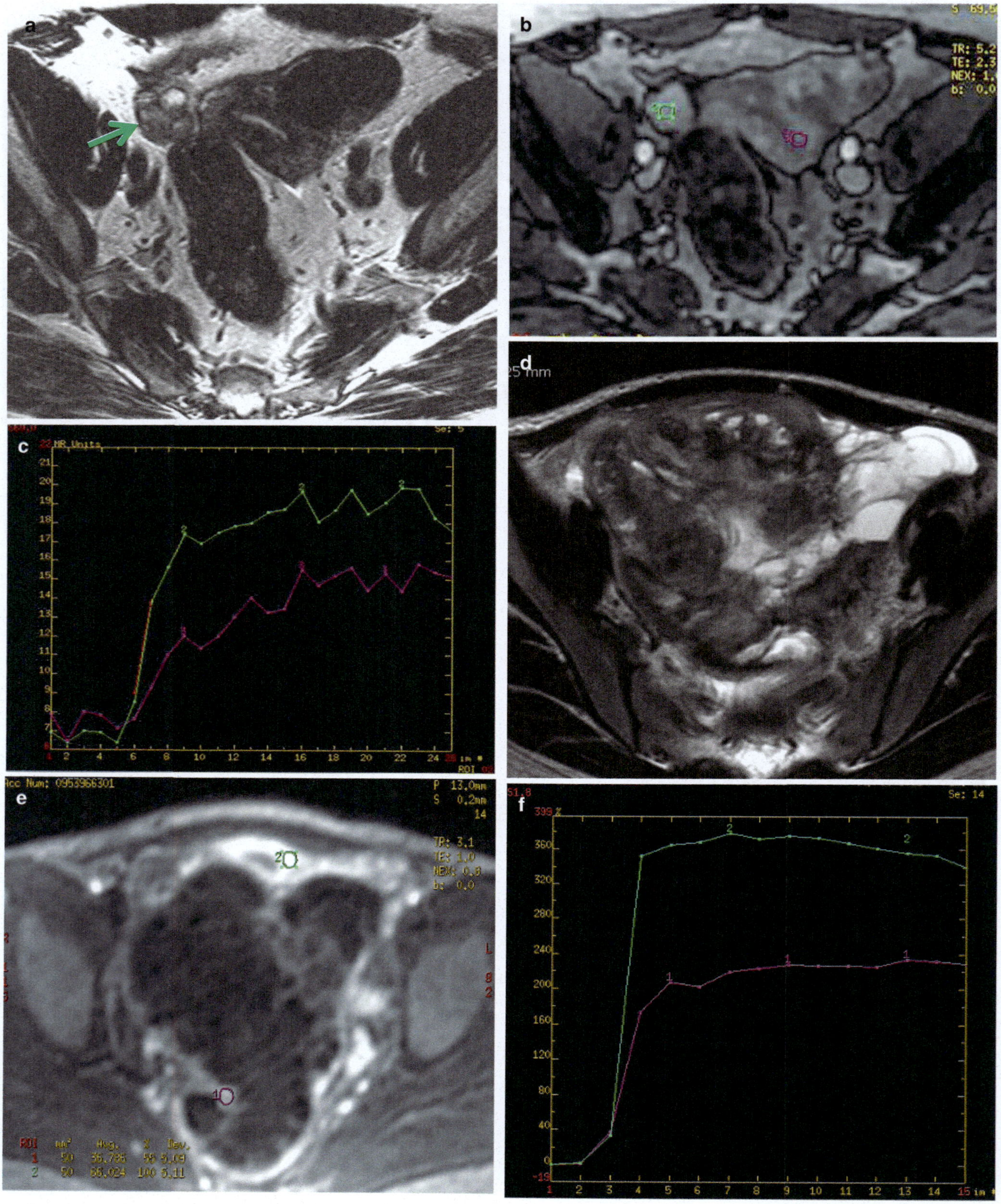

Fig. 3.14 Case 1: Sertoli-Leydig tumor in the right ovary. A permeability study with gadolinium shows a rapid initial increase, more intense than that of the myometrium, with a type 3 curve. (**a**) Small nodule in the right ovary. (**b**) Permeability study (ROI in green in the ovarian lesion and pink in the uterus). (**c**) Enhancement curve. Case 2: Choriocarcinoma. Large, rapidly growing complex cyst in a 14-year-old female displacing the uterus. Rapid increase of the enhancement, although smaller than the myometrium, with a type 2 curve (ROI in green in the uterus and pink in the lesion). (**a, d**) T2-weighted sequences. (**b, e**) Permeability study (T1 with gadolinium). (**c, f**) Enhancement curve, intensity x time. Axial plane

3.3.3 Associated Inflammatory Process Identification

There is an association between endometriosis and the pelvic inflammatory process. In the peritoneal fluid of patients, there are increased concentrations of cytokines and growth factors, generating an inflammatory process that probably contributes to the progression of the disease.

MRI can show thickening and diffuse peritoneal enhancement, especially near the ovarian fossa. This type of change usually occurs in patients with advanced deep endometriosis with a prominent glandular tissue and ovary and peritoneal endometriosis association (Fig. 3.15) [8, 9].

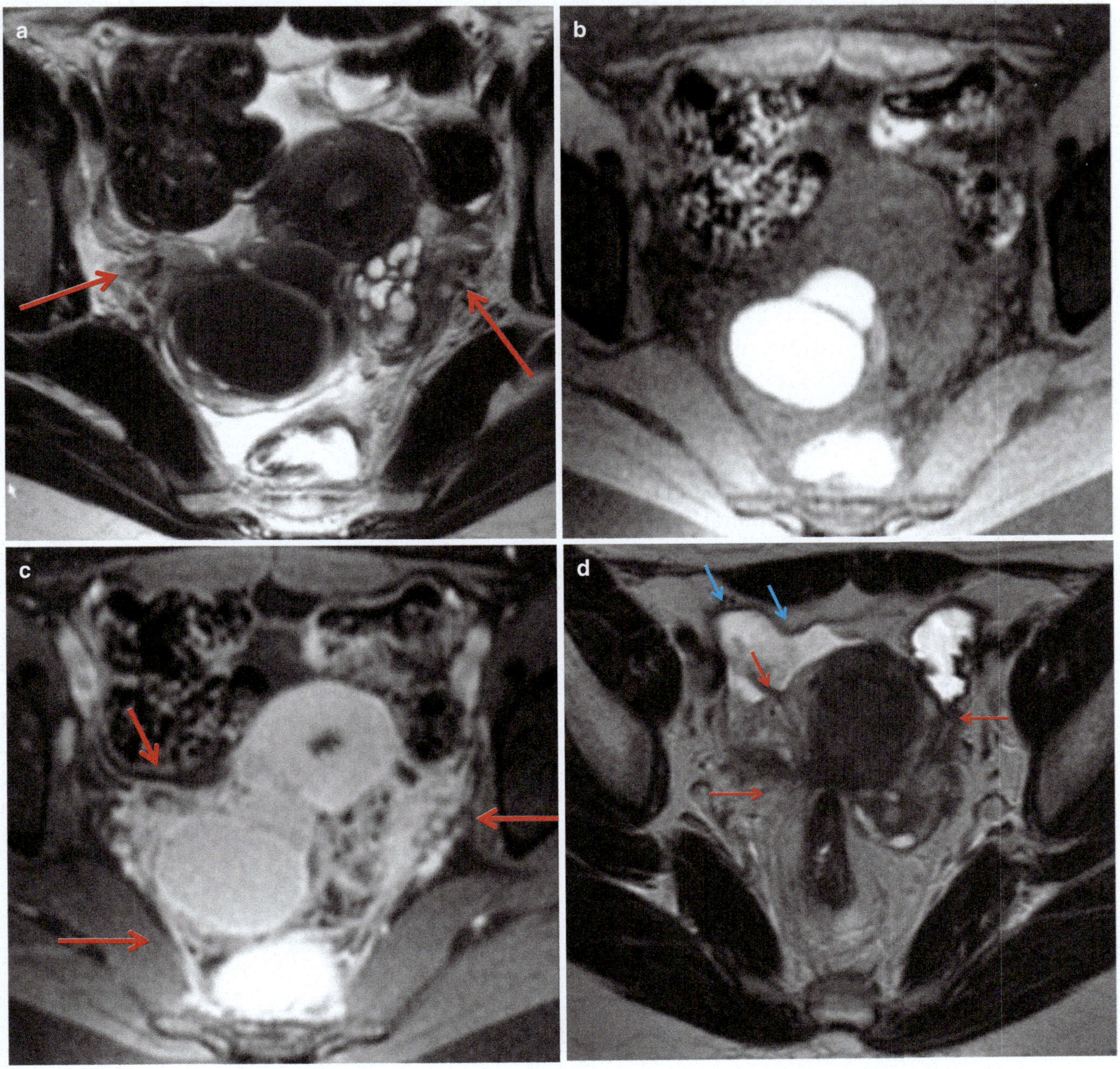

Fig. 3.15 Thickening and diffuse peritoneal enhancement, notably bilateral periadnexal and left tubal (red—**a**–**e**), in addition to free fluid (blue—**d**–**f**). Notice endometriomas on the right (**a**–**c**, **f**). T2-weighted sequences (**a**, **d**, **f**), T1 with fat saturation (**b**), and gadolinium (**c**, **e**). (**a**–**e**) Axial. (**f**) Sagittal

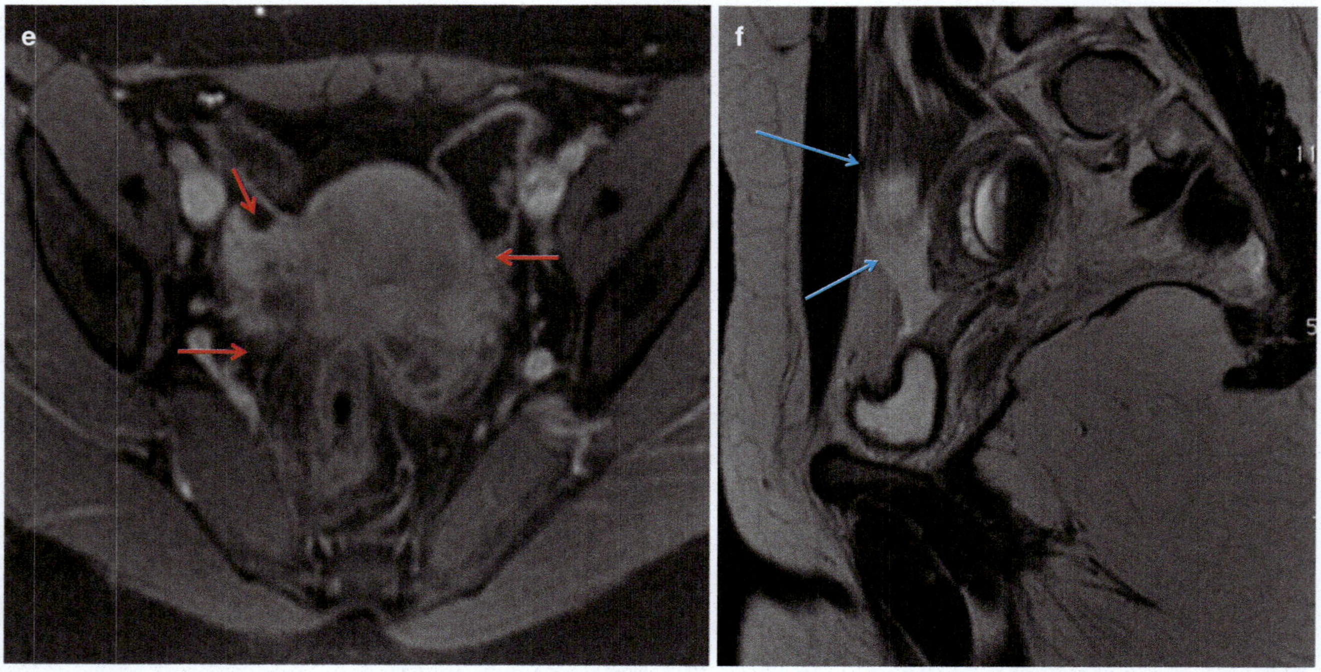

Fig. 3.15 (continued)

3.3.4 Improved Identification of a Small Non-hemorrhagic Abdominal Wall Deep Endometriosis

These lesions, when predominantly muscular, may share similar signal intensity to the muscle belly, intermediate in the T1-weighted sequence and hypointense in the T2-weighted sequence, due to the predominance of fibrosis and absence of glandular tissue, making them very subtle. As there is usually an associated inflammatory process, these lesions will be enhanced by the administration of gadolinium, making their identification easier.

Desmoid tumors can have similar signal intensity and enhancing behavior in MRI; however the clinical history and the age of the patient may suggest a diagnosis of endometriosis (Fig. 3.16).

3.3.4.1 Abdominal Adhesions

Deep endometriosis is an infiltrative disease often complicated by adhesions. In one study, pelvic adhesion was identified in 66.7% of cases, and partial or total obliteration of the cul-de-sac was observed in 60% of women [10].

The predominantly fibrous lesions induce interstitial fibrosis and penetrate tissues or adjacent organs, distorting and displacing them, accentuating pelvic pain. Interstitial fibrosis is sometimes so prominent that it can be difficult to identify ectopic endometrial tissue in the pathology [11].

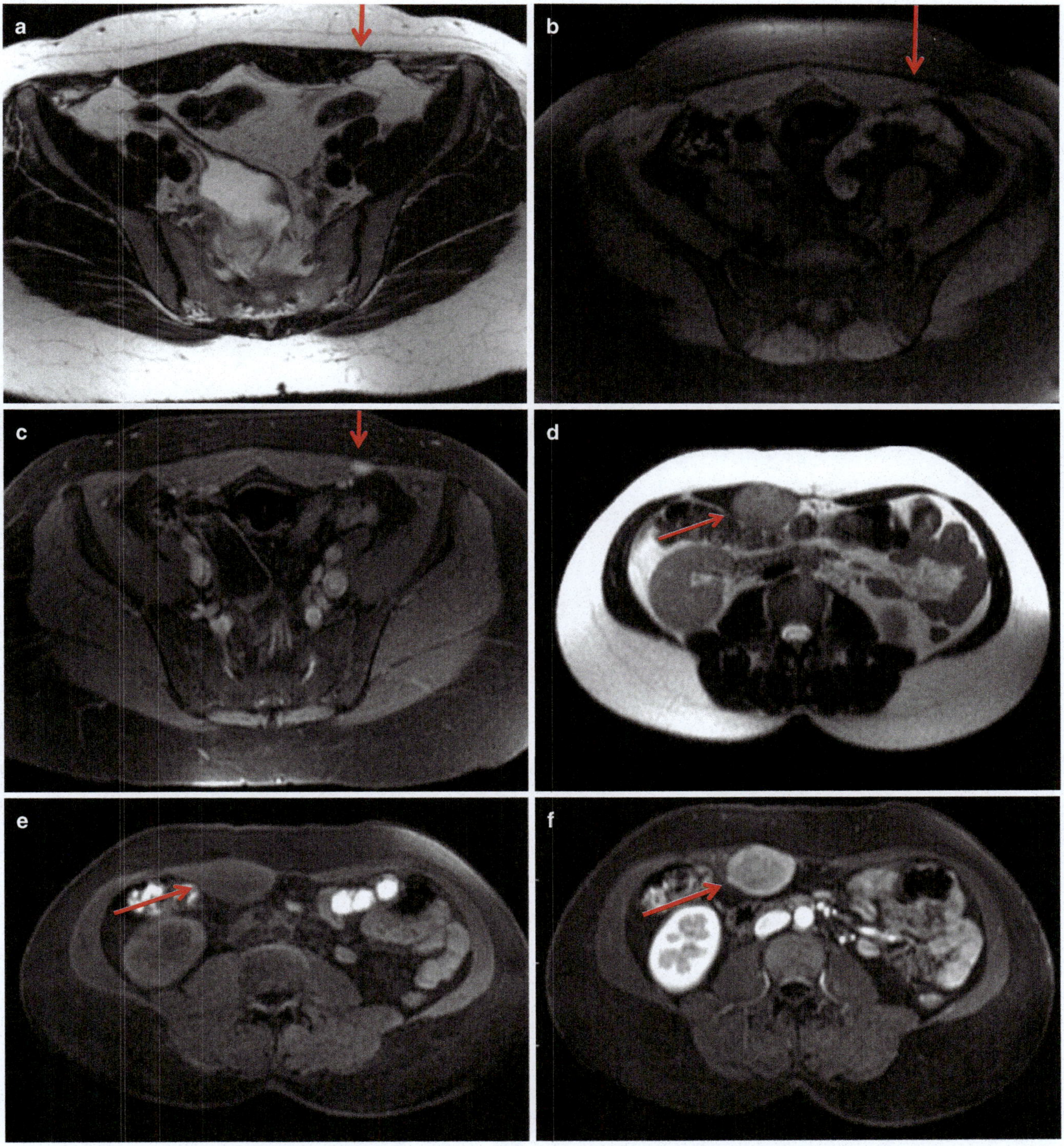

Fig. 3.16 Endometriosis of the abdominal wall. Importance of gadolinium. Case 1: (**a–c**) Lesion with muscle-like sign in T1-weighted T2-weighted sequences and enhancement after administration of gadolinium (**c**). Clinical history and age of the patient suggested the diagnosis. Case 2: (**d–f**) Desmoid tumor. Similar lesion, located in the right rectum, expanding, well delimited, hyperintense in T2, and slightly hypointense in T1, with intense enhancement (**f**). (**a**, **d**) T2-weighted sequences. (**b**, **c**, **e**, **f**) T1-weighted with fat saturation, (**c**, **f**) being after administration of intravenous gadolinium. (**a–f**) Axial

This process may join pelvic organs, promoting displacement of the uterus and ovaries, tubal distortion and dilation, vaginal fornix retraction, obliteration of the cul-de-sac, and bowel hyperangulation (Table 3.2). The position and shape of the uterus can change, with retroflexion, severe lateral flexion of the body and/or cervix, as well as posterior medial and inferior adnexal deviation, sometimes with retroversion of the uterus. When bilateral, the ovaries are fixed together at the midline, which is called "kissing ovaries" (Fig. 3.17).

Table 3.2 Signs of pelvic adhesion

Displacement of uterus and ovaries
Tubal distortion and dilation
Posterior vaginal fornix retraction
Cul-de-sac obliteration
Bowel hyperangulation
Focal accumulation of peritoneal fluid

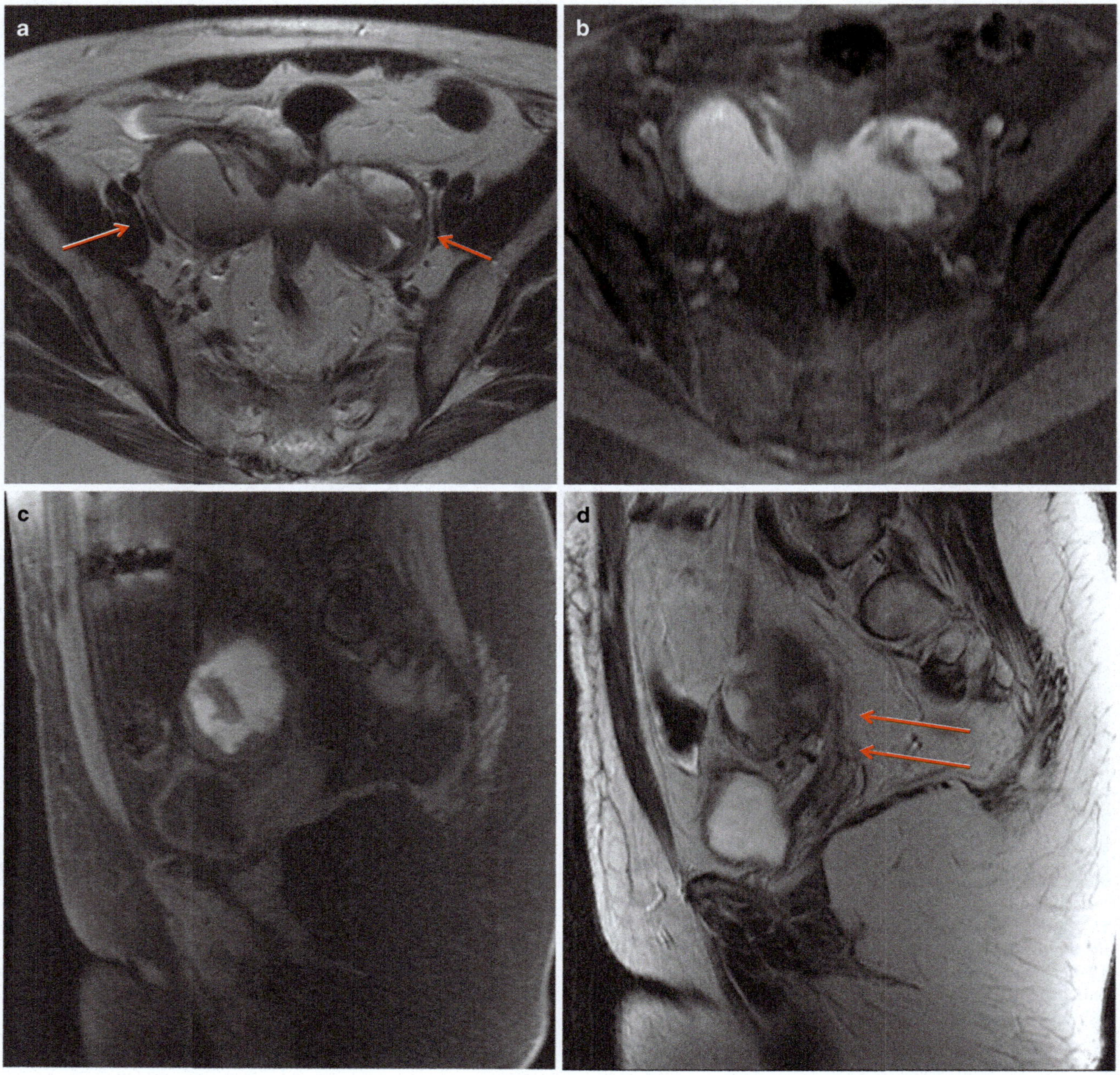

Fig. 3.17 Adherence promoting displacement of the ovaries fixed in the midline above the uterus, an aspect called "kissing ovaries." Bilateral ovarian endometriosis with thick wall endometriomas, with septa and clots. Notice increased enhancement in the subtraction image (**g**). There is proximity of the left endometrioma with the ureter (**d**). (**a**, **d**, **e**) T2-weighted sequence. (**b**, **c**, **f**) T1-weighted with fat saturation. (**g**) Subtraction. (**a**, **b**, **f**, **g**) Axial. (**c**, **d**) Sagittal. (**e**) Coronal. (**h**) Laparoscopy

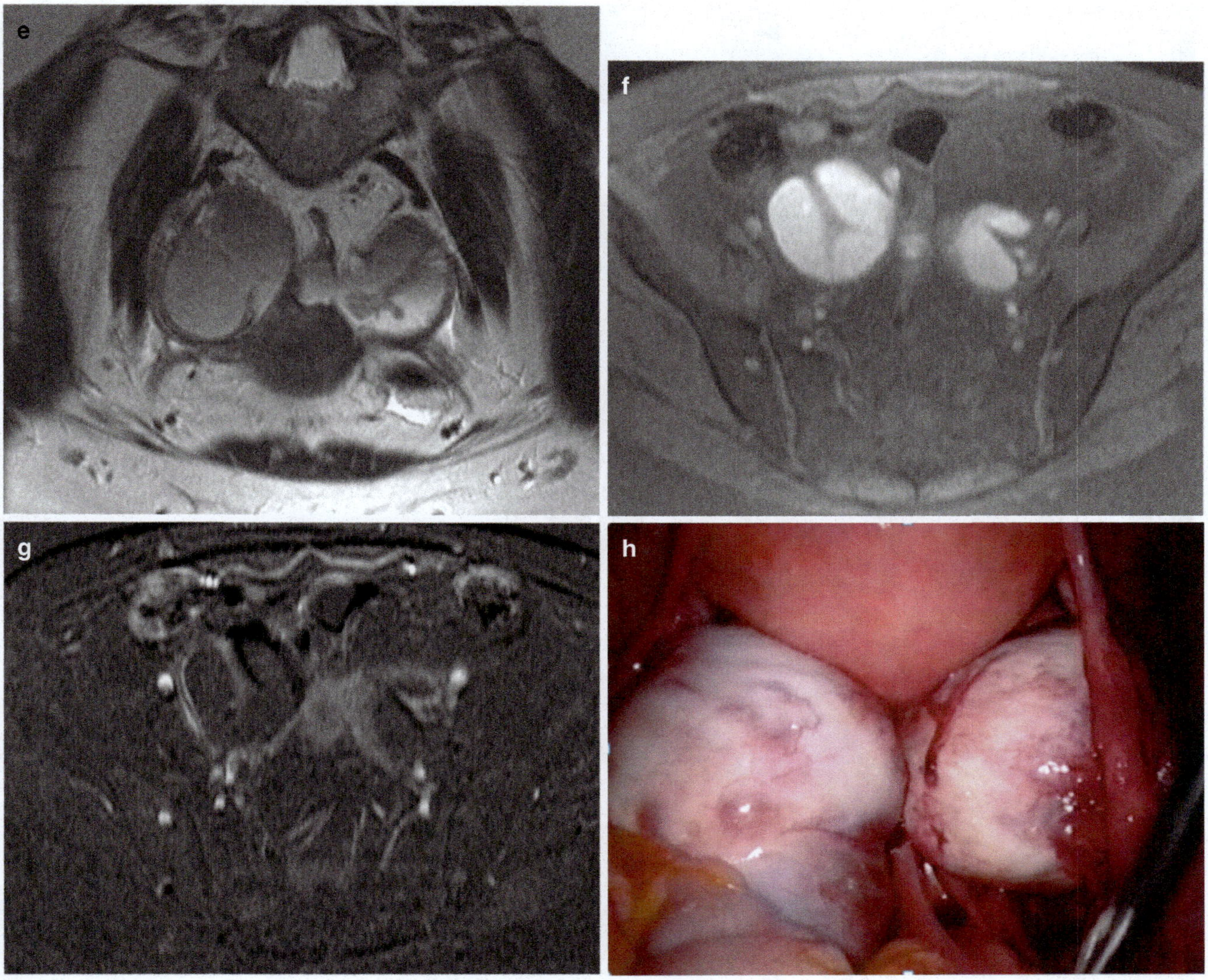

Fig. 3.17 (continued)

Moreover, this process involves both the rectum and sigmoid in the posterior compartment, the sigmoid at the ovarian fossa, and the cecum, the appendix, and the terminal ileum in the right parieto-colic gutter or in the anterior compartment (Fig. 3.18).

Another consequence of abdominal adhesions is focal accumulation of peritoneal fluid, which, associated with peritoneal endometriosis, promotes the formation of peritoneal pseudocysts (Fig. 3.19).

When there is parametrial or ovarian fossa infiltration, the resulting fibrosis may promote extrinsic ureteral involvement with stenosis and sometimes hydronephrosis (Fig. 3.20).

The adhesion process at an early stage can be difficult to identify in MRI and may even not be visible. On the other hand, peritoneal reflection or normal anatomical situations, such as contact of the small bowel with the uterus in the cul-de-sac and of the sigmoid with the superior face of the left ovary, should not be misinterpreted as adherence (Fig. 3.21).

Surgery is dictated by the depth of invasion and the topographic distribution of the disease, and the laparoscopic pro-

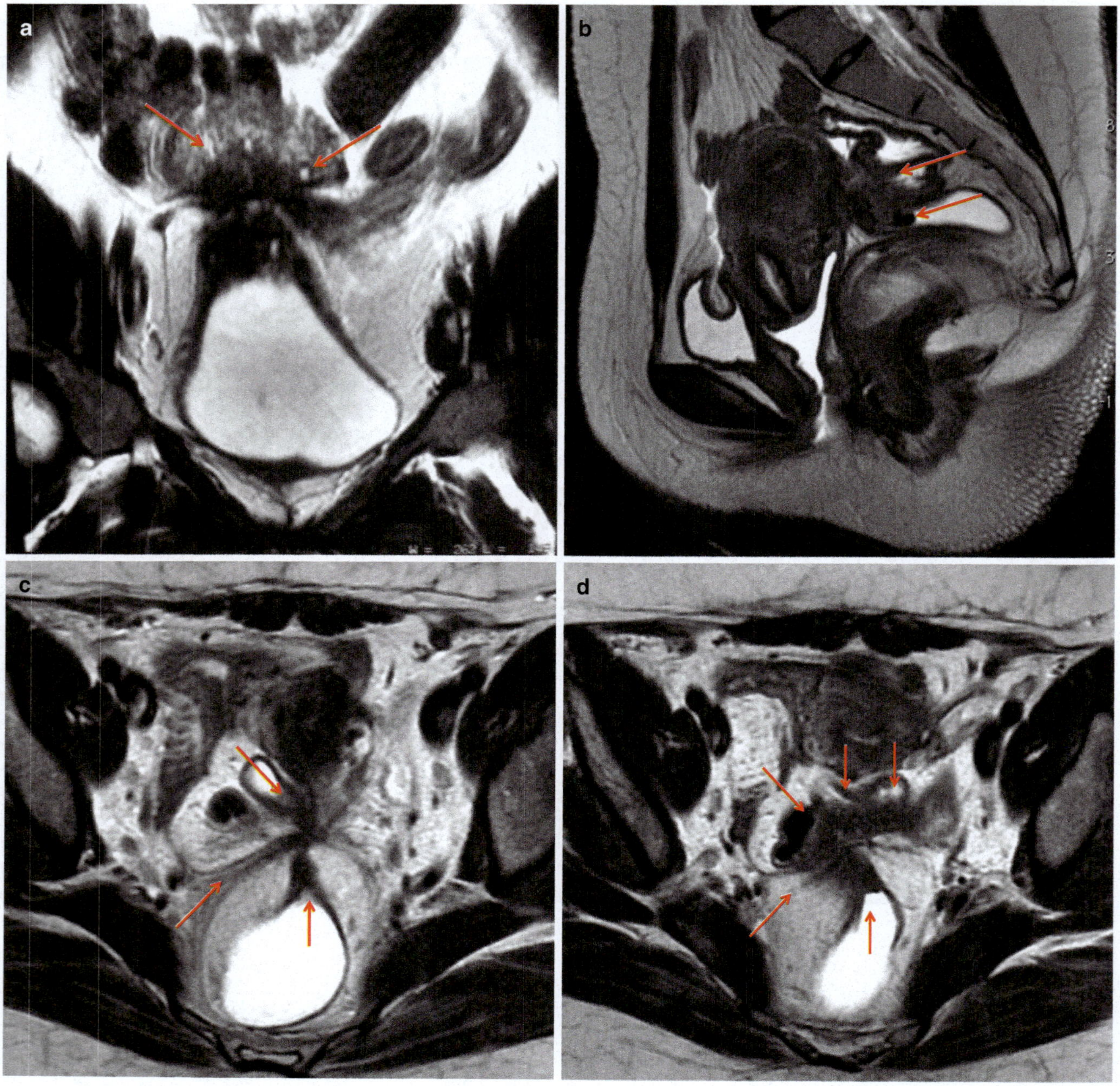

Fig. 3.18 Adherence determined by deep endometriosis, promoting hyperangulation of the loops. (**a**) Medial and inferior deviations of the cecum by extension of the lesion from the bladder ceiling to the cecal base, valve, and distal ileum (arrows). (**b**) Anterior retraction of the rectum, related to the retrocervical lesion. (**c–f**) Hyperangulation of the redundant sigmoid and posterior cul-de-sac by the retrocervical lesion. T2-weighted sequences. (**a**) Coronal. (**b**, **e**, **f**) Sagittal. (**c**, **d**) Axial. (**g–j**) Laparoscopy of the case (**b**) demonstrating complete blockage of the posterior cul-de-sac by adhesion and endometriosis (**g**) and resection of the retrocervical and intestinal lesion (**h–j**)

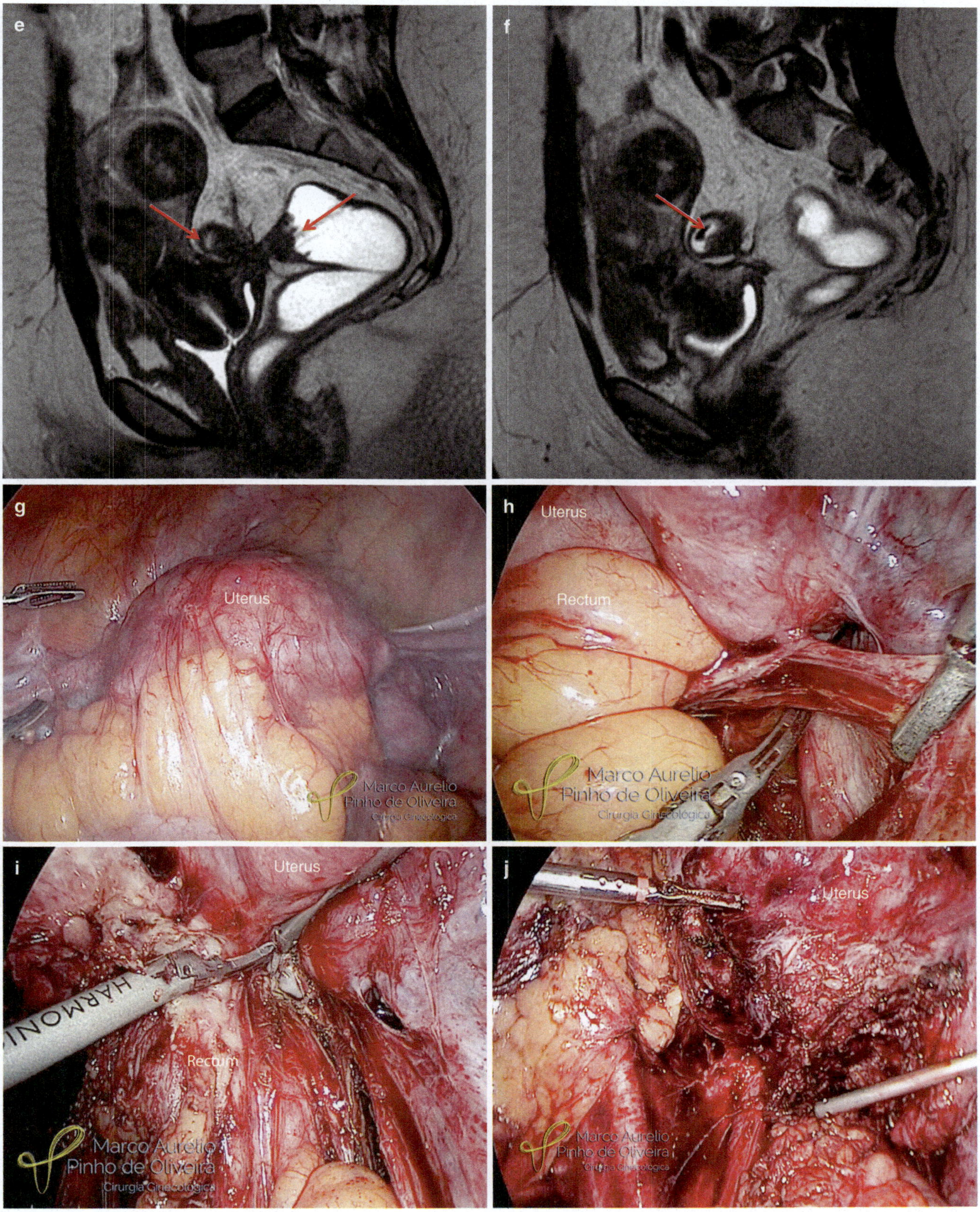

Fig. 3.18 (continued)

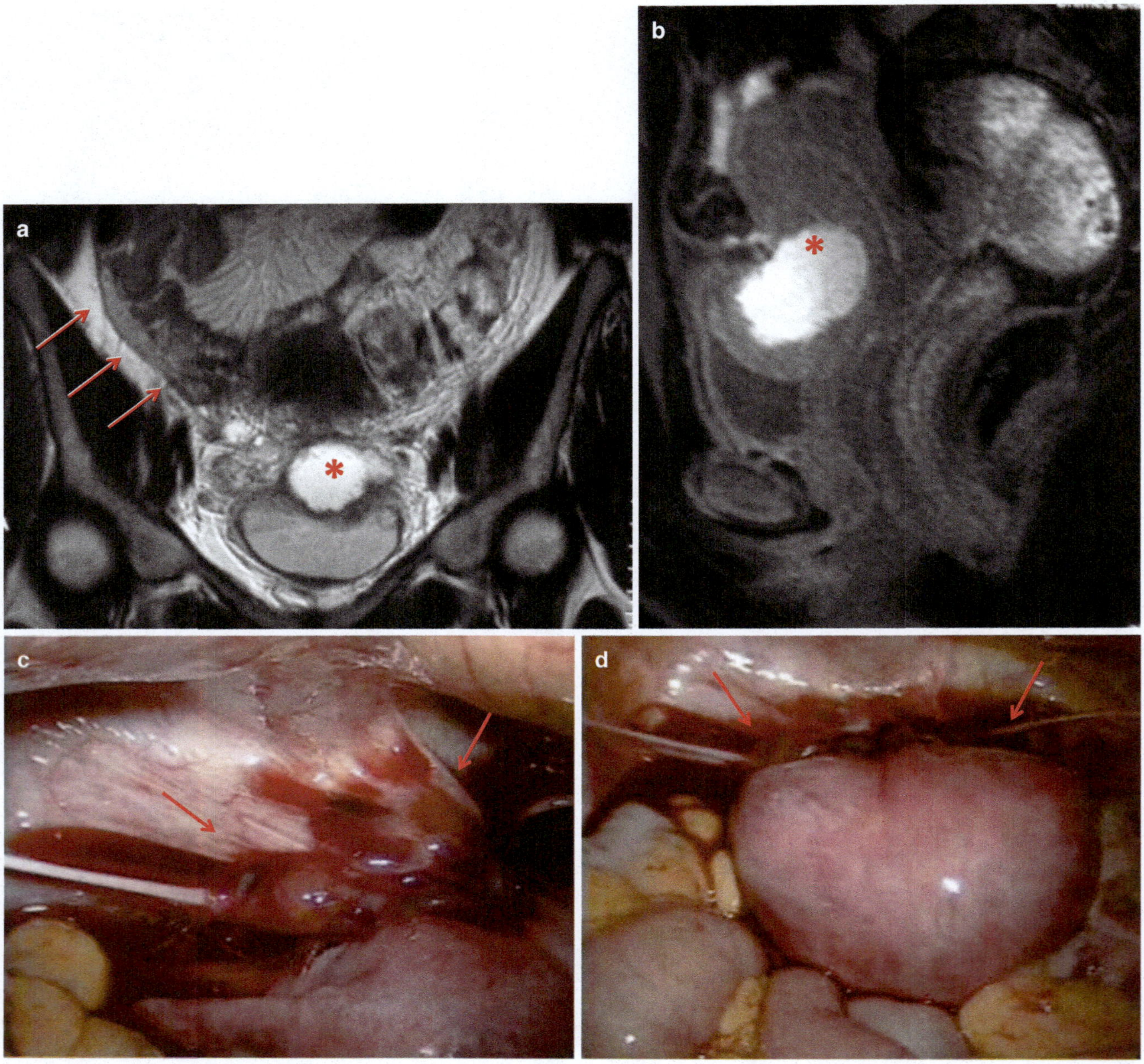

Fig. 3.19 Extensive adherence in the anterior compartment. Note the focal accumulation of blood (*) hyperintense in the T2- (**a**) and T1-weighted sequences (**b**) in the midline between the uterus and bladder, associated with peritoneal endometriosis (hematic liquid and peritoneal thickening in the right iliac fossa—arrows). (**a**) Coronal. (**b**) Sagittal. (**c**, **d**) Laparoscopy

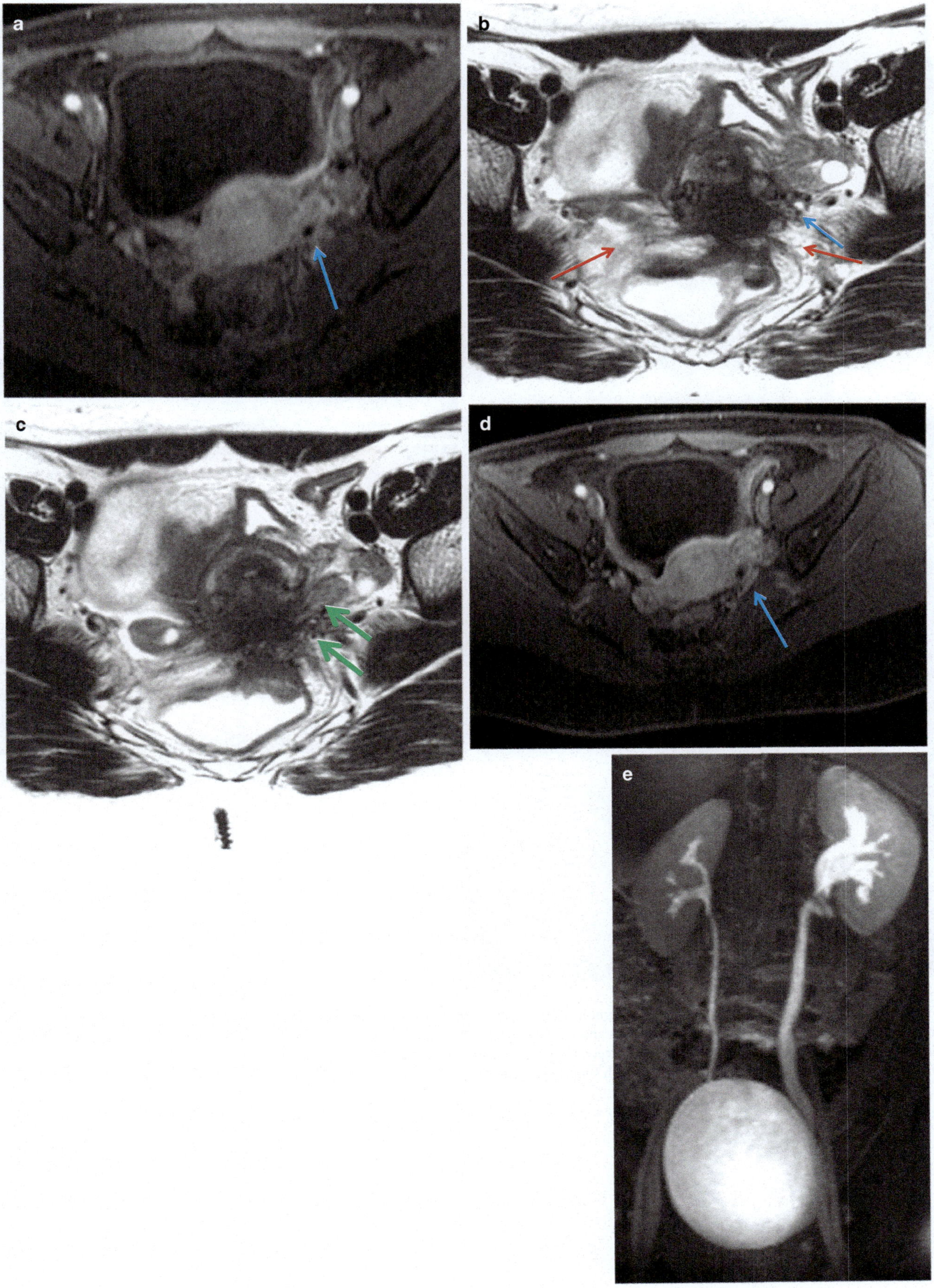

Fig. 3.20 Lesion in the posterior compartment (arrows), forming mass with parametrial infiltration, upper left (red arrows), determining ureteral stenosis (blue arrow) and light hydronephrosis. Note the proximity of the lesion to the internal iliac vessels and hypogastric plexus (green arrow). (**b**, **c**) T2-weighted sequences. (**a**, **d**) T1-weighted with gadolinium. (**e**) MR urography with MIP

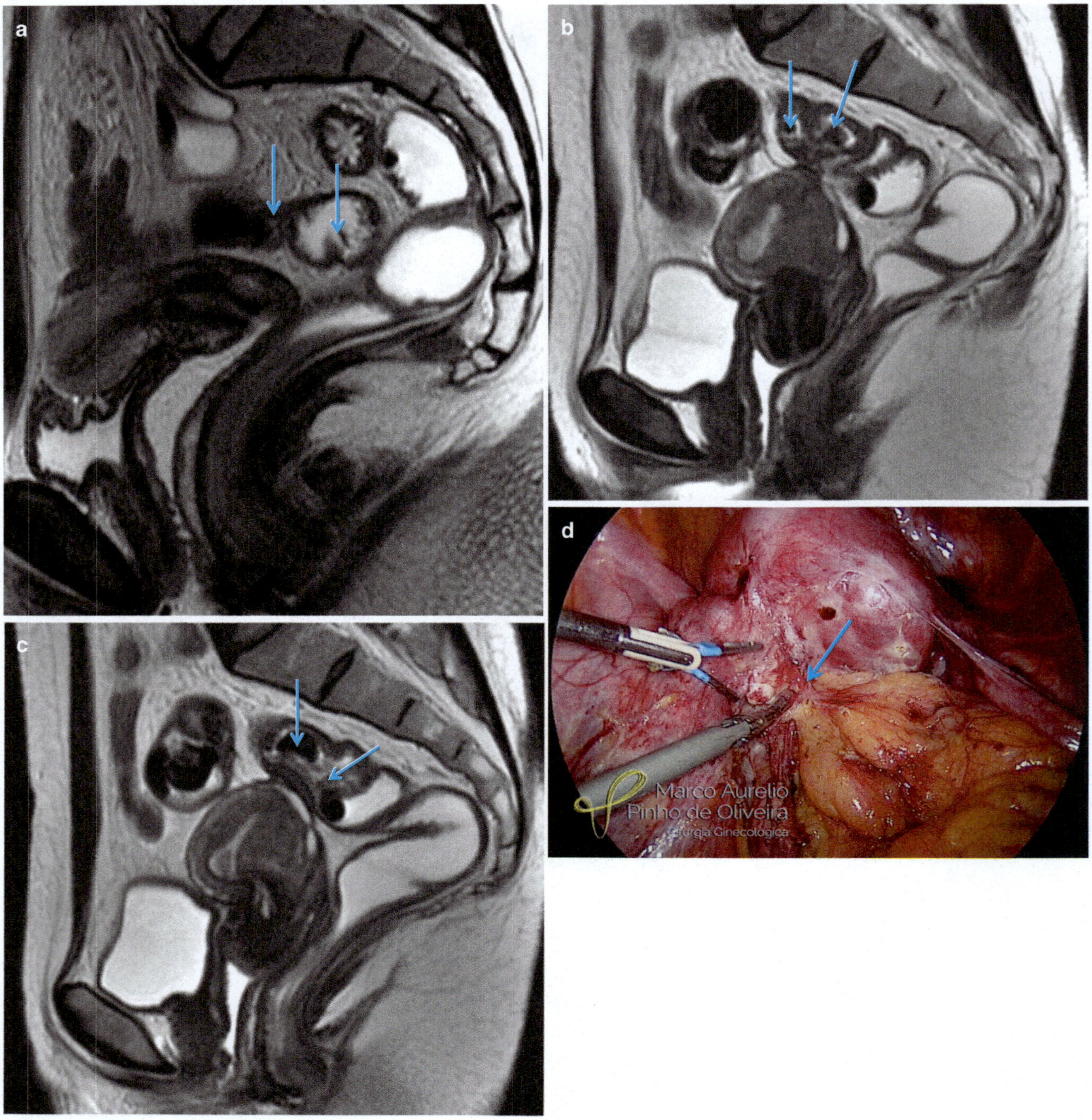

Fig. 3.21 (**a**) Normal contact of the redundant sigmoid with the uterus in the posterior fornix, preservation of fatty planes and without angulation of the loop. (**b**) Note endometriotic tissue between the sigmoid and the uterus, promoting adherence with the loop, with superficial penetration (5 mm). (**a**–**c**) T2-weighted sequences. Sagittal. (**d**–**g**) Laparoscopy demonstrating adherence of the sigmoid to the posterior wall of the uterus and left attachment

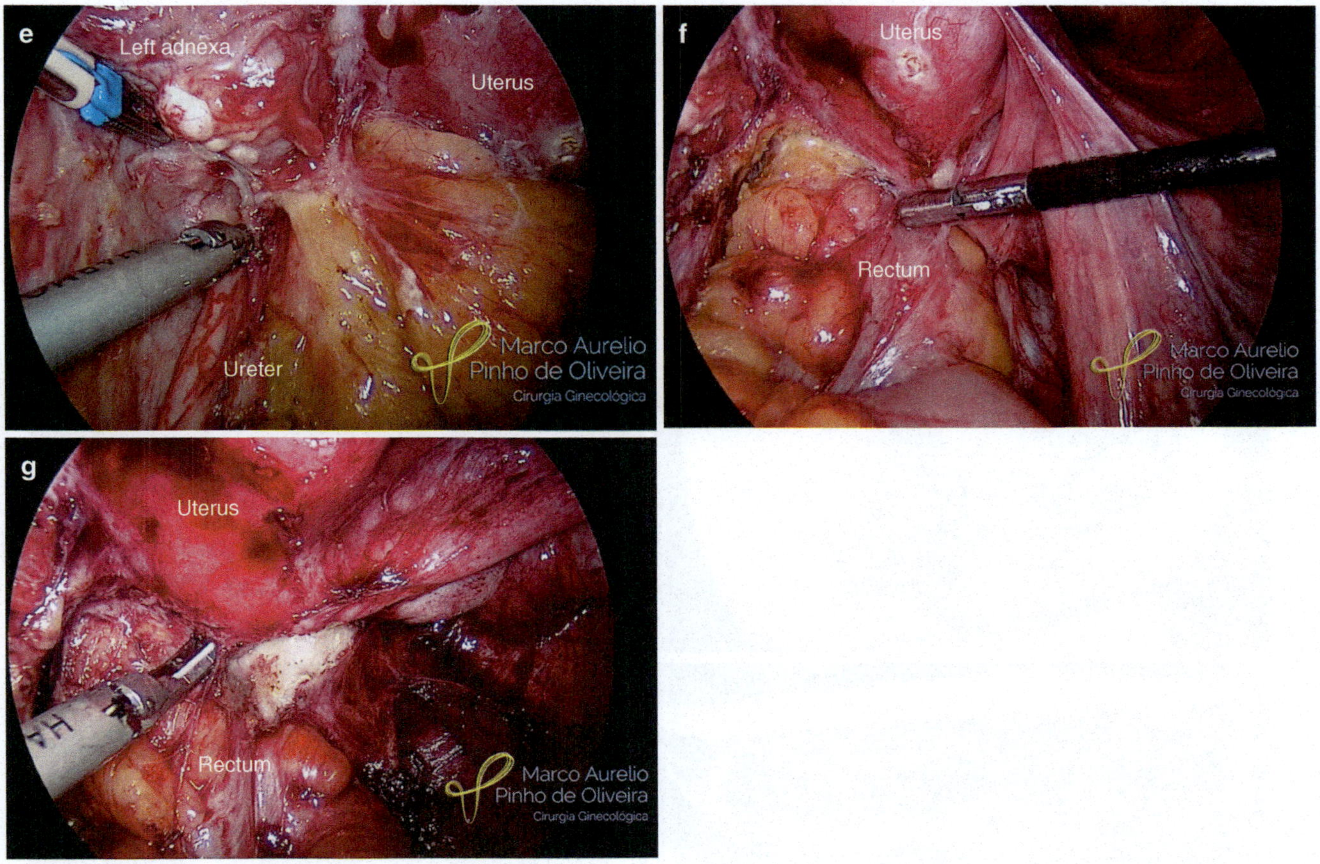

Fig. 3.21 (continued)

cedure usually begins with adhesiolysis. As a consequence, in an advanced endometriosis with extensive pelvic adhesions, initial surgical visual assessment may be insufficient. In this situation, MRI is excellent, since in addition to allowing a proper assessment of the distortion of the anatomy, it identifies the deep endometriosis associated lesions, at typical and atypical locations, as well as ureteral, nerve, and vascular involvement (Fig. 3.22) [12].

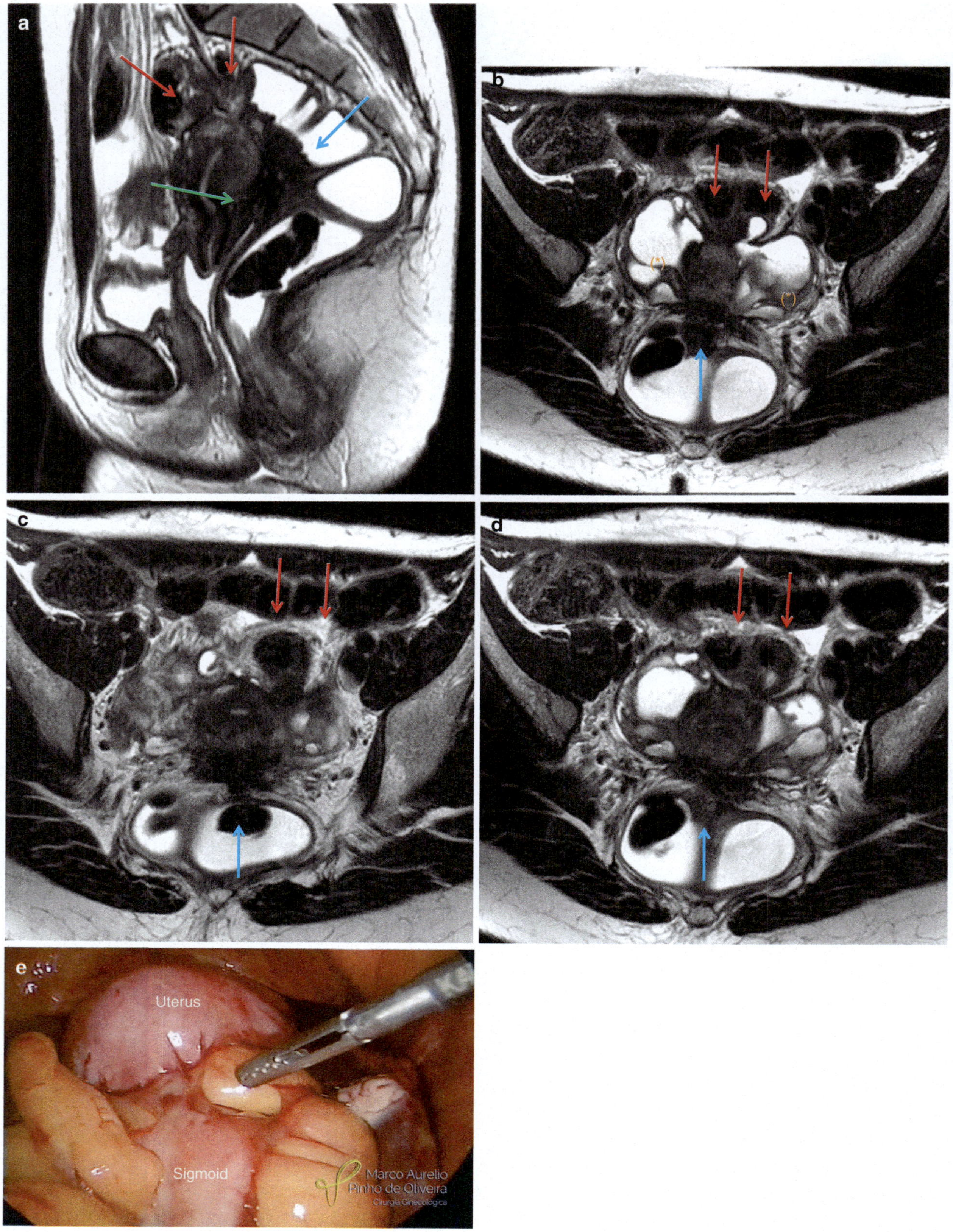

Fig. 3.22 Posterior deep endometriosis, from the fundus to the rectovaginal septum with extensive adhesions and deep commitment of the sigmoid (red arrows) and rectum (blue arrows), uterus and vagina (green arrow), and medial deviation of the appendages (*). Note the associated ovarian endometriosis, as well as bilateral parametrial extension. (**a**, **b**) T2-weighted sequences. (**a**) Sagittal. (**b-d**) Axial. (**e**) Laparoscopy showing lesion adhered from the fundus to the retrocervical region, with extensive adhesion between the rectum, sigmoid, appendages, and uterus

References

1. Bennett G, Slywotzky C, Cantera M, Hecht E. Unusual manifestations and complications of endometriosis—spectrum of imaging findings: pictorial review. Am J Roentgenol. 2010;194:WS34–46.
2. Anaf V, Simon P, Fayt I, Noel J. Smooth muscles are frequent components of endometriotic lesions. Hum Reprod. 2000;15:767–71.
3. Kondi-Pafitis A. Pathological aspects of endometriosis. In: Chakravarty B, Chaudhury K, editors. Endometriosis—basic concepts and current research trends. Hampshire: Intech; 2012. p. 101–12.
4. Koyama T. MR spectrum of benign endometriomas and malignant transformation in endometriomas: correlation with pathologic findings. Educational Exhibit at the 2007 European Congress of Radiology, Poster N: C-319.
5. Brandão A, Silva A. Diseases of the female pelvis: advances in imaging evaluation. Magn Reson Imaging Clin N Am. 2013;21:447–69.
6. Thomassin-Naggara I, Bazot M, Daraï E, Callard P, Thomassin J, Cuenod C. Epithelial ovarian tumors: value of dynamic contrast-enhanced MR imaging and correlation with tumor angiogenesis. Radiology. 2008;248:148–59.
7. Varma R, Rollason T, Gupta J, Maher E. Endometriosis and the neoplastic process. Reproduction. 2004;127:293–304.
8. Ryan I, Taylor R. Endometriosis and infertility: new concepts. Obstet Gynecol Surv. 1997;52:365–71.
9. Crispi C. Tratado de Videoendoscopia e Cirurgia minimamente invasiva em Ginecologia. 5th ed. Rio de Janeiro: Revinter; 2011.
10. Kondo W, Ribeiro R, Trippia C, Zomer M. Deep infiltrating endometriosis: anatomical distribution and surgical treatment. Rev Bras Ginecol Obstet. 2012;34:278–84.
11. Novellas S, Chassang M, Bouaziz J, Delotte J, Toullalan O, Chevallier E. Anterior pelvic endometriosis: MRI features. Abdom Imaging. 2010;35:742–9.
12. Piketty M, Chopin N, Dousset B, Millischer-Bellaische A, Roseau G, Leconte M, Borghese B, Chapron C. Preoperative work-up for patients with deeply infiltrating endometriosis: transvaginal ultrasonography must definitely be the first-line imaging examination. Hum Reprod. 2008;24:602–7.

4 Deep Endometriosis by Location

Deep endometriosis presents predominantly as a multifocal disease, and knowledge of its anatomical distribution is extremely important for the planning of therapeutic and surgical procedures. Furthermore, surgical treatment aims at completely removing all deep endometriosis lesions; thus the precise lesion description in the radiology report determines the choice of the technique and the associated surgical procedures [1].

According to Kondo, the average number of deep endometriosis lesions per patient is 4, and of these 45.4% presented bowel involvement, 8.4% bladder involvement, and 6.3% ureteral infiltration. A similar finding was obtained by Piketty, who found bowel, bladder, and ureteral involvement in 56%, 5.4%, and 6.7% of patients, respectively (Fig. 4.1) [1, 2].

The literature suggests that the anatomical distribution of these lesions in the abdominal cavity can be explained by the regurgitation theory and the pattern of peritoneal flow, with preferred location in the posterior and left compartments. According to Vercellini, the left uterosacral ligament was affected in 64.5% of the cases, the left ureter in 64%, and the rectosigmoid in 74%. Chapron noted that 93.4% of the lesions were posteriorly located (Fig. 4.2) [3–5].

There are also specific characteristics according to the location of the organ affected by the deep lesion. Intestinal deep lesion present a pattern of multifocal distribution in 30–50% of the patients, the most common locations being the rectum (96%), sigmoid colon (38%), cecum (22%), omentum (10%), ileum (7%), and appendix (7%) according to Piketty (Fig. 4.3) [2].

The location of the deep endometriosis lesion may also be related to the disease severity. Obliteration of the posterior cul-de-sac; bowel, bladder, and ureter involvement; involvement of the lateral wall or pelvic floor, and extension into pelvic nerves are considered severe forms of the disease (Fig. 4.4) [6].

The extension of deep lesion in a compartment may vary between patients and also be asymmetrical. There may be a predominant involvement in an organ, such as the myometrium or the bowel. This extension pattern can impact on surgical planning. Thus, the authors conclude that the measurement of the deep endometriosis lesion should include the following parameters:

(a) The entire lesion
(b) The lesion within the involved organs
(c) The relationship of the lesion with muscle and mucosa

On Table 4.1, we detail these parameters by organ.

A. Brandão et al., *Atlas of Deep Endometriosis*, https://doi.org/10.1007/978-3-319-71697-8_4

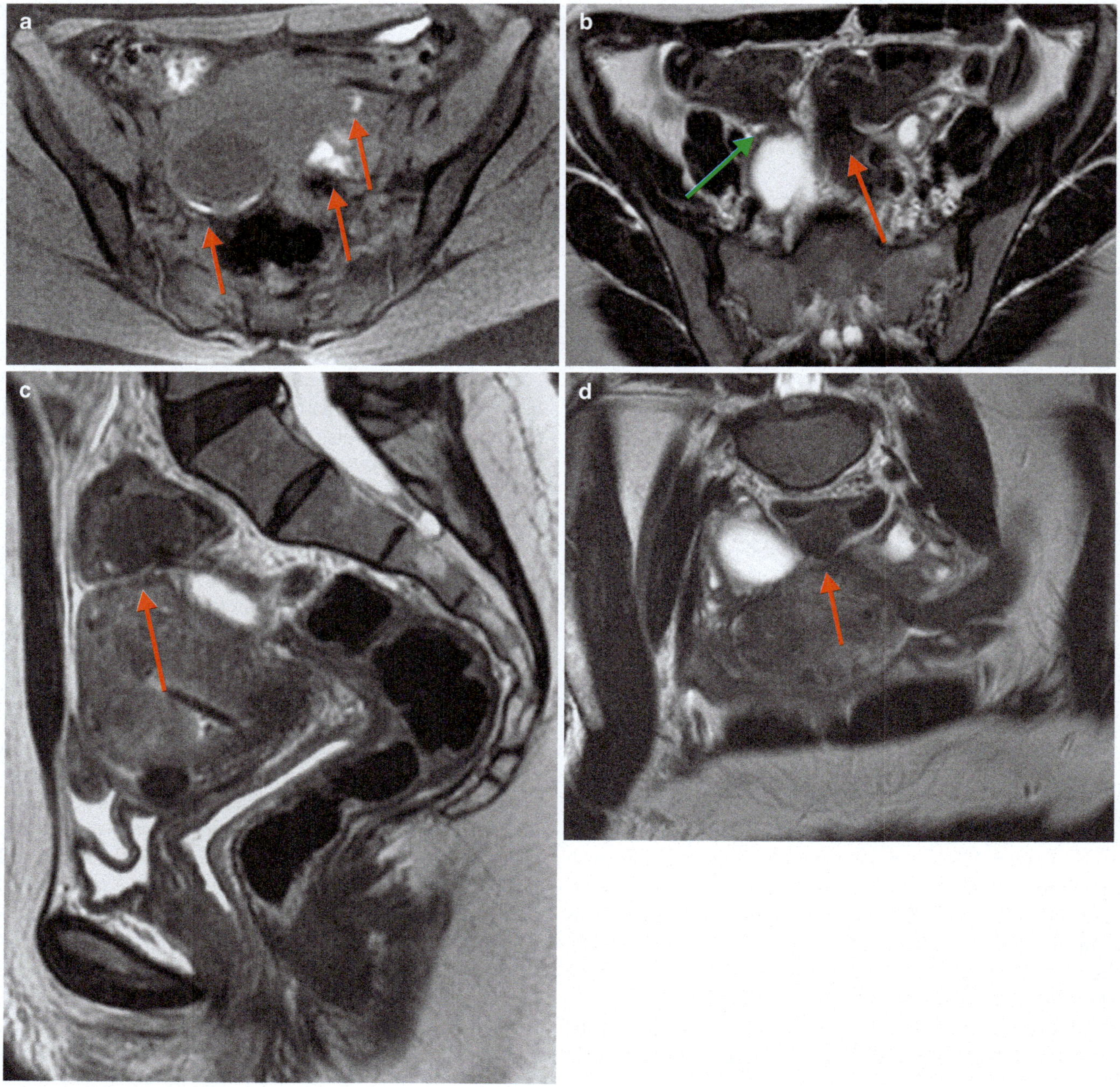

Fig. 4.1 Bilateral ovarian endometriosis with superficial bleeding on the right, endometriomas on the left (arrows in **a**), deep involvement of the sigmoid (red arrows **b–d**) and cecum (green arrow **b**), and deep retrocervical lesion with involvement of the rectum and ligaments (arrows in **e**, **f**). (**a**) T1-weighted sequence with fat suppression. Axial. (**b–f**) T2-weighted sequences. (**b**, **f**) Axial. (**c**) Sagittal. (**d**, **e**) Coronal short axis

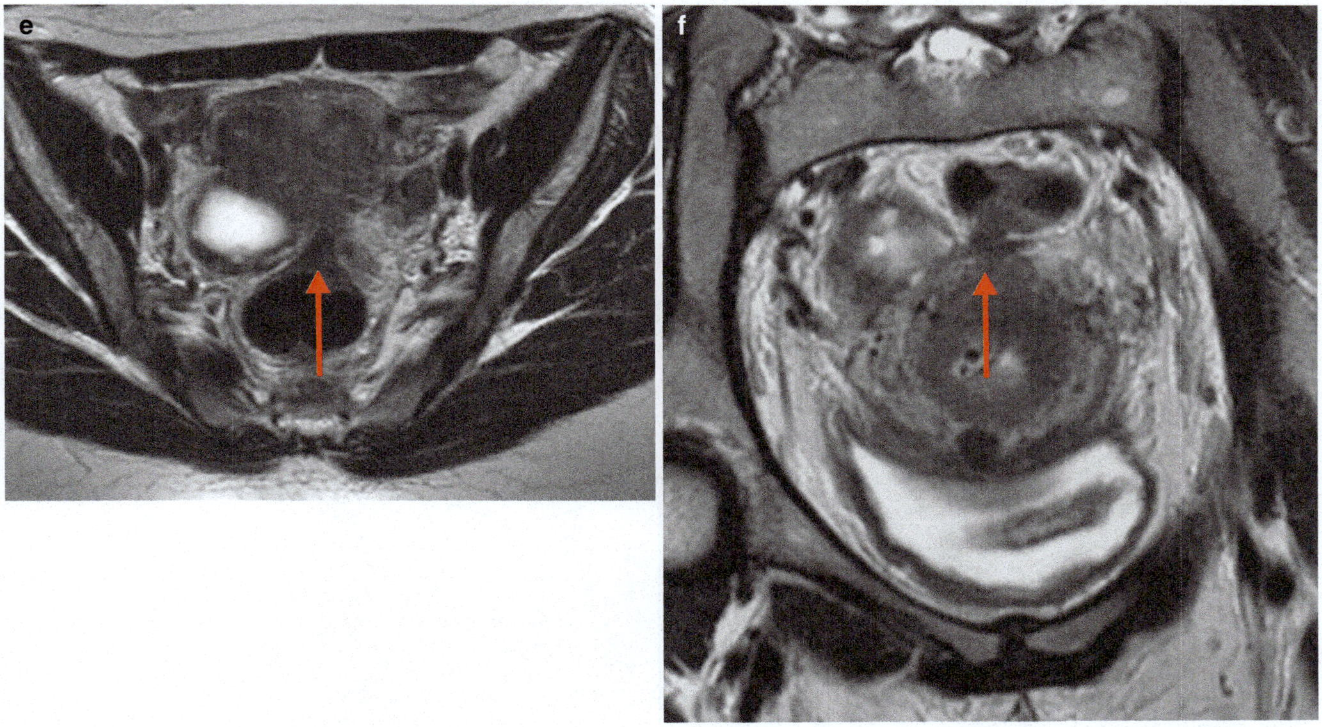

Fig. 4.1 (continued)

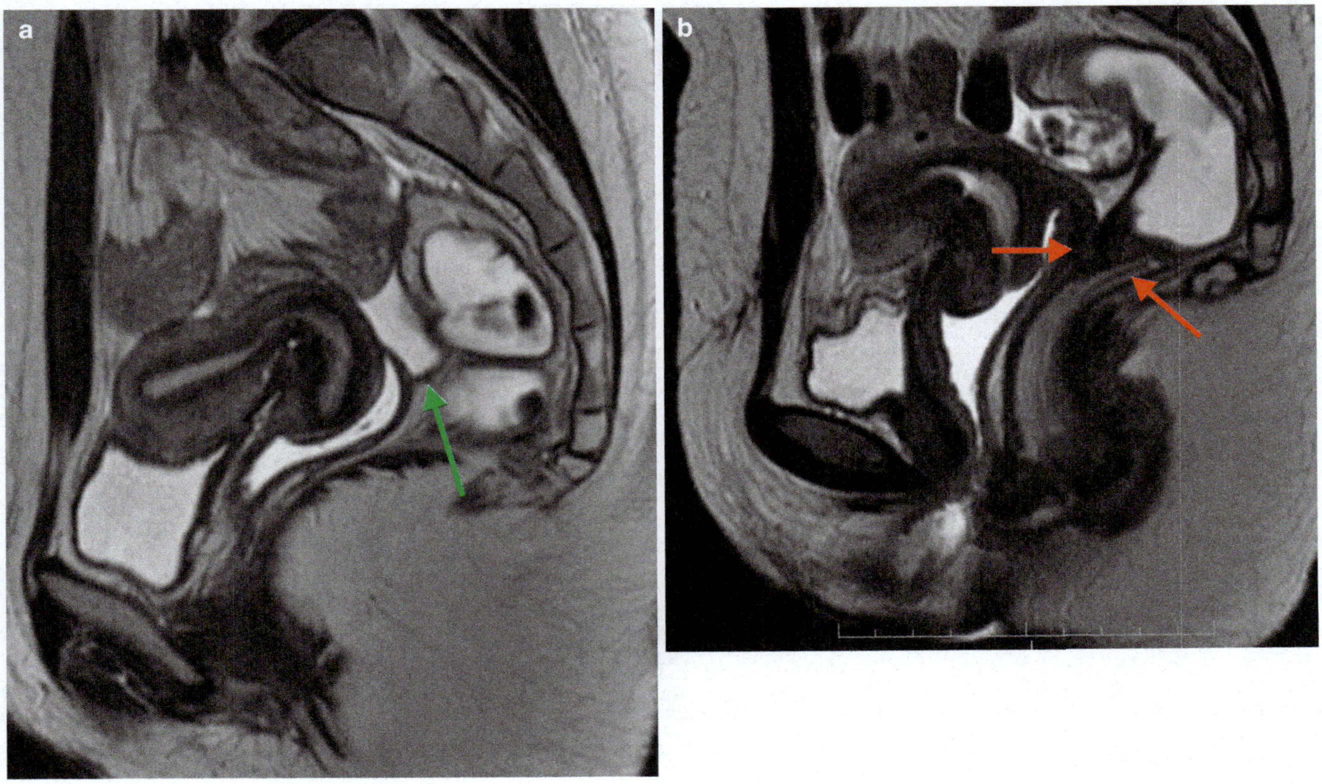

Fig. 4.2 The posterior lower fornix (green arrow in **a**) provides a greater number of lesions in the posterior compartment (**b**). In the left lateral compartment, the sigmoid blocks diffusion of the menstrual reflux by proximity to the left ovary (**c**, **d**). (**b**) Rectovaginal septum endometriosis with vaginal and lower rectal extension. (**e**–**h**) Deep endometriosis of the sigmoid and left ovarian fossa. Note in relation to ovary (blue). (**a**–**h**) T2-weighted sequences. (**a**, **d**–**h**) Sagittal. (**c**) Axial

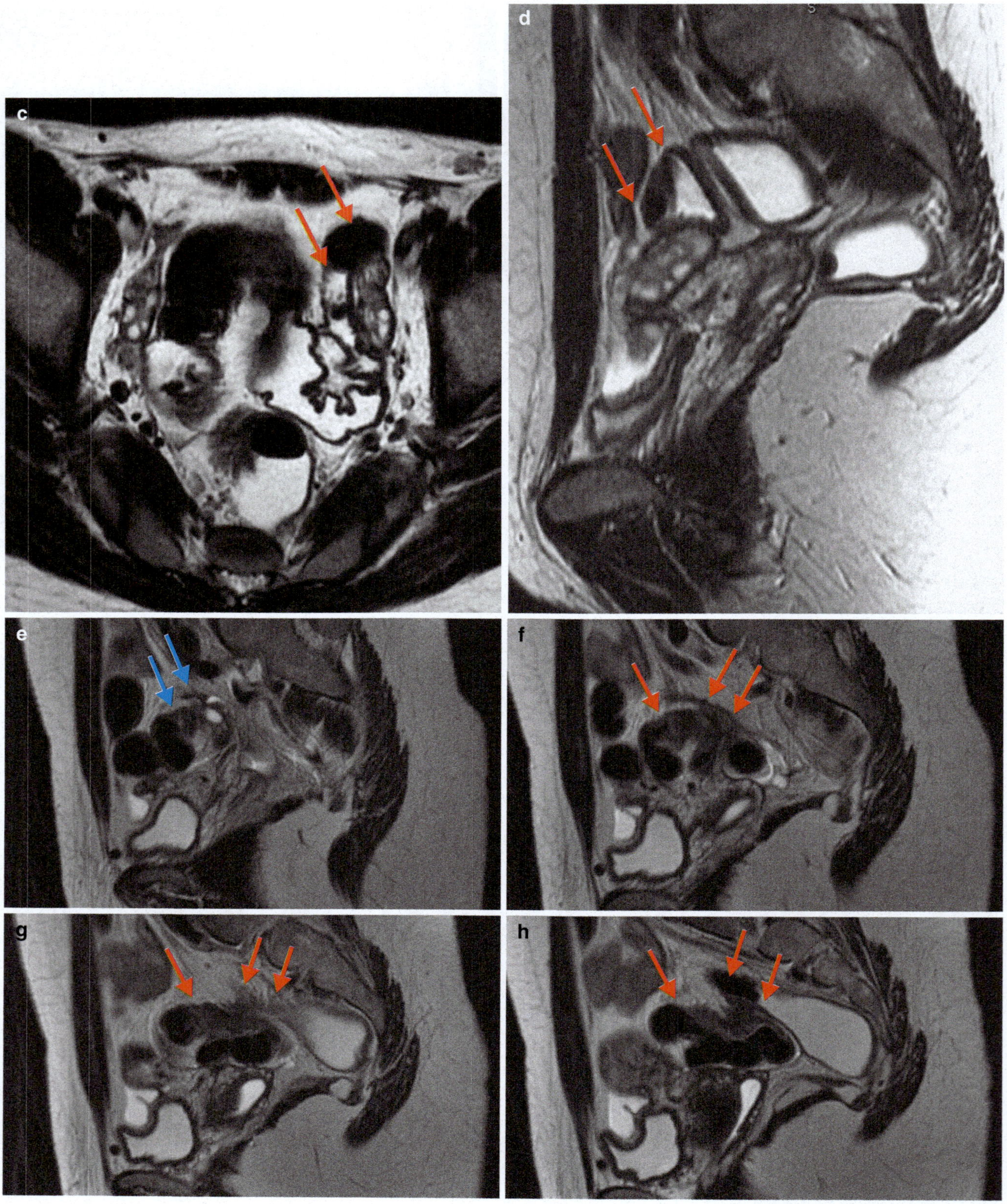

Fig. 4.2 (continued)

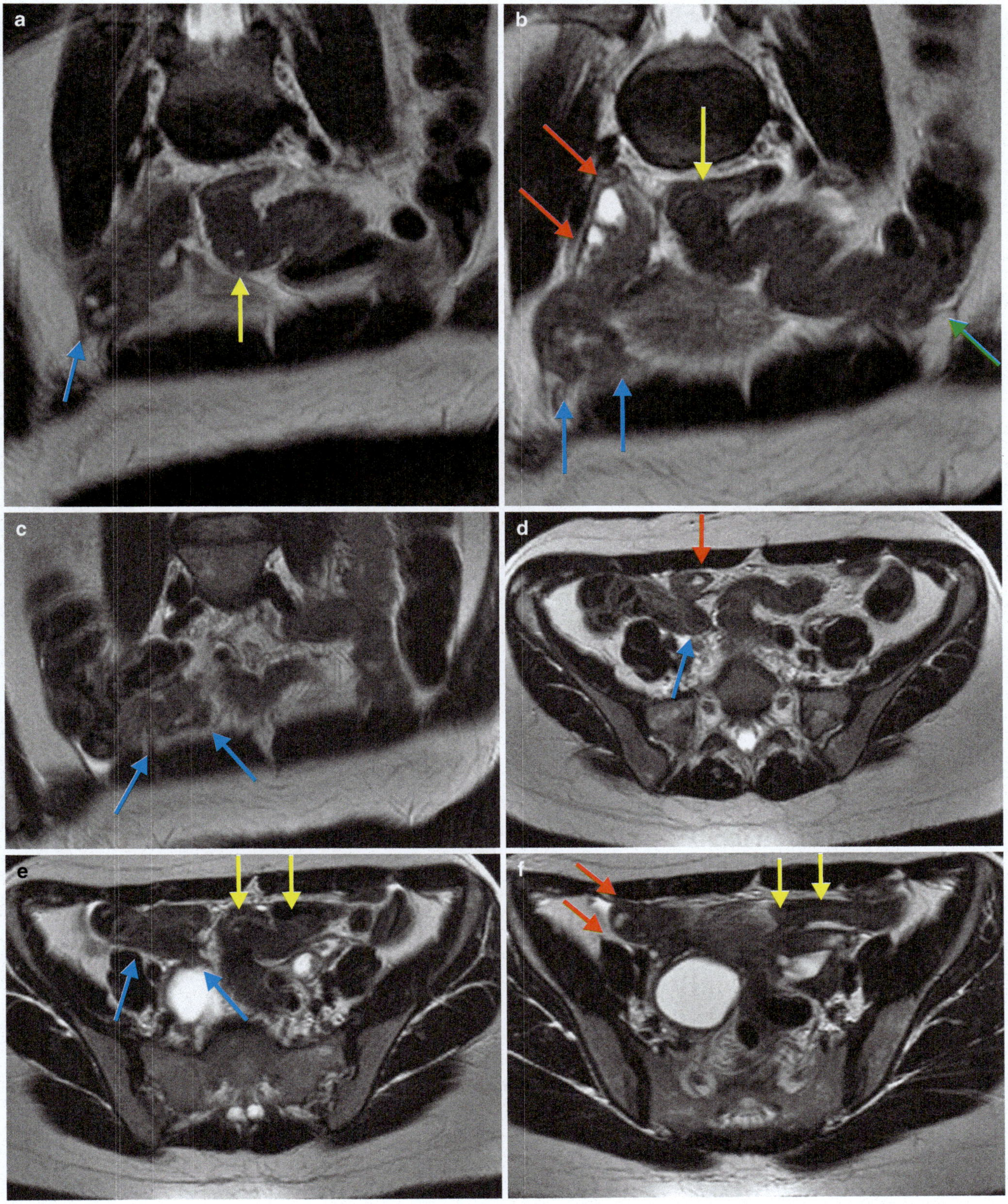

Fig. 4.3 The same case as Fig. 4.42. Infiltrative multifocal intestinal endometriosis with six lesions, including the rectum, sigmoid (yellow) and cecum (blue), and descending colon (green) and ileum (red). (**b**) T2-weighted sequences. (**a–c**) Coronal. (**d–f**) Axial

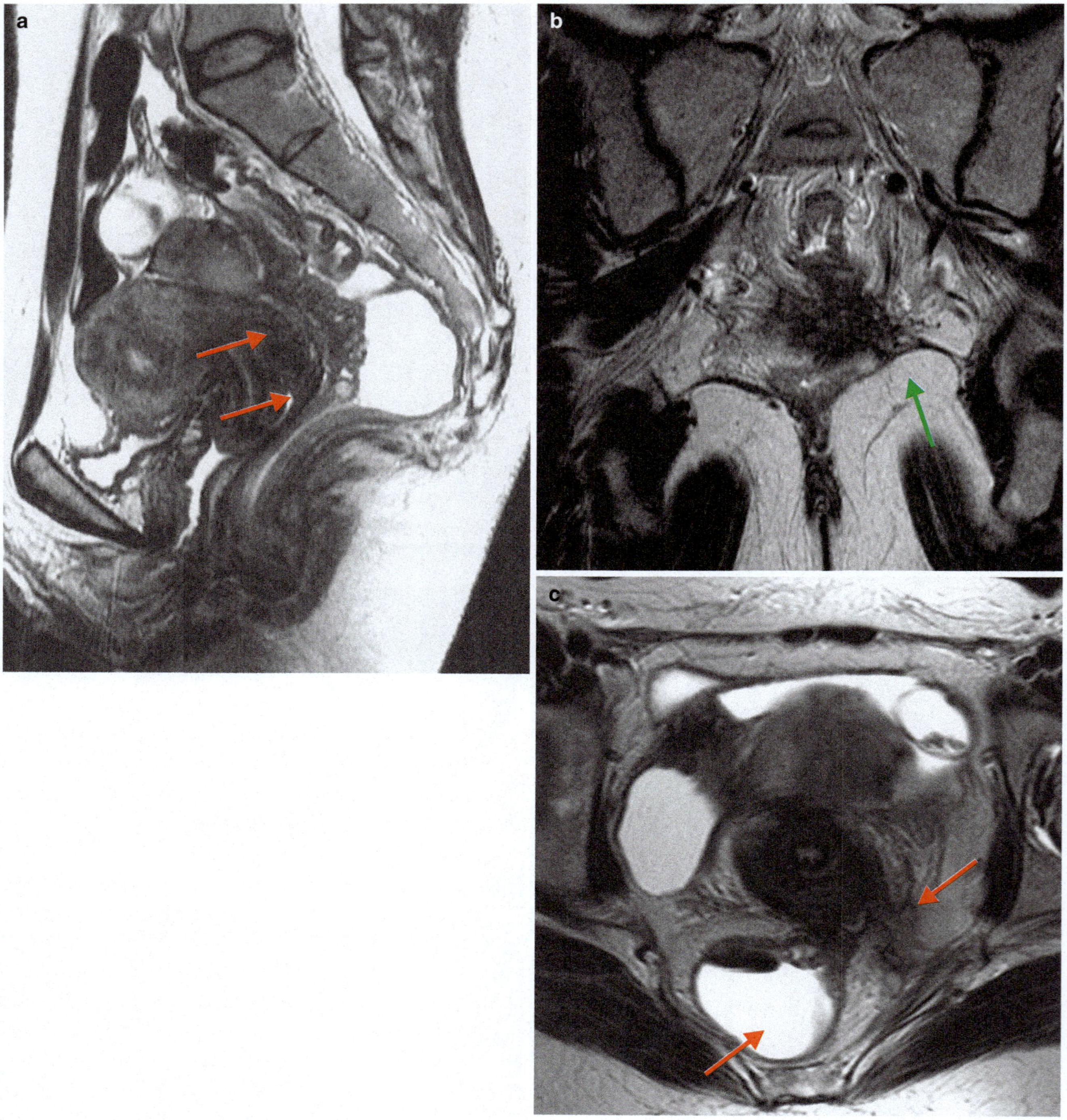

Fig. 4.4 Retrocervical lesion determining obliteration of the posterior fornix, rectal, vaginal, ligament, and left parametrial involvement (red arrows), and affecting the levator ani muscle (green arrow). (**a**–**c**) T2-weighted sequences. (**a**) Sagittal. (**b**) Coronal. (**c**) Axial

Table 4.1 Main lesions descriptors

Uterosacral ligament	Length and diameter
Myometrium	Extent and depth Distance from the uterine cavity
Bowel	Length, depth, mucosa involvement circumference location, stenosis, distance to the anal verge
Bladder	Length, muscle and mucosa involvement ureteral ostium involvement
Vaginal fornix	Length, mucosal involvement
Parametria	Length, uterine artery, and ureter involvement
Paracolpo	Inferior hypogastric plexus involvement and levator ani extension

4.1 Anterior Compartment

Anterior compartment deep endometriosis involvement presents a multifocal penetration pattern with lateral extension to the round ligaments, anterior extension to the bladder (usually superior and posterior surfaces), and posterior extension to the myometrium. Usually there is no vaginal involvement (Figs. 4.5, 4.6, 4.7, and 4.8).

Eventually, the disease also extends to the tube, ovary, and broad ligaments, due to proximity with these organs. The cecum and peri-cecum region may be affected by the adhesions with right side anterior compartment deep endometriosis (Fig. 4.9).

Thus, for didactic purposes, we will cover separately the affected organs, the urinary tract, the myometrium, and the ligaments.

Before proceeding, it is worth remembering some protocol imaging acquisition details. An empty bladder improves the identification of small lesions, especially in superficial bladder lesions, as well as in myometrial and ligamentous nodules. In addition, large lesions may be missed by bladder distension, since it can be displaced posteriorly and superiorly, and also by motion artifacts related to the bladder fluid as well as by its proximity to the small bowel (Fig. 4.10).

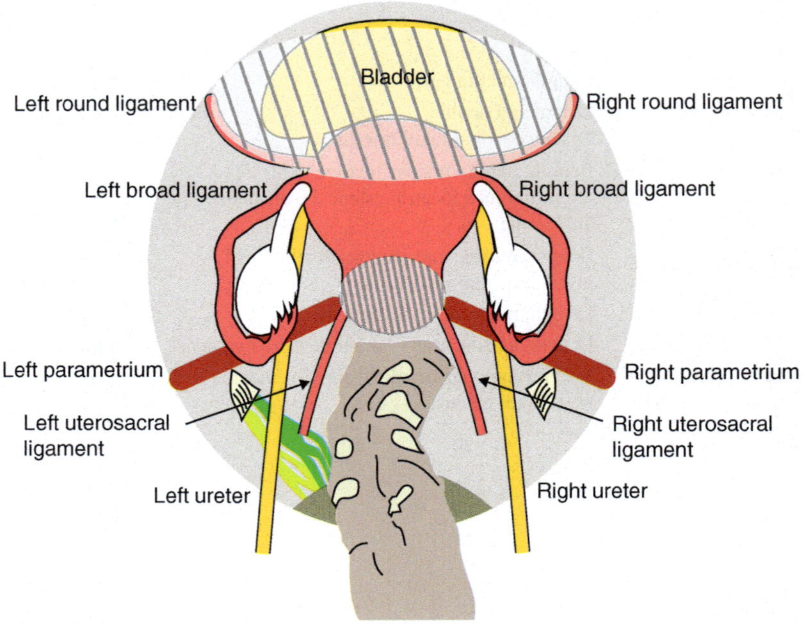

Fig. 4.5 Extension pattern of deep endometriosis of the anterior compartment: (1) Laterally: involvement of the round ligaments. (2) Anteriorly: bladder. (3) Posteriorly: musculature of the anterior wall of the uterus (anterior myometrium). Note that the right side of the laparoscopy corresponds to the left side of the MRI

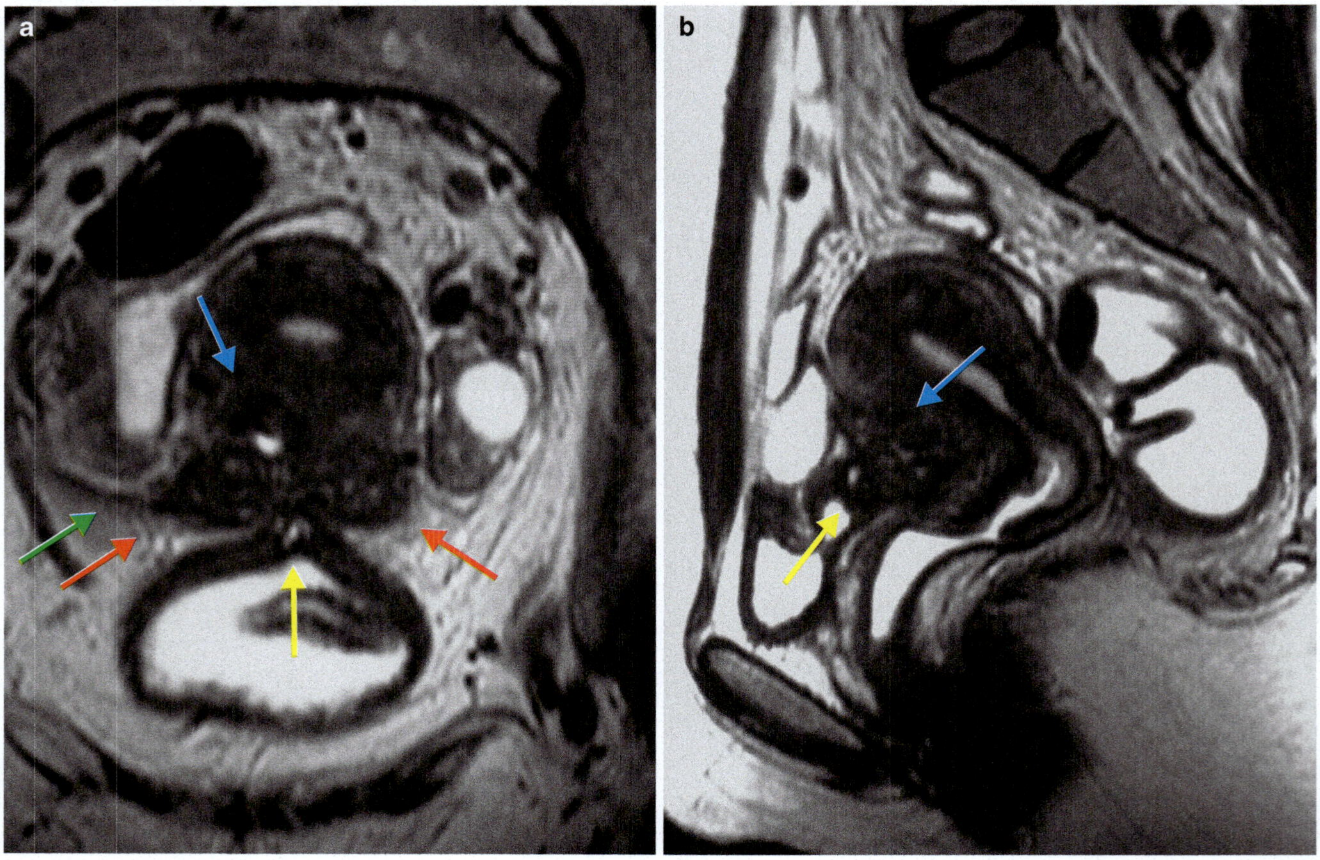

Fig. 4.6 Deep lesion in the anterior compartment with multifocal penetration (red arrows) and with lateral extension to the round ligaments (green arrow), anteriorly to the bladder roof (yellow arrow) and posteriorly in the myometrium (blue arrow). (**a**) Coronal. (**b**) Sagittal. T2-weighted sequences. (**c**) Laparoscopy. Lesion in the bladder and anterior myometrium

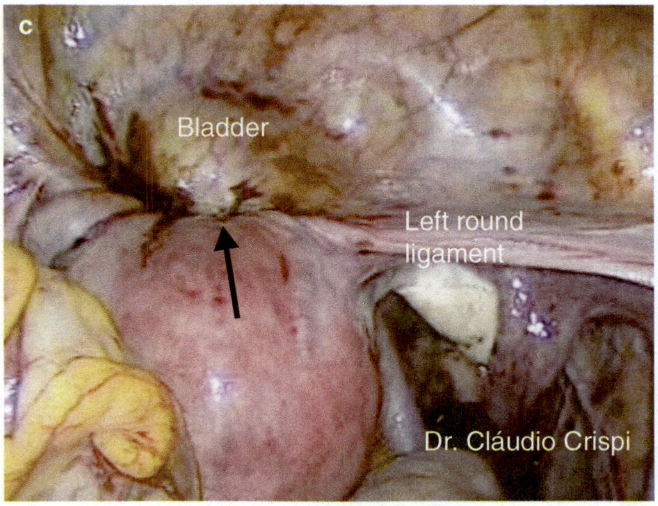

Fig. 4.6 (continued)

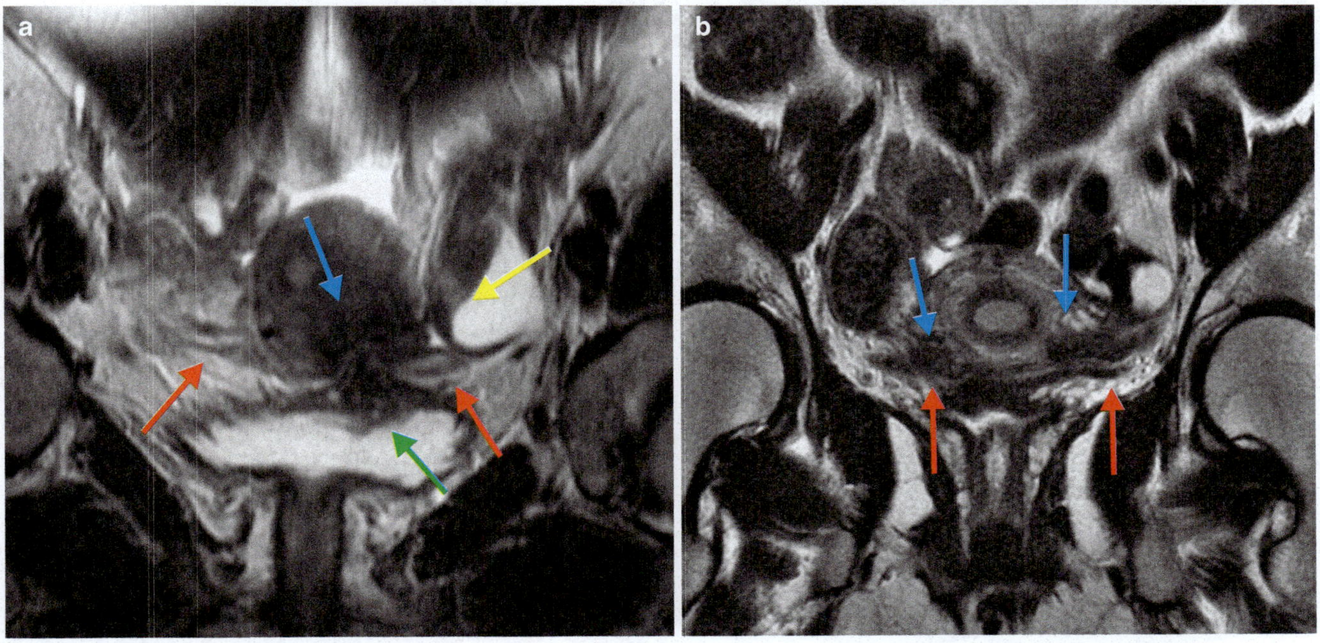

Fig. 4.7 (**a**) Deep bladder lesion (green arrow), with median predominant location, myometrial extension (blue arrow), and the round ligaments (red arrows), with adherence with the sigmoid on the left (yellow arrow). (**b**) Deep lesion with ligament predominance, with thickening of the round ligaments (red arrows) and bilateral myometrial penetration (blue arrows). T2-weighted sequence. Coronal

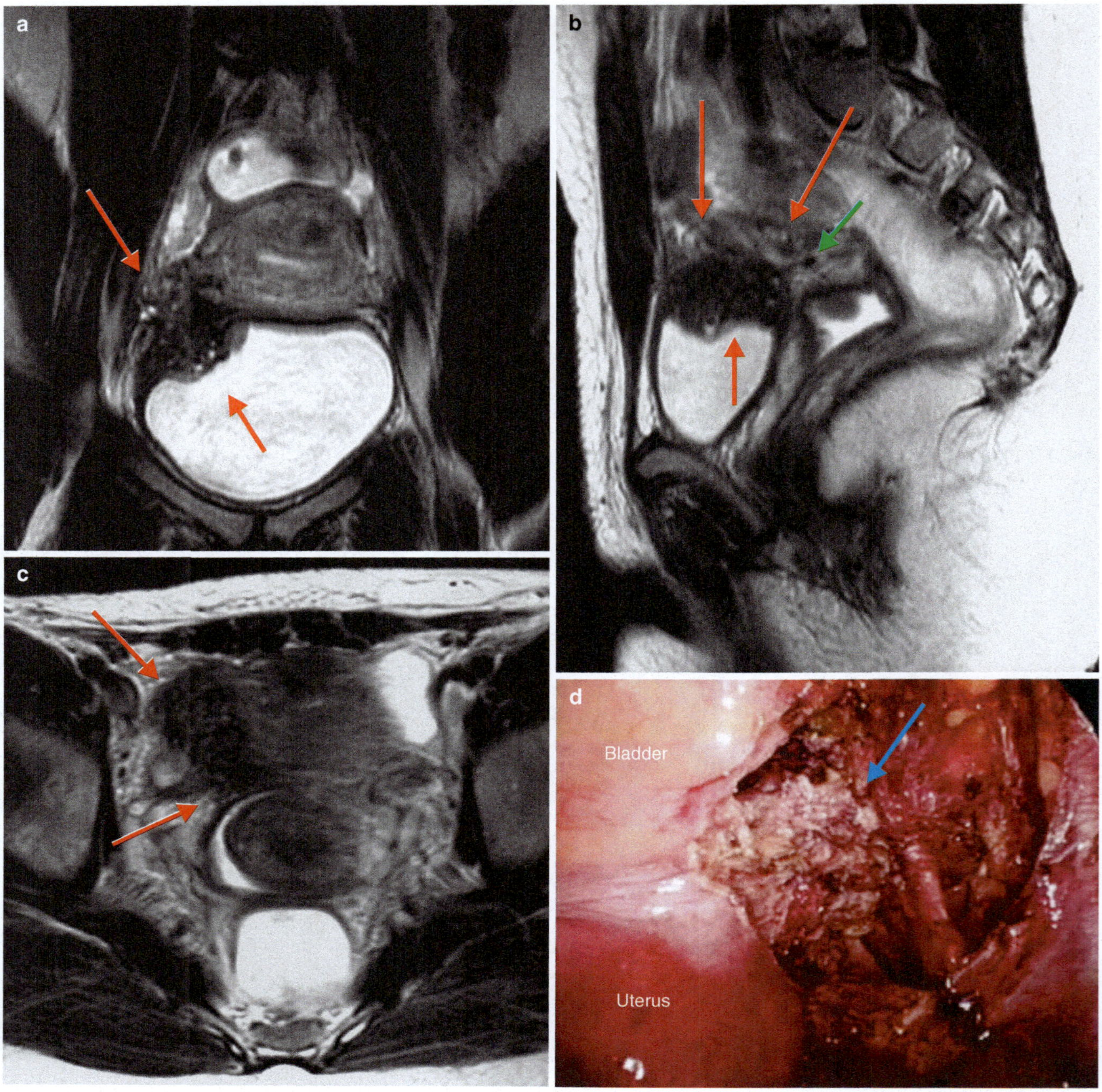

Fig. 4.8 Deep bladder lesion with right lateral localization in the anterior compartment, with extension to the broad and round ligaments. Note the proximity of the uterine artery lesion (green arrow in **b**). (**a**–**c**) T2-weighted sequences. (**a**) Coronal. (**b**) Sagittal. (**c**) Axial. (**d**) Laparoscopy. Lesion of the right lateral compartment (arrow)

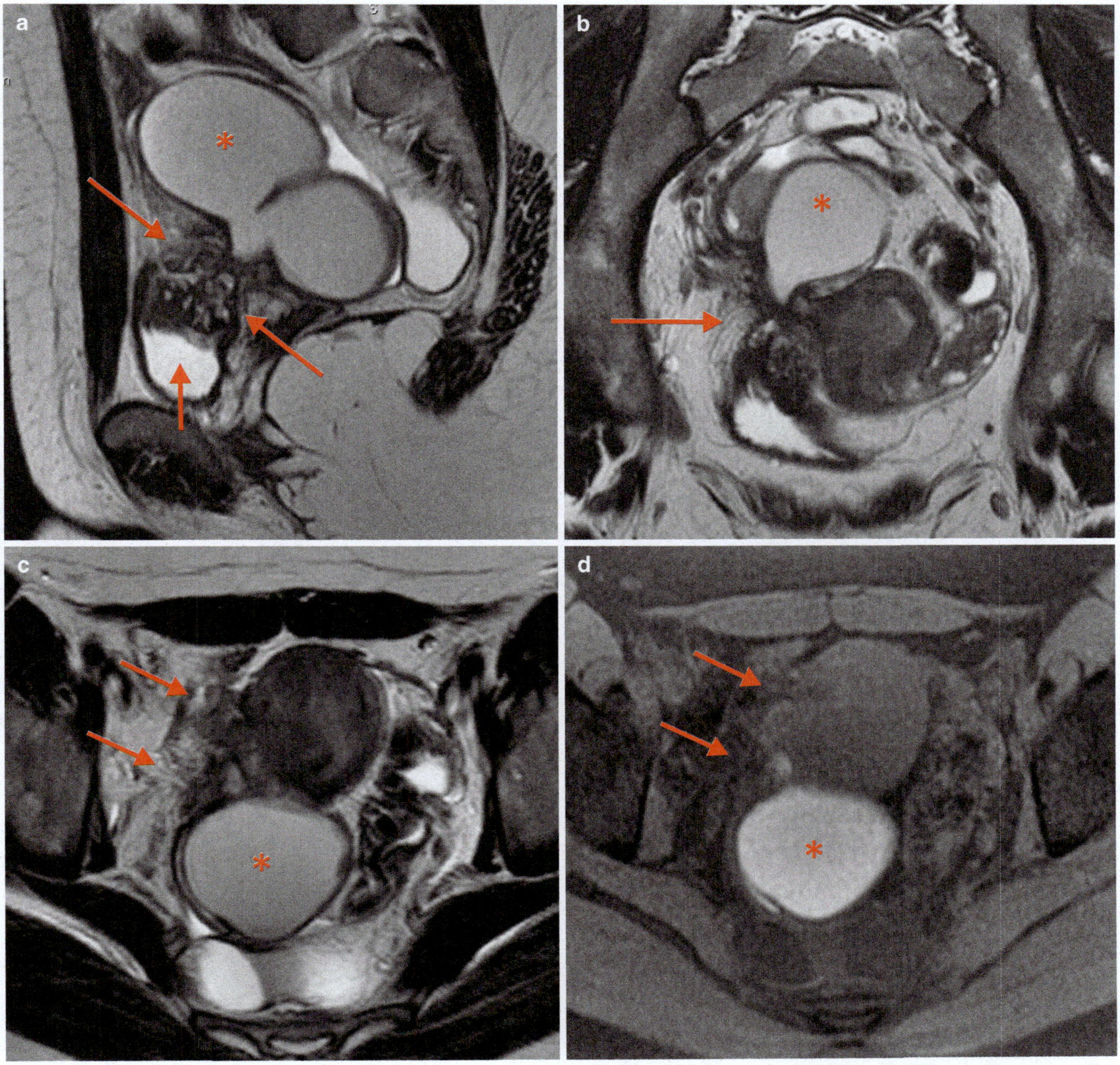

Fig. 4.9 Deep bladder endometriosis. Right lateral extension to the large and round ligaments, determining adhesion between the bladder, uterus, and attachment (arrows). Deviation of the right ovary, medially, with endometrioma (*). (**a–c**) T2-weighted sequences. (**a**) Sagittal. (**b**) Coronal. (**c**) Axial. (**d**) Endometrioma and bleeding foci (arrows) in the deep lesion, both hyperintense. T1 weighted with fat suppression. Axial

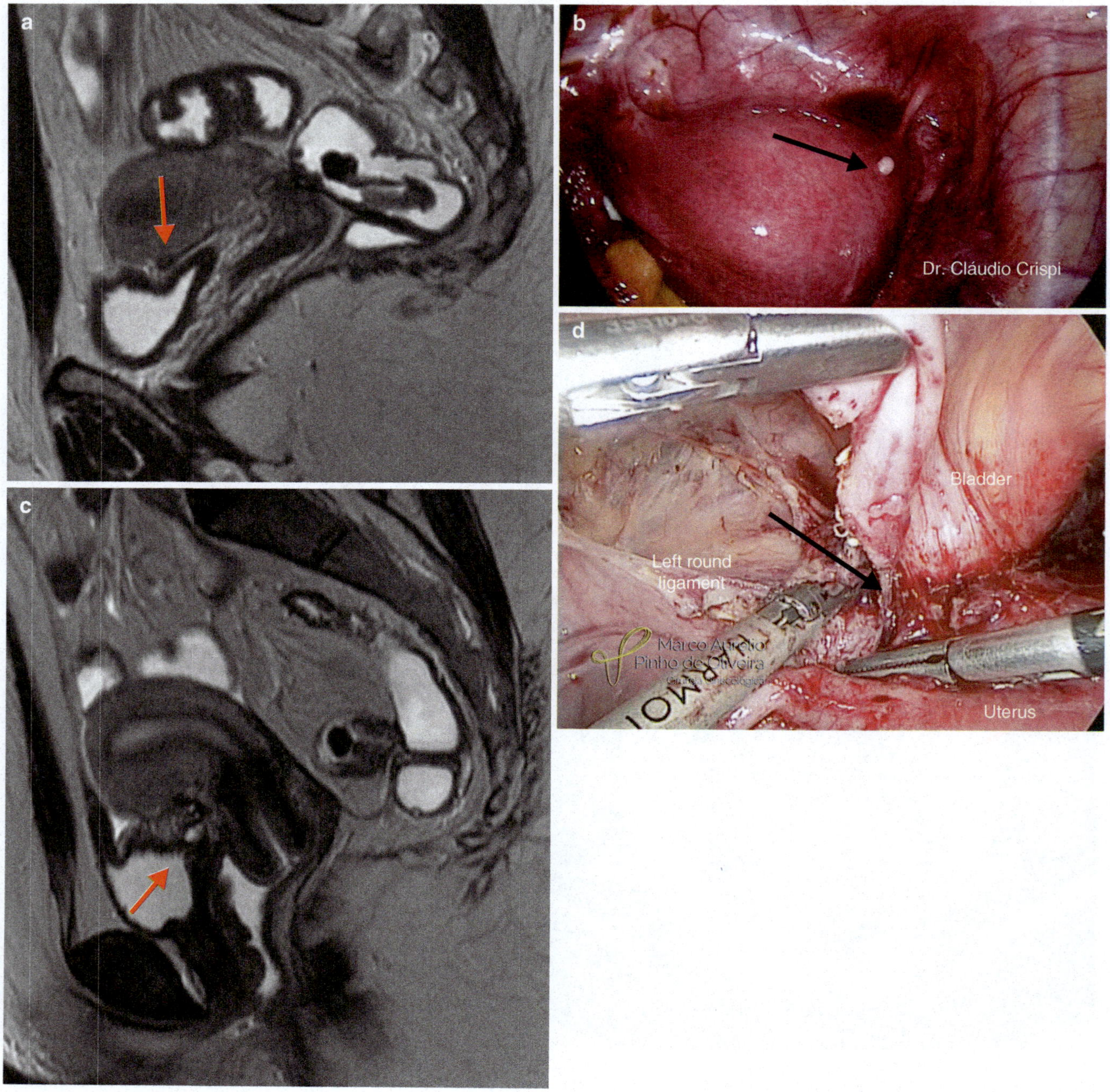

Fig. 4.10 The best technique for bladder study: empty bladder. Allows the identification of small lesions, including superficial lesions (**a**), as well as bladder involvement in the initial stage (**c**). (**a**, **b**) Glandular secretion. (**c**, **d**) Penetration of the detrusor in the midline. (**a**, **c**) T2-weighted sequences. Sagittal. (**b**) Laparoscopy demonstrating glandular excrescence on the uterine surface. (**d**) Laparoscopy during resection of the bladder node and the round ligament

4.1.1 Urinary Tract (Bladder and Distal Ureter)

Deep endometriosis involvement in the urinary tract is uncommon, involving about 1–2% of the patients. However, its incidence has increased in recent years, ranging from 0.3 to 12% of all women affected by endometriosis. The bladder is the most affected organ, involving about 11% of patients with deep endometriosis [3, 5, 7, 8].

Although the ureter is more affected by deep lesions of the posterior compartment, for didactic purposes, we will cover this in this section [9].

4.1.1.1 Bladder Anatomy

The bladder has an extraperitoneal location (retroperitoneal) in the pelvis. The peritoneum covers its superior surface, as well as the uterus anterior surface, forming the vesicouterine pouch (Fig. 4.11).

The following extraperitoneal pelvic spaces, important in surgical management, are located around the bladder:

1. The vesicocervical and vesicovaginal spaces: located between the lower urinary tract and genital tract, being separated by a thin septum, the supravaginal septum. It is bound by the bladder, the cervical and vaginal adventitia, and laterally by the bladder pillars. The ureters have a lower path in relation to the pillars, before entering the ostium. This space is rarely affected by endometriosis [9].
2. The Retzius or retropubic space: between the pubis and the anterior bladder surface; it contains veins and supporting ligaments (Fig. 4.12) [10].

The bladder has three layers: the adventitia (a fat layer, covered by the peritoneum on the superior surface), the detrusor muscle, and the mucosa (the urothelium and lamina

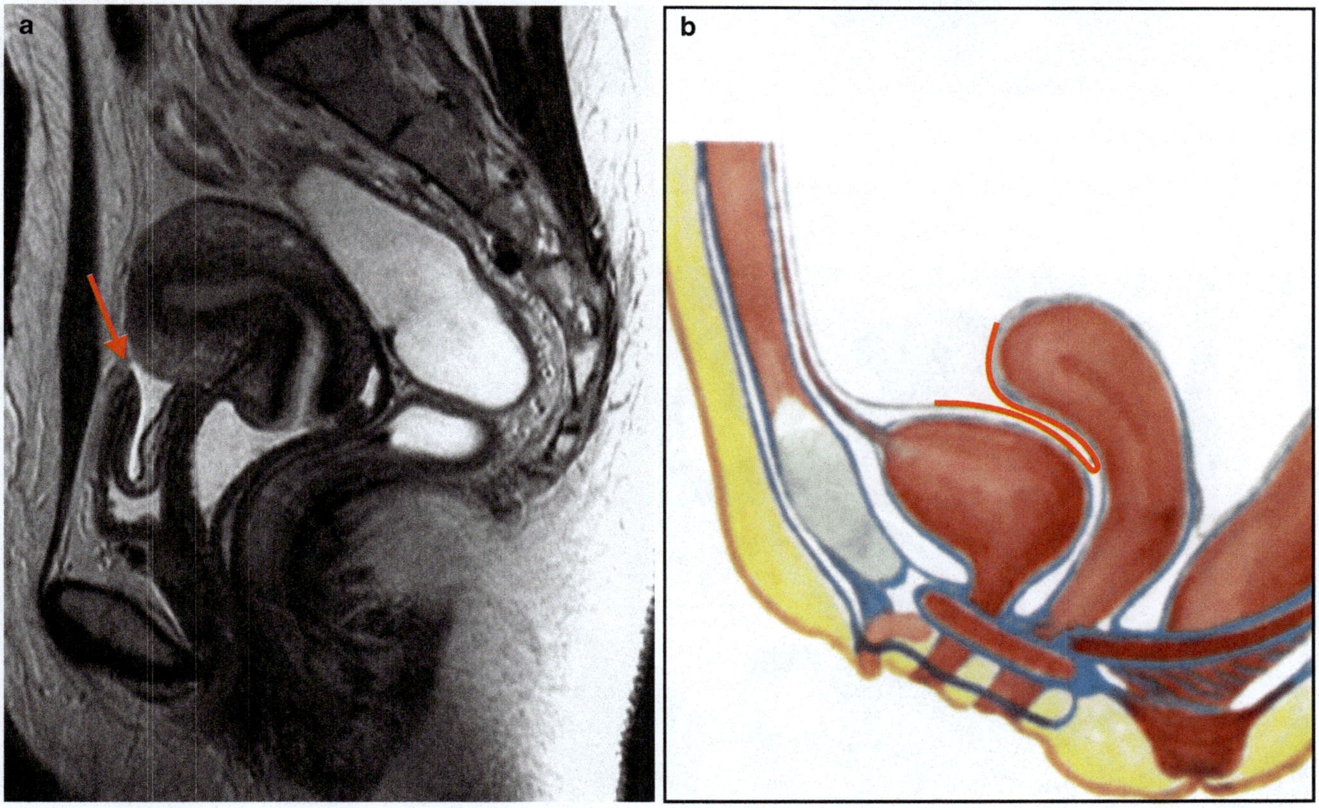

Fig. 4.11 The bladder has an extraperitoneal location. The free liquid enhances the coverage of the peritoneum in the bladder ceiling and the anterior aspect of the uterus (arrow in **a**), forming the vesicouterine recess (red outline in **b**). Note the usual signal of the bladder wall: an internal hyperintense layer with discrete enhancement by gadolinium, a hypointense hypofunctional detrusor, and a hyperintense outer layer without enhancement, the ceiling being the peritoneum (red line in the diagram) and the remaining endopelvic fascia—blue line in the diagram. (**a**, **c**) T2-weighted sequence. Sagittal. (**b**) Diagram. (**d**) T1-weighted sequence with suppression of fat and gadolinium

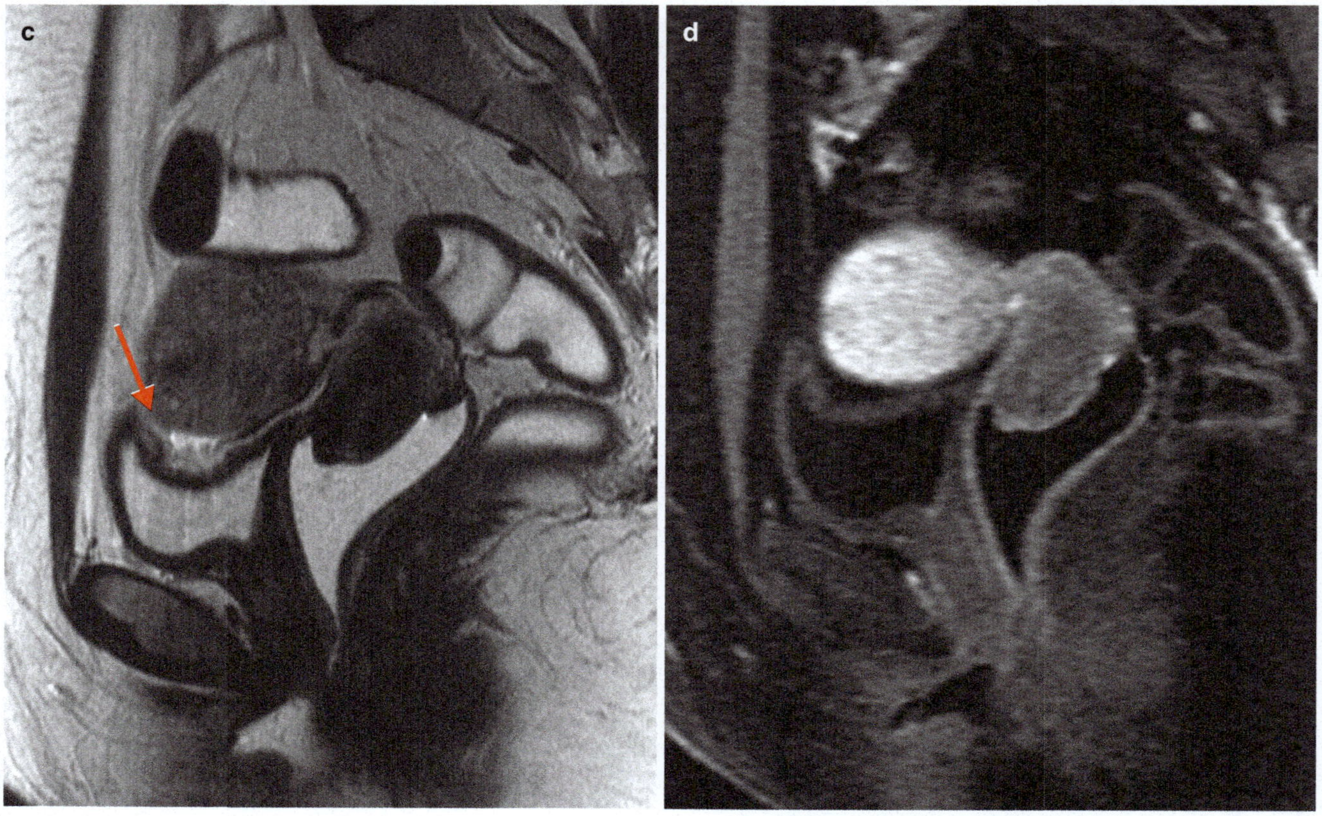

Fig. 4.11 (continued)

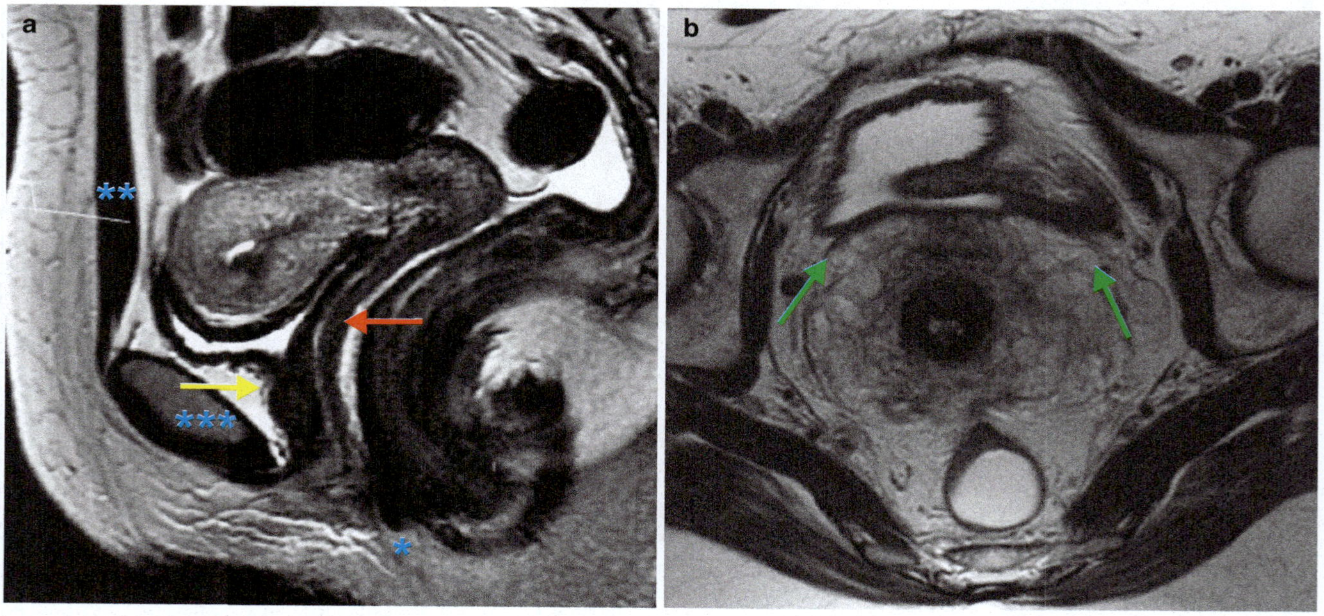

Fig. 4.12 Retropubic (orange arrow between the pubis (***) and the anterior surface of the bladder) and vesicovaginal spaces (red arrow—between the vagina, the posterior wall of the bladder, and the urethra). Note ureteral ostia (green arrows in **b**) and urethral support ligaments (yellow arrows). (**a**–**c**) T2-weighted sequences. (**a**) Sagittal. (**b**–**f**) Axial

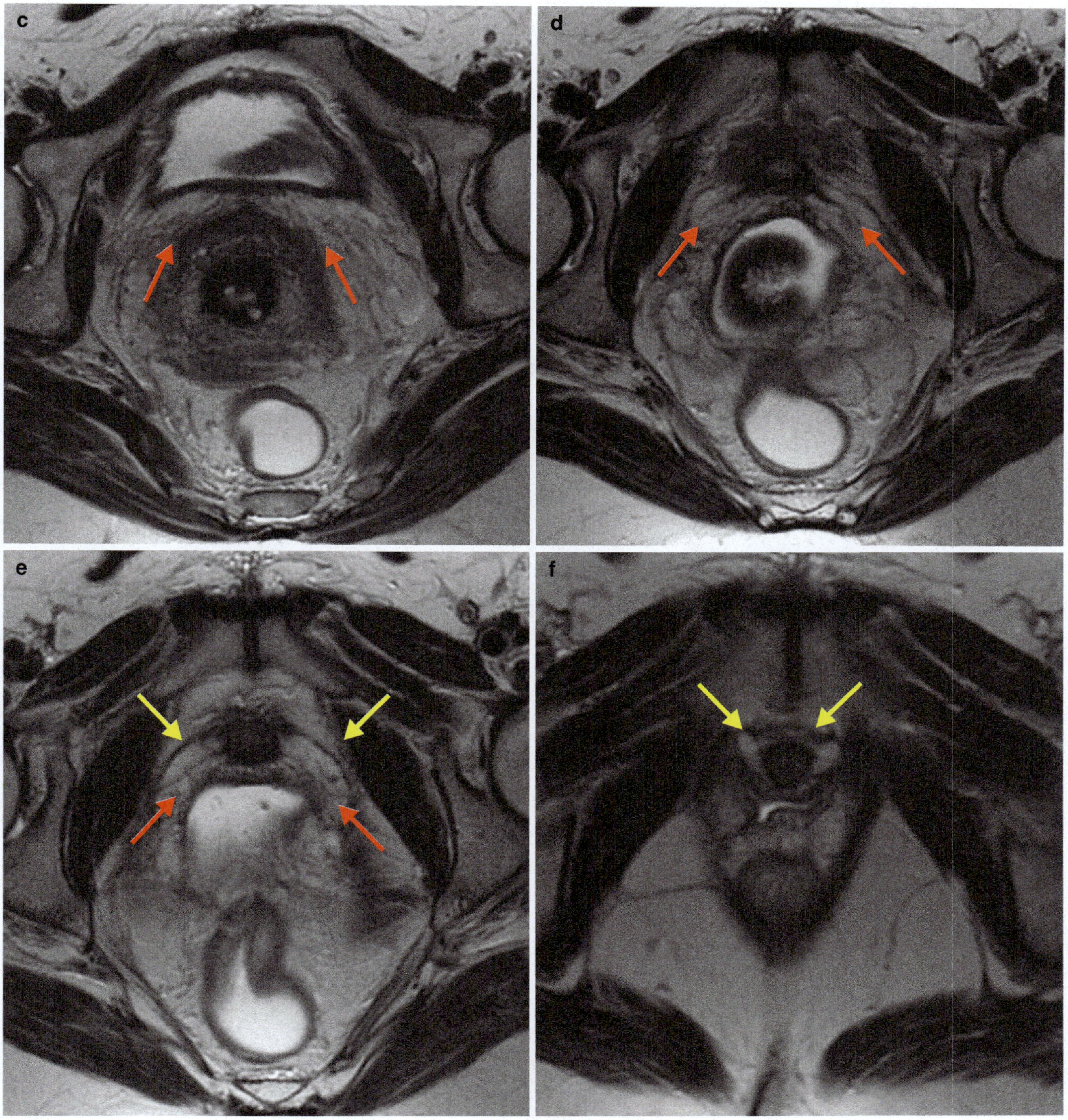

Fig. 4.12 (continued)

propria). The detrusor is the bladder muscle layer, being very important for the continence mechanism, as well as in deep endometriosis surgery planning.

TIP

The bladder is held in place by ligaments attached to the pelvic bones. The median umbilical ligament is located on the superior bladder surface, in the midline. It is a fibrous cord, an urachus vestige between the bladder and the umbilicus. When the bladder is empty, it may appear slightly thickened and should not be confused with deep endometriosis. Furthermore, a diverticulum from the remaining urachus can present as a high protein content cyst, hyperintense in T1-weighted, and hypointense in T2-weighted sequences, simulating endometriosis with atypical location (Figs. 4.8, 4.9, 4.13, and 4.14).

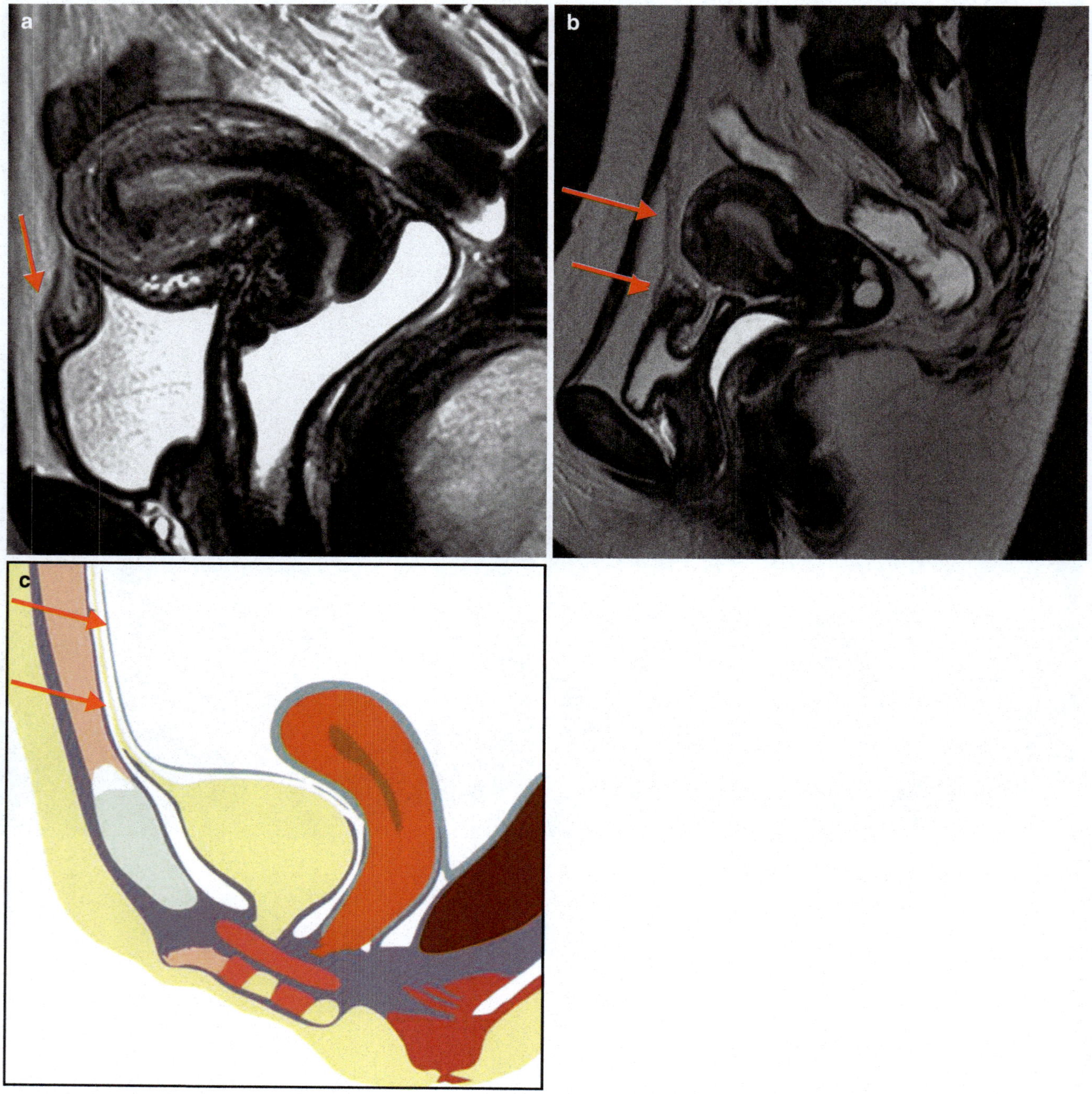

Fig. 4.13 Median umbilical ligament insertion (arrows). (**a**, **b**) Normal aspect of the bladder ceiling. It may become more prominent with the bladder empty. (**a**, **b**) T2-weighted sequences. Sagittal. Different patients. (**c**) Diagram

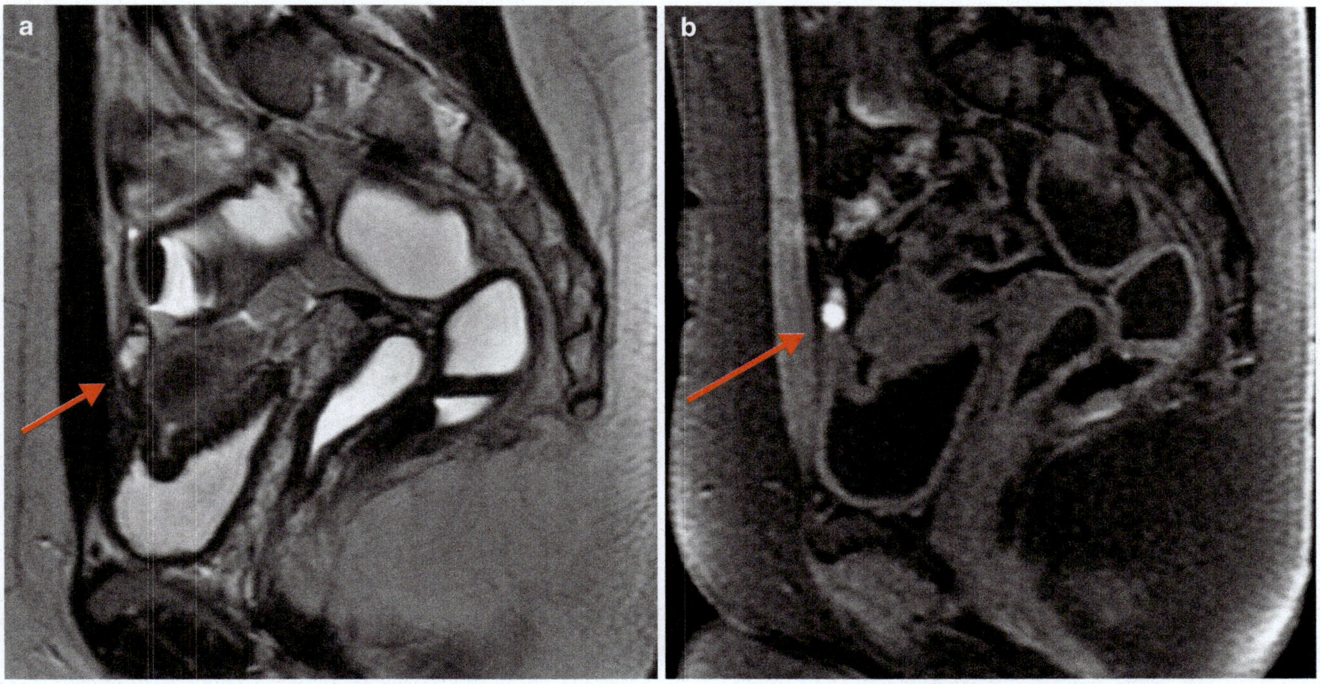

Fig. 4.14 Diverticulum of the urachus. Lobulated, circumscribed, supravesical cyst with septations at the median umbilical ligament insertion, with a hypersignal in the T2-weighted (**a**) and T1-weighted sequences with fat suppression (**b**), suggesting a high protein or hematic content. (**a**, **b**) Sagittal

4.1.1.2 Common Aspects of Bladder Deep Endometriosis

By definition, there is penetration by the endometrial implant into the muscle (detrusor), and occasionally it can reach the mucous membrane, projecting into the lumen of the bladder. Thus, cystoscopy may be negative in some cases (Fig. 4.15).

Deep bladder disease has a unifocal pattern, or isolated injury, usually affecting the posterior wall (above the trigone) and the bladder dome (superior surface). A study by Chapron found nodules in the posterior wall in 56 patients (74.7%) and in the dome in 19 (25.3%) (Fig. 4.16) [11].

From our experience, the location is predominantly at the midline, but it can be observed laterally. It commonly extends into the myometrium and the round ligaments, as described below. Moreover, the lesion can advance into the bowel, involving the cecum, ileum, appendix, and sigmoid (Figs. 4.8 and 4.9).

As in the posterior compartment, the lesion can promote adhesions, with partial or complete anterior cul-de-sac obliteration. It is usually associated with multiple site involvement. Chapron noted that in 64% of patients, a bladder nodule was associated with deep posterior lesions, involving the uterosacral ligament, vagina, and intestine (Fig. 4.17) [11].

Deep endometriosis usually does not affect the trigone, being involved in only 10% of the cases.

It can also extend to the ureteral ostium. It is important to emphasize that the distance from a bladder lesion to the ureteral ostium may be falsely reduced in relation to the empty bladder MRI protocol. The most accurate distance is obtained through cystoscopy. The involvement of the ureter ostium can change the surgical planning, as it may result in reimplantation or segmental resection of the affected ureter (Fig. 4.18) [11].

Another aspect of lower urinary tract endometriosis is the observation of different behaviors of bladder and ureteral lesions. Abrão observed patients with ureteral endometriosis, related to retrocervical deep endometriosis extension but with no bladder lesions. According to Gabriel, the ureteral involvement is usually asymptomatic, whereas bladder involvement manifests itself most often with dysuria, hematuria, and urinary tract infection [12, 13].

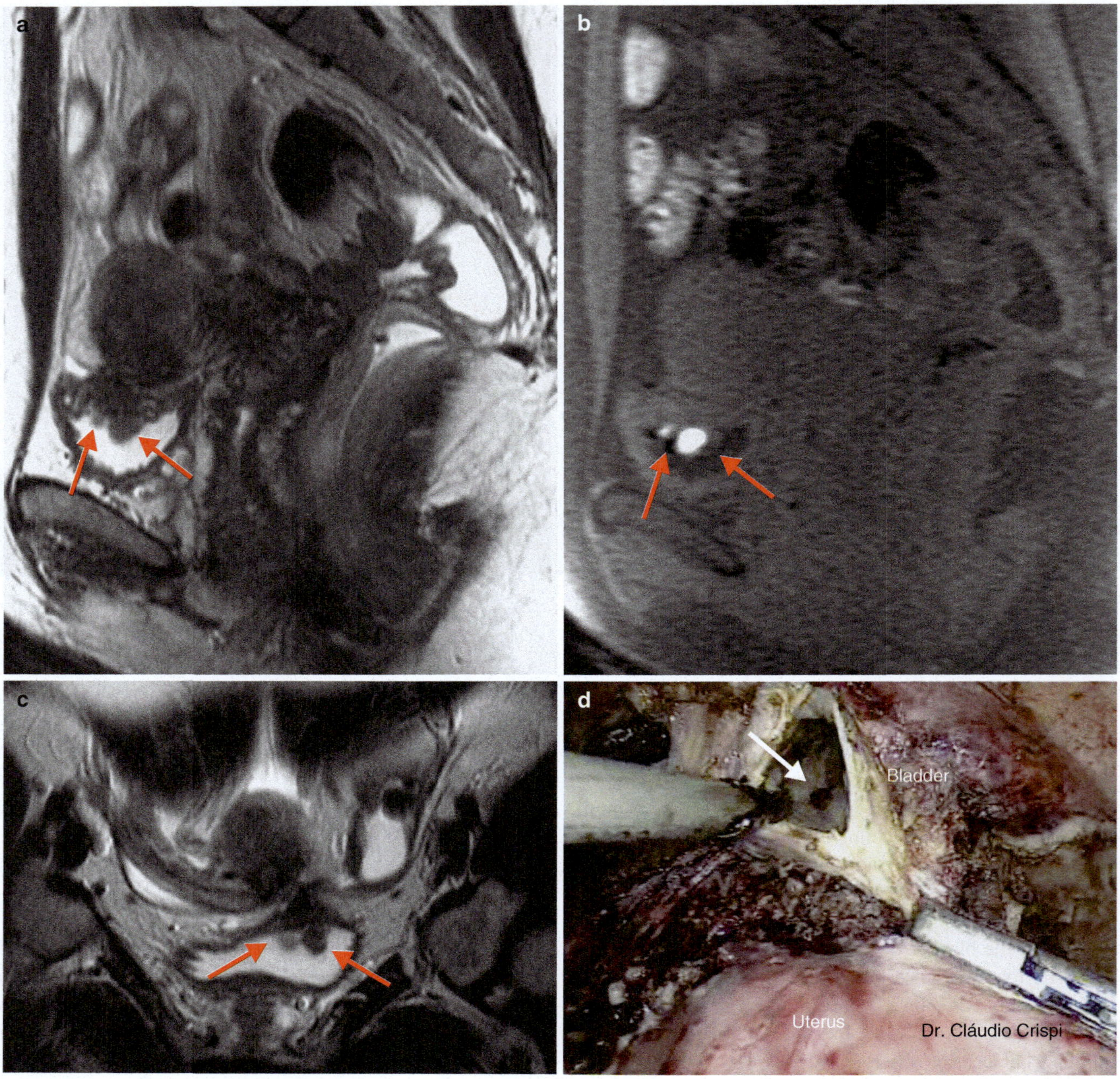

Fig. 4.15 Deep disease in the bladder roof, with penetration of the muscle and mucosal layers, projecting into the lumen of the bladder. Positive cystoscopy. (**a**, **c**) T2-weighted sequences. (**b**) T1-weighted sequence with fat suppression. (**a**, **b**) Sagittal. (**c**) Coronal. (**d**) Laparoscopy. Start of bladder opening

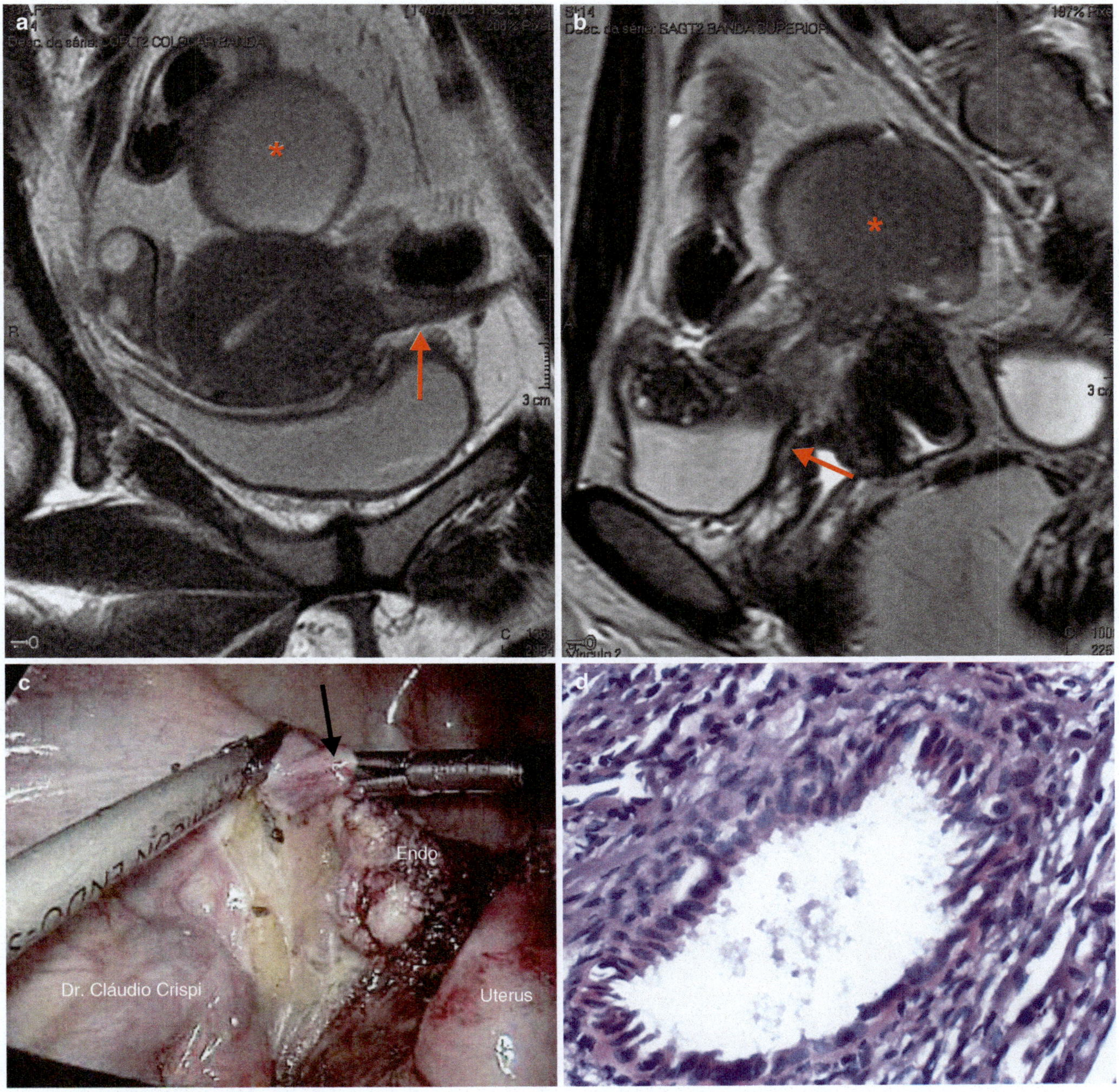

Fig. 4.16 Deep lesion in the bladder roof without compromising the trigone (arrow **b**), extending to the left round ligament (arrow **a**). Note endometrioma (*). T2-weighted sequences. (**a**) Coronal. (**b**) Sagittal. (**c**) Laparoscopy. Start of resection of ligament endometriosis. (**d**) Pathology (100× increase) showing endometriotic cyst in lesion in the vesicouterine fold

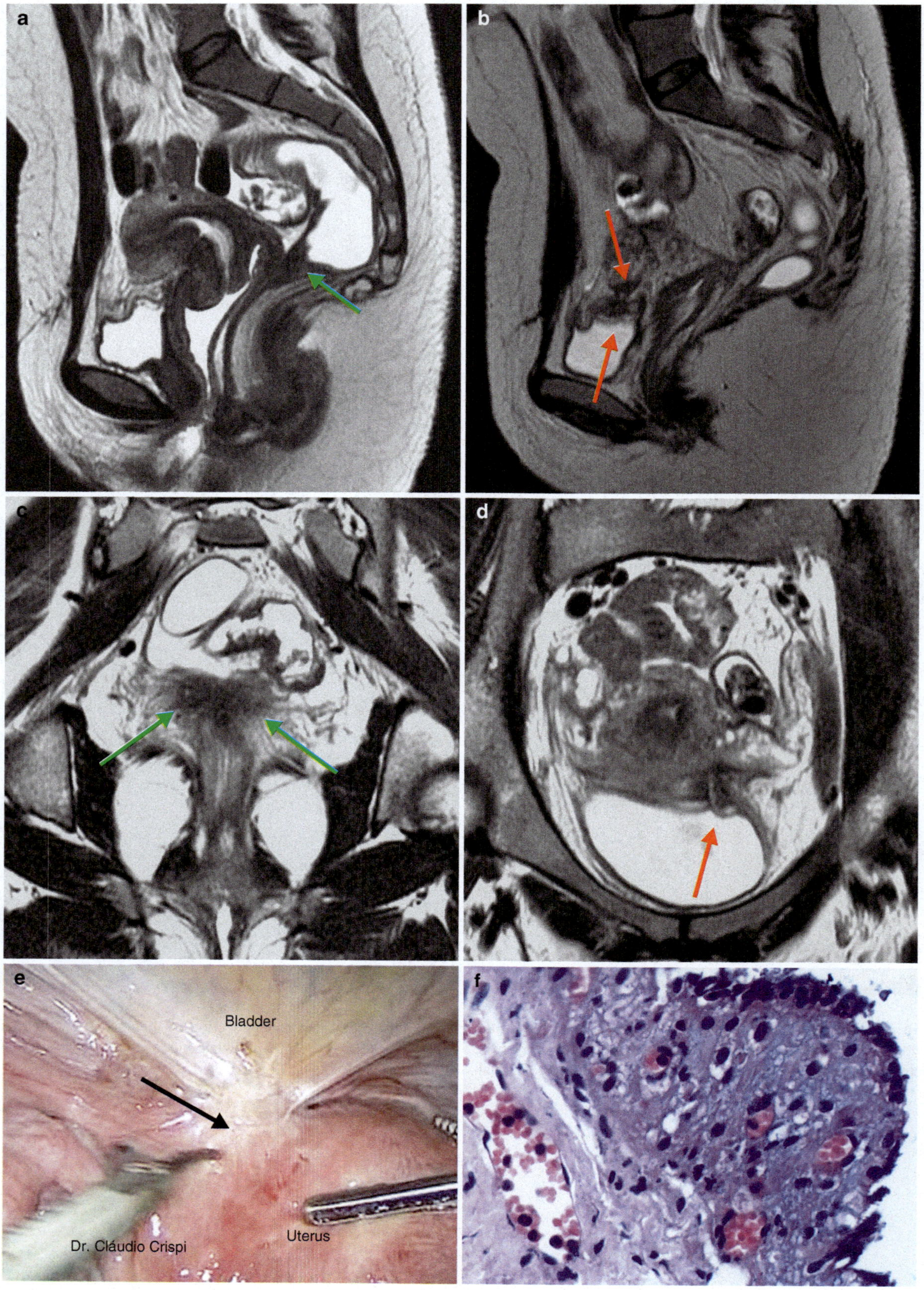

Fig. 4.17 Two deep lesions in the same patient. In the anterior compartment, vesical, being superficial myometrial (red arrow) and posterior in the rectovaginal septum, with involvement of the uterosacrals, vagina, and inferior rectum (green arrow). (**a**–**d**) T2-weighted sequences. (**a**, **b**) Sagittal. (**c**, **d**) Coronal. (**e**) Laparoscopy and pathology (**f**) demonstrating endometriotic bladder node

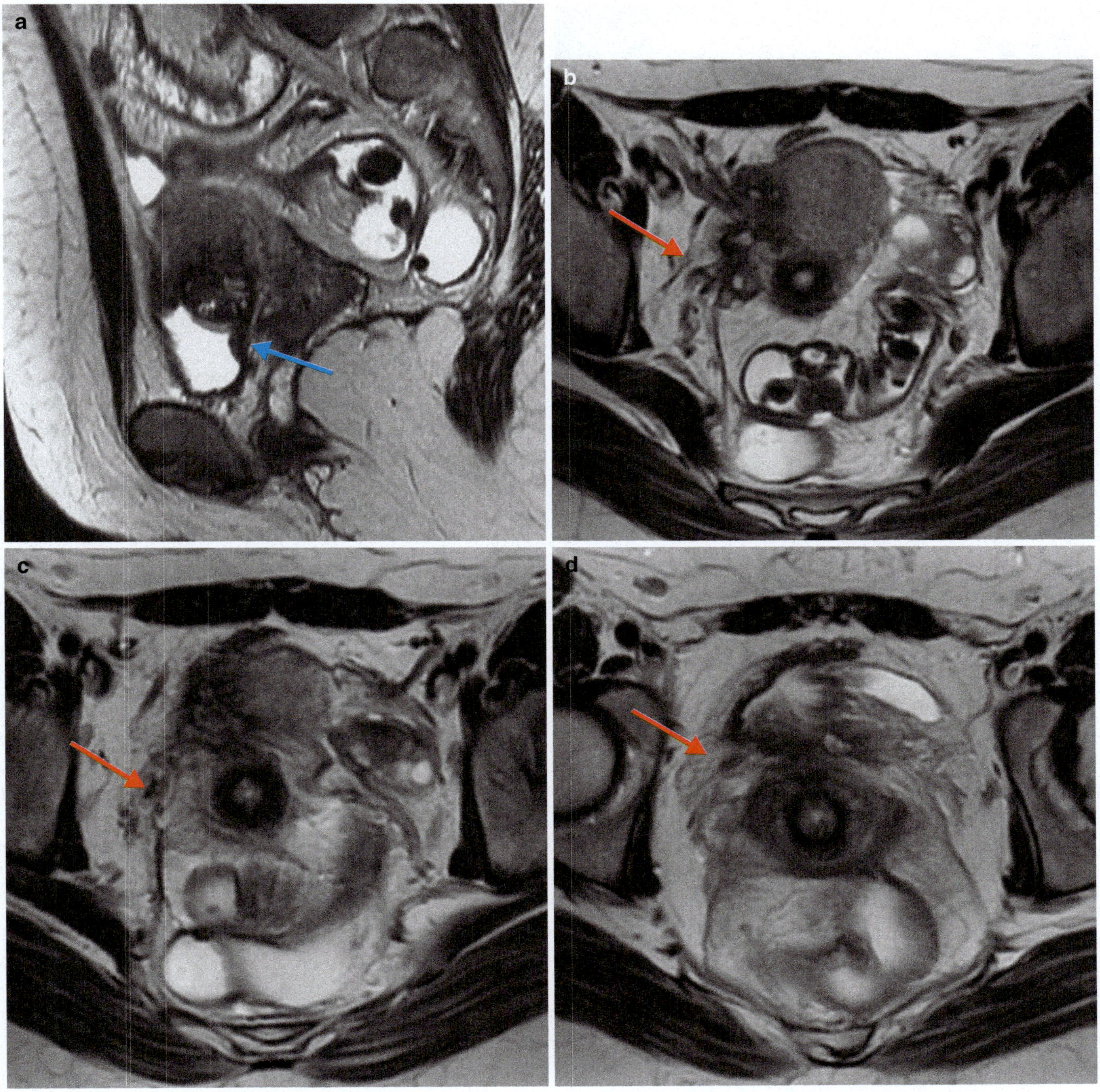

Fig. 4.18 The bladder involvement has no cleavage plane with the right ureteral ostium (blue arrow). The ureter above the bladder is preserved (red arrows). (**a–d**) T2-weighted sequences. (**a**) Sagittal. (**b–d**) Axial. (**e**) Cystoscopy with large bladder node, close to the bladder trigone. Same case as in Fig. 4.50 after hormonal blockade

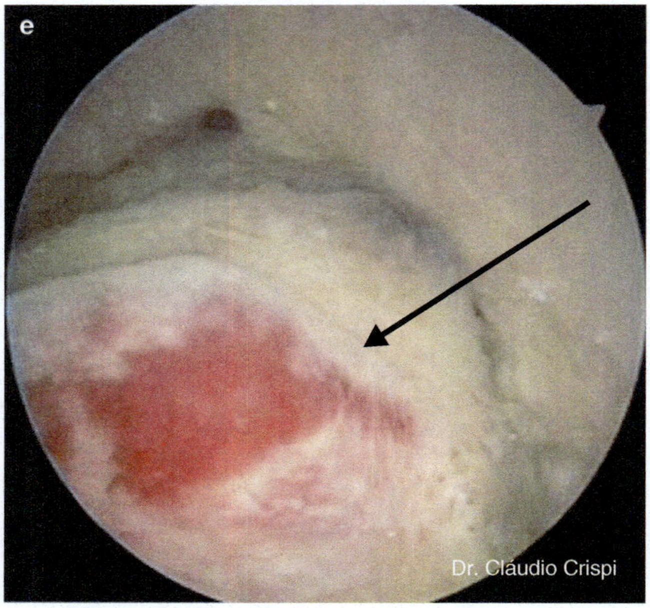

Fig. 4.18 (continued)

4.1.1.3 Clinical Manifestations

Typical symptoms are cyclical urgency, increased urinary frequency, suprapubic pain, hematuria, and dyspareunia in reproductive-age women. There may be exacerbation of the symptoms during menstruation.

Despite cyclical gross hematuria being pathognomonic, it is present in only 20% of the patients [14].

4.1.1.4 MRI and Laparoscopic Findings

Deep bladder endometriosis lesion usually presents in MRI as a poorly delimited nodule, irregular, with variable size, in the posterior wall or in the bladder dome. There may be an extension to the vesicouterine pouch and infiltration of the myometrium and round ligaments (Fig. 4.19).

Thickening and retraction of the round ligaments are common, pointing to the bladder injury, and may be considered an indirect sign of bladder injury, according to Crispi (Fig. 4.20) [15].

Muscle penetration can be inferred by the MRI, since there is a signal intensity difference between the hypointense endometriosis lesion and the hyperintense normal submucosa in the T2-weighted sequence. Moreover, continuous muscle gadolinium enhancement suggests muscle integrity (Fig. 4.21).

The lesion signal intensity can vary in relation to the predominance of fibrous or glandular tissue. Fibrotic lesions present with a hypointense signal in the T2-weighted sequence and an isointense one in the T1-weighted sequence. Lesions with prominent glandular tissue can present hyperintense foci in the T1- and T2-weighted sequences (Fig. 4.22) [15].

Busard identified cysts and bleeding in 59% of bladder lesions, predominantly in the submucosal, where the tissue is less compact compared to the muscular layer (Fig. 4.22).

The median umbilical ligament insertion or an urachal remnant should not be misinterpreted as a bladder lesion. The ligament insertion at the bladder dome presents a fine linear structure at the midline, extending superiorly to the umbilicus (Fig. 4.13). The urachal remnant is usually a cystic and well-defined lesion. A high signal intensity cyst content in the T1-weighted sequence is related to high protein content. The cyst does not penetrate into the myometrium or extend to the round ligament (Fig. 4.14).

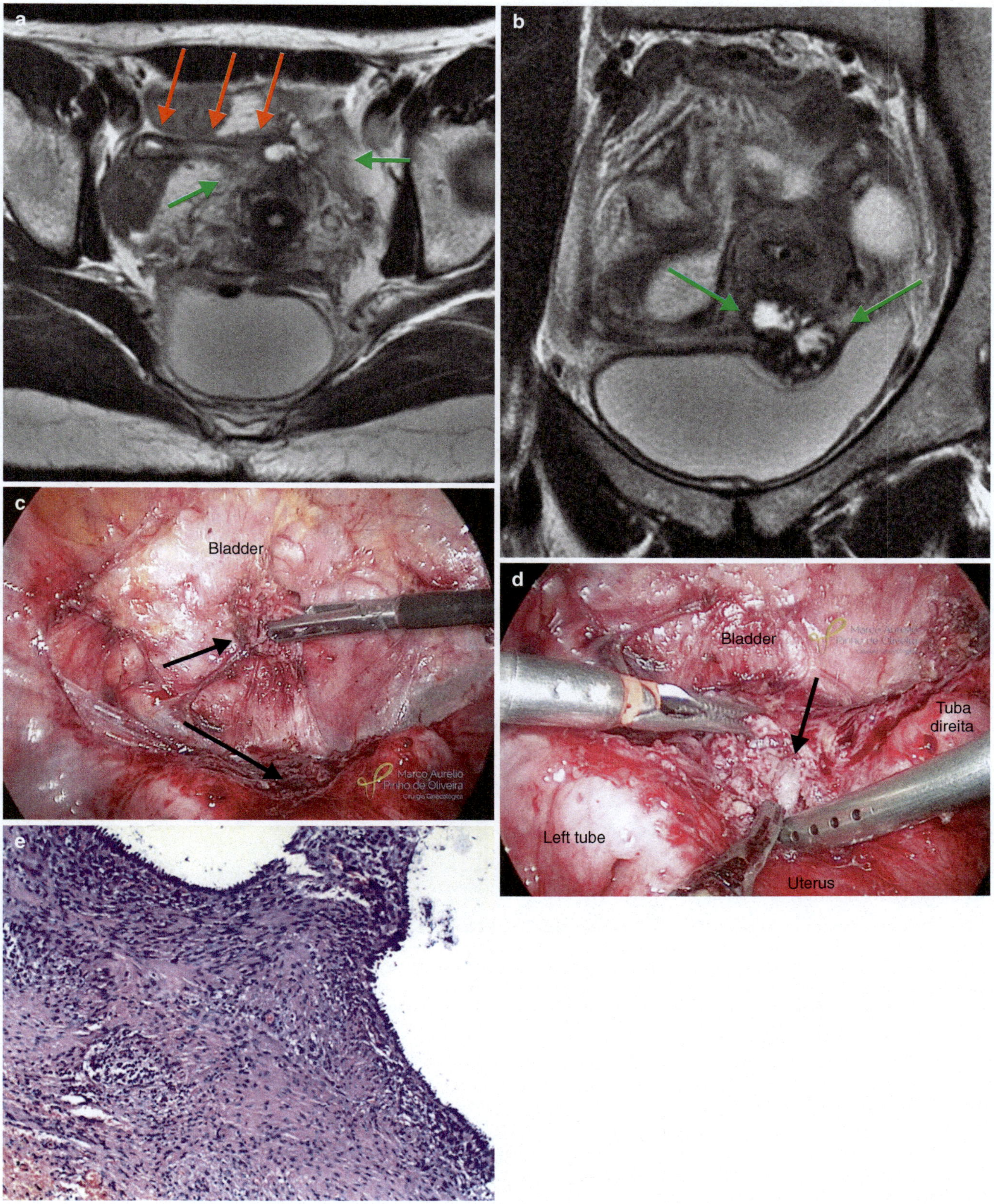

Fig. 4.19 Poorly delimited, irregular, heterogeneous nodule predominantly hyperintense in T2, in the posterior wall, with important component in vesicouterine recess and myometrial extension (green arrows). It also determines adhesion with right ovary (red arrows). (**a**, **b**) T2-weighted sequence. (**a**) Axial. (**b**) Coronal. (**c**, **d**) Laparoscopy. (**c**) Bladder node adhered to the myometrium. (**d**) Note relation with adnexa. (**e**) Pathology demonstrating two endometriotic cysts on top of the bladder musculature

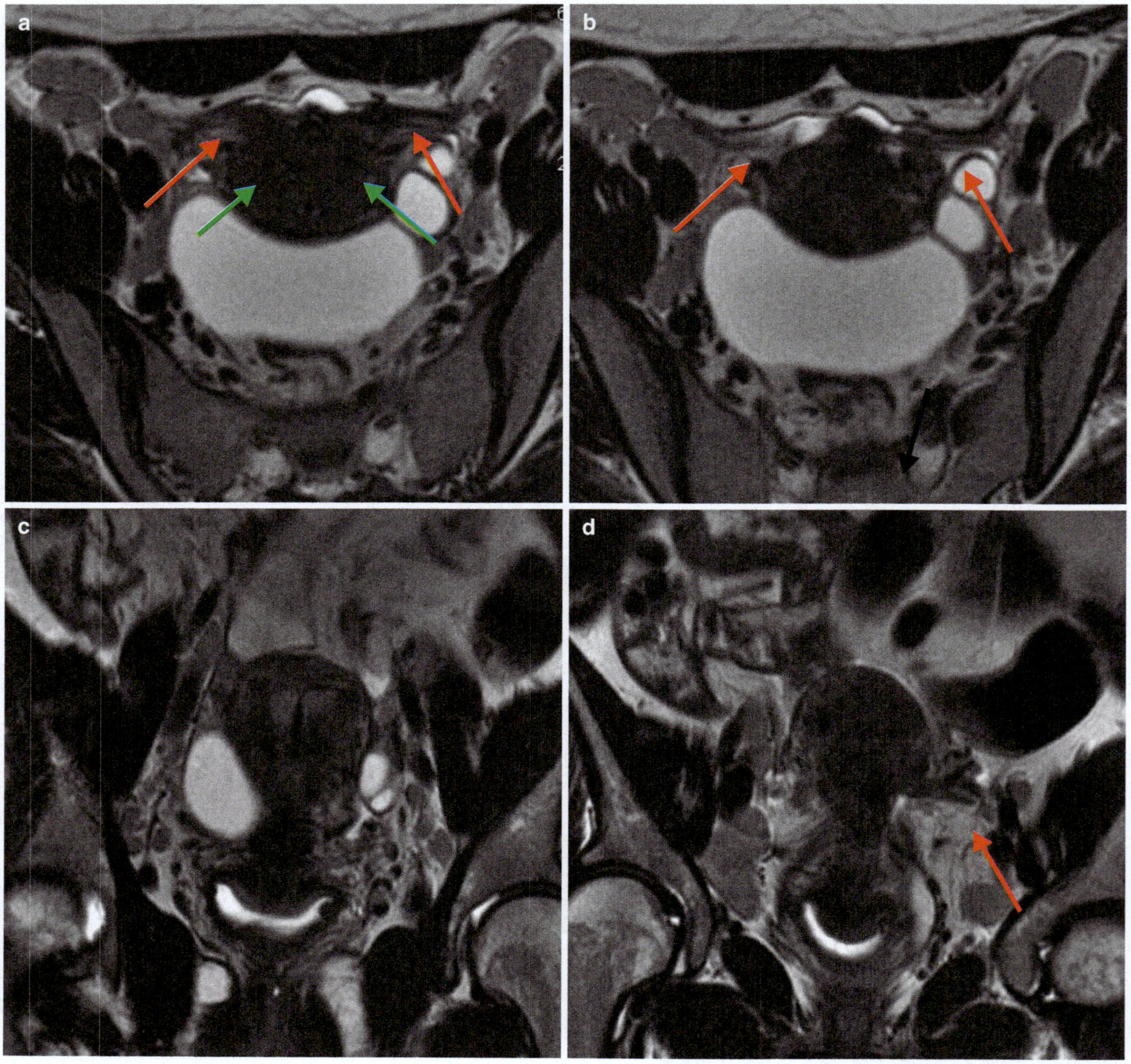

Fig. 4.20 Thickening and retraction of the round ligaments (red arrow), which points to bladder and myometrial lesions (green arrows). Note lymph node enlargement. Patient with antiphospholipid antibody syndrome. (**a**, **b**) T2-weighted short-axis coronal. (**cf**) Long axis. (**g**). (**hj**) Laparoscopy. Note the retraction of the round ligament and resection of the nodule in the anterior myometrium

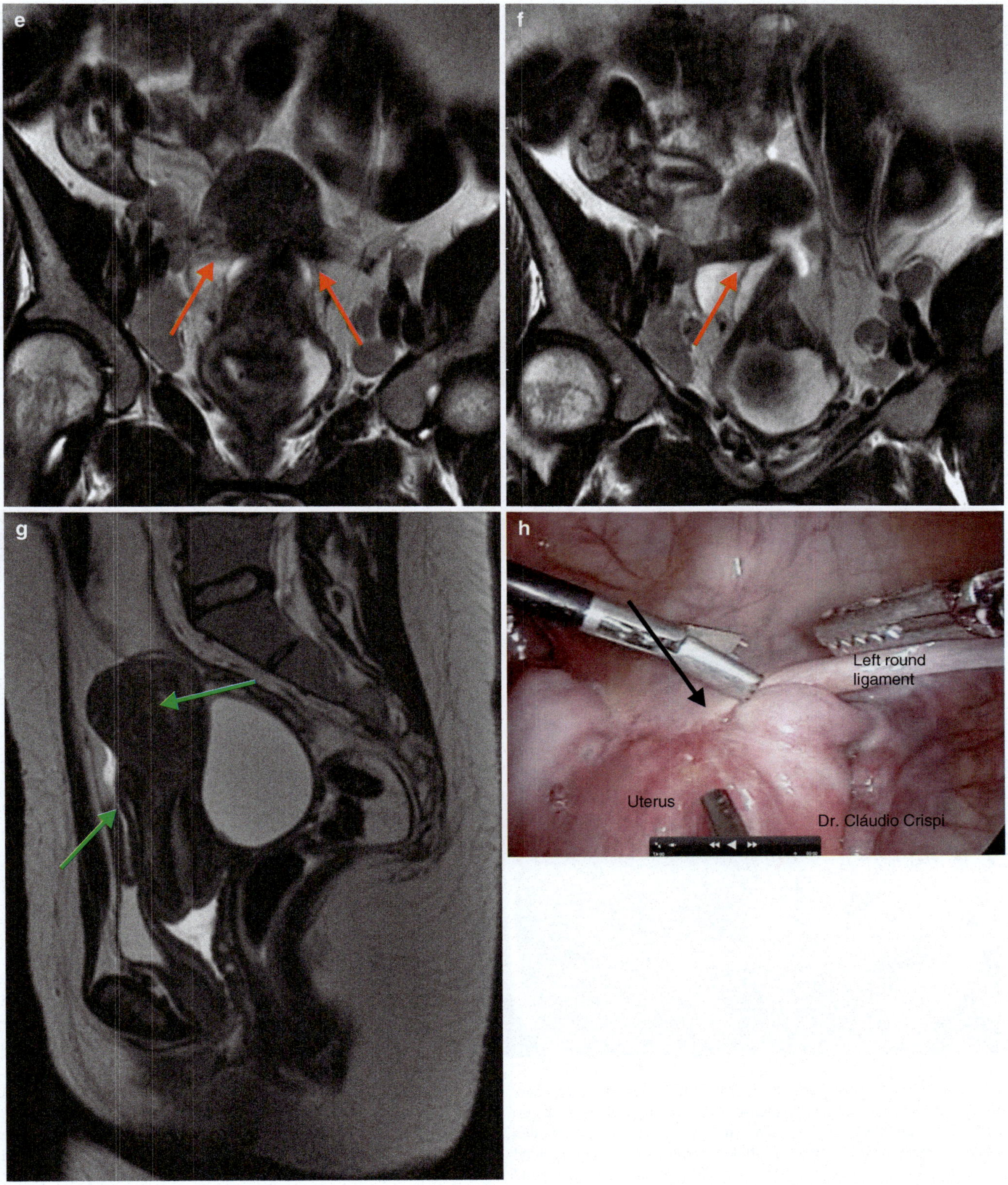

Fig. 4.20 (continued)

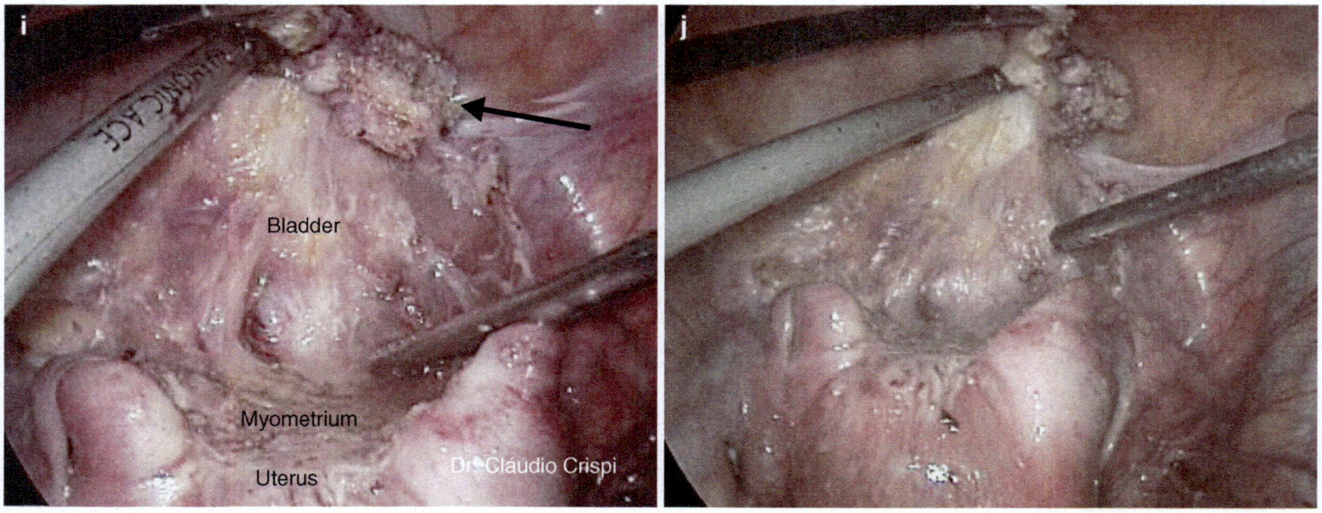

Fig. 4.20 (continued)

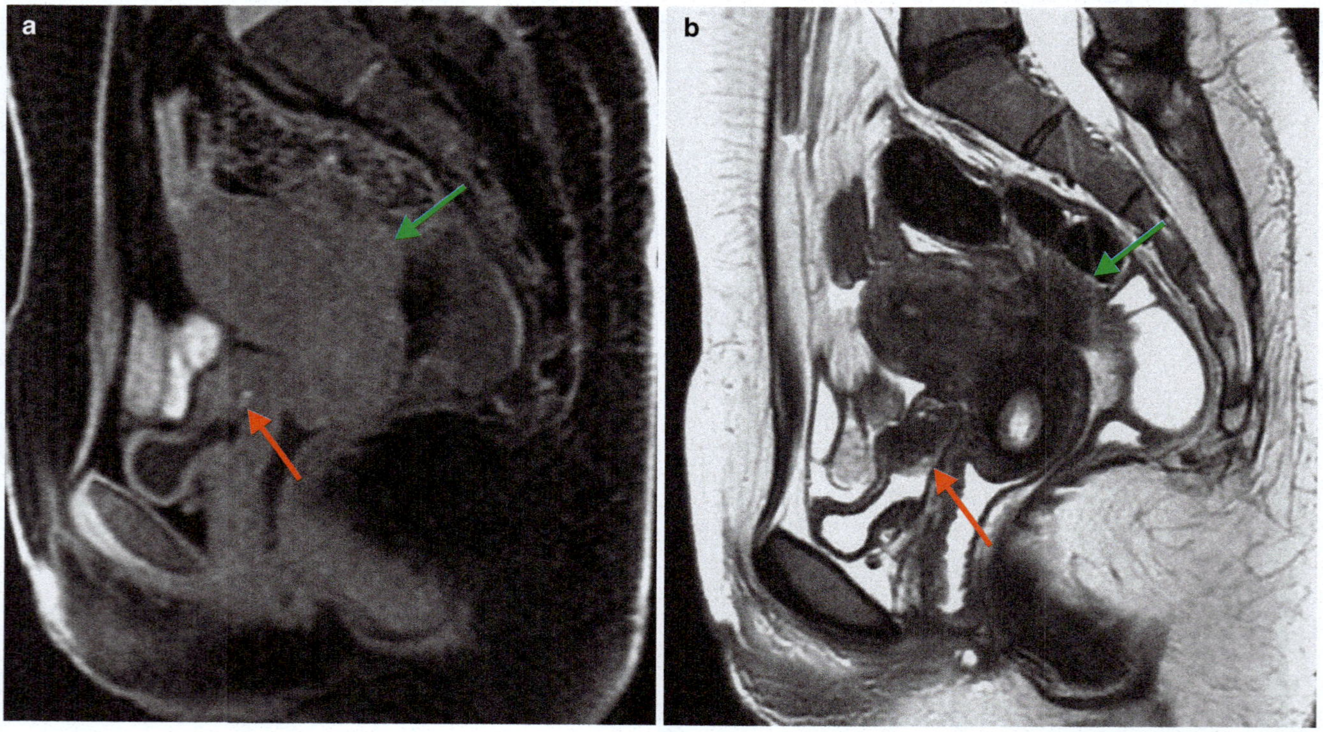

Fig. 4.21 Lesion in the posterior portion of the ceiling bladder, deep, sparing the mucosa. The hypointense lesion on T2-weighted images (**bd**) does not reach the mucosa, slightly thickened and swollen (arrows). Bleeding focus on T1 (**a**). It does not compromise the ureteral ostia (**d**). Note simultaneous retrocervical lesion in the sigmoid and uterosacrals (green arrow), in addition to endometrioma in the left ovary (*). (**a**, **b**) Sagittal. (**c**) Coronal. (**d**) Axial. (**e**) Laparoscopy. Resection area of bladder endometriosis, allowing visualization of the detrusor muscle. (**f**) Microscopy demonstrating secretory endometrial gland limited by edematous striated muscle (400×)

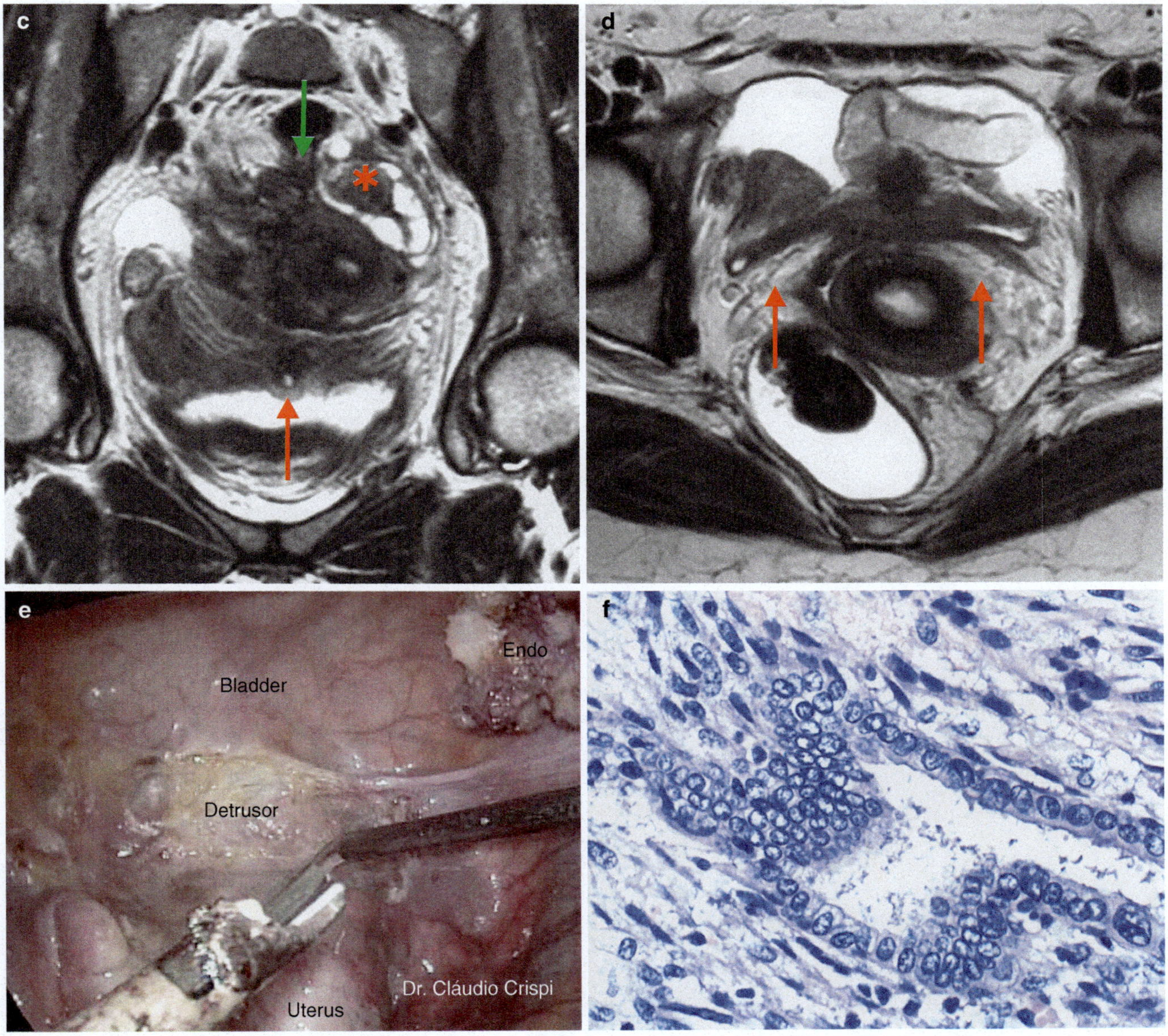

Fig. 4.21 (continued

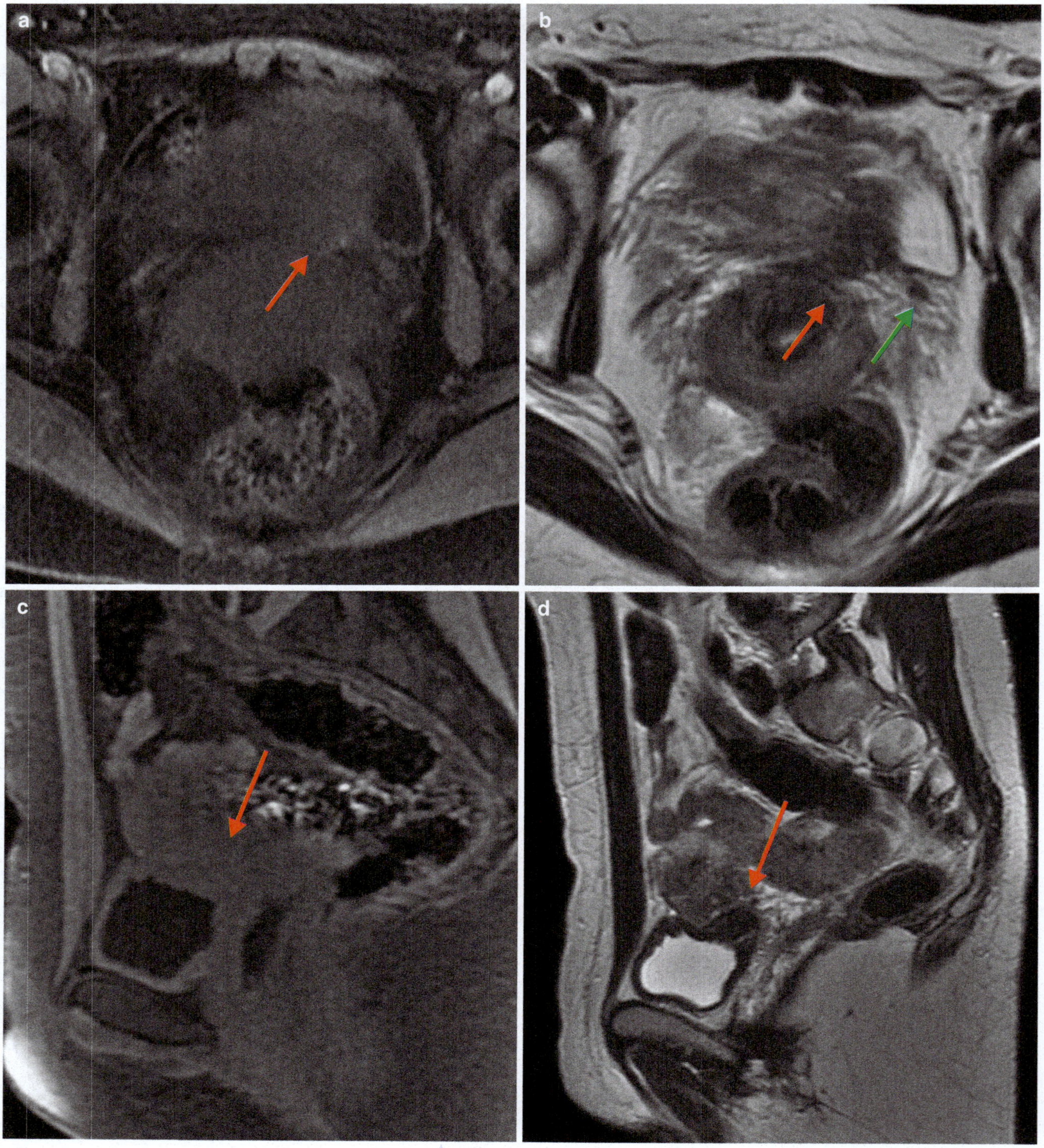

Fig. 4.22 Case 1: (**ad**) lesion with hypointense on T2-weighted sequences (**b**, **d**) and isosignal T1 (**a**, **d**) by a predominance of fibrotic tissue (red arrows). Note proximity to the ureter (green arrow). Case 2: (**e–h**) lesion with associated glandular component, hyperintense in the T2-weighted sequences (**f**, **h**), and with multiple bleeding foci in T1 with fat suppression (**e**, **g**) (red arrows). Blue arrow. (**a**, **b**, **e**, **f**) Axial. (**c**, **d**, **g**, **h**) Sagittal

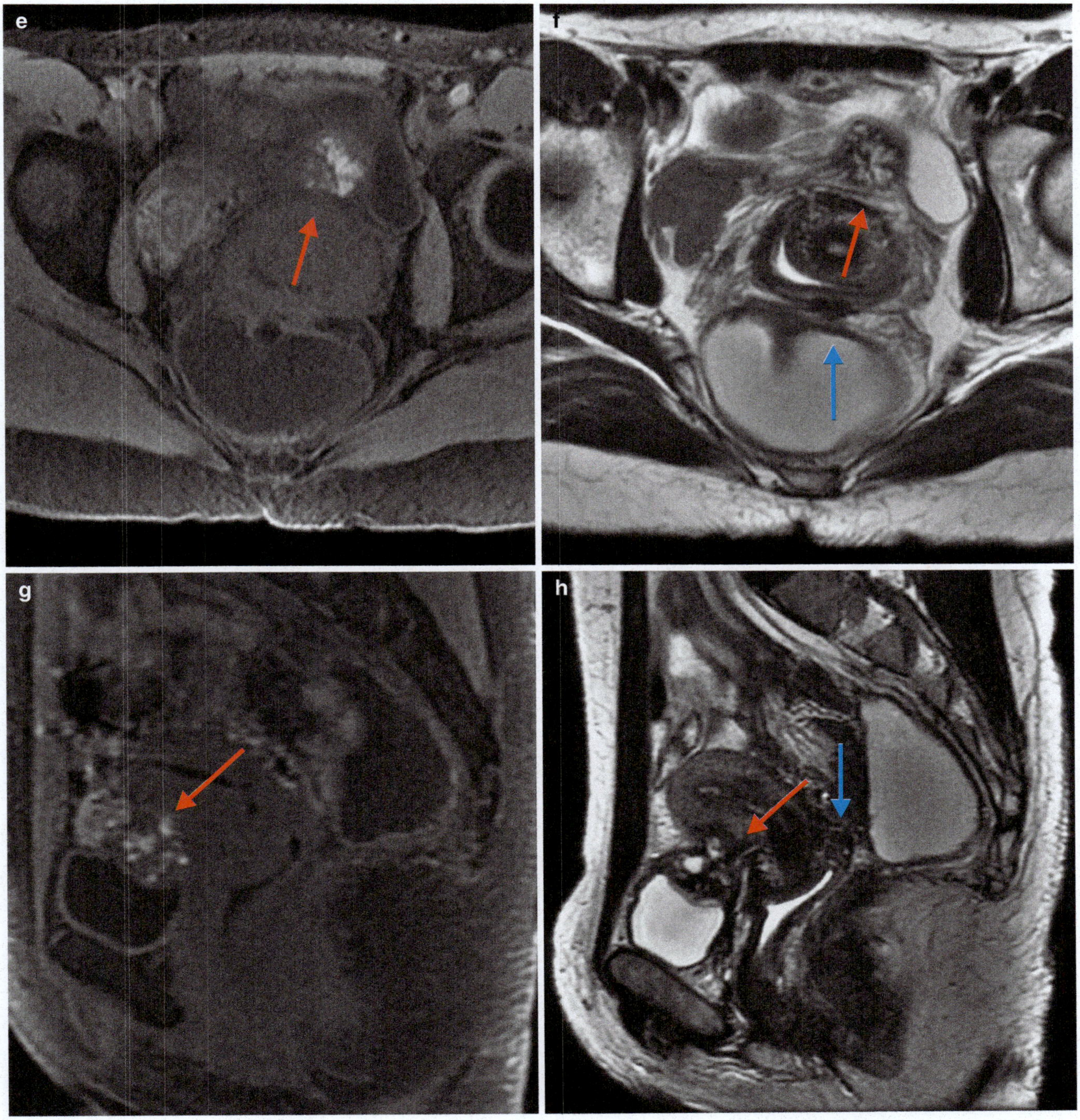

Fig. 4.22 (continued)

4.1.1.5 Comments About the Treatment

Surgical treatment of bladder endometriosis varies according to the location of the lesion reported by MRI and the following factors: (a) involvement of the submucosa/mucosa, (b) the distance from the ureteral ostium, (c) the extension of the ureter involvement, (d) size, and (e) myometrial involvement (Table 4.2).

When there is no involvement of the mucosa/submucosa, nodulectomy is the chosen procedure; for large lesions with involvement of these layers, the ideal surgical treatment is partial cystectomy (Fig. 4.23).

If there is extensive ostium involvement, it may be necessary to reimplant the ureter (Figs. 4.18 and 4.24).

The myometrial component of the lesion should be resected, as it is one of the most frequent causes of recurrence in this compartment.

We discuss myometrial involvement in subsequent sections below (Fig. 4.19) [9, 16].

Table 4.2 Important information for surgical treatment of bladder endometriosis

Involvement of the submucosa/mucosa
Distance from the ureteral ostium
Quantification of the involvement of the ureter
Size
Myometrial involvement

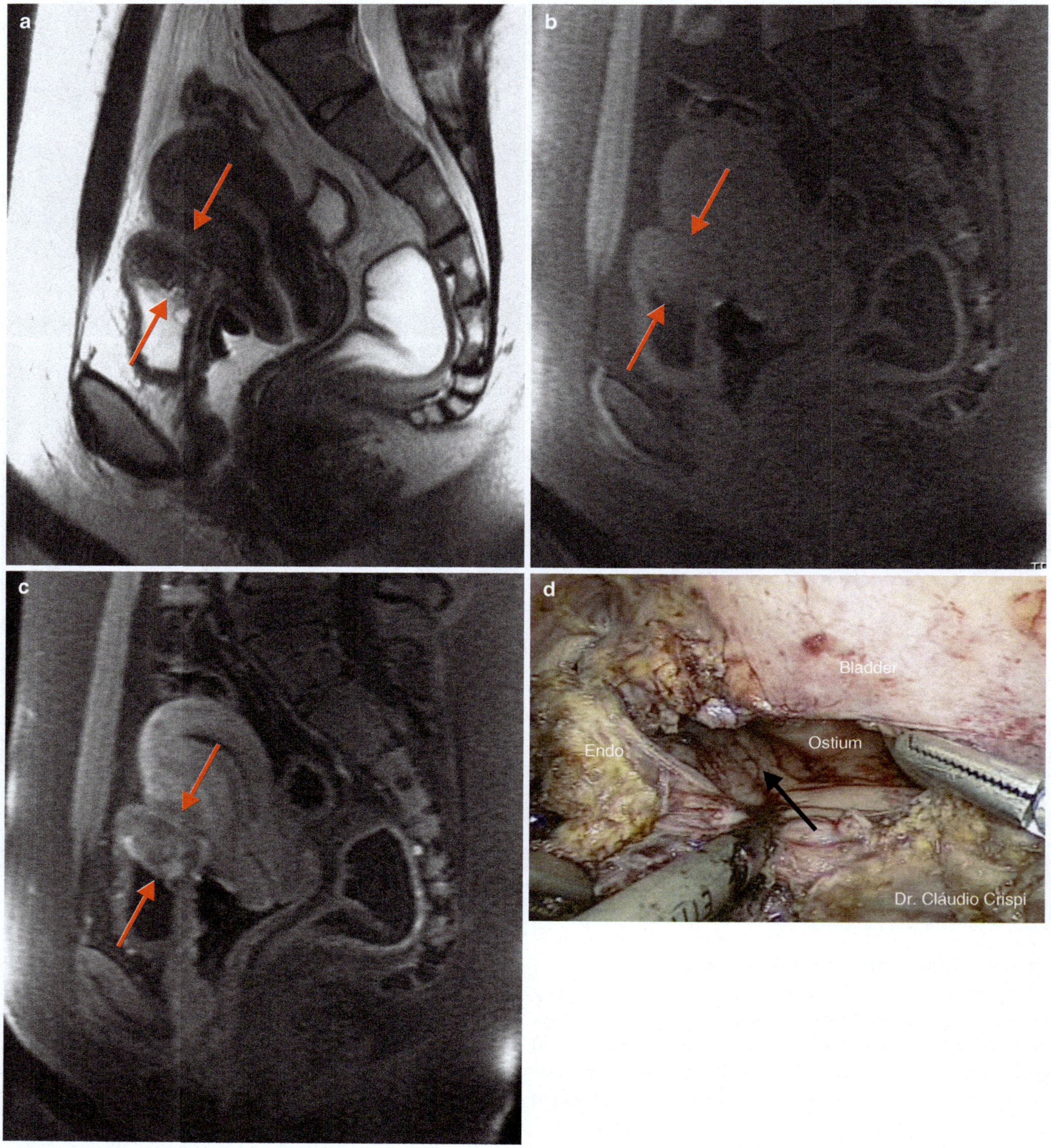

Fig. 4.23 Bladder lesion in the posterior, median wall. Notice penetration into the muscle. Note that the swollen mucosa is emphasized by the contrast medium continuously (**c**). (**a**) T2-weighted sequence. (**b**, **c**) T1 weighted with fat suppression. (**c**) With intravenous gadolinium. (**a**–**c**) Sagittal. (**d**) Beginning of partial cystectomy. We can observe the nodule compromising the region of the trine and the left ureteral ostium

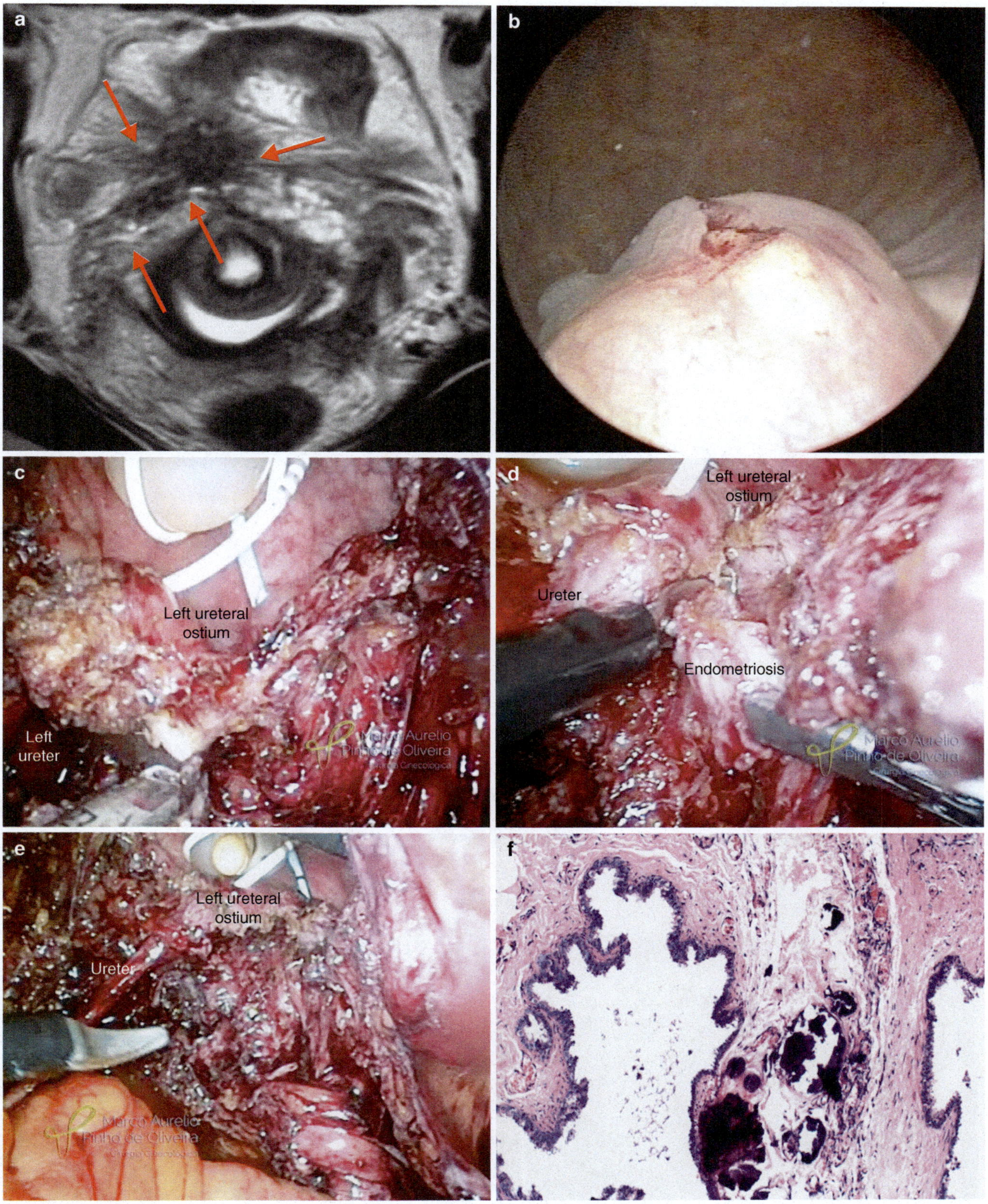

Fig. 4.24 (**a**) Lesion extension to the ureteral orifice and distal ureter right. (**a**) T2-weighted sequence. Axial. (**b**) Cystoscopy. Compromised. (**ce**) Laparoscopy. (**f**) Pathology demonstrating endometriotic implant with ciliated glands, in addition to foci of calcification

4.1.1.6 Ureter Anatomy

The ureter is an important anatomic reference point, especially for deep endometriosis surgery.

The ureter has a caudal course through the retroperitoneum from the kidney junction in the abdomen to the posterior bladder wall. The pelvic ureter can be segmented for didactic purpose in vertical and horizontal segments.

Initially the pelvic course is vertical, after crossing the iliac vessels, following the lateral wall with posterior and inferior direction, between the parietal peritoneum and the internal iliac artery. In this segment, it is related to the ovary, bordering the posterior surface of the ovarian fossa, and laterally to the uterosacral ligament.

At the level of the ischial spine, the trajectory changes to oblique horizontal, with forward and medial direction, crossing the broad ligament and the uterine artery, bordering laterally the uterine cervix and the fornix of the vagina, toward the posterior bladder base. The lateral nerve fibers originating at the inferior hypogastric plexus run beneath the ureter, before reaching the trigone of the bladder (Fig. 4.25) [17, 18].

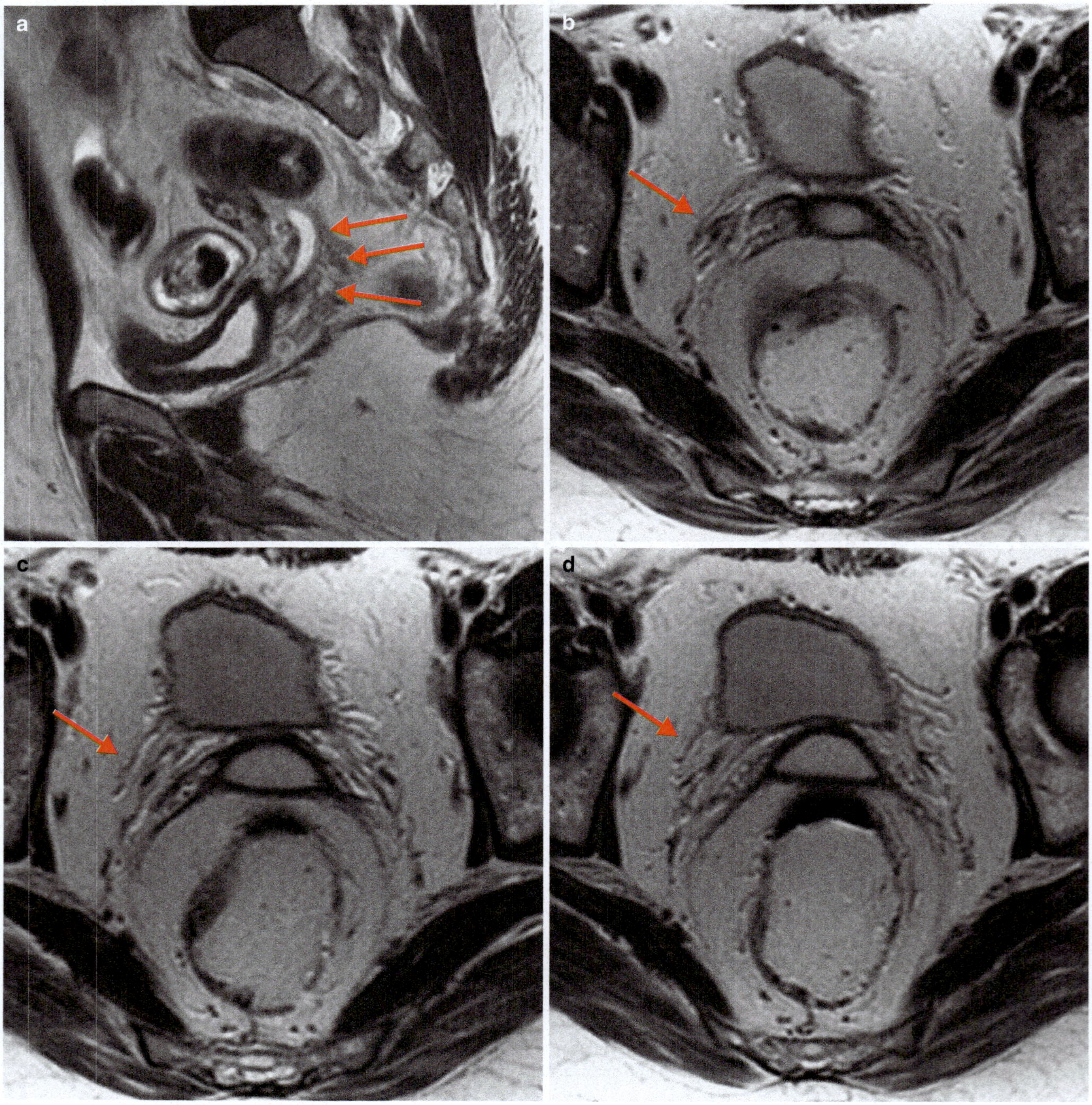

Fig. 4.25 (**a**–**e**) Ureter anatomy. T2-weighted sequences. Case 1: (**a**) sagittal plane. Identify trajectory change to horizontal oblique, anterior direction, crossing inferiorly the uterine artery, near the cervix, marking the vaginal fornix up to the posterosuperior vesical angle. Ureter lesion, with dilation (arrows). Case 2: axial plane, (**b**–**e**) identify anterior and medial trajectory change, crossing near the cervix, marking the vaginal fornix, to the ureteral ostium (arrows). (**f**) Laparoscopy demonstrating the location of the ureter (arrow)

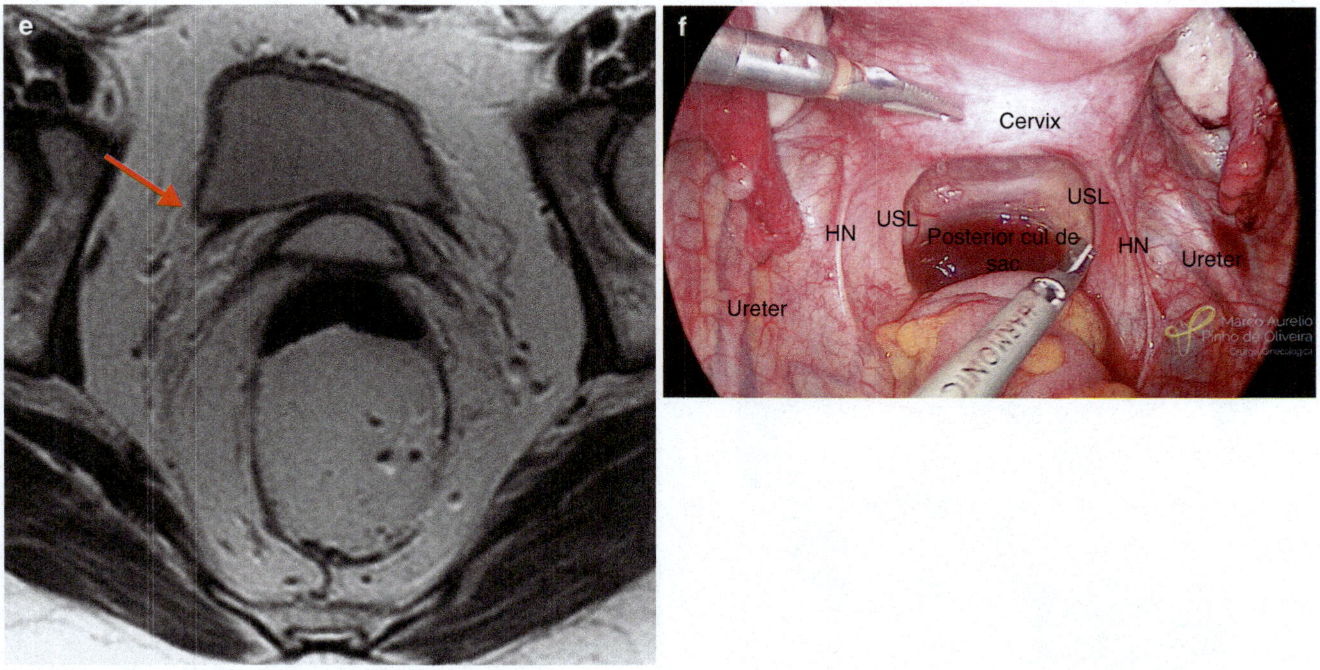

Fig. 4.25 (continued)

4.1.1.7 Common Aspects of Ureteral Endometriosis

Ureteral endometriosis is a serious condition which can lead to a silent renal loss function. The ureter is the second most common location in the urinary tract, with an increasing incidence due to improvements in diagnostic methods, as well as awareness and skill among physicians to recognize this type of lesion [13].

Endometriosis most commonly involves the pelvic ureter 3–4 cm above the ureterovesical junction and usually by lateral extension of a posterior compartment nodule. The involvement is unilateral in 80–90% of patients, with a slightly higher proportion on the left side. Some lesions may not lead to stenosis (Fig. 4.26) [19, 20].

Ureteral involvement may be extrinsic or intrinsic, depending on the histological degree of wall infiltration by the endometriosis. The ureteral wall is composed of three distinct layers: the mucosa, muscularis, and adventitia. The extrinsic form is the most common, accounting for 80% of cases, and is characterized by the involvement of the adventitia or the surrounding ureter connective tissue, without histological evidence of endometric gland or stroma in the ureter wall. The intrinsic disease infiltrates the muscularis propria or even the mucosa. Preoperatively, differentiation can be difficult. However, there are some clues in MRI, with thickening and parietal irregularity suggesting intrinsic involvement. Furthermore, both forms can cause luminal narrowing, ureteral dilation, and hydronephrosis [13, 18, 21, 22].

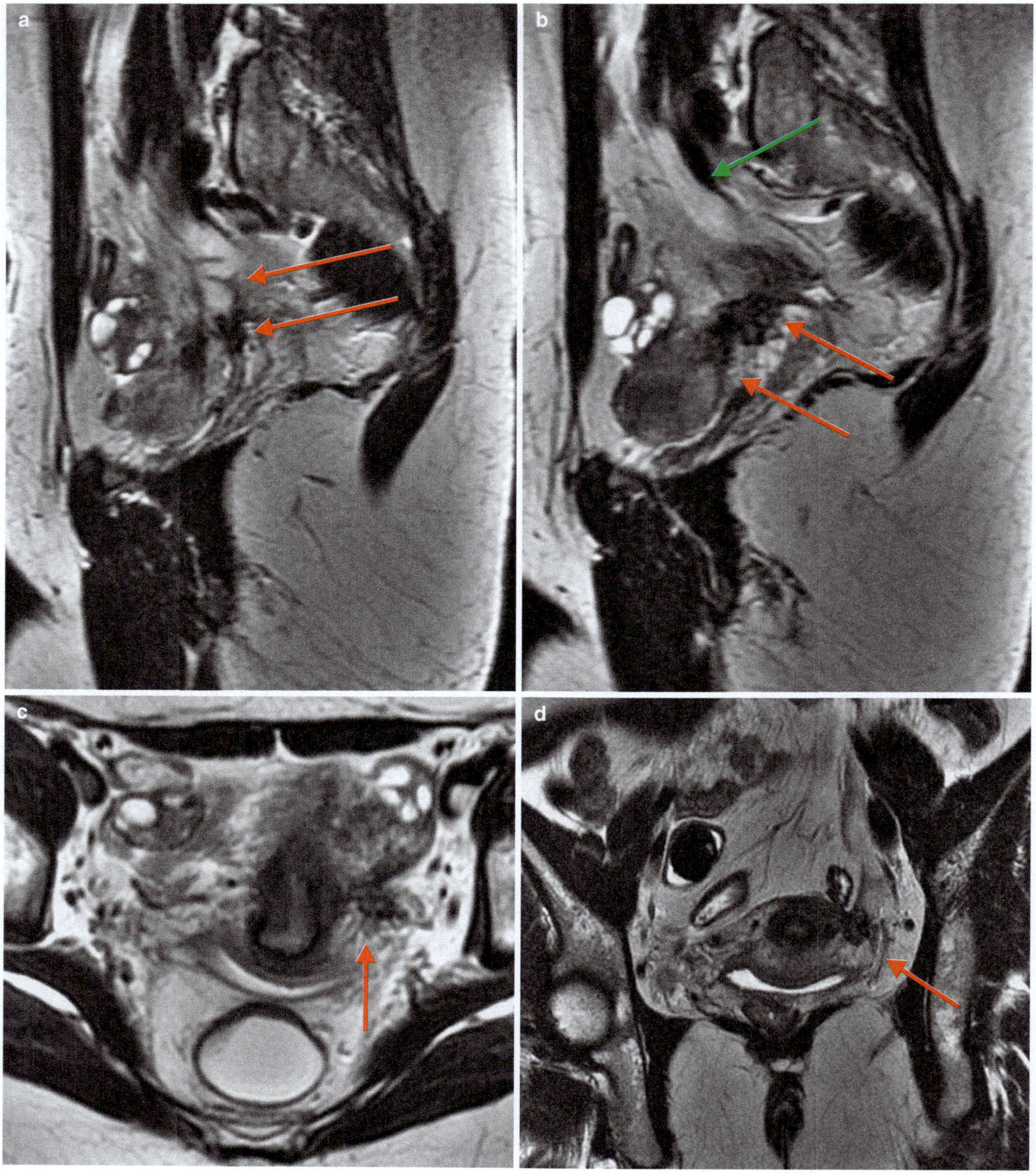

Fig. 4.26 Lesion left parametrial (red arrow), compromising the distal ureter to 3 cm above the ureterovesical junction, causing expansion (green arrow). T2-weighted sequences. (**a**, **b**). (**c**) Axial. (**d**) Coronal. (**e**) Laparoscopy. (**f**) Microscopy of the lesion (100×). Parametrium with endometriotic focus and connective tissues and peripheral nervous

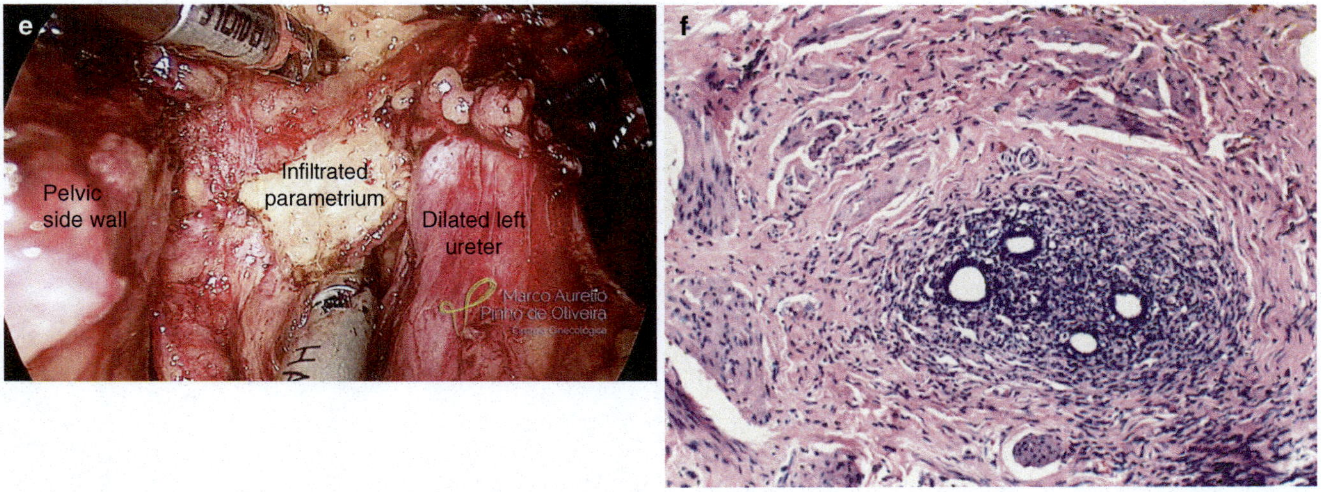

Fig. 4.26 (continued)

4.1.1.8 Clinical Manifestations

As mentioned previously, in most cases ureteral involvement is asymptomatic and consequently can lead to a silent loss of renal function. Early detection with imaging is crucial as it allows kidney preservation.

4.1.1.9 MRI and Laparoscopic Findings

Knowledge of the anatomy and high spatial MRI resolution are fundamental for presurgical identification of the ureteral endometriosis.

It is possible to identify the pelvic ureter without contrast or a urographic study in MRI. We suggest the use of T2-weighted high-resolution images, with long coronal axis and short-axis imaging planes, as well as the use of these anatomical markers: the uterine artery, parametria, uterosacral ligament, and posterior base of the bladder. In the short-axis plane, start the search at the bladder posterior base. Following posteriorly, after the identification of the trigone, identify the ureter. The course follows posteriorly in the upper parametria crossing the uterine artery, running laterally along the uterosacral ligament, and superiorly along the posterior surface of the ovary fossa, reaching the intersection with iliac vessels in the pelvic infundibulum (Fig. 4.27).

Ureteral endometriosis lesions may present a variable signal intensity; however, the most common aspect is related to tissue fibrosis predominance, with a hypointense signal in the T2-weighted and an isointense signal in the T1-weighted sequences, with rare bleeding spots.

Ureteral involvement may occur along its course and can be related to some types of lesions:

1. **The uterosacral ligament with lateral parametrial extension**
   The lesion infiltrates the ureter wall or the surrounding tissue in its horizontal oblique course, between the parametrium and the obturator fossa. It can present as a thickened ligament, irregular and retracted, adhered to the adjacent structures, or as an irregular nodule. It can be small in size in some cases requiring secondary ureter dilation to facilitate lesion identification (Figs. 4.28 and 4.29).
2. **The rectovaginal septum with parametrial extension**
   The vast majority are larger median posterior nodules, with a unilateral or bilateral extension to the parametrium with periureteral involvement, infiltrating both the uterine artery and the ureter (Fig. 4.30).
3. **The vesical-ureteral junction involvement**
   Endometriosis mainly involves the dome and the upper posterior surface of the bladder. Vesical-ureteral junction involvement is unusual. The distance between the lesion and the ureter should be mentioned in the radiology report.
   On some occasions, it may extend to the distal ureter or to the ureteral ostium and can impact the surgical approach (Fig. 4.31). When there is extensive ostium involvement, ureteral reimplantation may be necessary (Figs. 4.18 and 4.24) [9].
4. **The ovarian fossa (compressive effect of endometrioma or deep involvement)**
   Infiltrative lesions in the ovarian fossa usually involve both the sigmoid and the ureter. A careful analysis should be made, since intestinal involvement can be more prominent than the ureteral one (Fig. 4.32).
   Large endometriomas (>5 cm) can mechanically compress the ureter at the horizontal posterior course at the ovarian fossa. Also, inflammatory process can affect the ovarian fossa and extend to the ureter (Table 4.3 and Fig. 4.33).

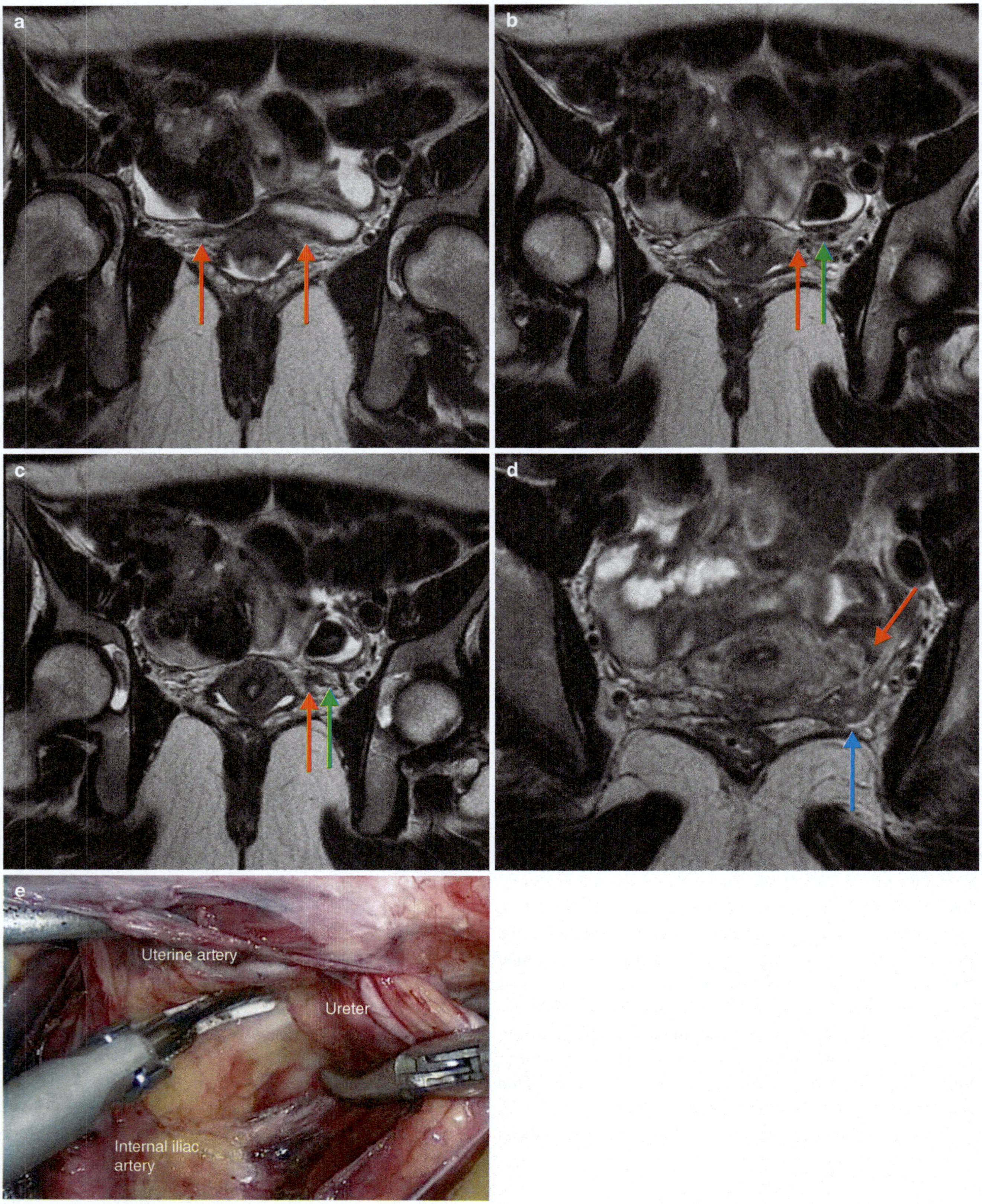

Fig. 4.27 Identifies up the ureter at the posterior base of the bladder (red arrows in **a**), after the identification of the trigone. From there, the pathway follows (red arrows), through the superior portion of the parametrium, where it crosses the uterine artery (green arrows in **b**, **c**), near the uterosacral ligament, accompanying the posterosuperior surface of the appendages (blue arrow on the ovary in **d**) to the junction with iliac vessels in the pelvic infundibulum. (**a–d**) T2-weighted sequences. Coronal. (**e**) Laparoscopy. Identification of the uterine artery at the junction over the ureter

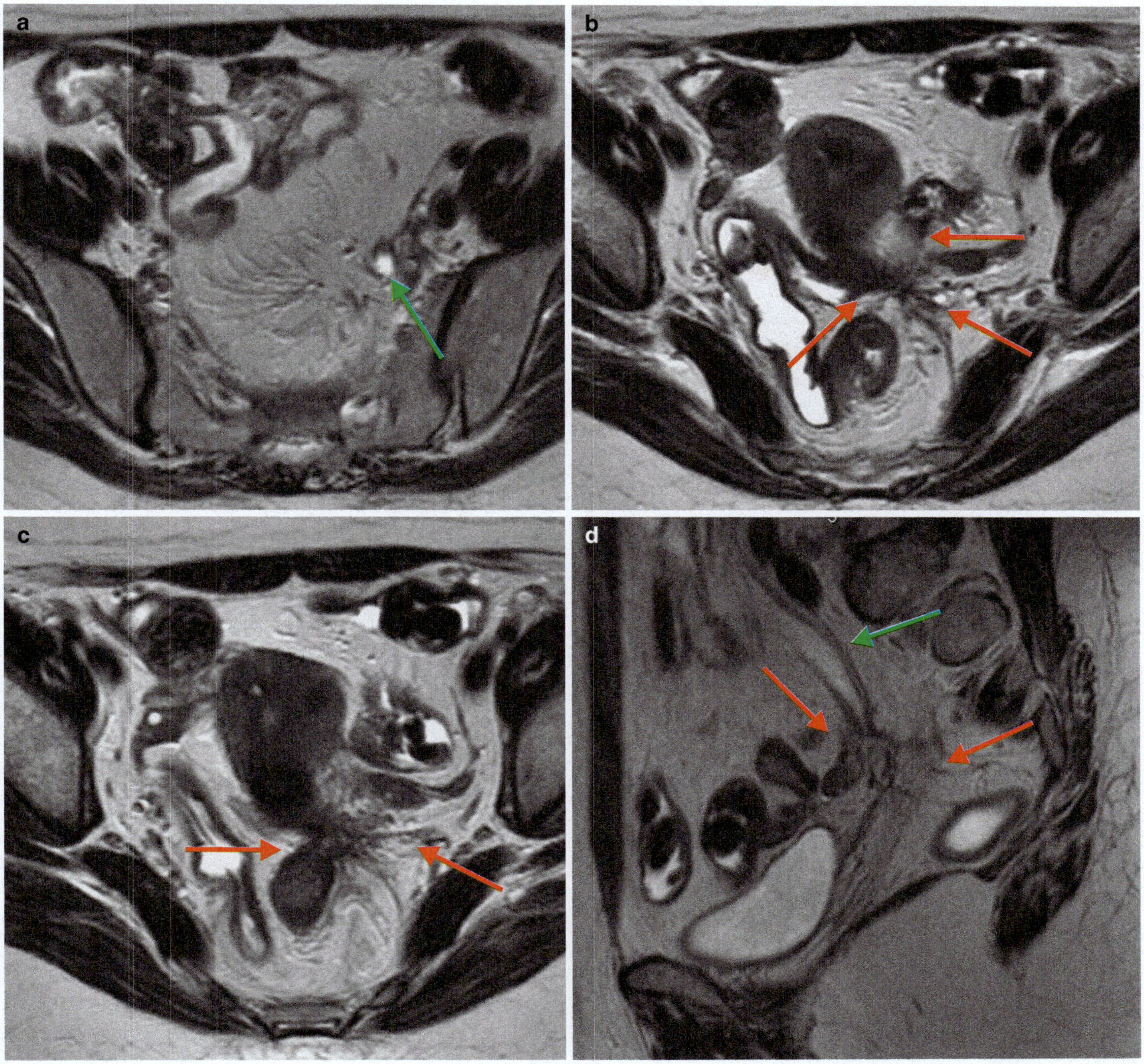

Fig. 4.28 Lesion in posterolateral compartment, centered on the left uterosacral ligament with parametrial extension (arrows **bg**). Note ligamentous, irregular, and retractile thickening, adhered to the rectum, redundant sigmoid, and attachment, infiltrating the parametrium, uterine artery, and ureter (green arrow in **e**, **k**), promoting medial deviation (**k**), dilation, and chronic obstructive nephropathy (**j**). (**ai**) T2-weighted sequences. (**ac**). (**df**) Sagittal. (**gi**). (**j**, **k**) MR Urography. (**j**) MIP reconstruction with gadolinium. (**k**) Axial. (**l**, **m**) Laparoscopy. (**l**) Beginning of the resection of the parametrium. (**m**) End of procedure

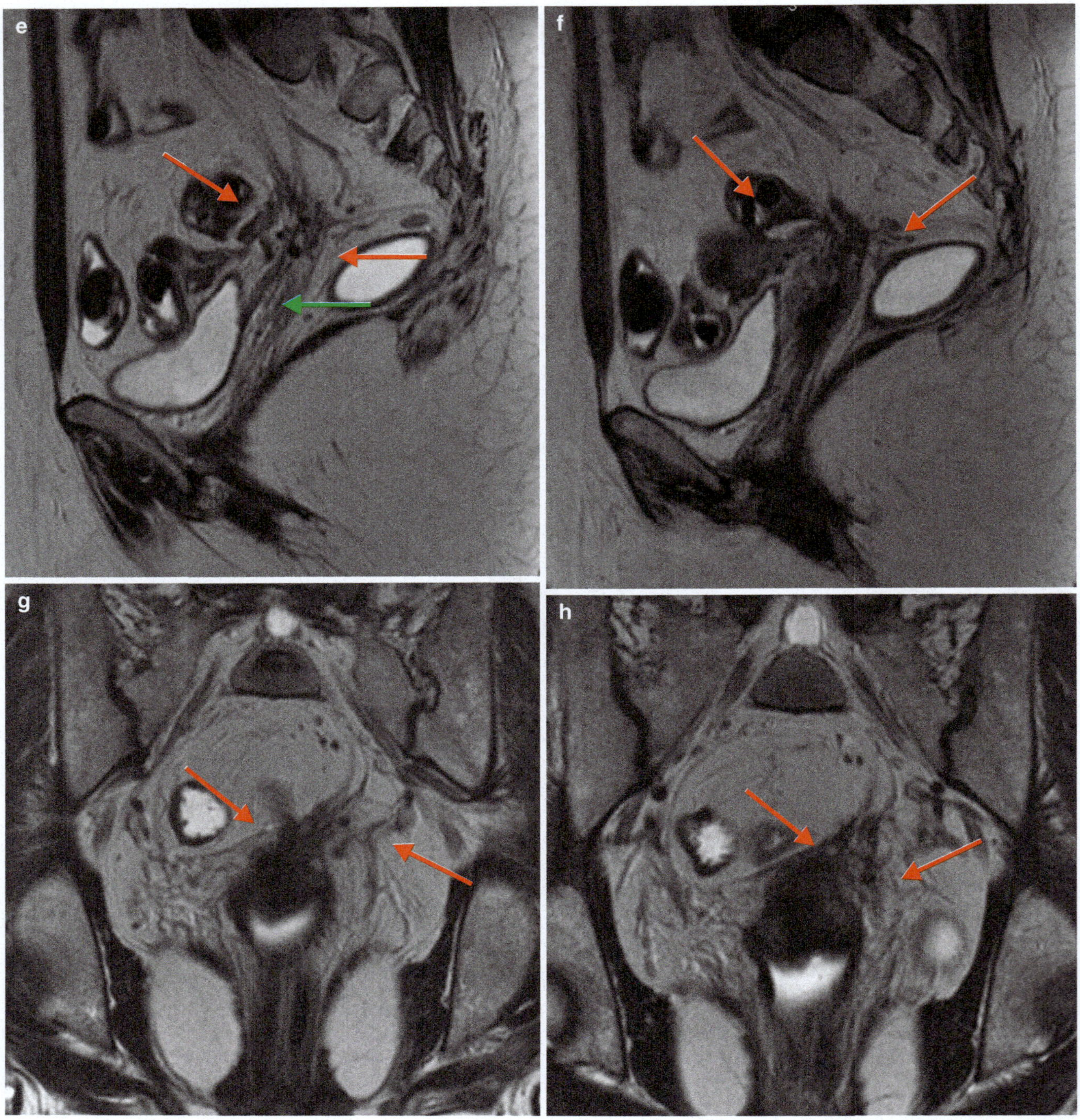

Fig. 4.28 (continued)

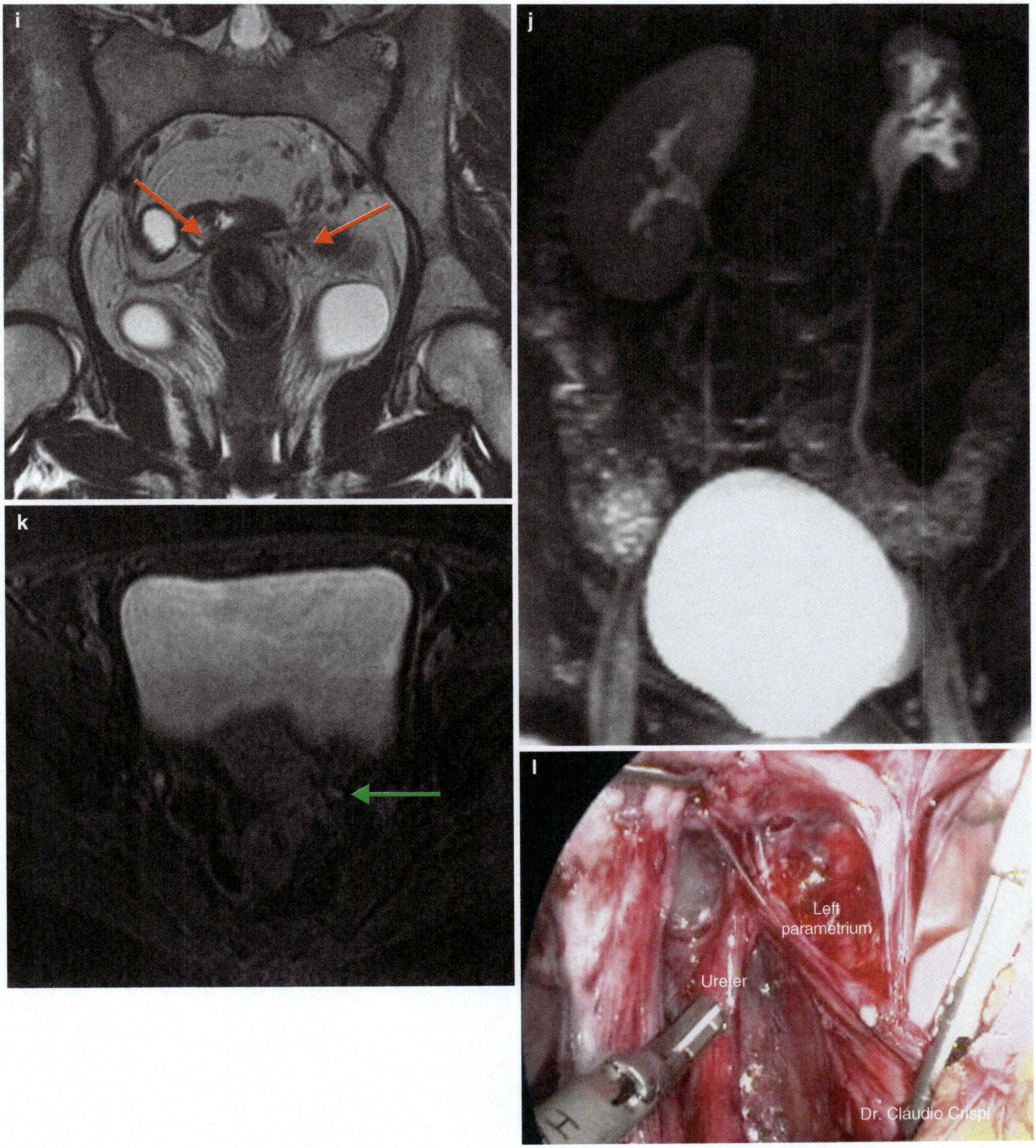

Fig. 4.28 (continued)

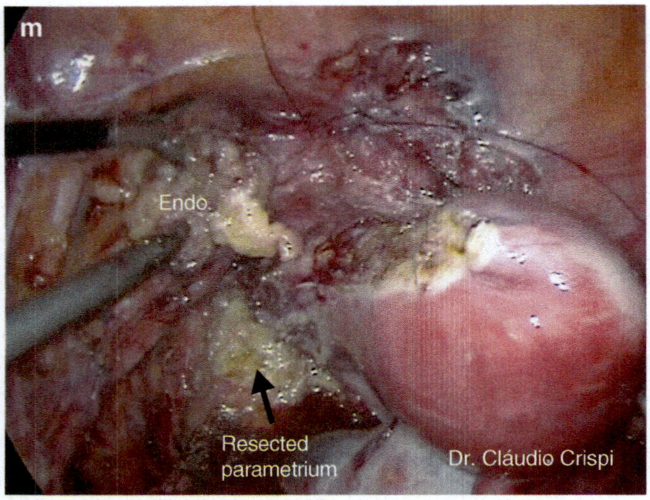

Fig. 4.28 (continued)

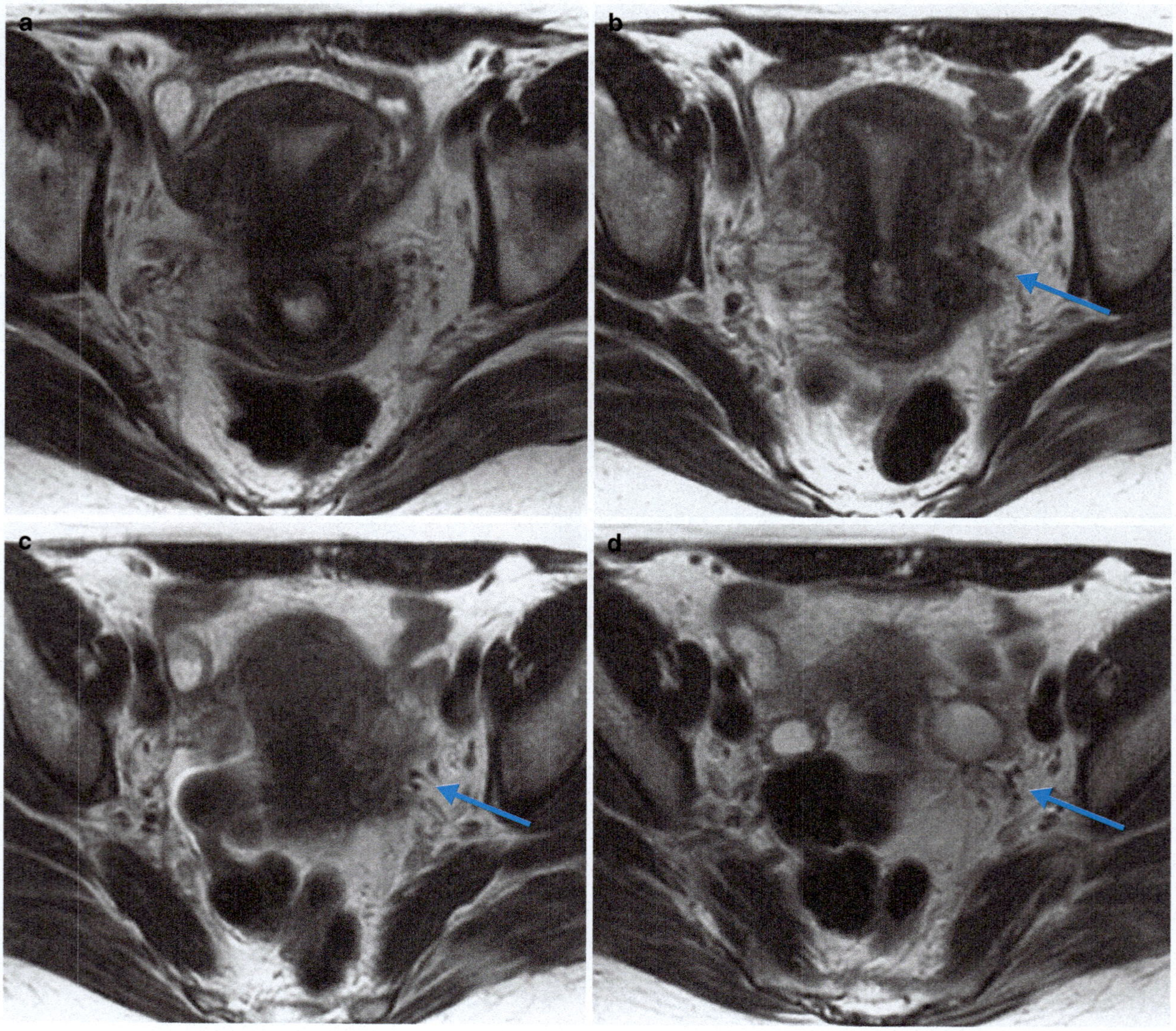

Fig. 4.29 Left parametrial nodule (blue arrows) irregular, causing stenosis of the ureter (red arrows—non-contrast-enhanced magnetic resonance urography) [**fk**]), in addition to involving the broad ligament (**b**, **e**) and ovarian fossa (**d**, **e**). (**ae**) T2-weighted sequences. (**ae**) Axial. (**fj**) Uro-resonance. Axial. (**k**, **l**) Laparoscopy. (**k**) Start of identification of the distal portion of the ureter after the stenosis area. Note dilated ureter. (**l**) Approximation of the proximal and distal stumps of the left ureter

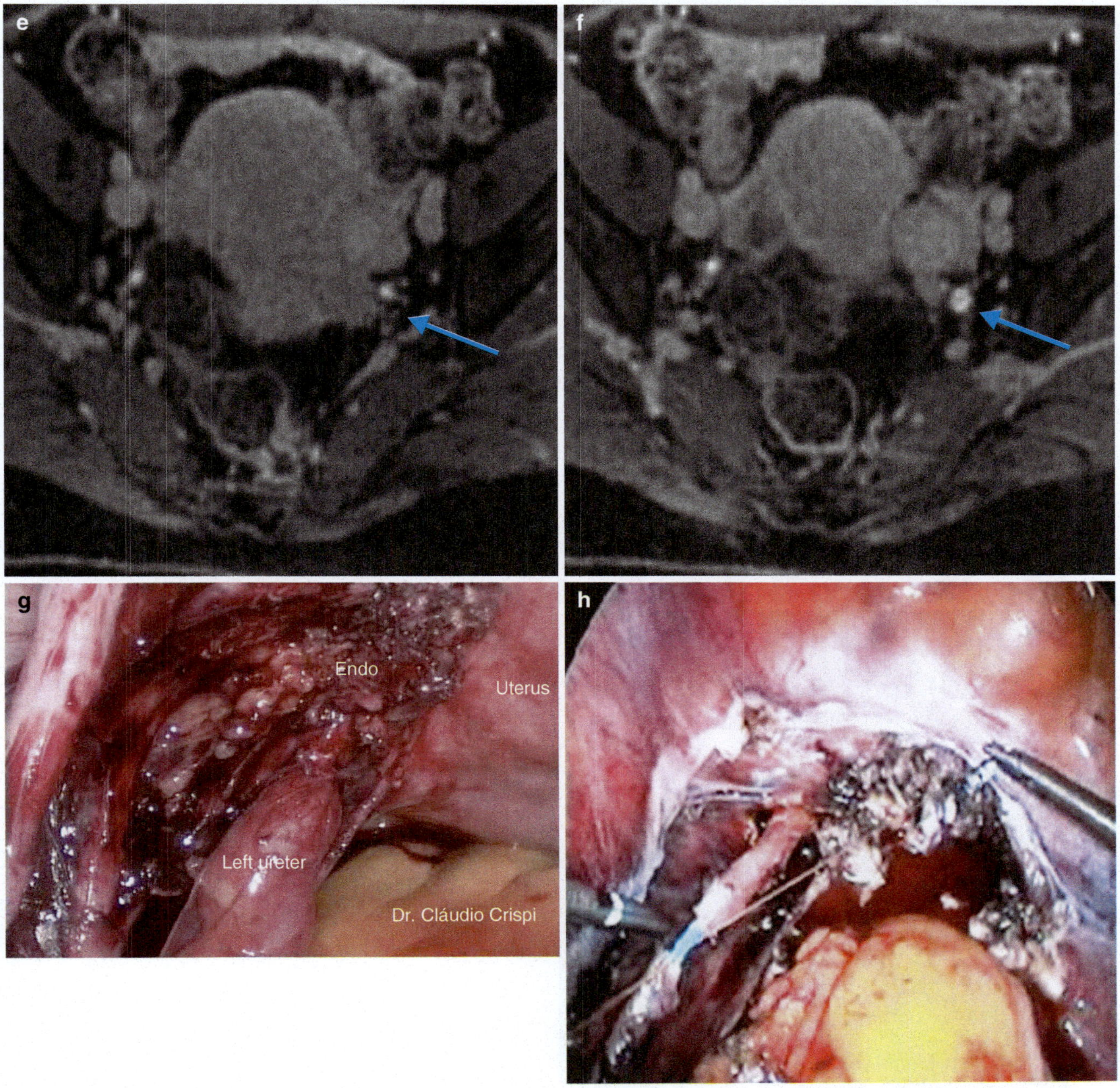

Fig. 4.29 (continued)

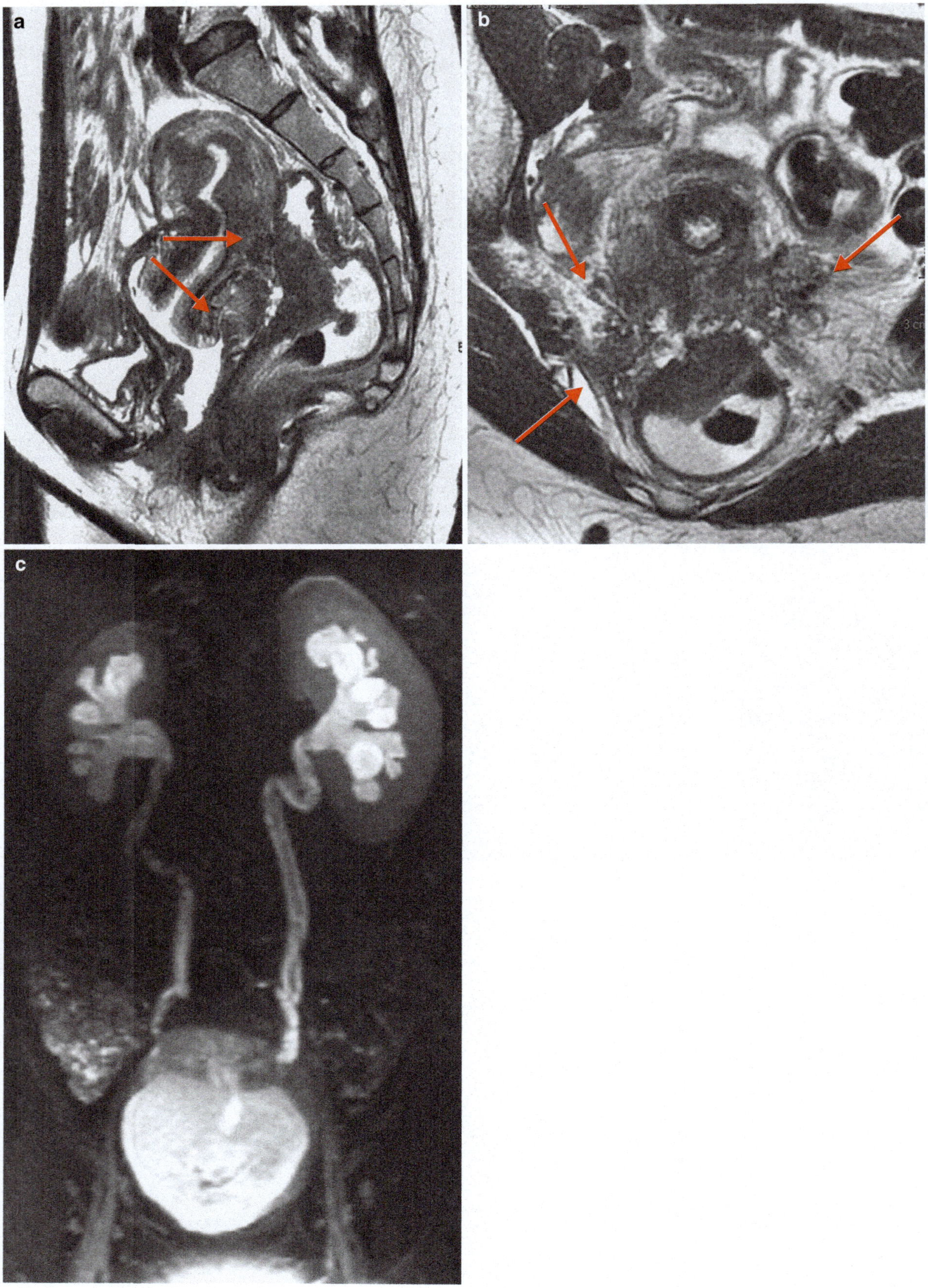

Fig. 4.30 Large node of the posterior compartment, retrocervical and rectovaginal septum (arrow **a**), with bilateral parametrial extension, infiltrating the uterine arteries and ureters (arrows **b**), promoting bilateral hydronephrosis, mostly on the left (**c**). Note also extensive ligament infiltration, greater on the right, in addition to intestinal. (**a**, **b**) T2-weighted sequences. (**a**) Sagittal. (**b**) Axial. (**c**) MR urography (MIP with gadolinium)

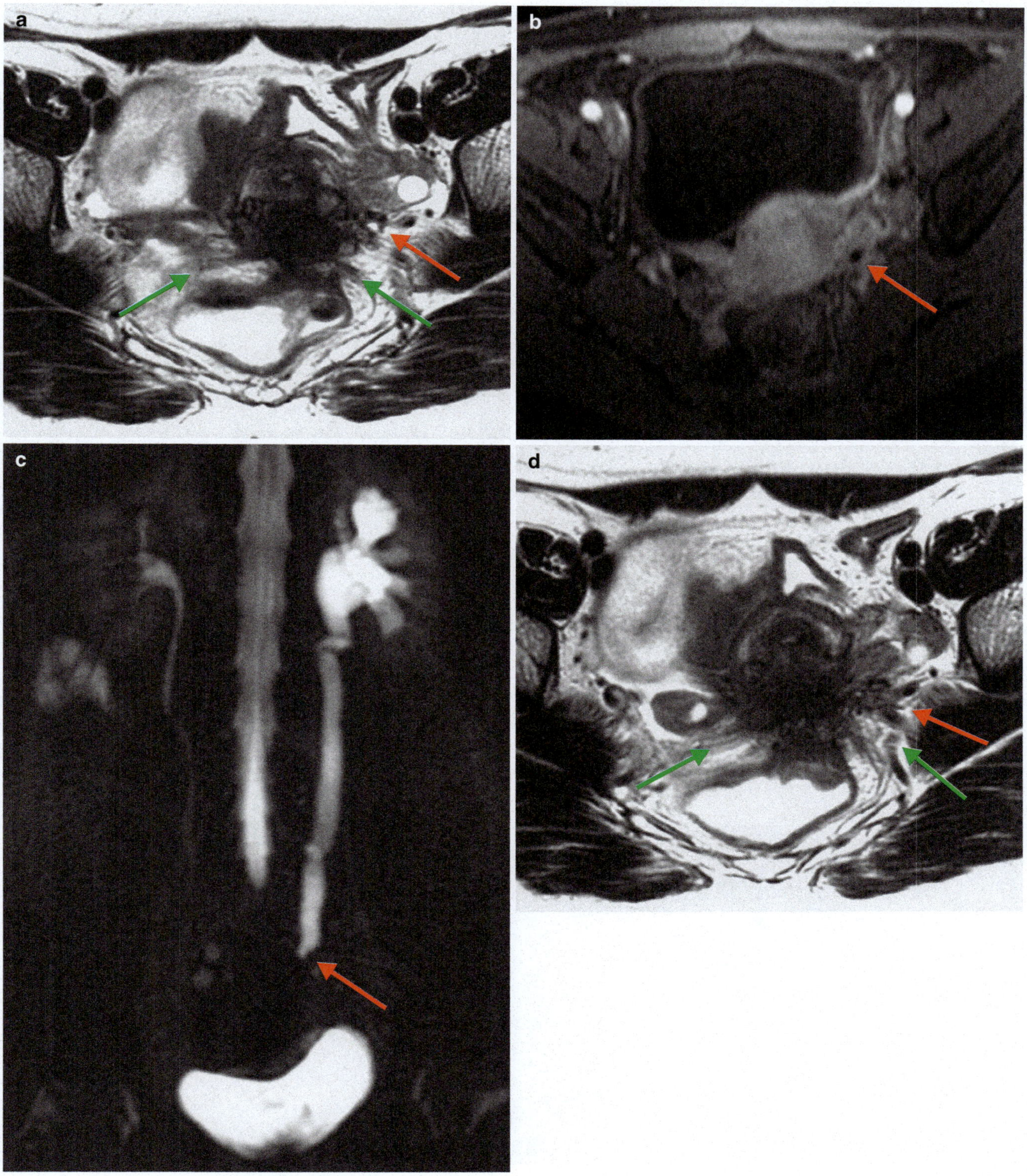

Fig. 4.31 Dilation of the left ureter. Extensive retrocervical lesion (green arrows in **a**, **b**, **d**) with bilateral parametrial extension, involving the distal portion of the urethus close to the ostium (red arrow in **a**, **c**, **e**, **f**). (**a**, **d**) T2-weighted sequences. Axial. MR urography images. (**b**, **e**). (**c**) T2 Projection. (**f**) MIP with gadolinium. (**gi**) Laparoscopy. (**g**) Enlarged left ureter, fully exposed (blue arrow). The beginning of the stenosis area is observed. (**h**) Beginning of the incision of the visceral peritoneum. Very dilated left ureter (blue arrow). (**i**) Isolated uterine artery (blue arrow)

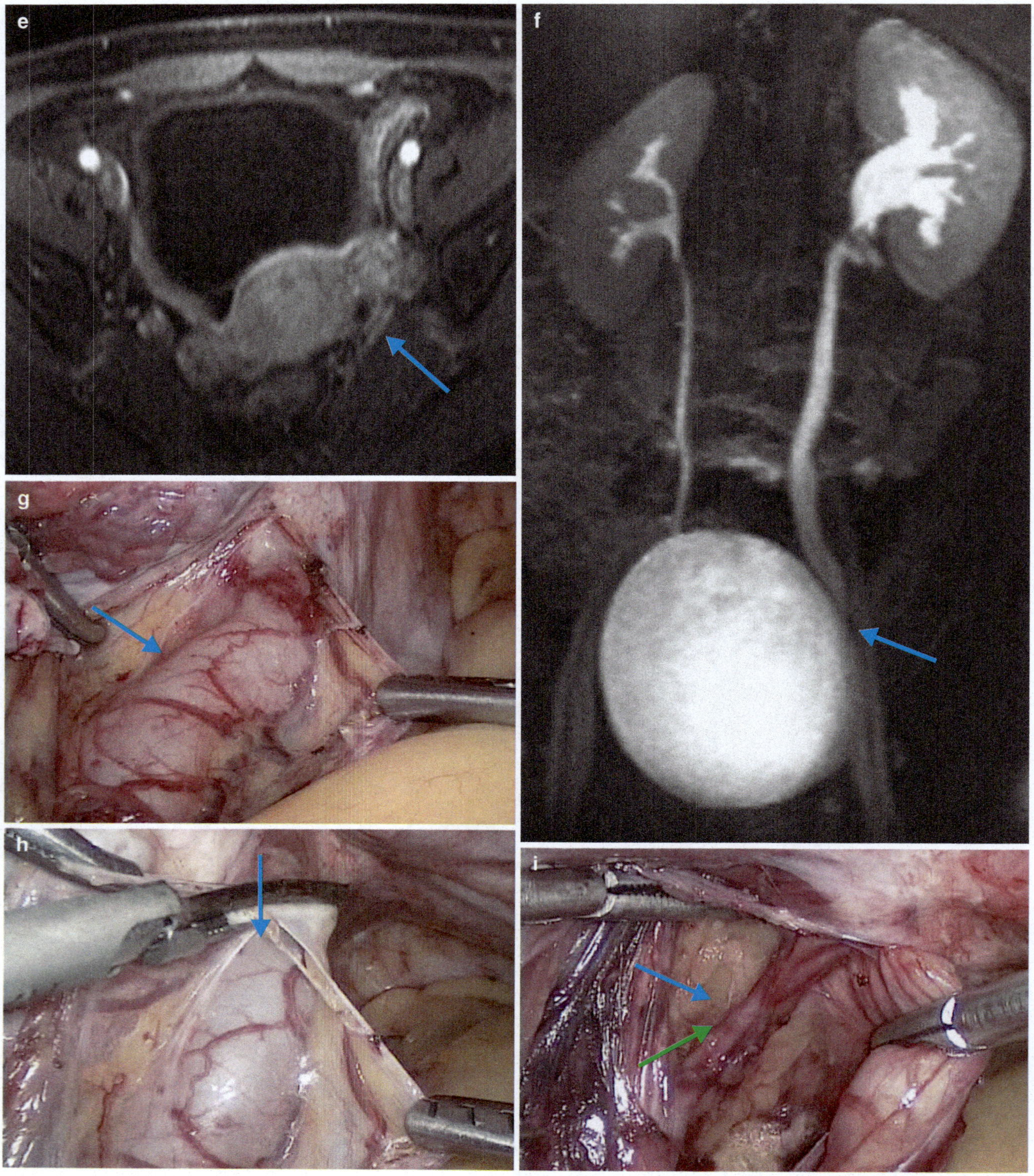

Fig. 4.31 (continued)

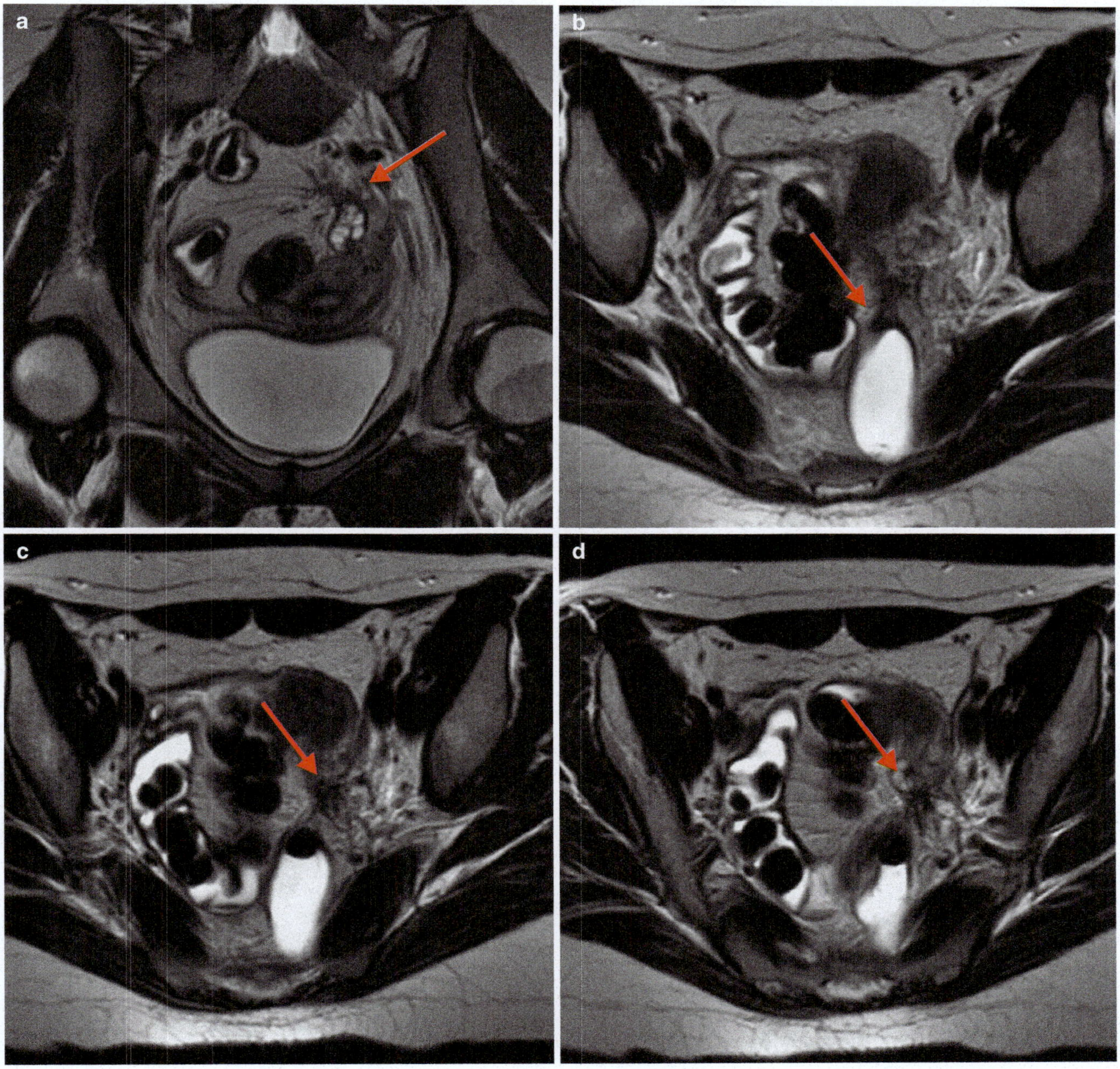

Fig. 4.32 Infiltrative lesion in the left ovarian fossa, although small, causes ureteral obstruction (arrows in **a**–**e**). (**a**–**e**) T2-weighted sequences. (**a**) Coronal plane. (**b**–**e**) Axial. (**f**, **g**) Laparoscopy. (**f**) Detail of the fibrotic ring surrounding the ureter (arrow). (**g**) Identification of the area of the clamping of the fibrotic ring (arrow)

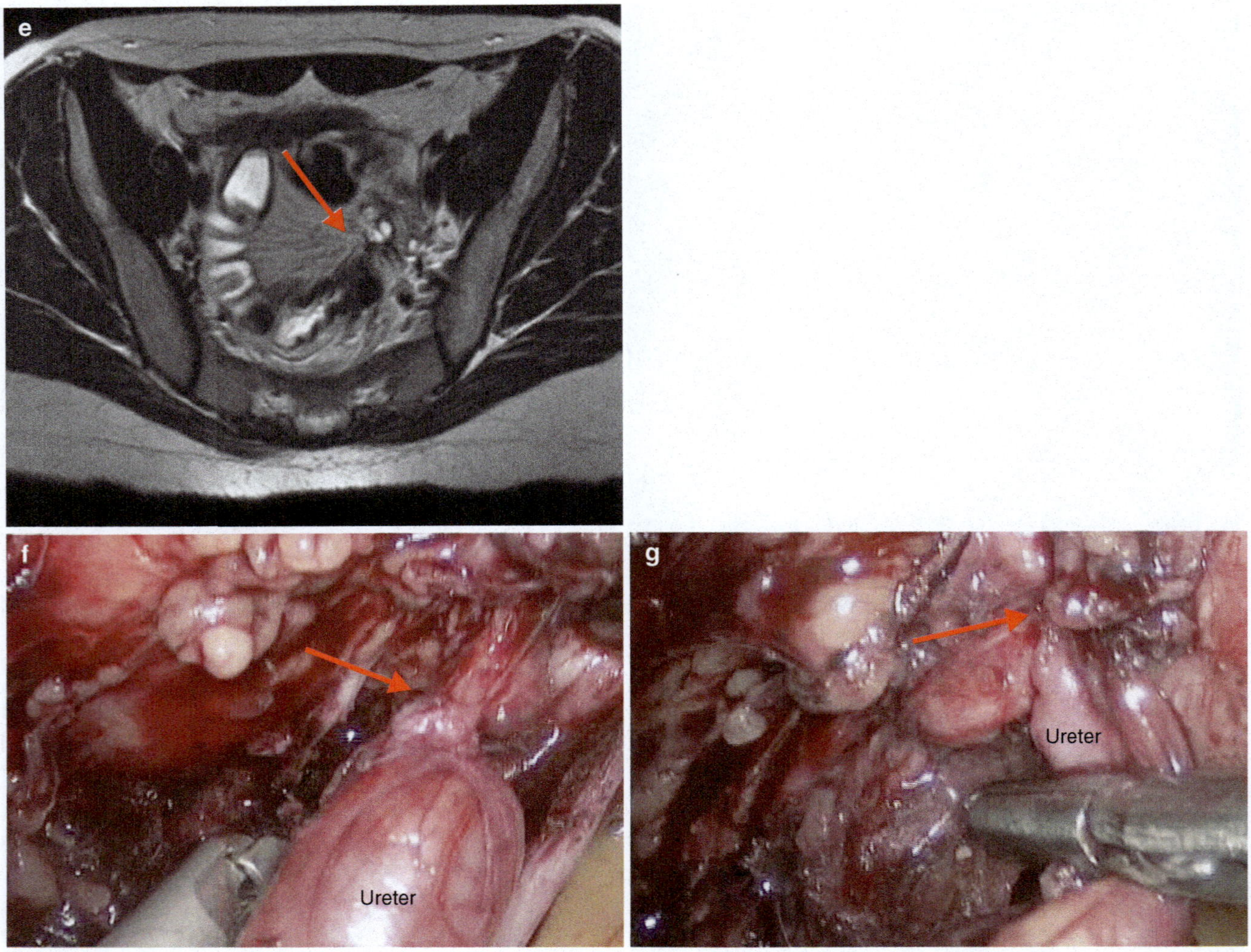

Fig. 4.32 (continued)

Table 4.3 Deep endometriosis ureteral involvement

A posterior and lateral compartment lesion, based on the uterosacral ligament with parametrial extension
A large posterior compartment nodule, retrocervical or rectovaginal septum with parametrial extension
An anterior compartment lesion infiltrating the ureterovesical junction
An infiltrative ovarian fossa lesion
Endometrioma compressive effect

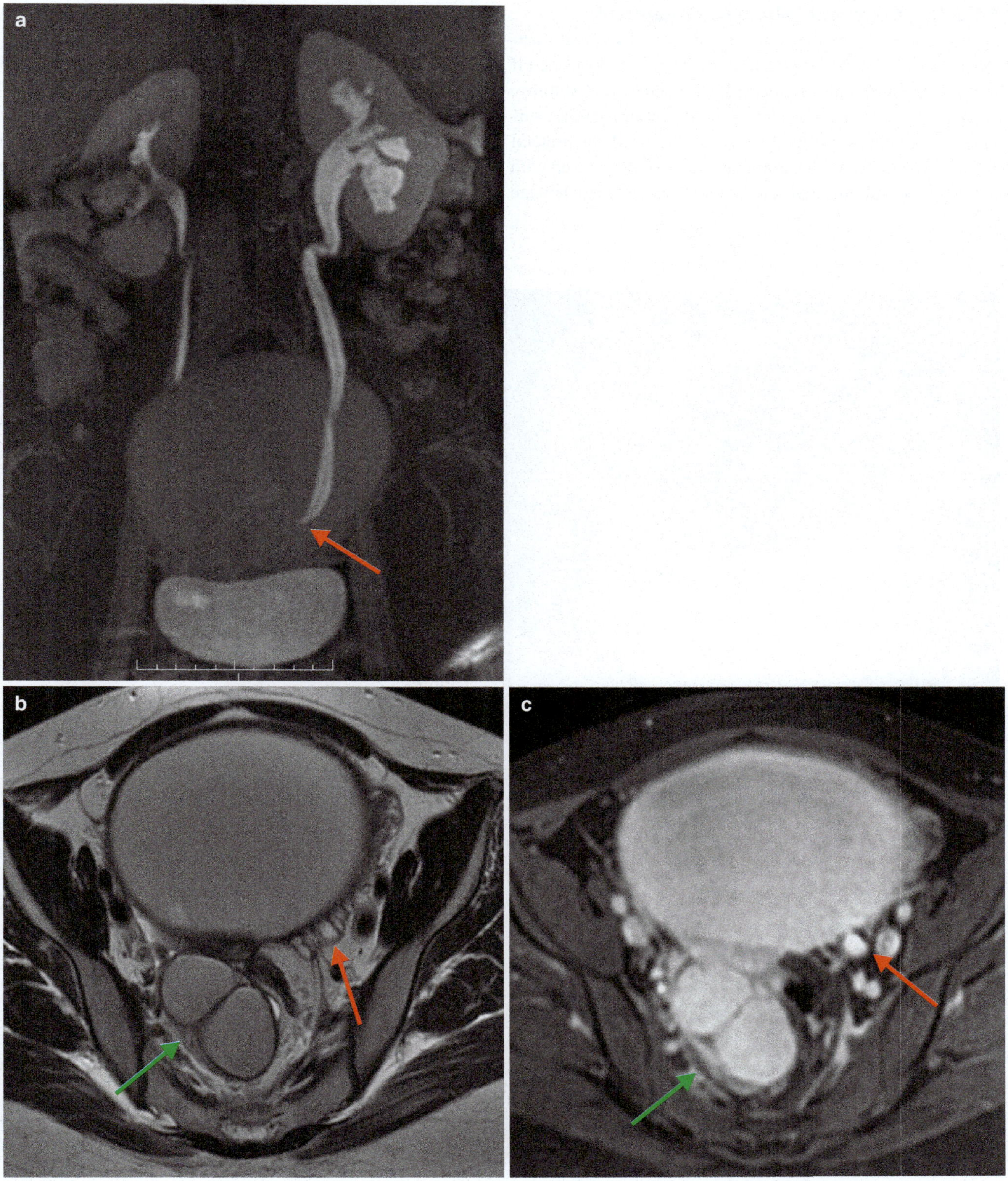

Fig. 4.33 Large endometrioma to the left (hyperintense cyst in T1 and hypointense in T2), causing ureteral compression, with hydronephrosis (red arrows in **a**–**c**). (**a**, **c**) T1-weighted sequences with fat and gadolinium suppression. (**a**) MR Urography with MIP. Note endometrioma in the right ovary, smaller (green arrow in **b**, **c**). (**b**) T2-weighted sequence. (**b**, **c**) Axial

4.1.1.10 Comments About the Treatment

Extrinsic ureteral involvement should prompt surgical treatment via ureterolysis. Segmental resection may be needed if intrinsic involvement is suspected, with ureteroureterotomy.

When the lesion extends to the ureter ostium, careful surgical evaluation is required to assess the need for ureteral reimplantation. Reimplantation may lead to reflux, even with the correct technique, and can lead to further kidney damage (Figs. 4.18 and 4.24). When there is extensive involvement of the ureteral ostium, resection of the lesion with the ureterocystostomy (reimplantation) should be performed (Fig. 4.34) [9].

From the authors' experience, there may be a discrepancy between the longitudinal extent of the ureteral lesion observed during laparoscopy and that identified by MRI. The longitudinal extent identified by MRI may be shorter.

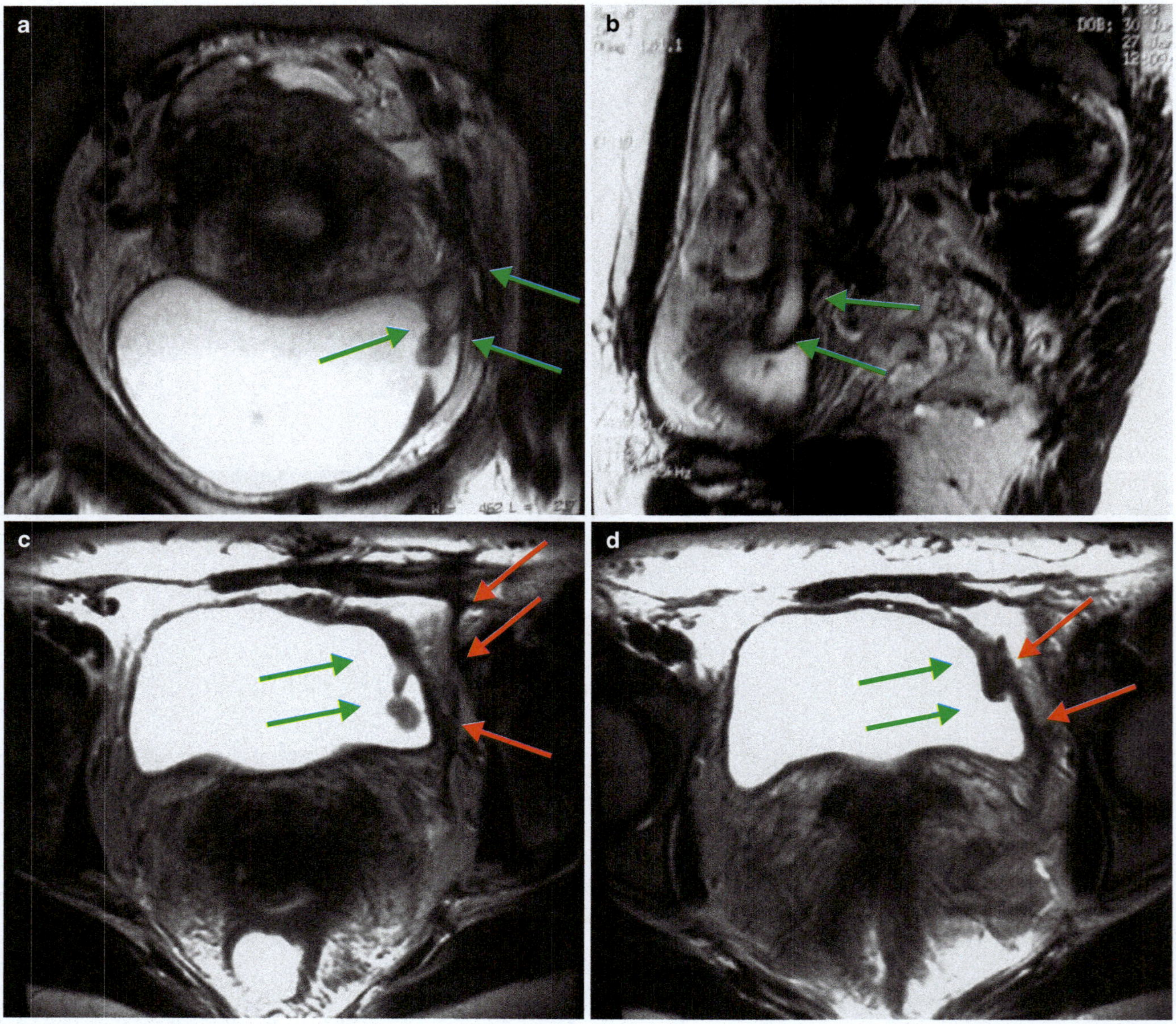

Fig. 4.34 View of ureterocystostomy after resection of the lesion affecting the left ureteral ostium. Note unusual positioning of the ureter on the lateral wall of the bladder (green arrows in **a**–**c**) and fibrocicatricial tissue on the perivesical fat (red arrows in **c**, **d**). (**a**–**d**) T2-weighted sequences. (**a**) Coronal. (**b**) Sagittal. (**c**, **d**) Axial

4.1.2 Round Ligament

4.1.2.1 Anatomy

The round ligament is a fibromuscular tissue originating in the gubernaculum, a cord embryo structure extending from the gonad, fixing them to the labioscrotal swellings. It measures 10–12 cm in length and consists of two portions, the intraperitoneal and the extraperitoneal.

The intraperitoneal portion starts at the anterior and lateral uterus surface, near the origin of the Fallopian tubes, and runs anteriorly through the broad ligament, above the iliac vessels, and exits the abdominal cavity by passing into the internal inguinal ring (Fig. 4.35).The extraperitoneal portion passes through the inguinal canal, adjacent to the canal of Nuck, and ends in the labium majus (Fig. 4.36) [9].

For didactic purposes, the female pelvis can be divided by the round and broad ligaments into anterior and posterior compartments, as mentioned in Sect. 4.1.

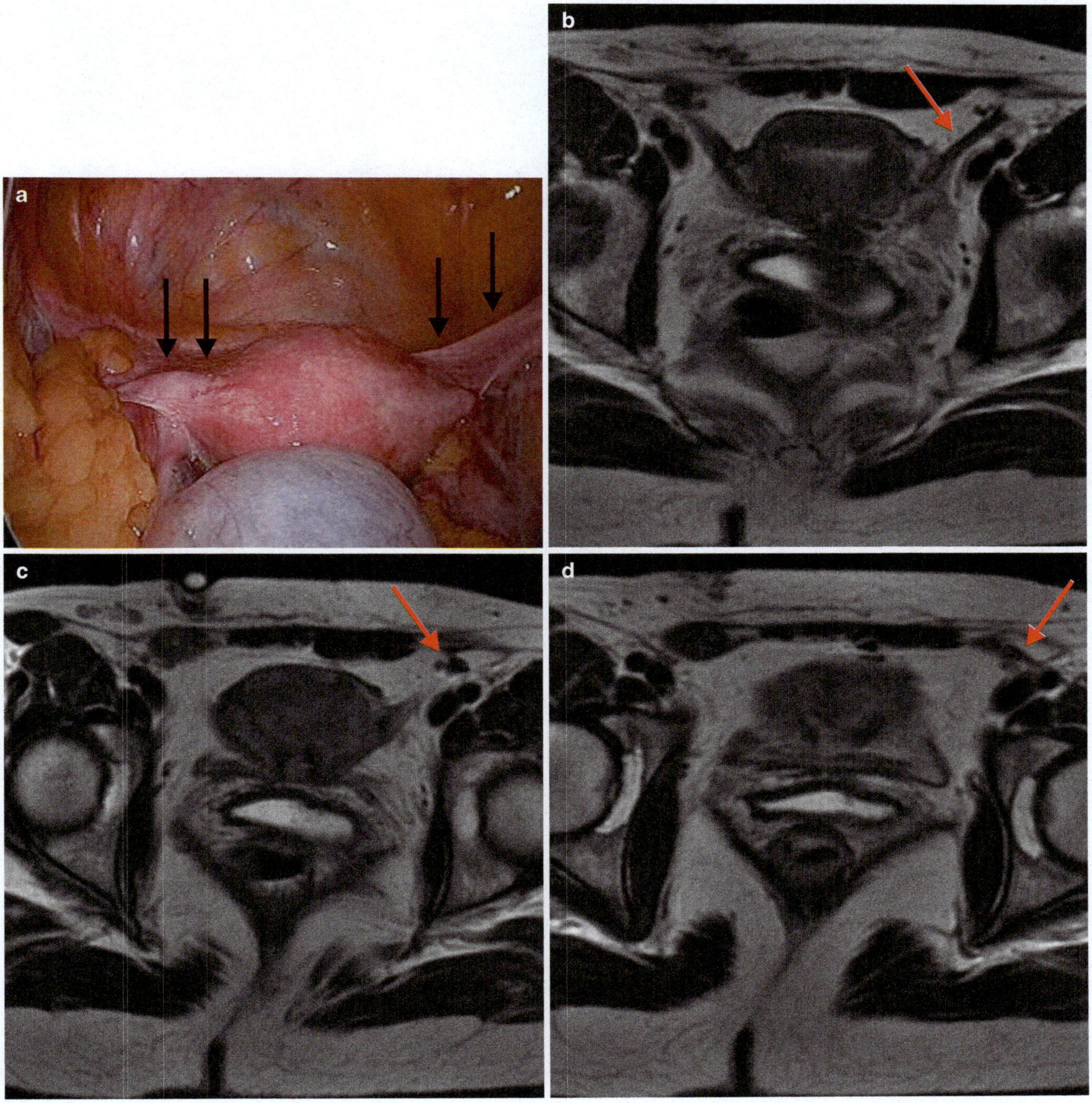

Fig. 4.35 Anatomy of intraperitoneal round ligament. Origin in the anterior and lateral faces of the uterine body (arrows in **a**), crosses the broad ligament and the tubes anteriorly and penetrates the inner inguinal ring (**b**–**k** arrows). (**a**) Laparoscopy. (**b**–**f**) T2-weighted sequences. Axial. (**g**–**k**) Coronal. Note normal aspect on the left and lesion on the right

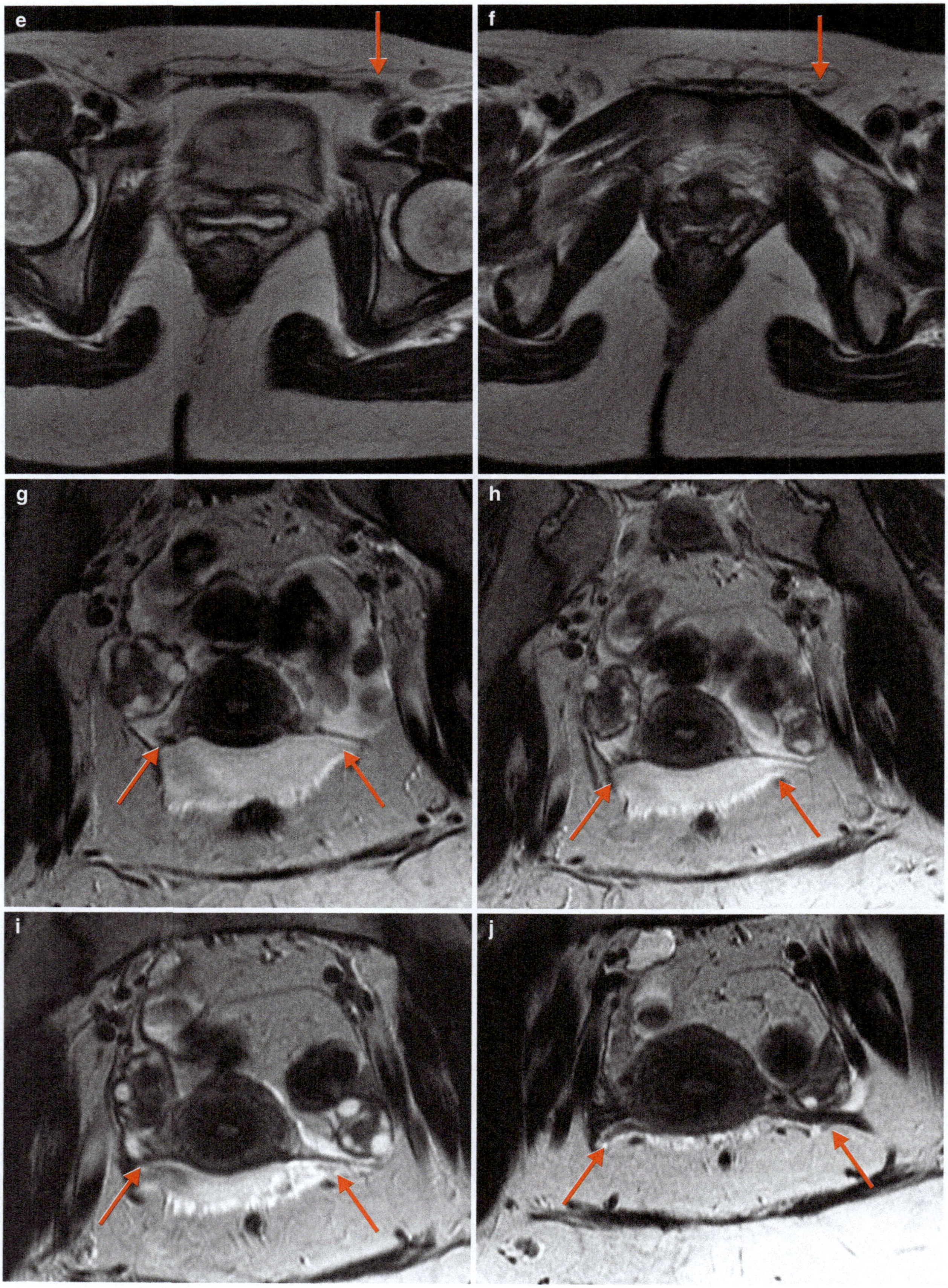

Fig. 4.35 (conrinued)

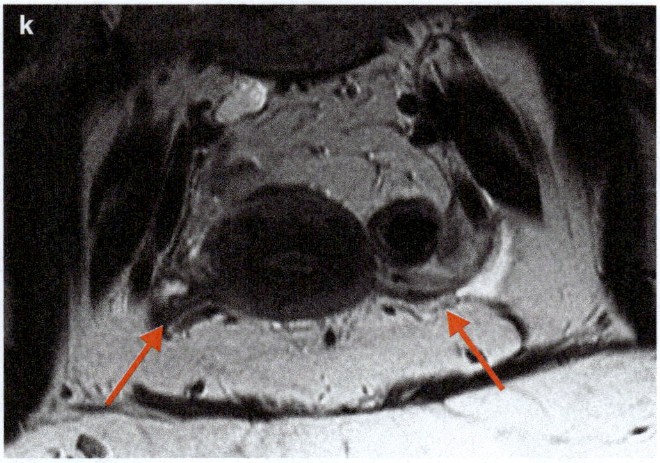

Fig. 4.35 (continued)

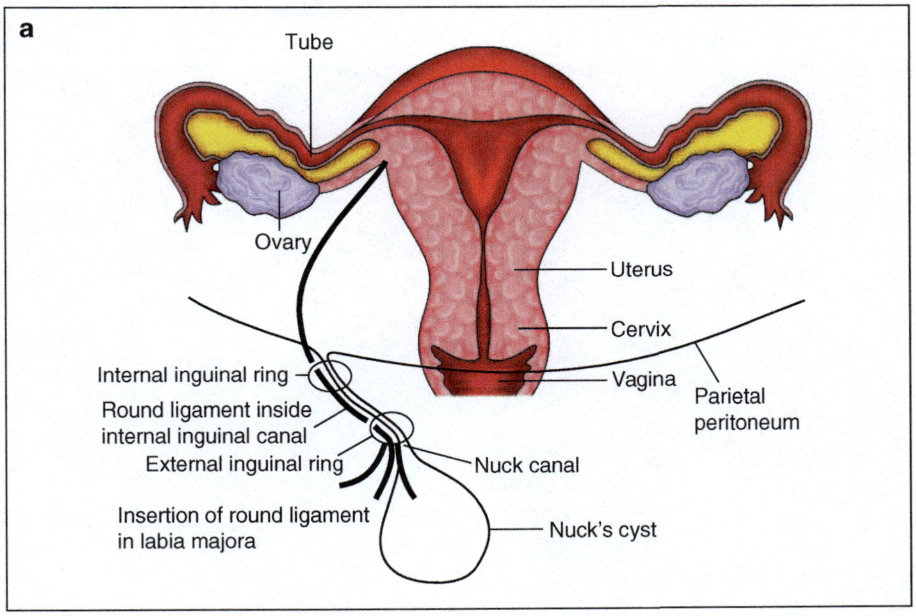

Fig. 4.36 Anatomy of extraperitoneal round ligament. It crosses the inguinal canal, adjacent to the canal of Nuck, with an inferior and medial path, until inserting itself in the labia majora (follows the arrows of **b–f**). (**a**) Diagram. (**b–f**) T2-weighted sequences. Axial

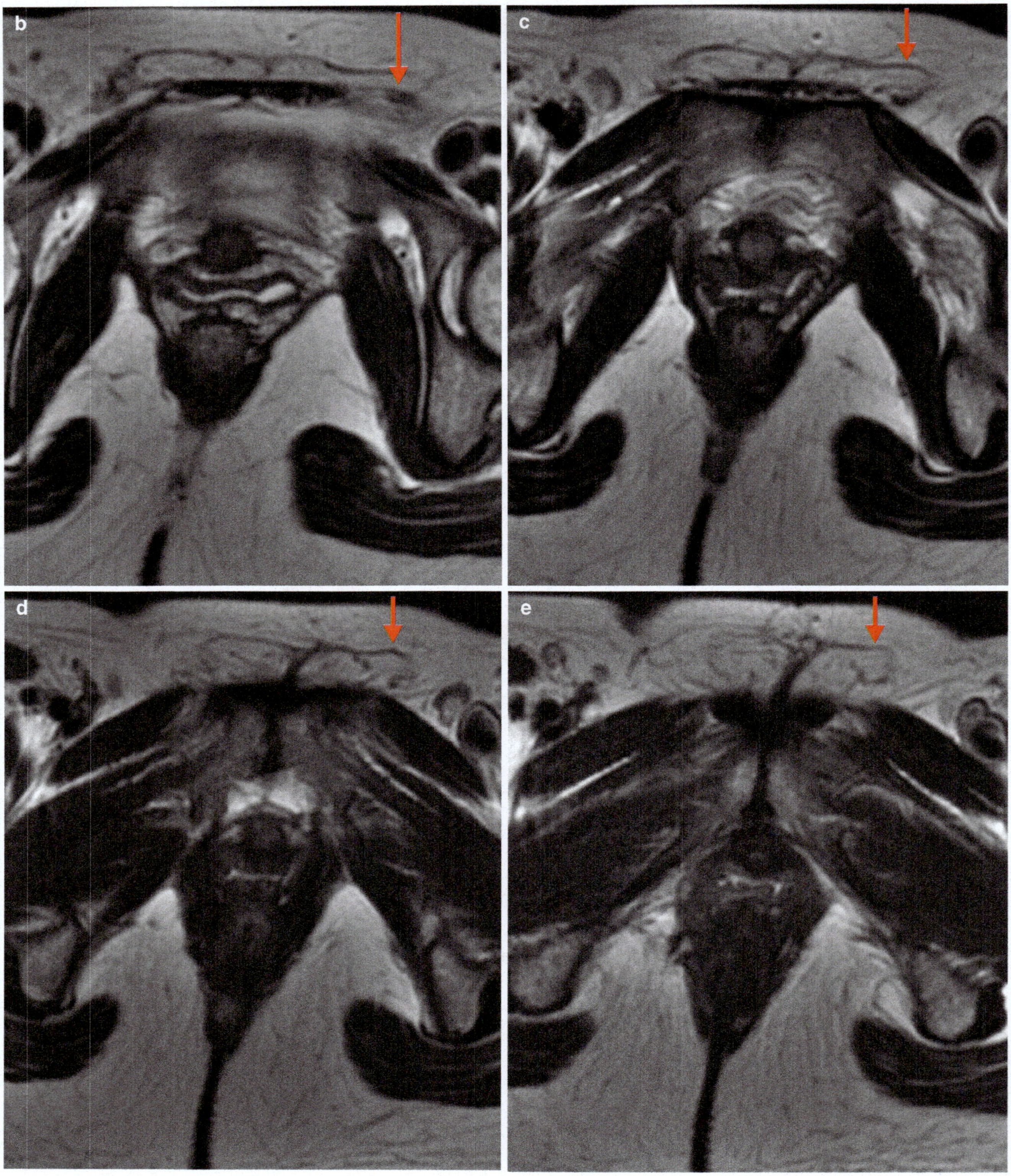

Fig. 4.36 (continued

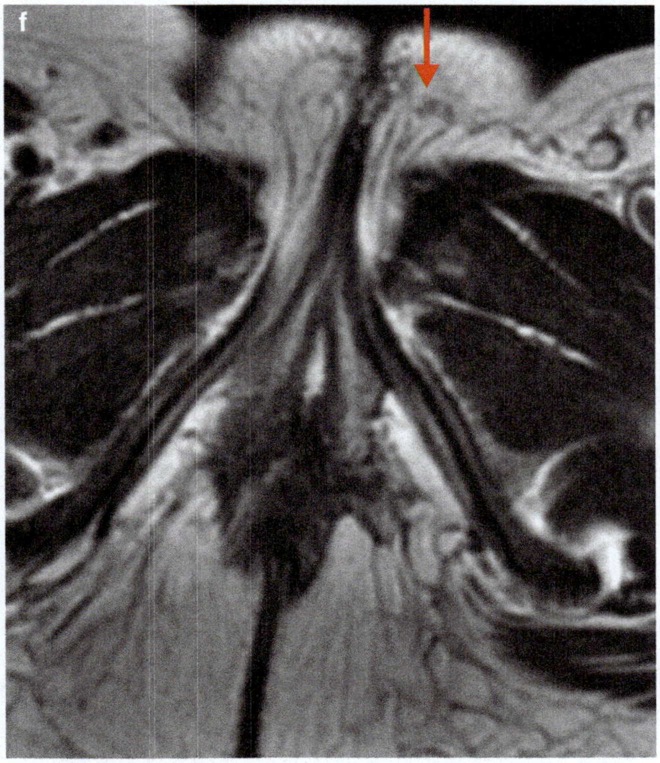

Fig. 4.36 (continued)

4.1.2.2 Most Common Aspects of Endometriosis

Endometriosis of the round ligament can involve the intra- and extraperitoneal portions, the intraperitoneal being the most common. Their involvement is underestimated by the literature. According to Crispi, involvement of the intraperitoneal round ligament occurred in 13.8% of the 174 women patients with infiltrative endometriosis submitted to surgical treatment [15].

4.1.2.3 Clinical Manifestations

Patients may experience pain and bladder discomfort and may complain of monthly vulvar swelling.

A physical examination may be able to diagnose the condition, especially in the case of extraperitoneal involvement.

4.1.2.4 MRI and Laparoscopic Findings

Typical laparoscopic aspects of deep endometriosis of the round ligament are thickening, deviation, and shortening of the ligament (Fig. 4.37).

The involvement of this ligament can occur along its course, be unifocal or diffuse, and may be associated with extension to other organ, as shown in Table 4.4, such as:

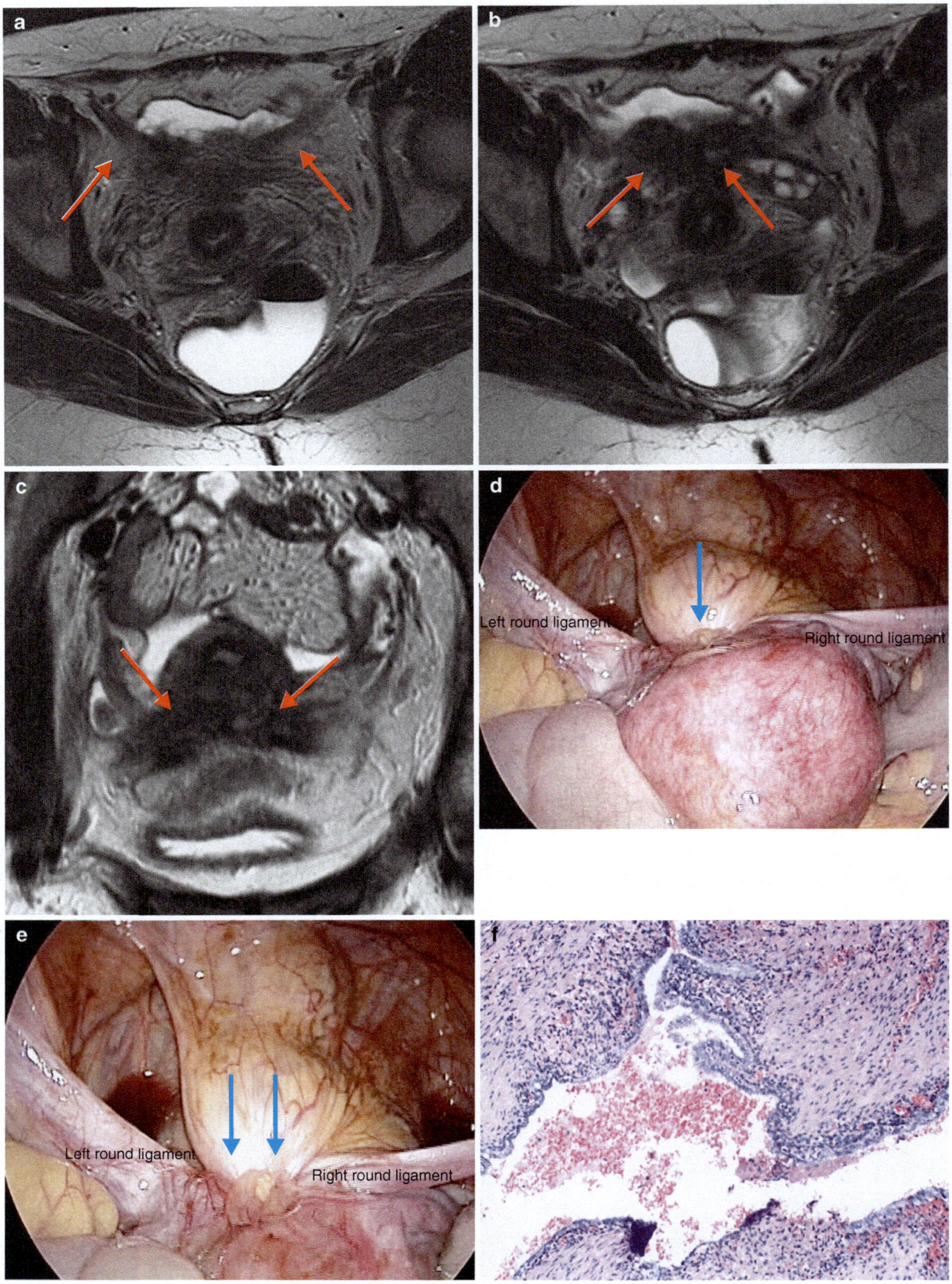

Fig. 4.37 Deep Endometriosis of the round ligaments with thickening, irregularity and hypointense bilateral (arrows). T2-weighted sequences. (**a**, **b**) Axial. (**c**) Coronal. (**d**, **e**) Laparoscopy. Note the thickening and retraction of the ligaments toward the lesion that infiltrates the anterior myometrium (arrow). (**d**) Panorama and (**e**) detail of the lesion. (**f**) Microscopy (100×). Endometriotic focus with interstitial edema of striated muscle

Table 4.4 Round ligament deep endometriosis involvement

Intraperitoneal lesion, predominantly ligamentous
Bladder injury with ligamentous extension
Intra and extra peritoneal lesion
Extraperitoneal lesion

1. **Intraperitoneal lesion, predominantly ligamentous**
   The ligament involvement can occur at the uterine attachment, laterally at the anterior compartment, causing thickening, irregularity, and ligament retraction. Signal modification can occur, with a hypointense nodule in the T2-weighted sequence and bleeding foci (Fig. 4.38).
   Larger lesions can extend posteriorly and penetrate the myometrium, anteriorly to the bladder dome, and also laterally to the broad ligament, causing adherence with the fallopian tube and ovary, as well as to the cecum and sigmoid, when the involvement is on the right and left sides, respectively (Fig. 4.39).
2. **Bladder injury with ligamentous extension**
   When the impairment is predominantly in the bladder, the lesion has a median location and extends laterally, thickening and retracting the round ligaments. The involved round ligament points to the bladder lesion (Fig. 4.40).
3. **Both intraperitoneal and extraperitoneal lesions**
   The involvement occurs along its course, intra- and extraperitoneal, extending through the canal of Nuck, an evagination of the parietal peritoneum that accompanies the round ligament through the inguinal ring in the inguinal canal (obliterated soon after birth). When present, it allows ectopic endometrial implants to spread from the peritoneal cavity to the inguinal canal.

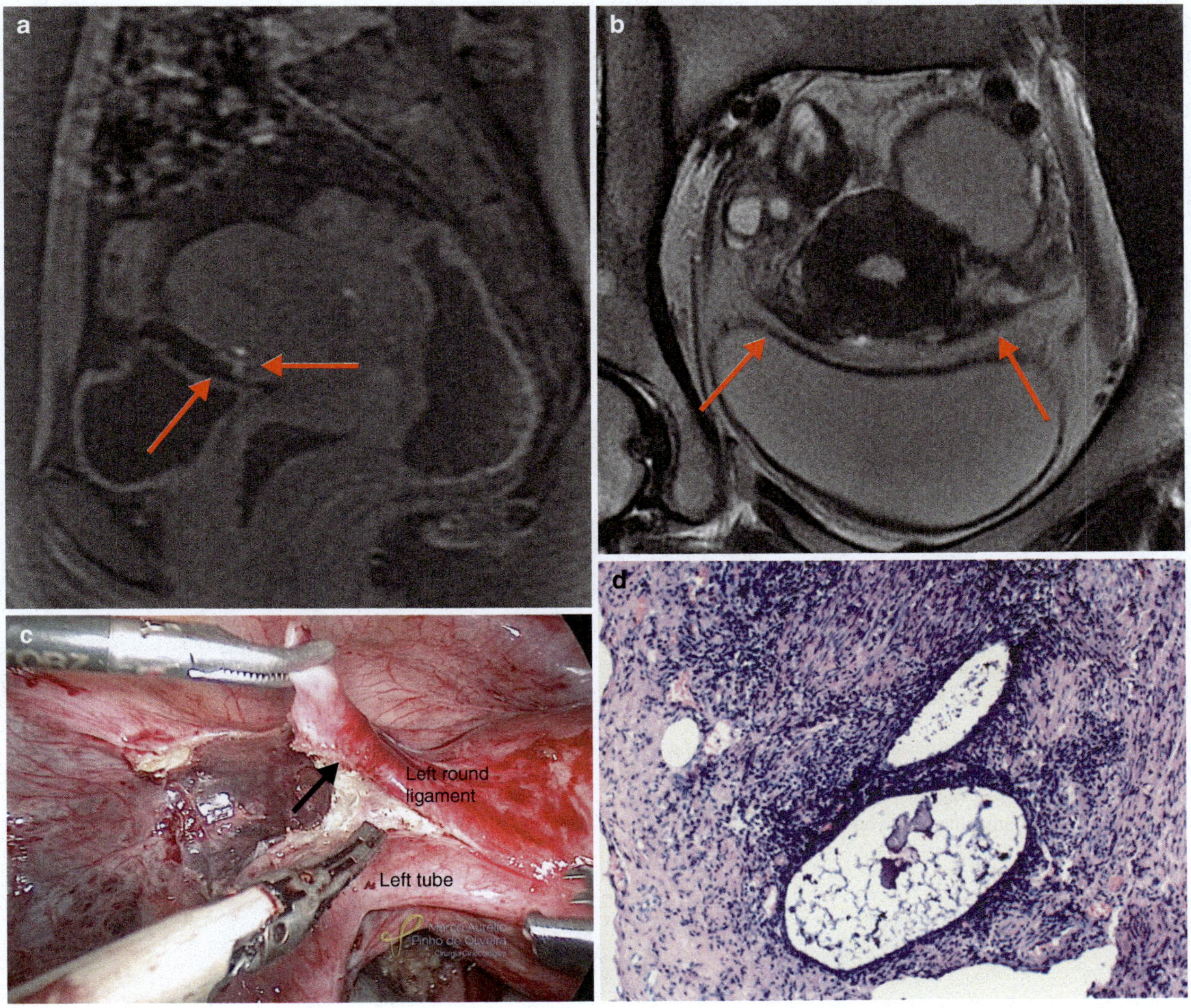

Fig. 4.38 Intraperitoneal ligament lesion, lateral in the compartment, causing thickening, irregularity, retraction and heterogeneous signal, hypointense in T2-weighted sequence (arrows **b**) with hyperintense foci, and bleeding in T1-weighted fat-suppressed sequence (arrows in **a**). Sagittal. (**b**) Coronal. (**c**) Laparoscopy. (**d**) Microscopy showing stroma and endometrial glands, with two ligamentous cysts

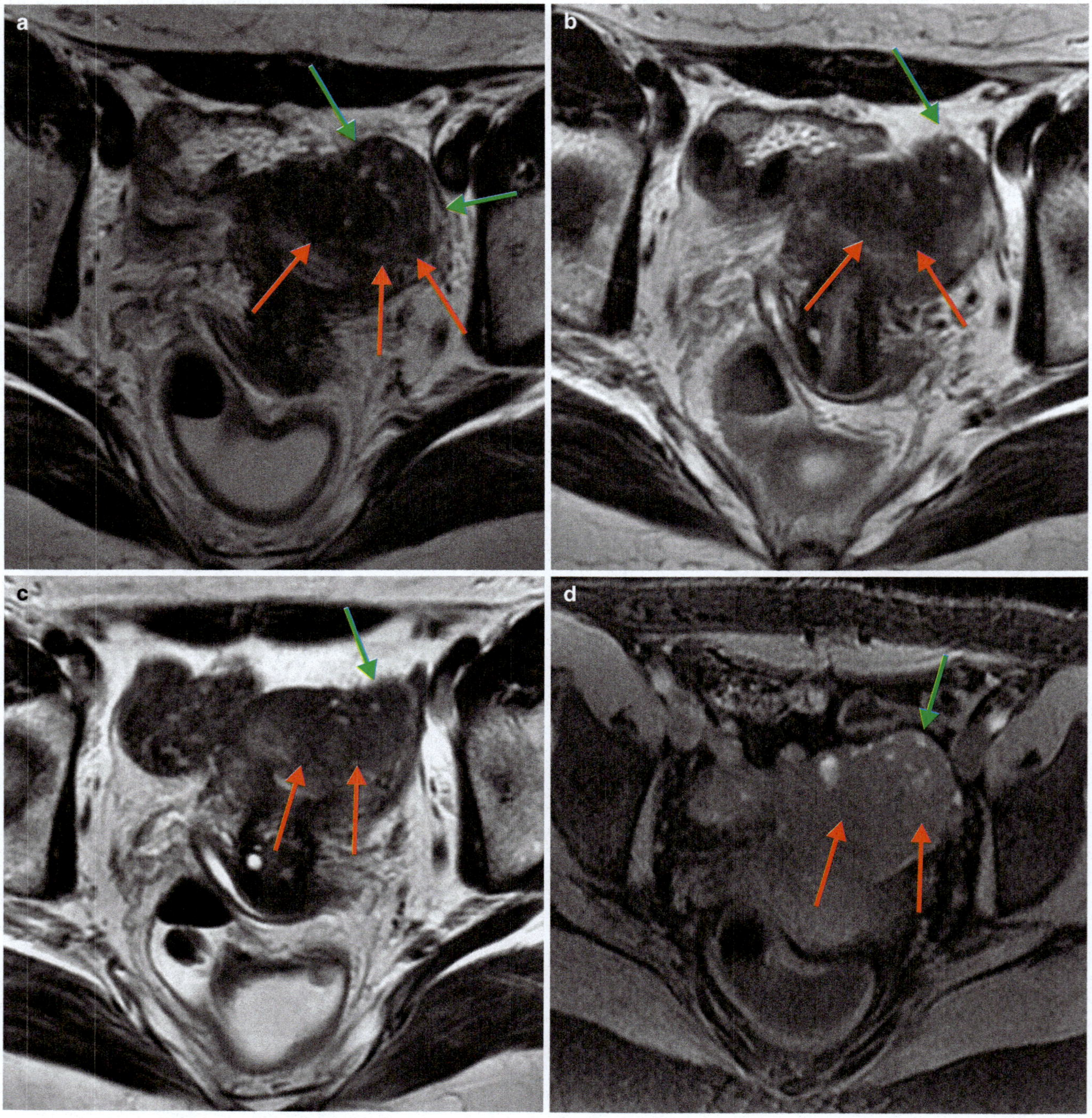

Fig. 4.39 Left round ligament lesion (green arrows **a–c**, **e**) with significant penetration in the anterior myometrium (red arrows), distorting and thickening the anterior wall of the uterus, with hyperintense foci, with bleeding (Note **d**), moving the myometrium. (**a–c**, **e**) T2-weighted sequences. (**d**) T1-weighted sequence with fat suppression. (**a–d**) Axial. (**e**) Coronal. (**f**) Pathology showing endometrioid cyst in the round ligament with necrotic content

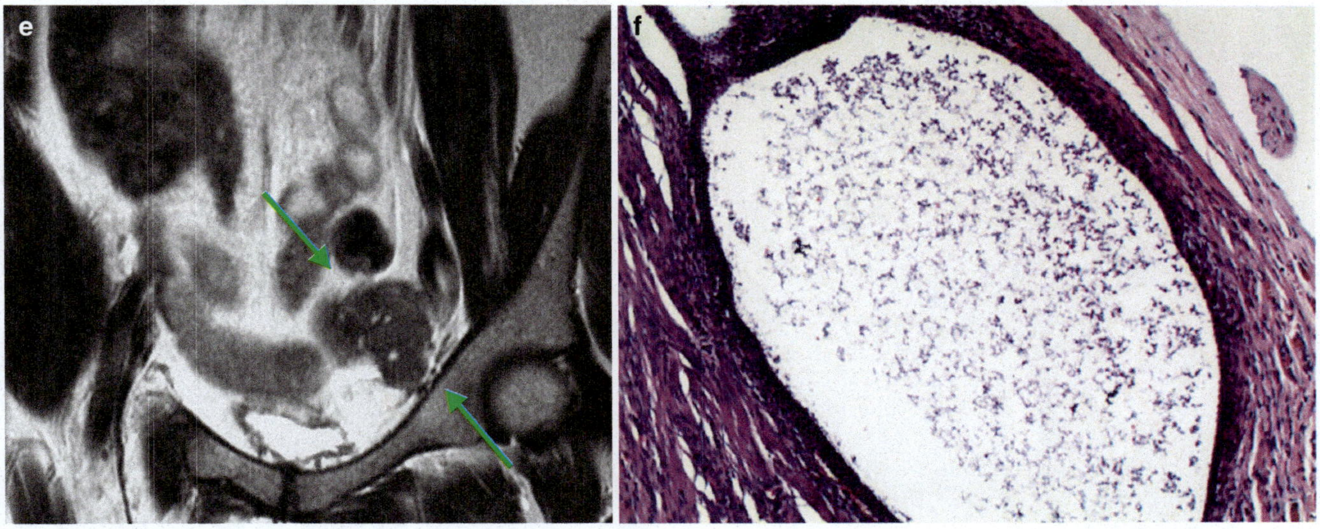

Fig. 4.39 (continued)

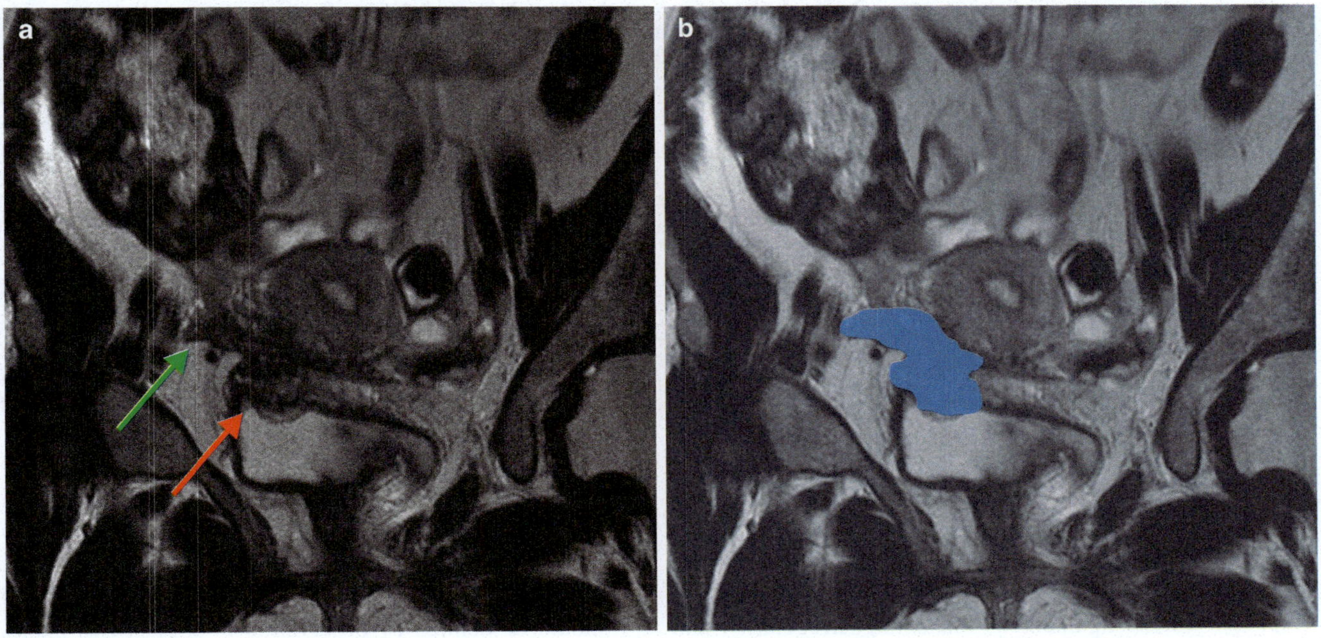

Fig. 4.40 Bladder lesion lateralized to the right (red arrow) with ligamentous extension. The round ligament involved (green arrow in **a** and blue diagram in **b**) points to the bladder lesion. Note the proximity of the lesion to the ureteral ostium in the sagittal plane (red arrows). (**a**, **b**) Coronal. (**c**) Sagittal. (**d**) Control after hormonal therapy with reduction of volume and modification of signal intensity of the lesion (green and red arrows). (**e**) Laparoscopy. Deviation and retraction of the round ligament (arrows). (**f**) Microscopy (400×). Endometriotic focus with compact cytotoxic stroma

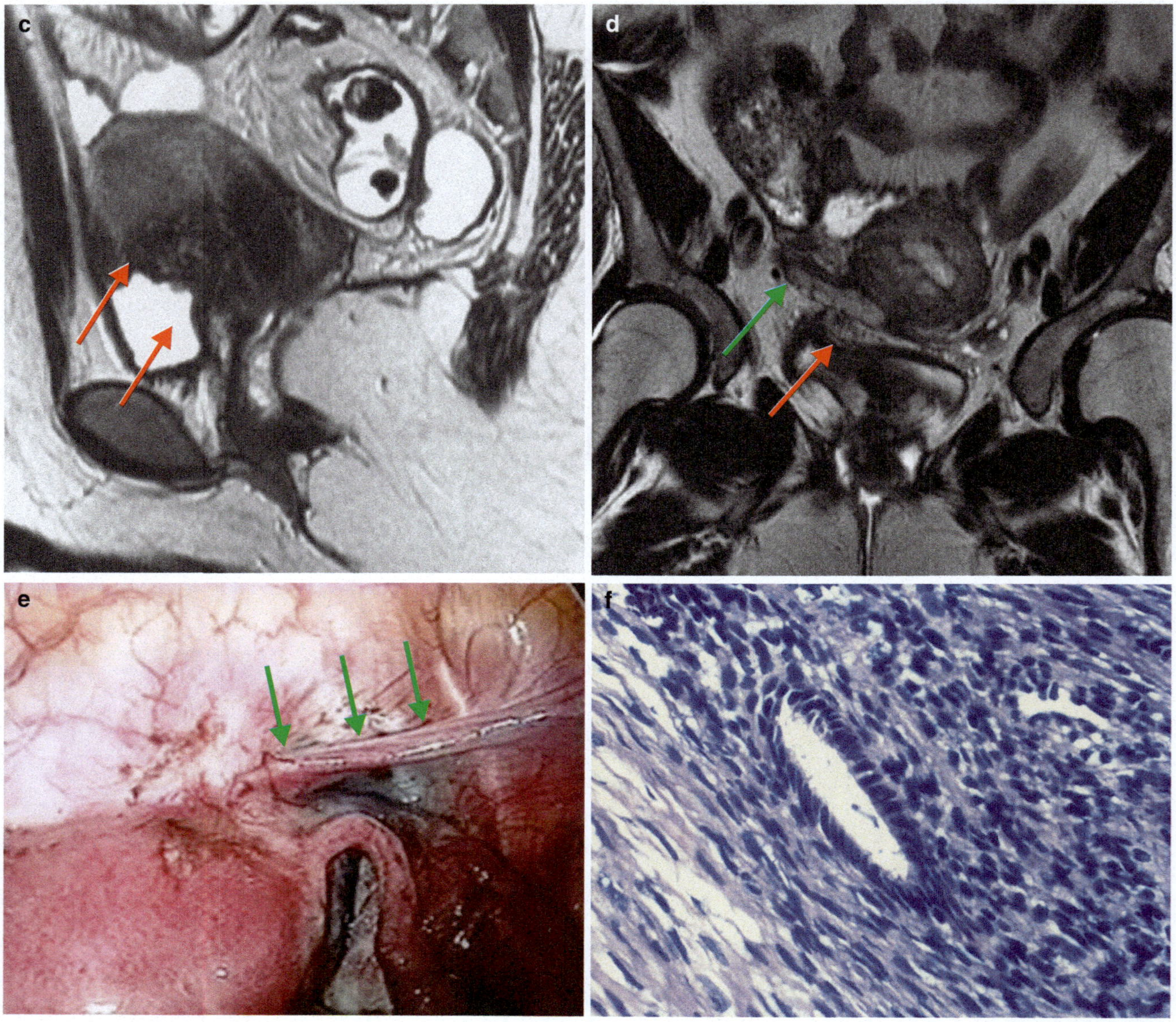

Fig. 4.40 (continued)

This is a rare form of ligamentous involvement and causes diffuse ligamentous thickening, irregularity, and signal intensity changes (Fig. 4.41).

4. **Lesion in the extraperitoneal portion**

   We describe this in the section on deep endometriosis lesions with atypical location [21].

   Unilateral ligament involvement may present a diagnostic challenge.

   The round ligament has a long and loose course, and sometimes its tortuosity simulates thickening in MRI. From the authors' experience, ligament thickening should be defined by observation in at least two planes (Fig. 4.42).

   Another differential diagnosis, when the lesion is isolated, is leiomyoma. Both can present as a small hypointense nodule in the T2-weighted sequence; however, the subserous leiomyoma is a well-defined nodule, and the endometriotic lesion has an ill-defined margin (Fig. 4.43).

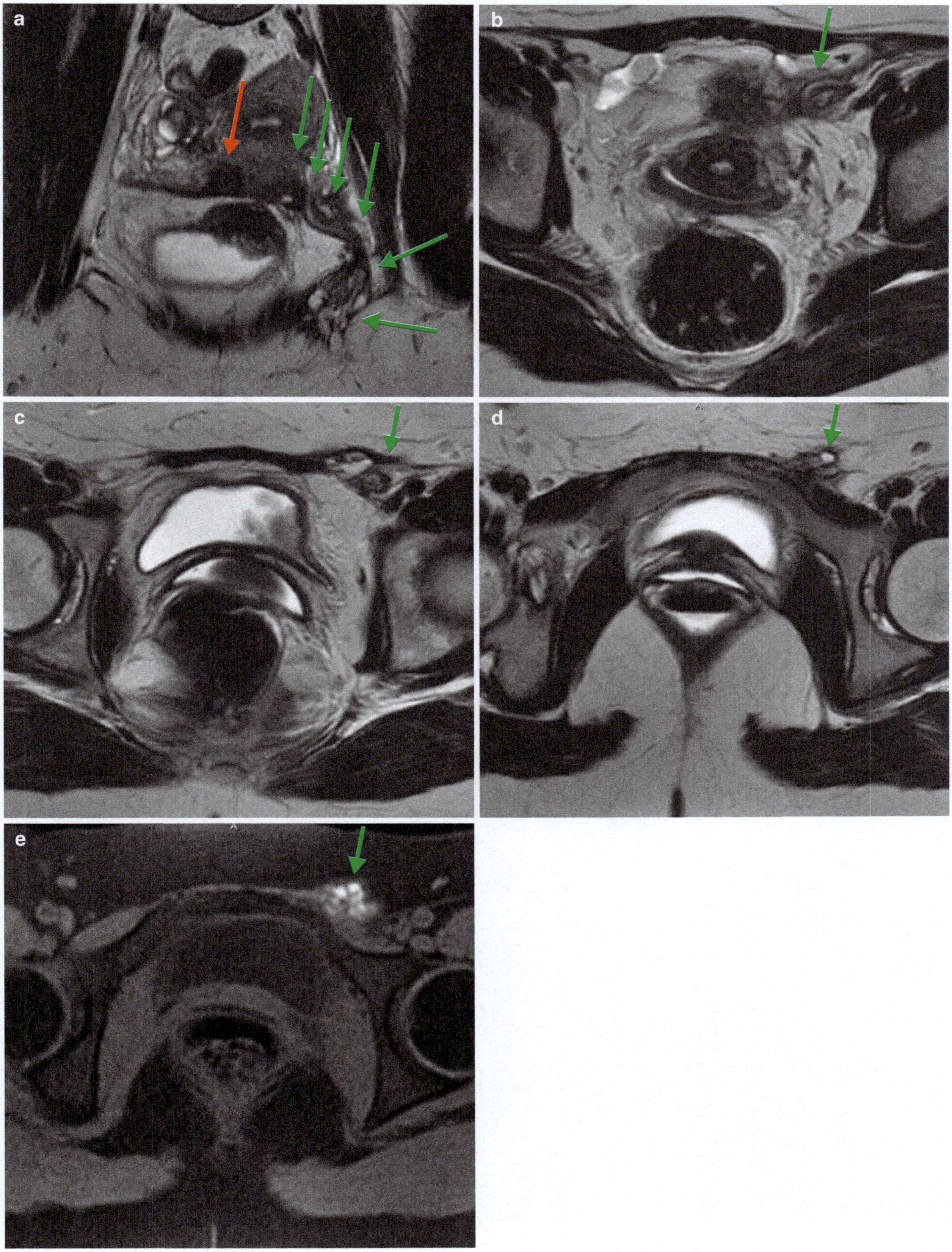

Fig. 4.41 Lesion of the intraperitoneal portion of the right round ligament (red arrows in **a**), intra- and extraperitoneal on the left (green arrows **a–e**) extending through the canal of Nuck to the inguinal canal (**ec**). Note bleeding in the lesion with hyperintense foci in T2 and T1 (**a**, **d**, **e**). (**a–d**) T2-weighted sequences. (**a**) Coronal. (**b–d**) Axial. (**e**) T1-weighted with fat suppression. Axial

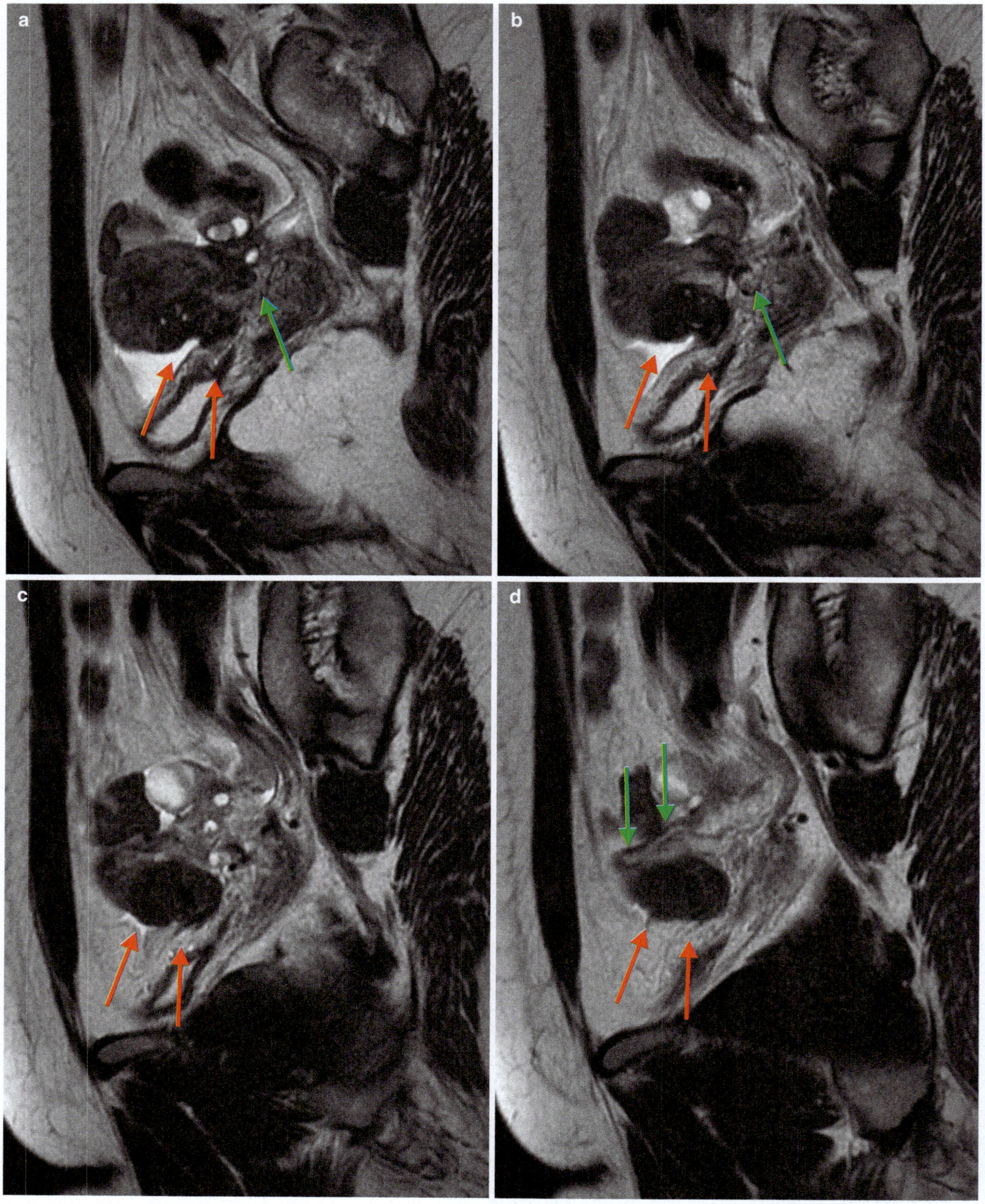

Fig. 4.42 Thickening with nodular aspect, retraction and change in the ligamentous signal observed in the three planes (red arrows). The lesion is hypointense in T2, with hyperintense foci (red arrows in **a**, **g**), with an intermediate signal in T1, and with slight bleeding (**e**) and enhancement (**f**), and has posterior extension to the broad ligament (arrows in **g**). (**a–d**, **g–l**) T2-weighted sequences. (**a–d**) Sagittal. (**g**) Axial. (**h–l**) Coronal. (**m**) Laparoscopy during resection of the ligament. Note the lesion in the ovarian fossa, endometrioma and discrete tubal dilation on the same side (green arrows in **a**, **b**, **d**, **l**), as well as a hyperintense T2 focus indicating superficial endometriosis in the sigmoid (yellow arrow in **k**)

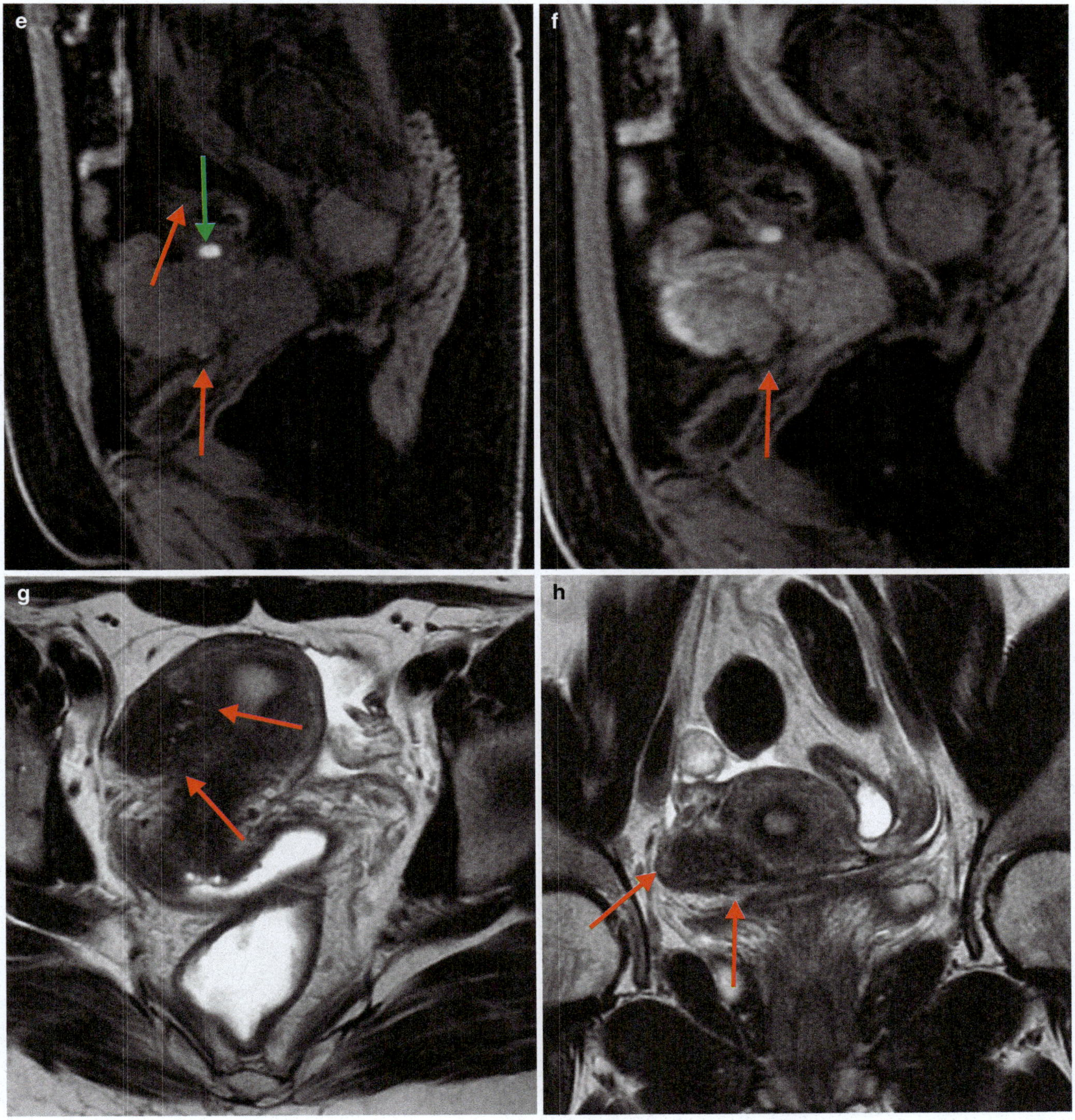

Fig. 4.42 (conitinued)

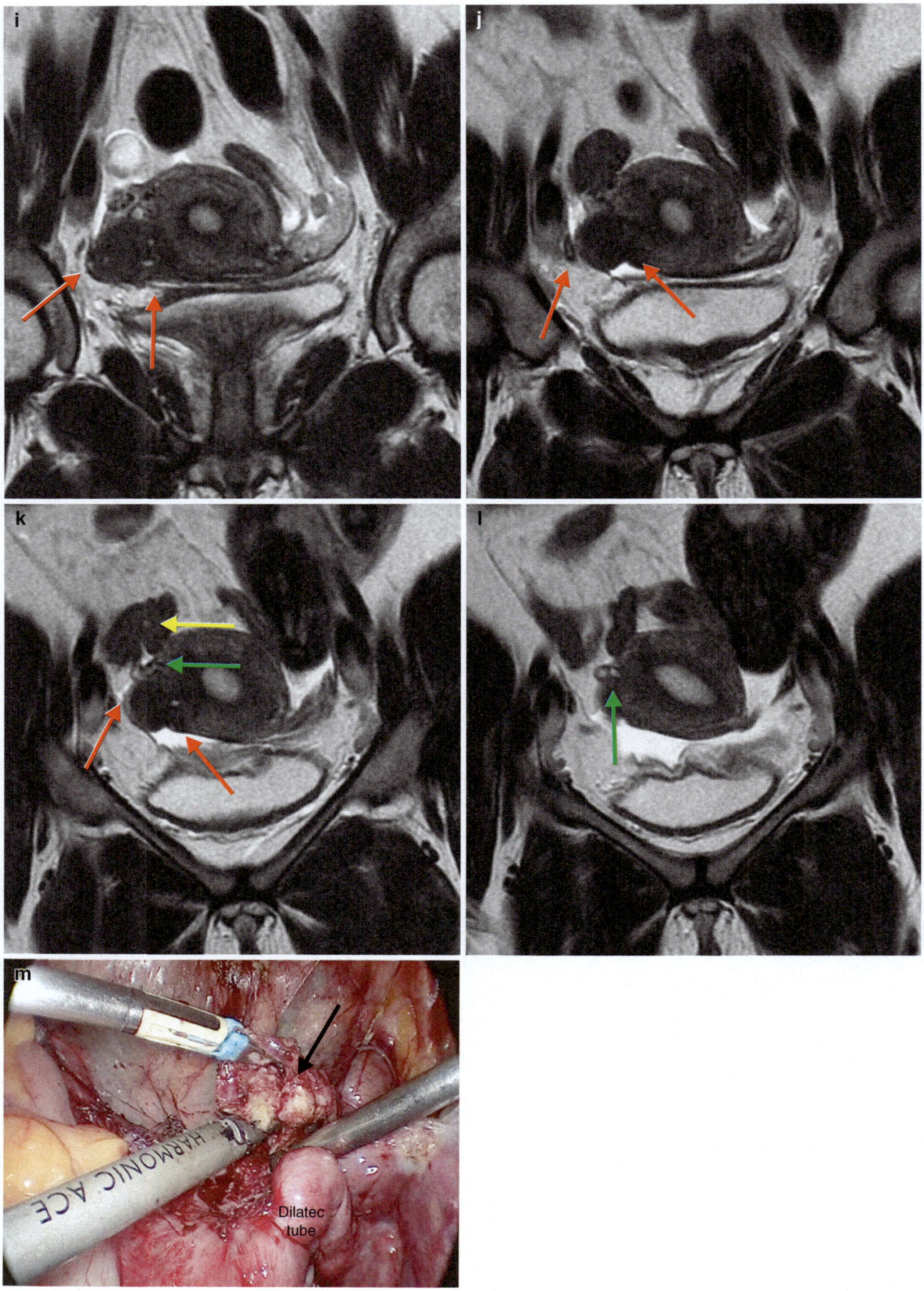

Fig. 4.42 (conitinued)

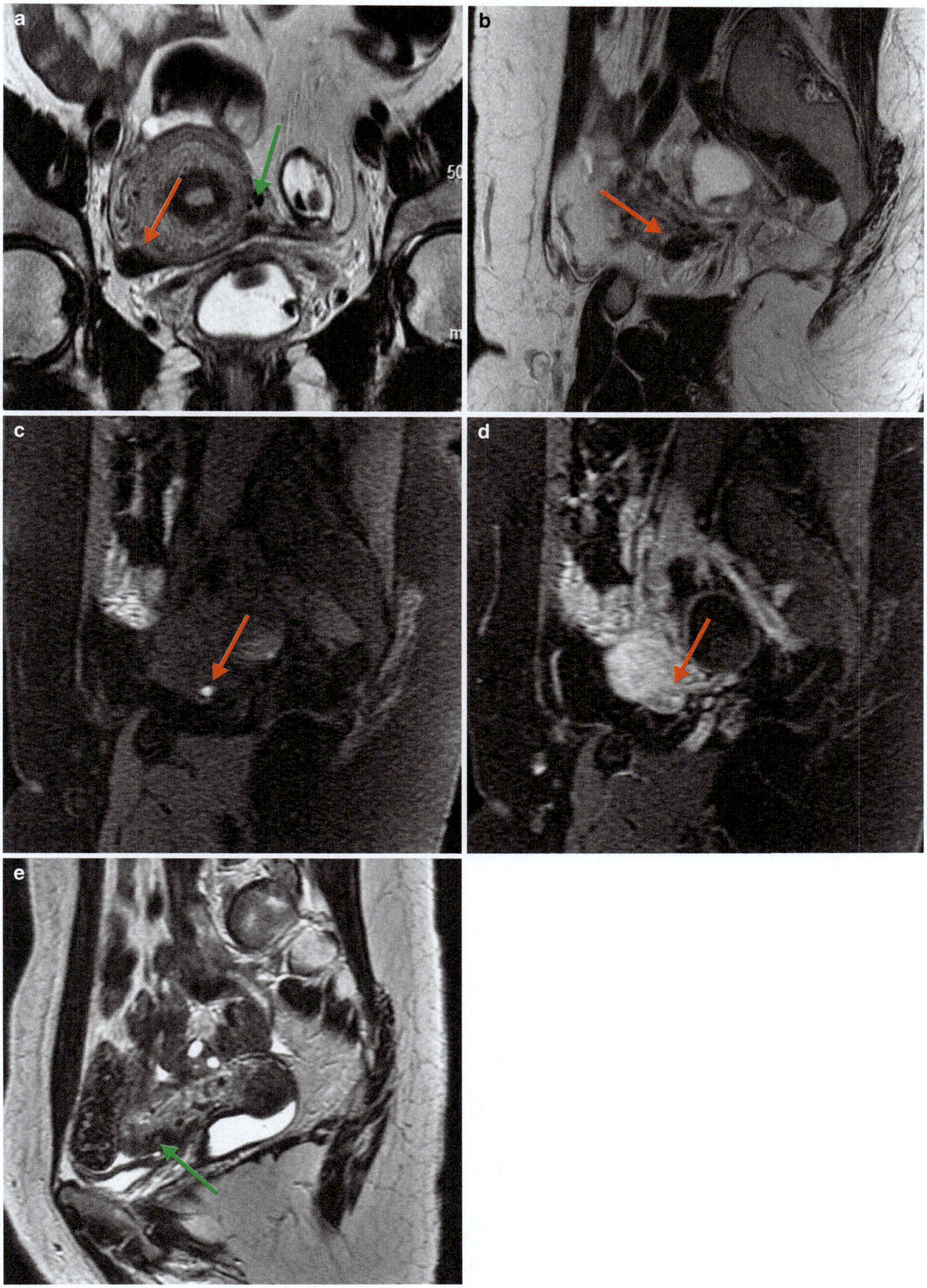

Fig. 4.43 (**a**) Sessile subserosal myometrial nodule in the topography of the right round ligament (red arrows), hypointense in T2-weighted sequences (**a**, **b**), bleeding in T1-weighted sequence with fat saturation (**c**), and gadolinium enhancement (**d**). The differential diagnosis is round ligament endometriosis and subserosal adenomyoma. In this case, it is ligamentous endometriosis. Note similar involvement in the left ligament, smaller but with a hyperintense focus (**a**, **e**—green arrow). (**a**) Coronal. (**b**–**e**) Sagittal

4.1.2.5 Comment About the Treatment

When ligament involvement is detected, the lesion should be resectioned. Its persistence can maintain pelvic symptoms.

4.1.3 Myometrium

4.1.3.1 Myometrium Anatomy

The myometrium forms the bulk mass of the uterus and consists of interlaced involuntary smooth muscle fibers. The smooth muscle bundles form three ill-defined layers: the "submucosum stratum," the "stratum vasculare," and the "subserosum stratum." The inner layer is thin with circular fibers running transversely, and the outer is formed by longitudinally running fibers, parallel to the major uterus axis. The "stratum vasculare" is the thickest layer of the myometrium, rich in blood vessels, and the muscle bundles run in all directions, mostly perpendicular [23].

The orientation and thickness of these fibers impact on the zonal uterus anatomy seen in MRI in women in the reproductive phase. In T2-weighted images, this fiber complex will appear as:

(a) An inner layer with a longitudinal fiber arrangement, referred to as the junctional zone, hypointense
(b) A thicker central portion with circular arrangement, with a variable signal intensity, usually hyperintense with a gradual increase in signal intensity from the follicular phase to the secretory menstrual cycle phase
(c) A more external, thin layer with longitudinal fibers, hypointense (Fig. 4.44) [24].

The characterization of the zonal anatomy is important to define the extent of the penetration of deep endometriosis into the myometrium.

The external myometrium layer is covered by the peritoneum, the outermost coat or serous layer. It covers the anterior surface of the uterus, from the fundus to the body, until the anterior peritoneal reflection. The anterior uterine cervix is not covered by the peritoneum, but by a loose connective tissue, the endopelvic fascia.

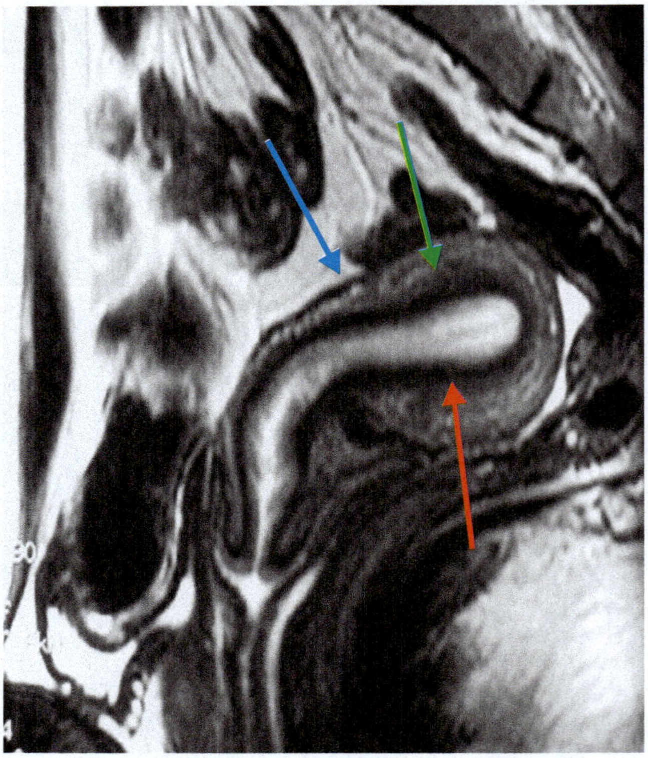

Fig. 4.44 Zonal anatomy: (**a**) the inner layer (junctional zone), longitudinal arrangement of fibers, hypointense (red arrow); (**b**) central portion, thicker, with circular arrangement of fibers, hyperintense (green arrow); **c**) outer layer, thin with longitudinal fibers, hypointense (blue arrow). T2-weighted sequence. Sagittal

4.1.3.2 Most Common Aspects of Endometriosis

Uterine involvement by endometriosis is a relatively new concept. The infiltrative process does not respect the uterine serous and penetrates into the myometrium, both in lesions of the anterior compartment and in lesions of the posterior and lateral compartments (Fig. 4.45).

Myometrial penetration can be prominent, coming close to the uterine cavity. However, the process is different from adenomyosis, which is considered a separate disease. In adenomyosis there is a direct extension of the endometrial tissue into the myometrium, near the basal endometrium (subbasal adenomyosis) or extending beyond the myometrium, associated with fibrosis, myometrial hypertrophy, and hyperplasia, therefore causing the thickening of the junctional zone. The adenomyosis process is centrally located, from the cavity to the serous. On the other hand, myometrial endometriosis occurs at the uterus periphery and starts at the serous. The external penetration of the ectopic endometrial tissue similarly induces changes in smooth muscle and myometrial fibrosis (Fig. 4.46) [25].

However, extensive endometriosis myometrium involvement can mimic adenomyosis, especially in patients on hormone suppression. The lesion outside the uterus reduces; however, the myometrial involvement does not change significantly due to the associated muscle hypertrophy and fibrosis (Fig. 4.47) [26].

Moreover, myometrial endometriosis involvement and adenomyosis may coexist in the uterus (Fig. 4.48) [27].

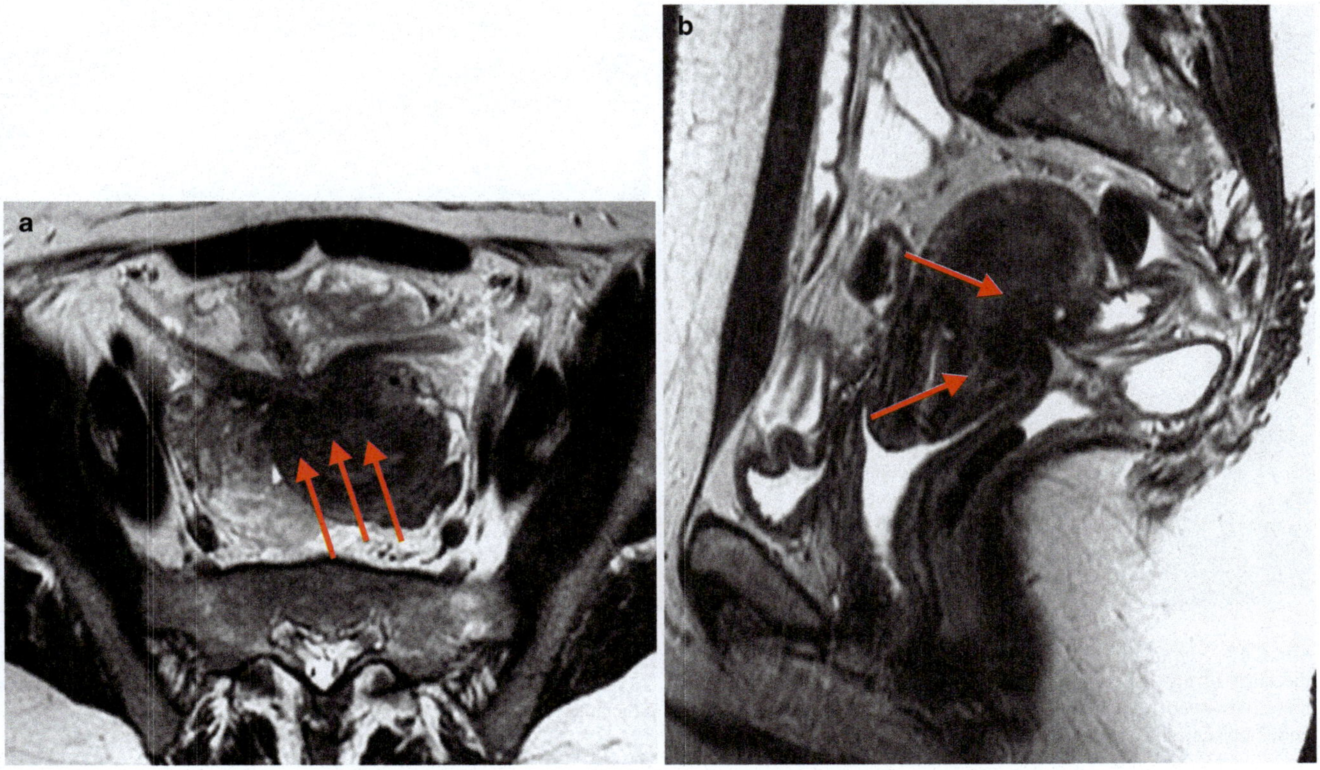

Fig. 4.45 Uterine compromised by endometriosis. Infiltrative lesions (arrows) in the anterior (**a**) and posterior (**b**) compartments, which do not respect the serosa and penetrate the myometrium. (**a, b**) T2-weighted sequences. (**a**) Axial. (**b**) Sagittal

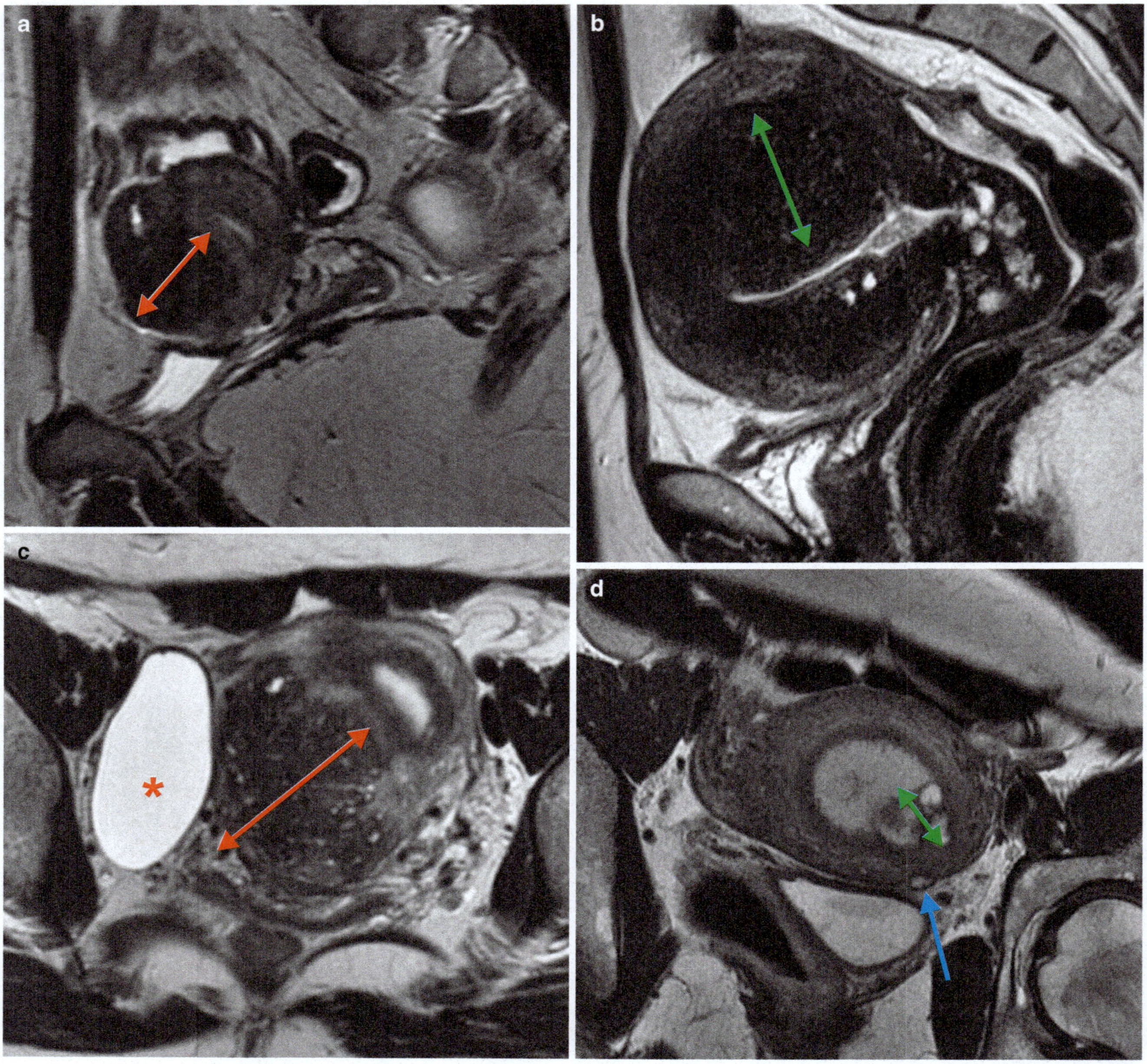

Fig. 4.46 Myometrial penetration. (**a**, **c**) In myometrial endometriosis, the onset of myometrial involvement is peripheral (from the serosa to the cavity—red line). (**b**, **d**) In adenomyosis, the penetration of the endometrial tissue is central (from the cavity to the serosa—green line). (**a**, **b**) T2-weighted sequences. (**a**, **b**) Sagittal. (**c**, **d**) Coronal with short axis. Note in (**c**) hydrosalpinx (*) and in (**d**) peritoneal endometriosis in the anterior compartment (blue)

Fig. 4.47 Lesion with significant penetration in the anterior myometrium (distortion and thickening with hyperintense foci, moving the myometrium—blue arrows in **b**) and smaller in the roof of the bladder (focal thickening of the posterior roof—green arrow). Note posterior extension of the ligaments (blue arrows in **b**). In addition, there is a lesion in the posterior compartment (red arrows). T2-weighted sequences. (**a**) Sagittal. (**b**) Axial. (**c**) Laparoscopy showing adhesions and anterior myometrial involvement. (**d**) Microscopy (400×). Island of endometrial tissue surrounded by smooth musculature

4.1.3.3 Clinical Manifestations

There is no specific symptom of myometrial involvement; however, dysmenorrhea and abnormal uterine bleeding can occur, classic symptoms of adenomyosis.

4.1.3.4 MRI and Laparoscopic Findings

The gross appearance of anterior myometrial involvement may have two morphologies, based on its relationship with the bladder lesion, according to Busard:

1. **A plaque-like myometrial lesion**, where there is contact on most of the surface of the bladder lesion with infiltration into the anterior uterine wall (Fig. 4.49)
2. **An hourglass-like lesion**, wherein only part of the bladder lesion is in contact with the anterior wall lesion of the uterus (Fig. 4.50) [27].

The myometrial lesion is ill defined and predominantly shows a hypointense signal in T2- and intermediate T1-weighted sequences. Hyperintense foci in the T2-weighted sequence, glands and ectopic endometrial cysts, as well as some bleeding spots, hyperintense on T1-weighted sequence, can be identified. Most of the time, there is an associated ligament or bladder lesion (Fig. 4.51).

The deepness and extension of the myometrial involvement may be underestimated during laparoscopy; thus it must be detailed in the MRI report. It is necessary to describe the length in the longitudinal and transverse axes, the myometrial penetration, as well as its distance from the uterine cavity (Table 4.5 and Fig. 4.52).

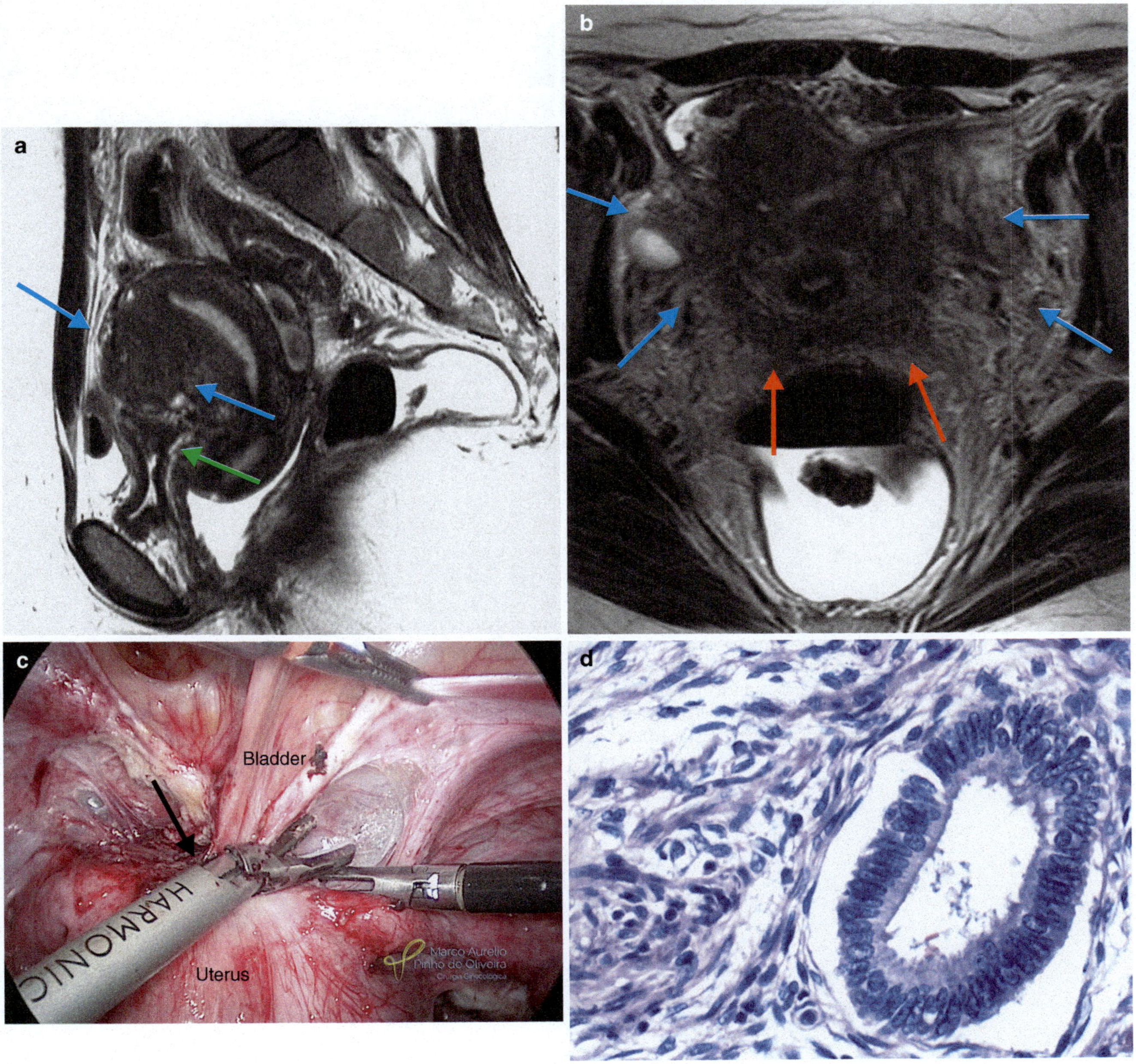

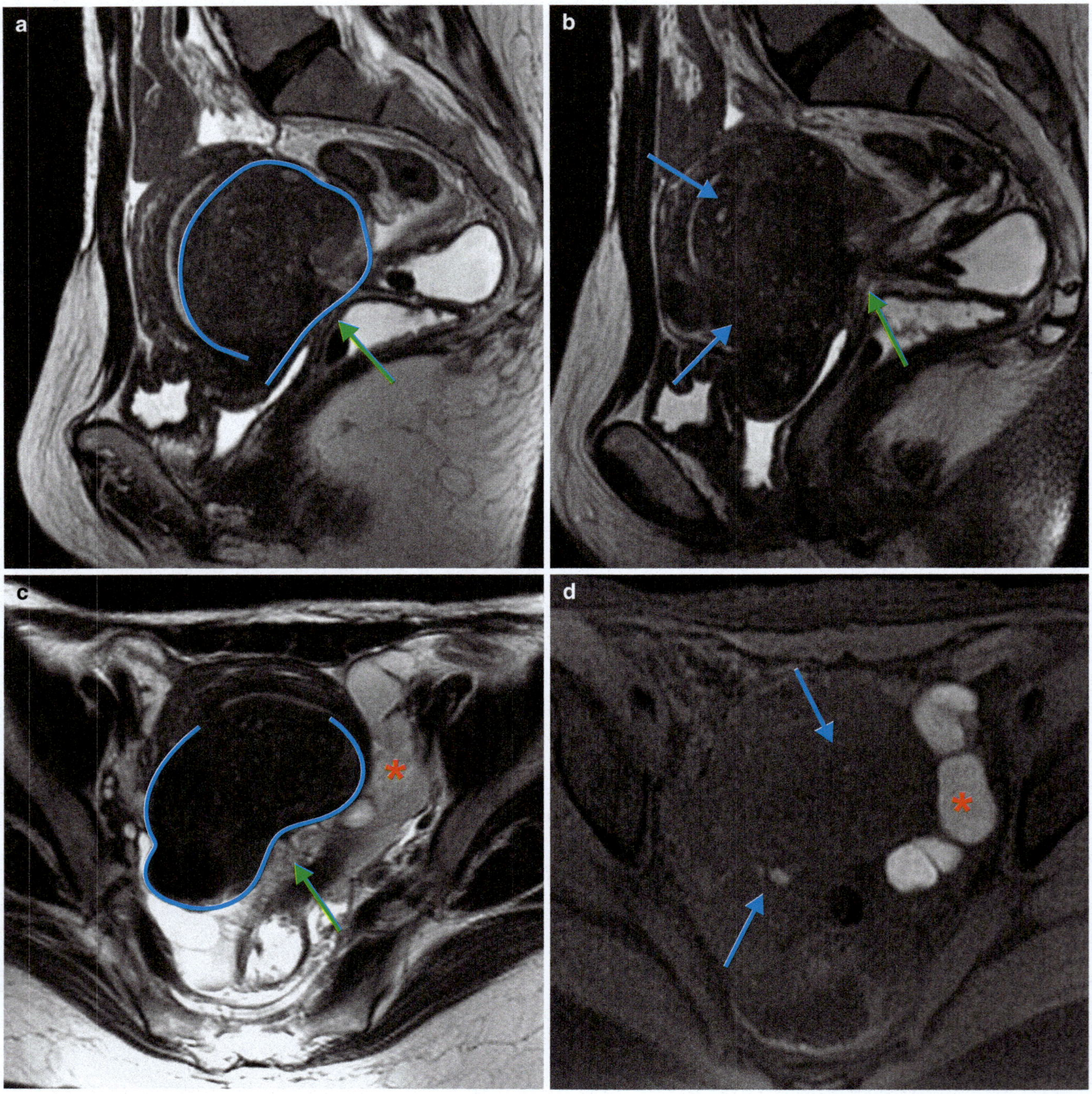

Fig. 4.48 Extensive posterior myometrial lesion (blue arrows and blue line) producing globular and asymmetric appearance of the uterus, wall thickening, with discrete areas of the myometrium spared the interface with the endometrium. Note rare bleeding foci in the lesion (**d**), in addition to deep retrocervical endometriosis (green), peritoneal (liquid with retrouterine blood), and left hematosalpinx (*). (**ac**) T2-weighted sequences. (**a**, **b**) Sagittal. (**c**, **d**) Axial

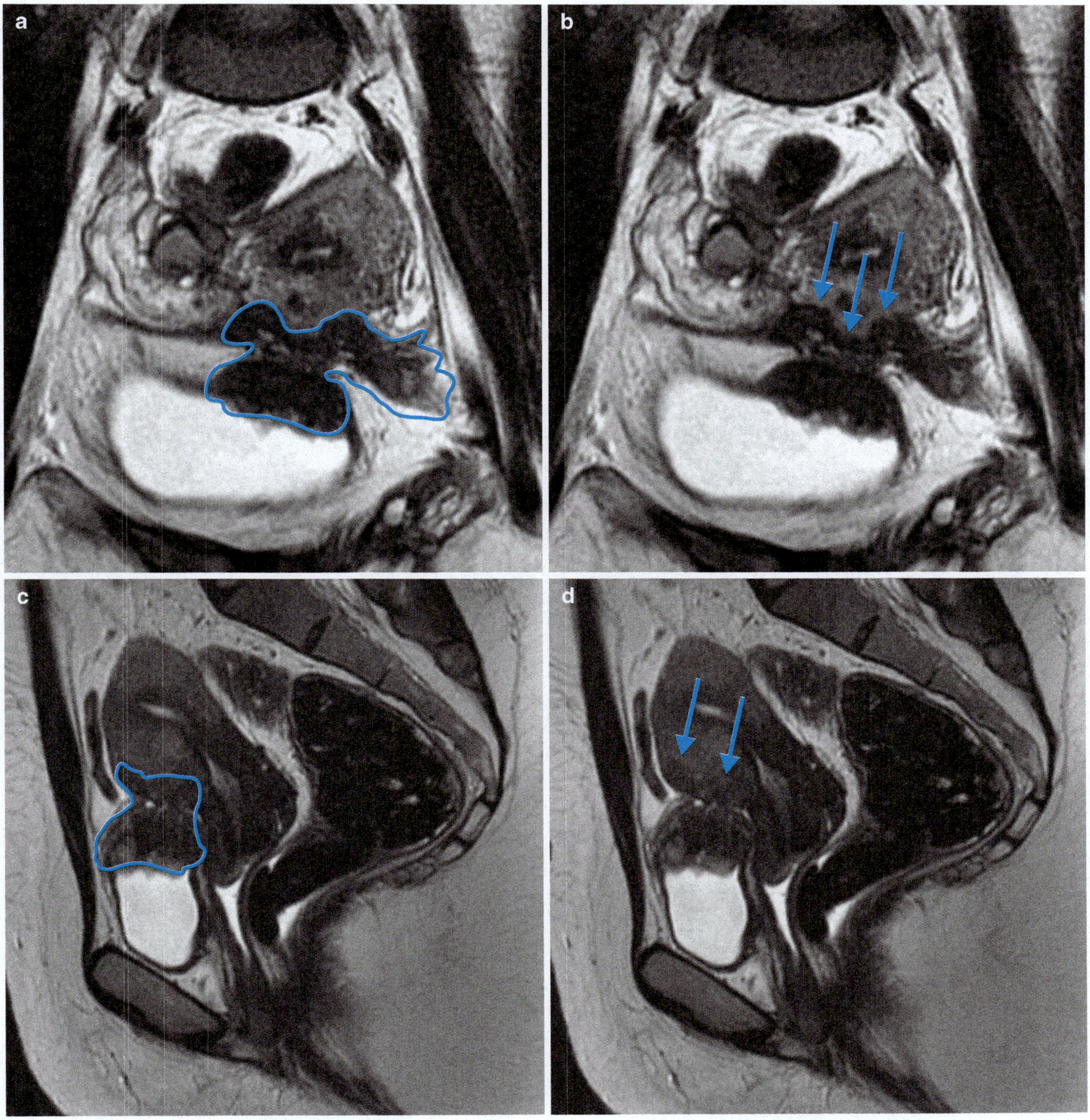

Fig. 4.49 Plaque-like involvement. Less common myometrial lesion in contact with the surface of the bladder for most of its extent (blue line in **a**, **c** and blue arrows in **b**, **d**). There is also involvement of the round ligaments, greater to the left, extending to the inguinal canal. Note right endometrioma and hematosalpinx (**a**, **b**) and small retrocervical lesion (**c**). (**a**–**d**) T2-weighted sequences. (**a**, **b**) Coronal. (**c**, **d**) Sagittal

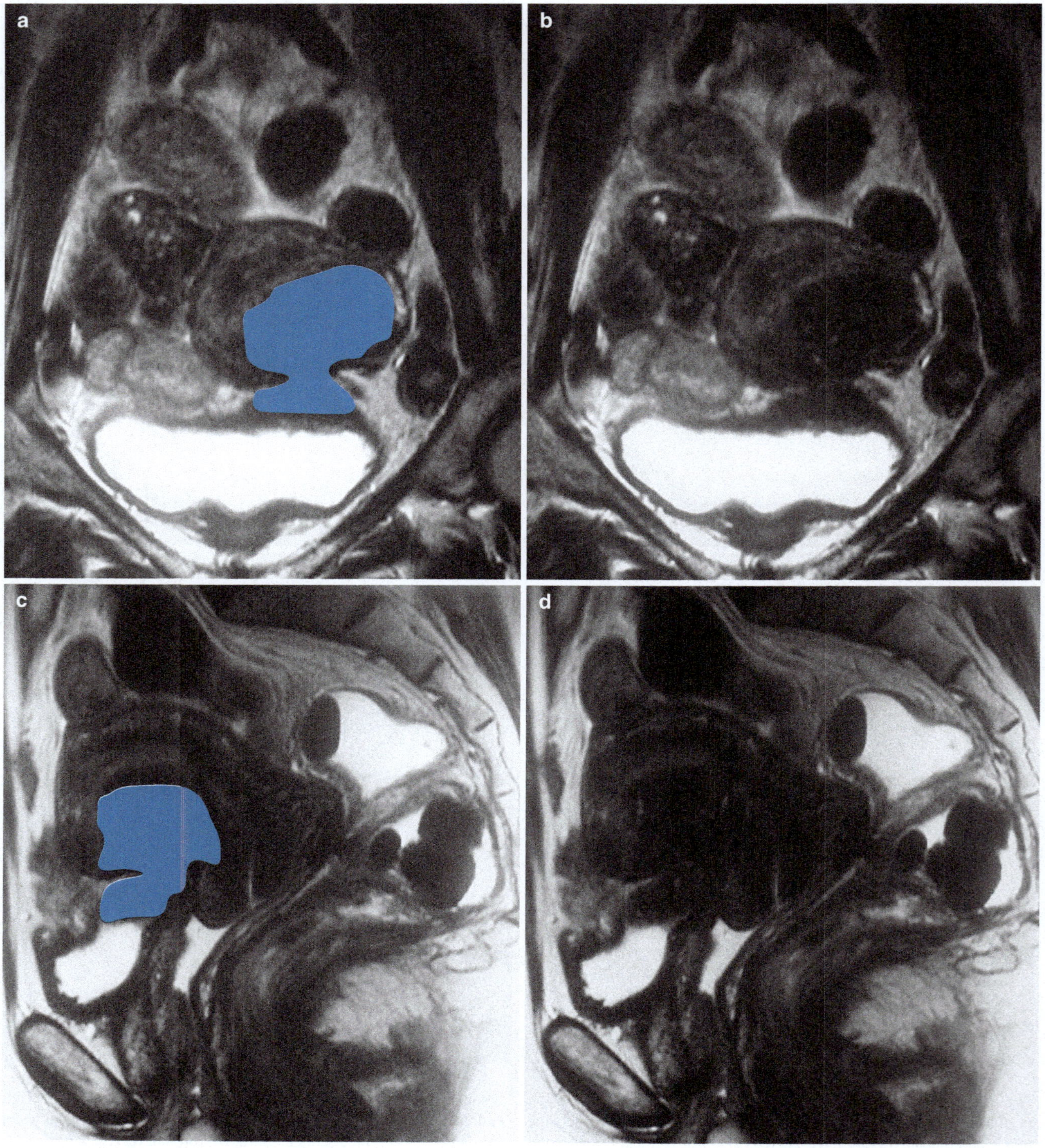

Fig. 4.50 Hourglass appearance (drawn in blue in **a**, **c** to figures **b**, **d**). Only part of the bladder lesion has contact and infiltrates the anterior wall of the uterus. (**a–d**) T2-weighted sequences. (**a**, **b**) Coronal. (**c**, **d**) Sagittal. (**e**, **f**) Laparoscopy showing anterior myometrial infiltration

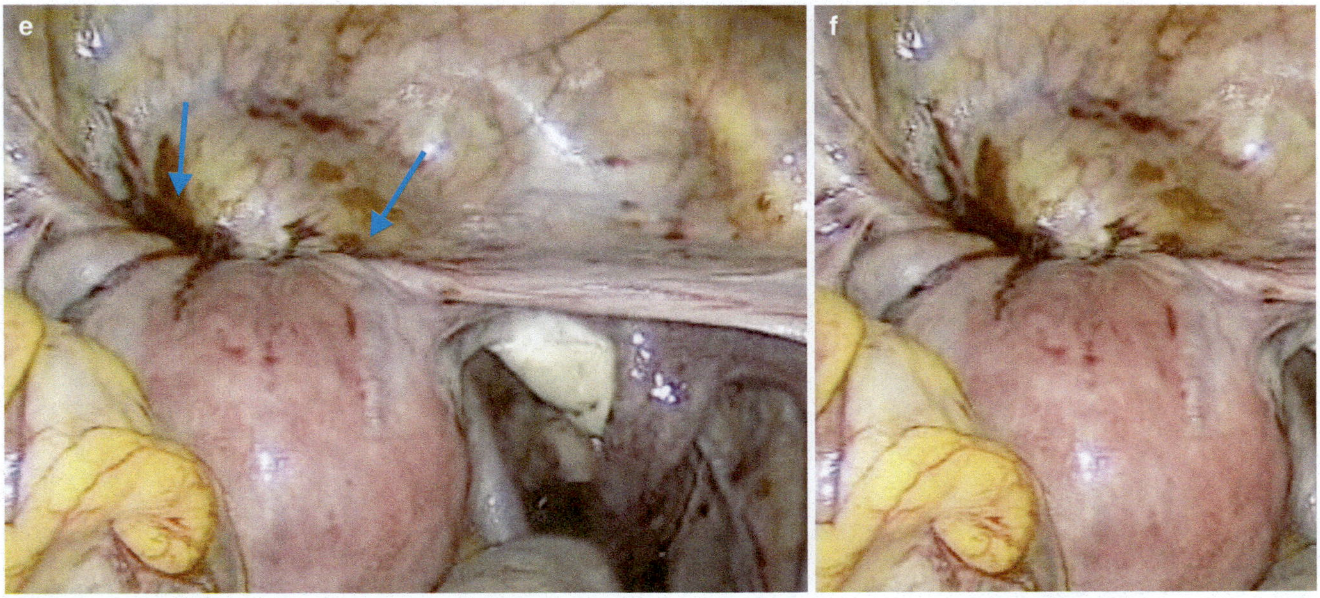

Fig. 4.50 (continued)

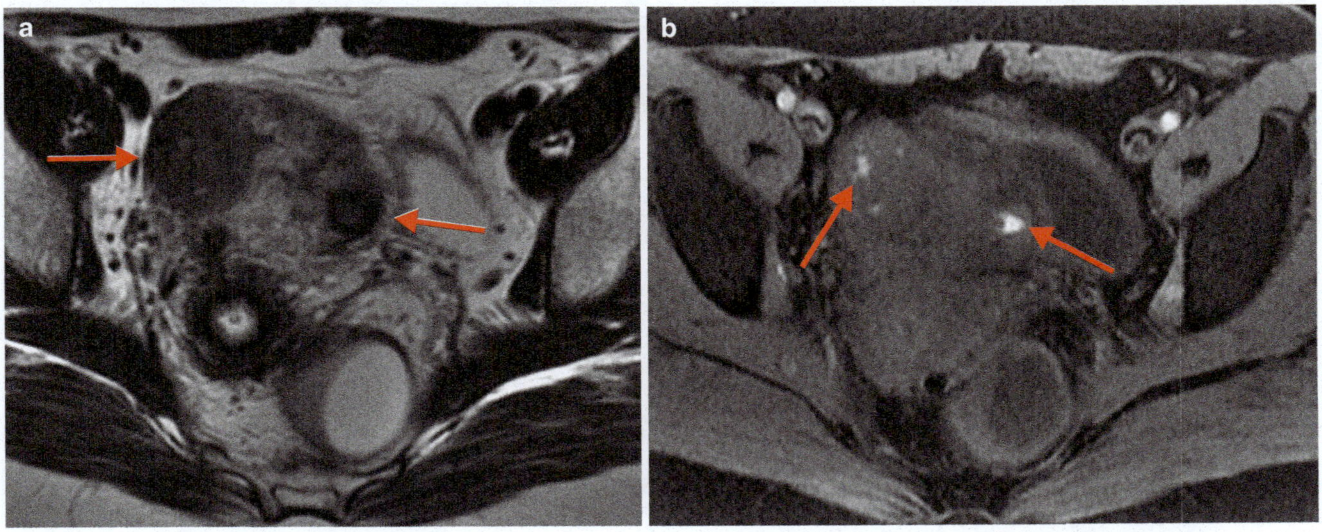

Fig. 4.51 Bilateral myometrial lesion (red arrows) in continuity with the round ligaments, ill-defined, predominantly hypointense in T2-weighted sequences (**a**, **c**, **e**), with hyperintense foci (ectopic endometrial glands and cysts) and bleeding in T1-weighted sequence (**b**, **d**). (**a**, **b**) Axial. (**c**, **d**, **e**) Sagittal. (**f**) Laparoscopy during resection of the lesion. (**g**) Lesion pathology (400×). Note only endometriotic glandular structure

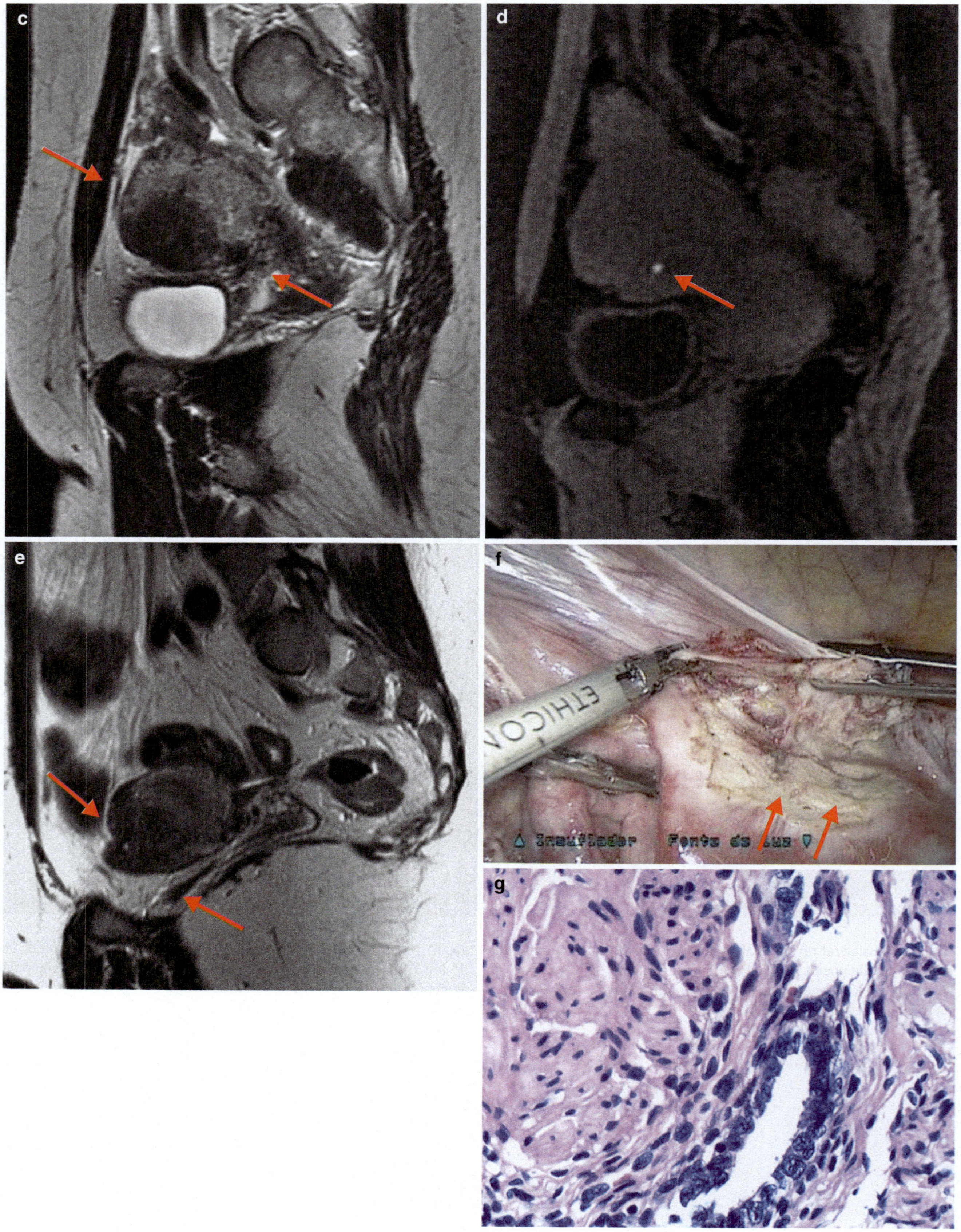

Fig. 4.51 (continued)

Table 4.5 Descriptor parameters of the myometrial lesion

Length of the involvement (longitudinal and transverse axes)
Myometrial penetration
Distance from the uterine cavity

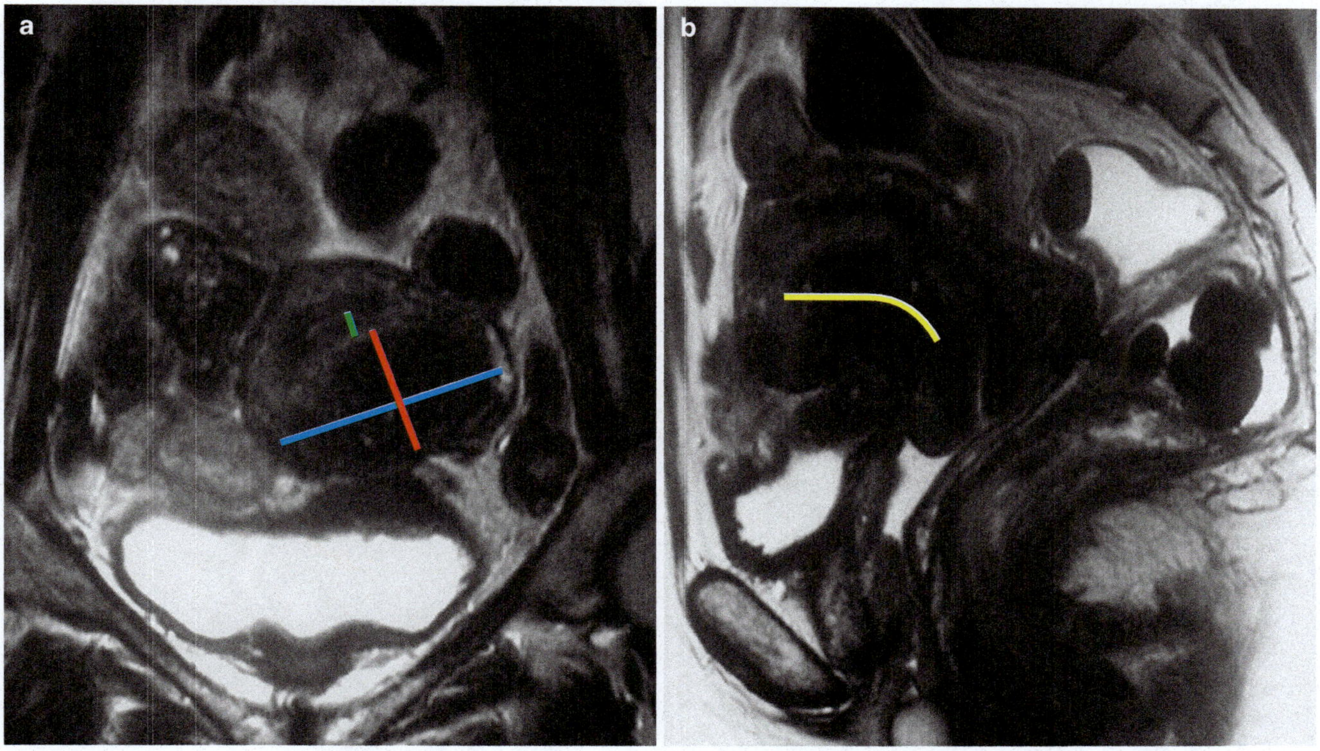

Fig. 4.52 Descriptive criteria. Length of extension in longitudinal (yellow) and transverse (blue) axes, penetration of the endometriotic process (red), and distance from the uterine cavity (green). (**a**, **b**) T2-weighted sequences. (**a**) Coronal. (**b**) Sagittal

4.1.3.5 Comments About Treatment

Accurate preoperative assessment of the extent of the uterine disease is required for a proper planning of surgical excision, since the success of the treatment depends on radical surgical removal. The myometrial involvement in the anterior compartment is considered a major cause of relapse after surgery for bladder endometriosis (Fig. 4.53) [16, 28].

Hence, resection of the uterine involvement should be performed when identified by MRI. However, when a lesion is large, the distance to the cavity is too small, leading to a complete resection that can result in hysterectomy. Thus, when considering a patient who wishes to get pregnant, it may become necessary to leave part of the deep myometrial disease (Fig. 4.54) [15].

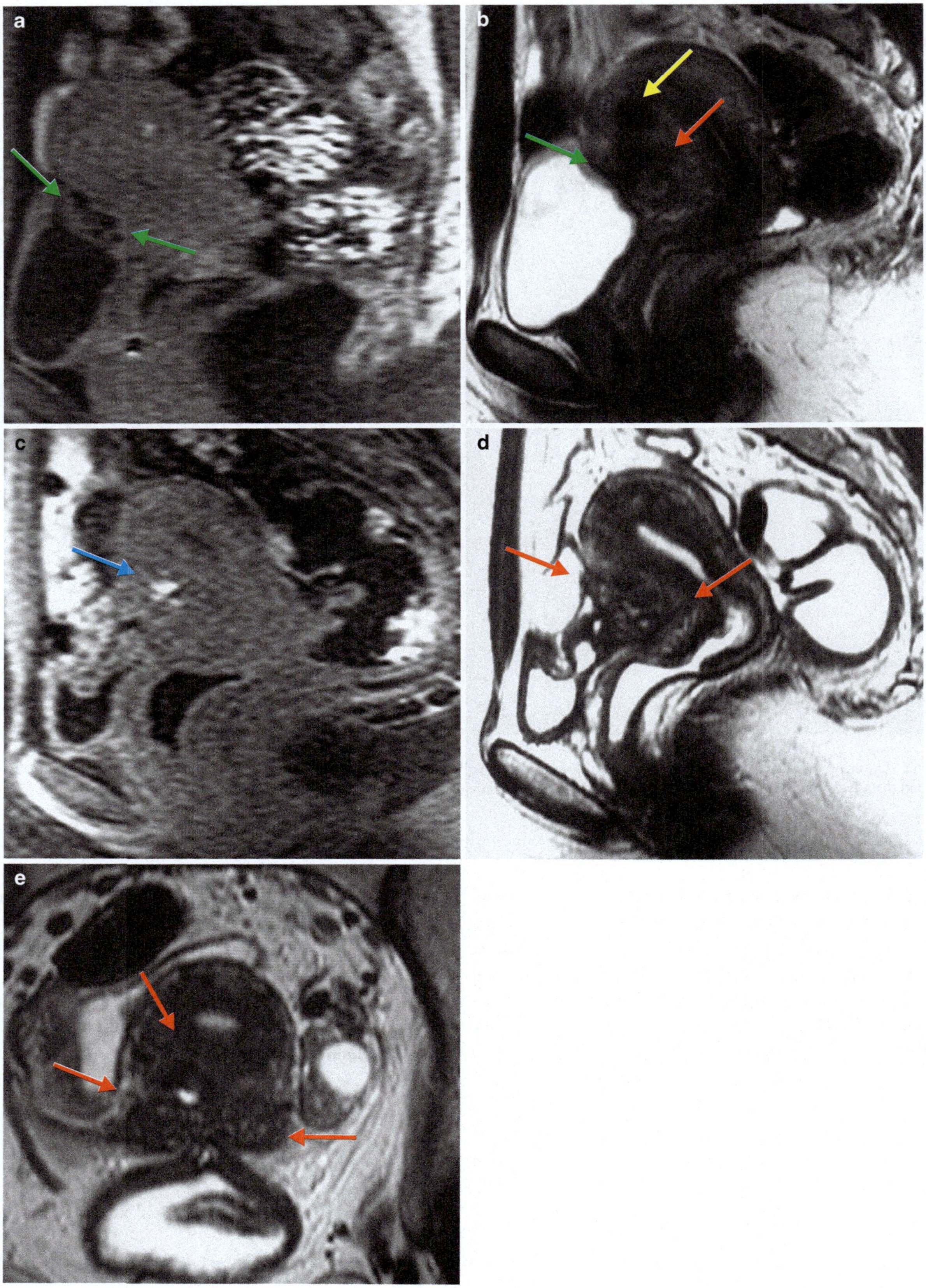

Fig. 4.53 Deep myometrial lesion in the anterior compartment, permeating the fibrocicatricial tissue. (**a**, **b**) First exam, asymptomatic. Note a discrete, poorly delimited hypointense area in T2 (red arrow in **b**) in the anterior myometrium, as well as leiomyoma (yellow arrow) and fibrocicatricial tissue with absence of signal foci in the vesicouterine recess (green arrows). (**e**–**c**) Second examination. Occasional pain when urinating during the menstrual period. Myometrial, bladder, and ligament infiltrative lesions with development of mass (red arrows) and hyperintense foci in T1 (blue arrow) and T2 (ectopic endometrial glands with bleeding). (**b**, **d**, **e**) T2-weighted sequences. (**a**, **c**) T1-weighted sequences. (**ad**) Sagittal. (**e**) Coronal short axis

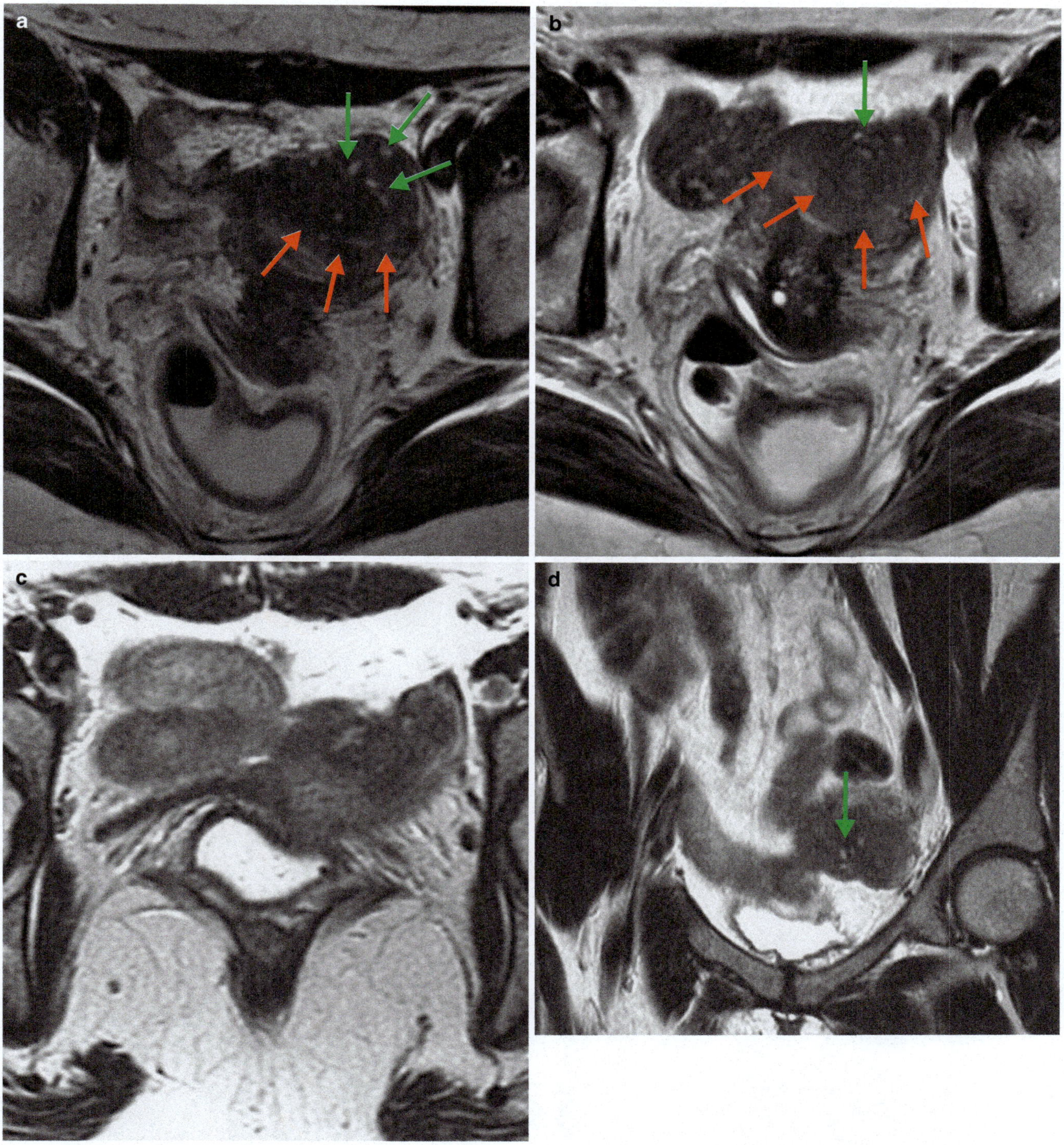

Fig. 4.54 Large anterior myometrial lesion, involving almost the entire anterior wall and body of the fundus extending to near the uterine cavity (red arrows). The lesion is infiltrative and has multiple hyperintense foci in T2 (green arrows). T2-weighted sequences. (**a–c**) Axial plane. (**d**) Short-axis coronal plane

4.2 Posterior Compartment

The most common deep endometriosis location is the posterior compartment. Peritoneal endometriosis in the cul-de-sac and chronic inflammation by cyclical bleeding result in infiltration of adjacent organs and obliteration of the cul-de-sac (Fig. 4.55).

Knowledge of the anatomical distribution and detail of the presurgical diagnosis of the extent of the deep endometriosis lesions in this compartment are highly important, as it has a complicated access, and relationship with vital pelvic structures. In this compartment, a lesion can infiltrate the uterosacral ligaments, retrocervical region and rectovaginal septum, and posterior vaginal fornix (Fig. 4.56).

These lesions may extend laterally, near the ureter, and require ureterolysis. Moreover, large centrally located lesions (retrocervical and rectovaginal septum) may affect the parametrium, paracolpos, hypogastric nerves, inferior hypogastric and lumbosacral plexus, and uterosacral ligaments and ureter (Figs. 4.57 and 4.58).

Therefore, posterior compartment deep endometriosis is one of the greatest surgical challenges due to its complex and multifocal pattern. MRI mapping will provide fundamental information that will enable a thorough and a personalized therapeutic approach.

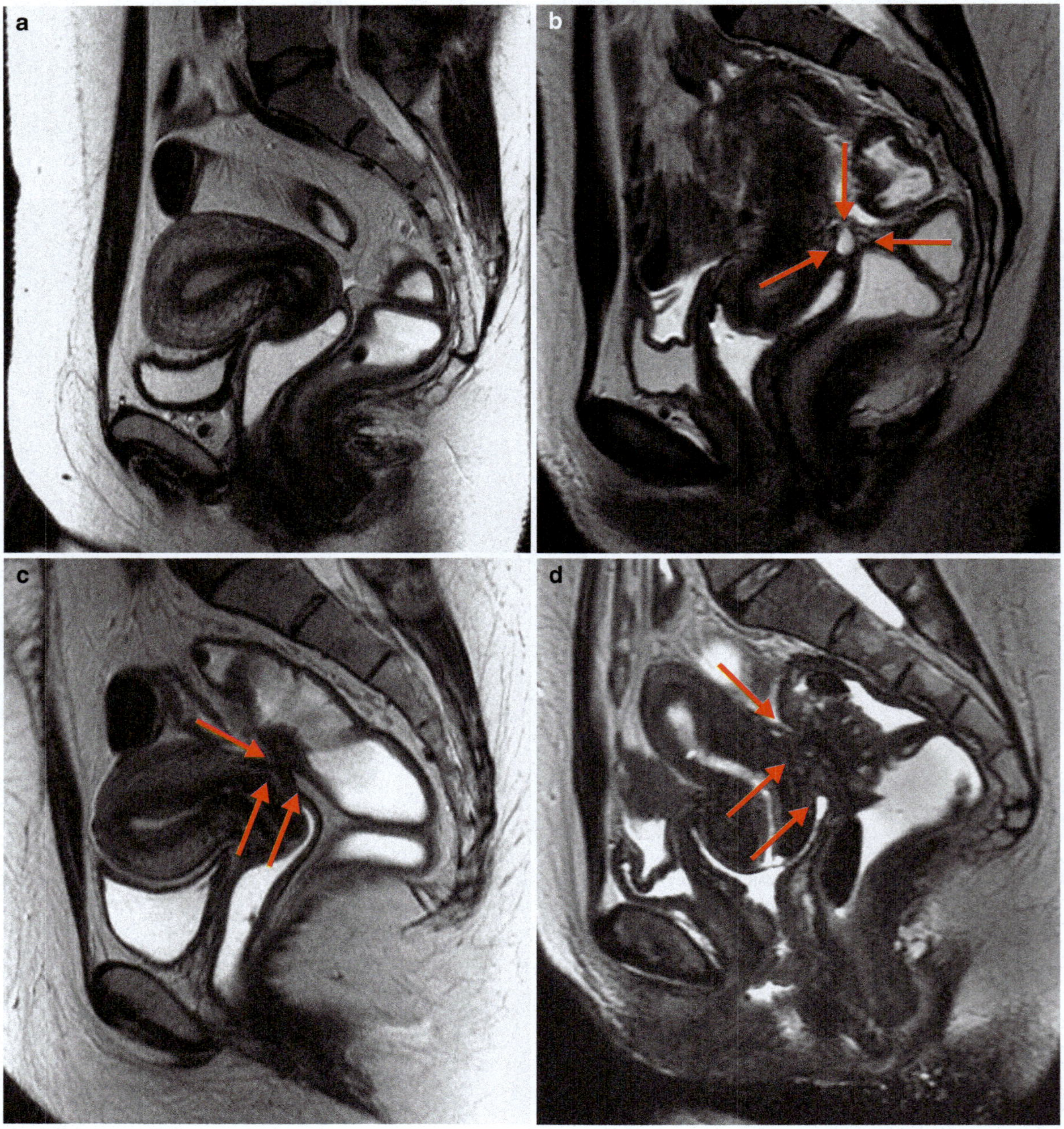

Fig. 4.55 Evolution of peritoneal endometriosis in the posterior cul-de-sac (arrows). (**a**) Normal posterior cul-de-sac. (**b**) Top of obliteration. (**c**) partial obliteration. (**d**) Complete obliteration. (**a–d**) Sagittal T2-weighted plane

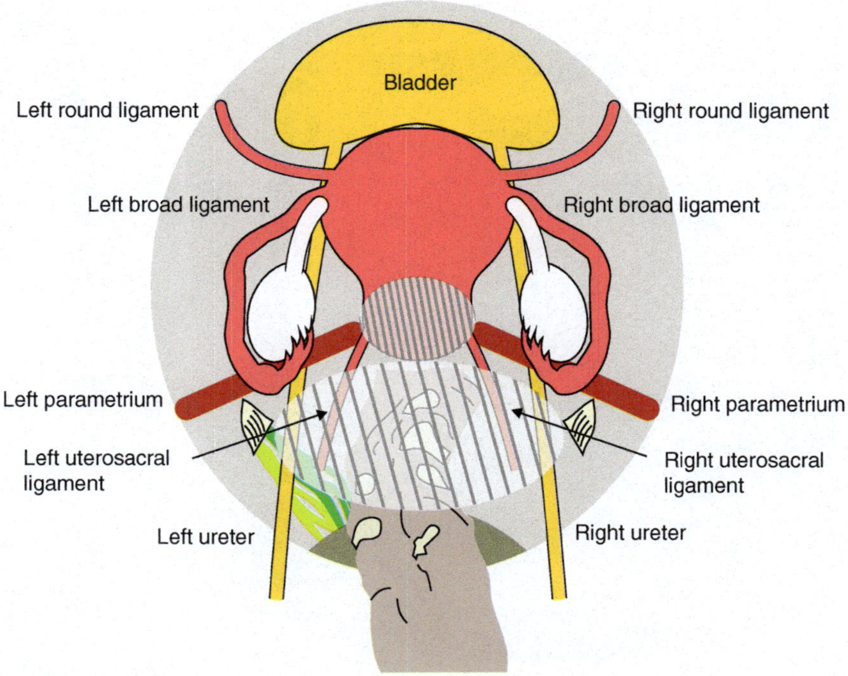

Fig. 4.56 Pattern of extension of deep endometriosis of the posterior compartment: (1) Lateral to the uterosacral ligaments, parametrium, and paracolpos. (2) Myometrium and vaginal fornix anteriorly. (3) Rectum and sigmoid posteriorly. Notice that the diagram was based on the laparoscopic view, where the left side corresponds to the right of an MR image and vice versa

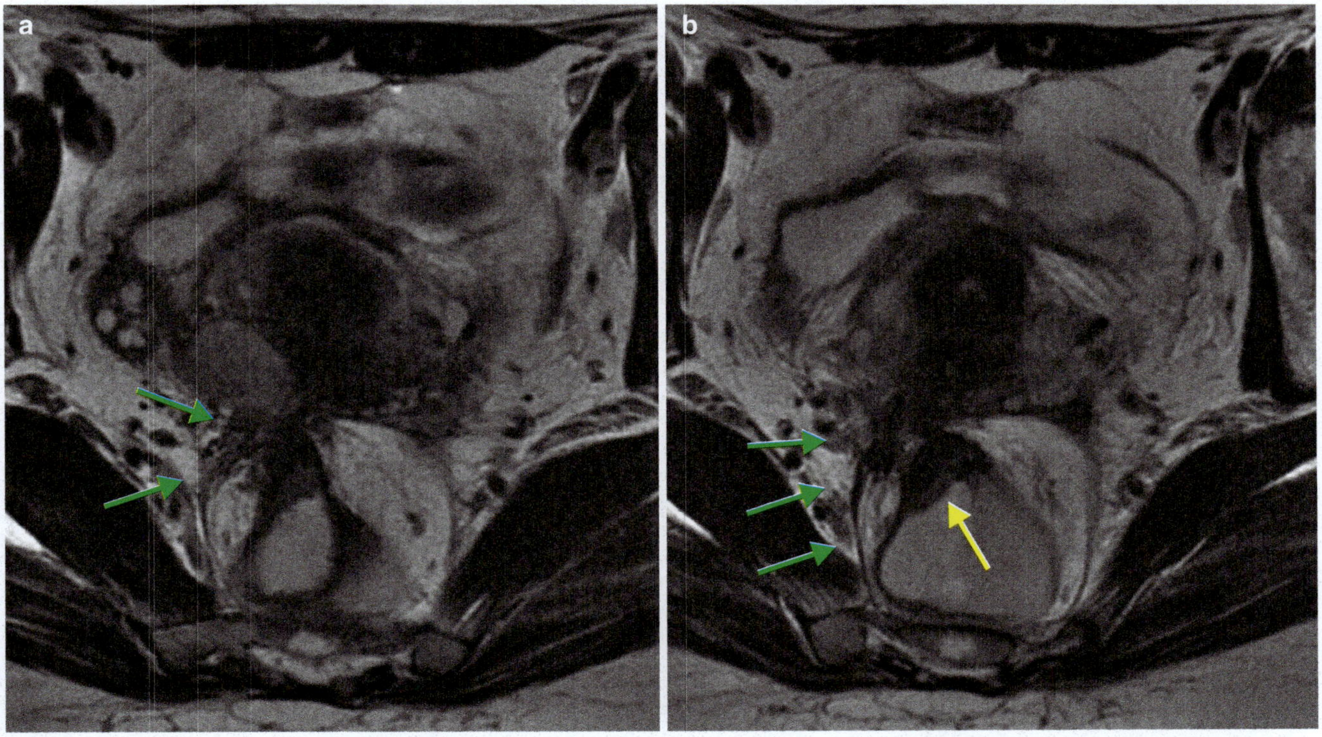

Fig. 4.57 (**a–d**) Lesion with lateral extension infiltrating the uterosacral ligaments, predominantly on the right (green arrows) to the parametrium, touching the ureter (blue arrows) and involving the hypogastric nerve (red arrow in **d**), requiring ureterolysis during the surgical procedure. Also notice further extension to the right (yellow arrows **a–c**)

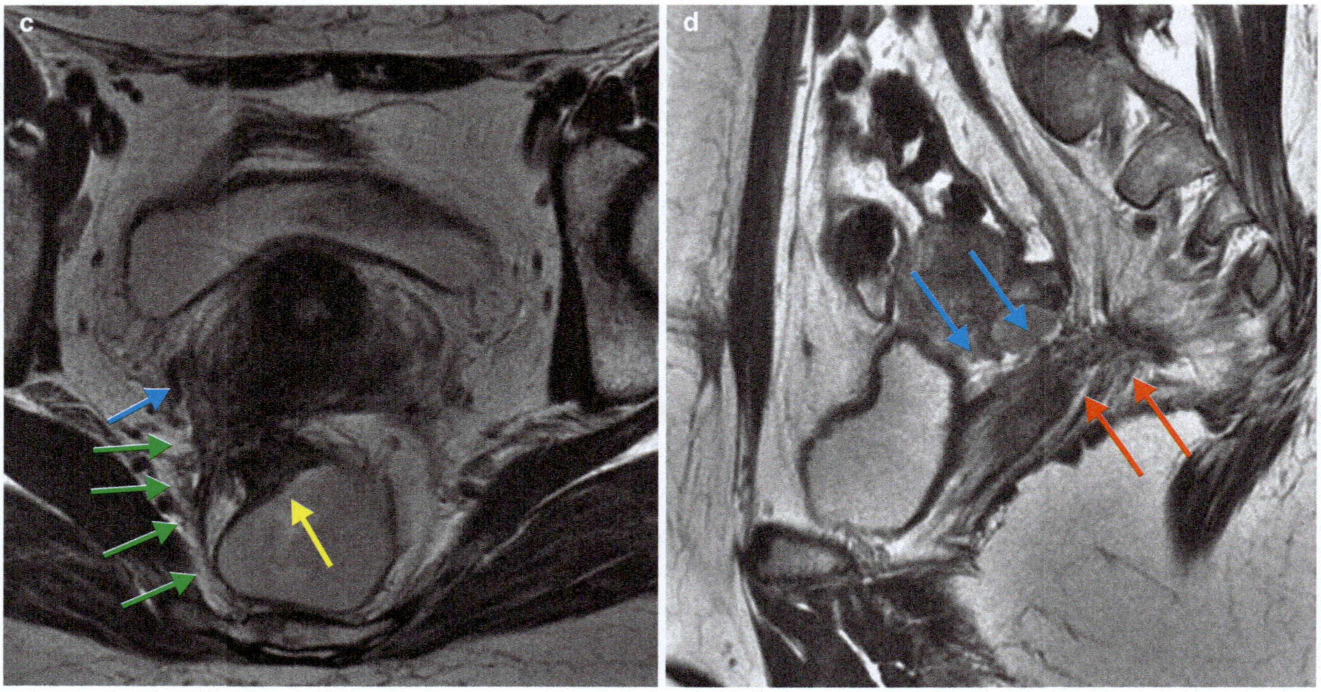

Fig. 4.57 (continued)

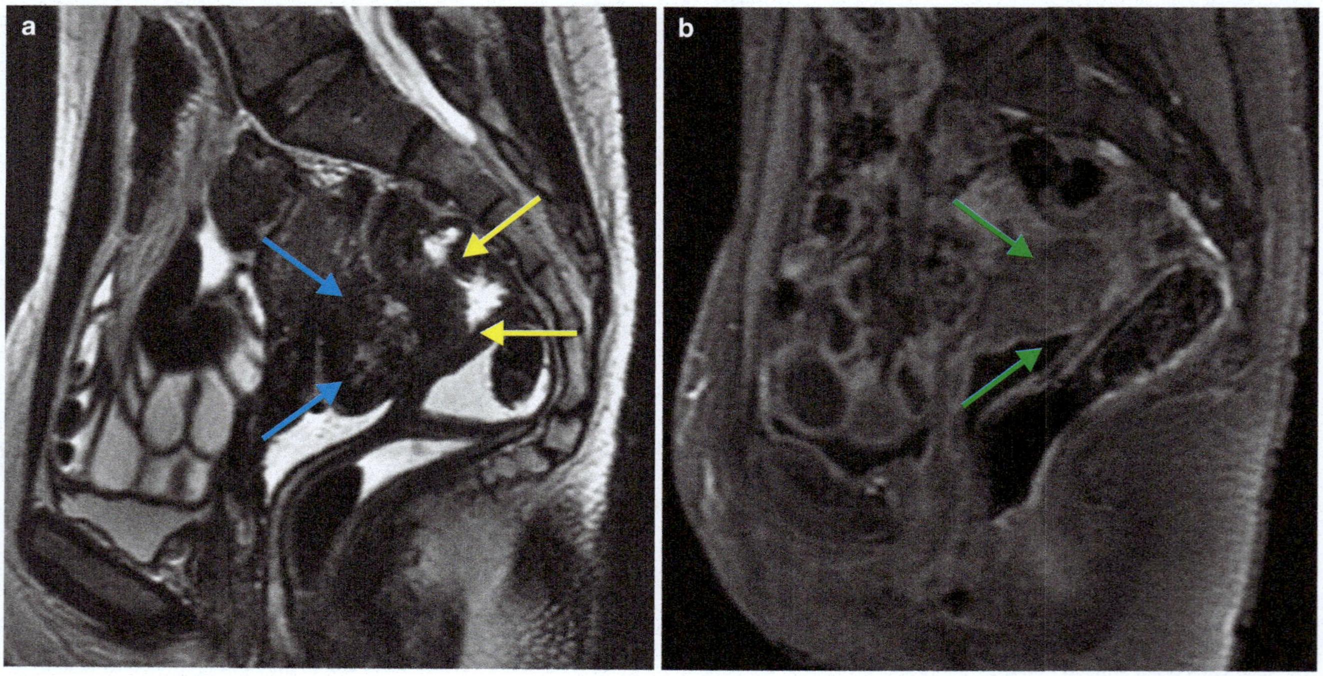

Fig. 4.58 Median lesion, retrocervical region, with great lateral extension to the uterosacral ligaments, parametrium (green), involving the uterine arteries (red), penetrating the rectum (yellow) and the myometrium (blue). (**b**, **d**) T1-weighted sequences with fat suppression and gadolinium. (**a**, **c**, **e**, **f**) T2-weighted sequences. (**a**–**c**) Sagittal plane. (**d**–**e**) Axial plane. (**f**) Long axis

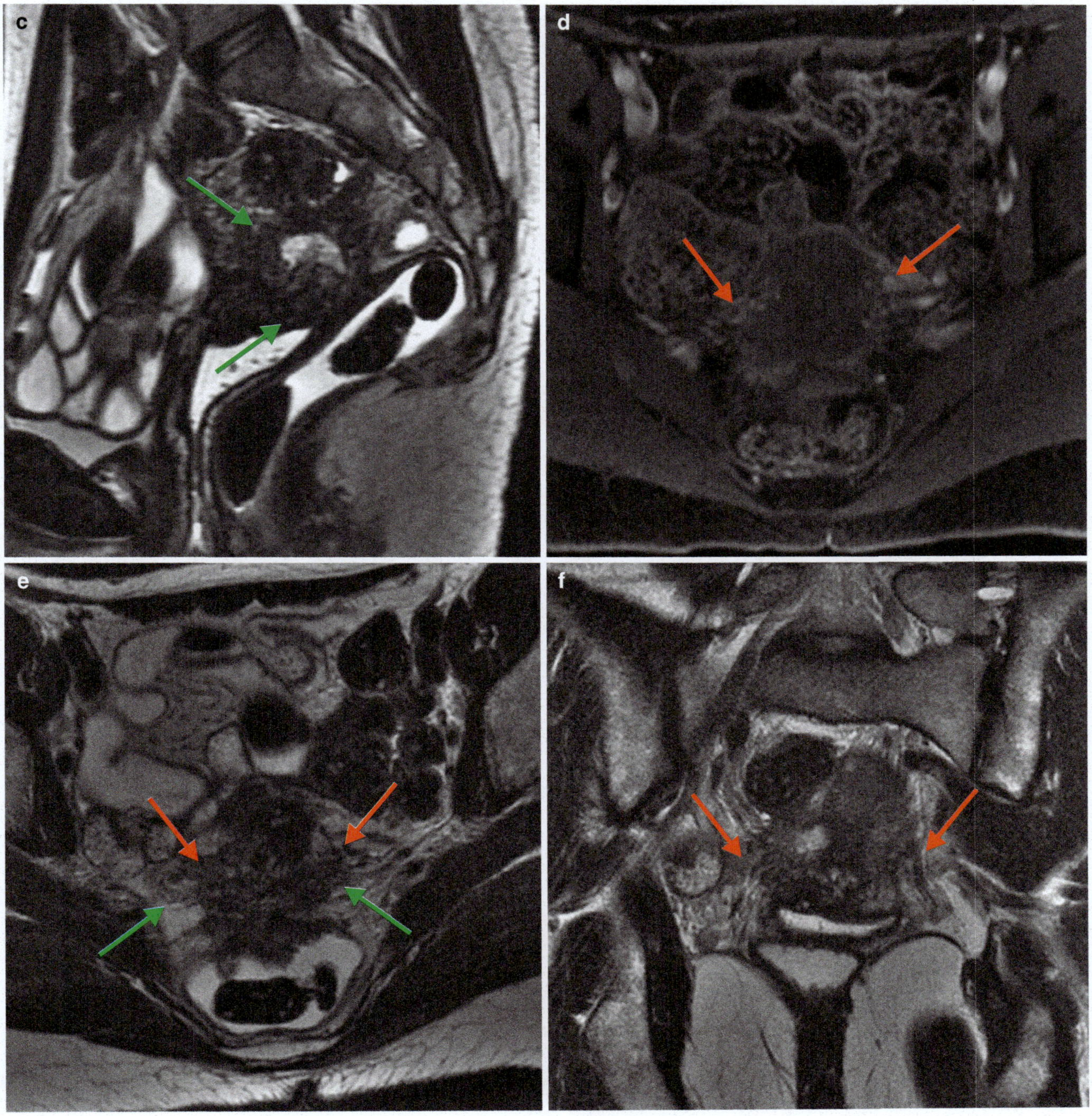

Fig. 4.58 (continued)

4.2.1 Retrocervical Region

4.2.1.1 Anatomy

The retrocervical region is an extraperitoneal space below the cul-de-sac, located between the uterine insertion of the uterosacral ligaments (torus uterinus) and the rectovaginal space (Fig. 4.59) [9, 29].

There is some confusion regarding the nomination of this region in the literature, especially in respect of the rectovaginal septum and the retrocervical region, probably related to the anatomic variation in the depth of the cul-de-sac. In some patients, the cul-de-sac is deeply located posterior to the vagina.

Authors have defined the retrocervical region as delimited cranially and laterally by the insertion of the uterosacral ligaments, inferiorly by the rectovaginal septum, anteriorly by the cervix and vaginal fornix insertion, and posteriorly by the rectum (Fig. 4.60).

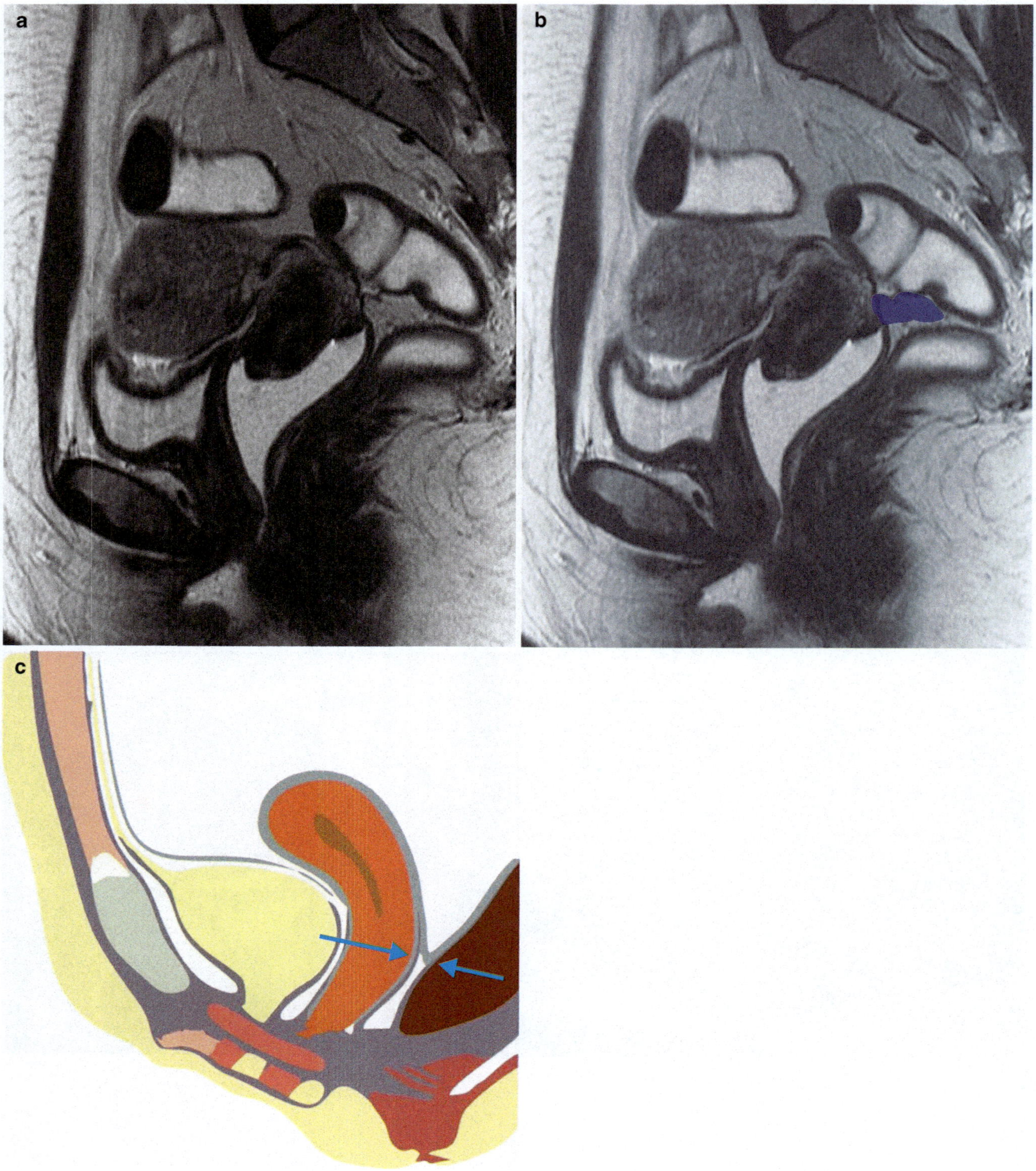

Fig. 4.59 (**a**, **b**) The retrocervical region is a virtual extraperitoneal space below the peritoneal reflection of the posterior cul-de-sac, between this and the rectovaginal septum, behind the isthmus and the cervix. Notice the drawing in blue in (**b**), reference in (**a**), and arrow in diagram (**c**). T2-weighted sequences. (**a**, **b**) Sagittal plane. (**c**) Diagram

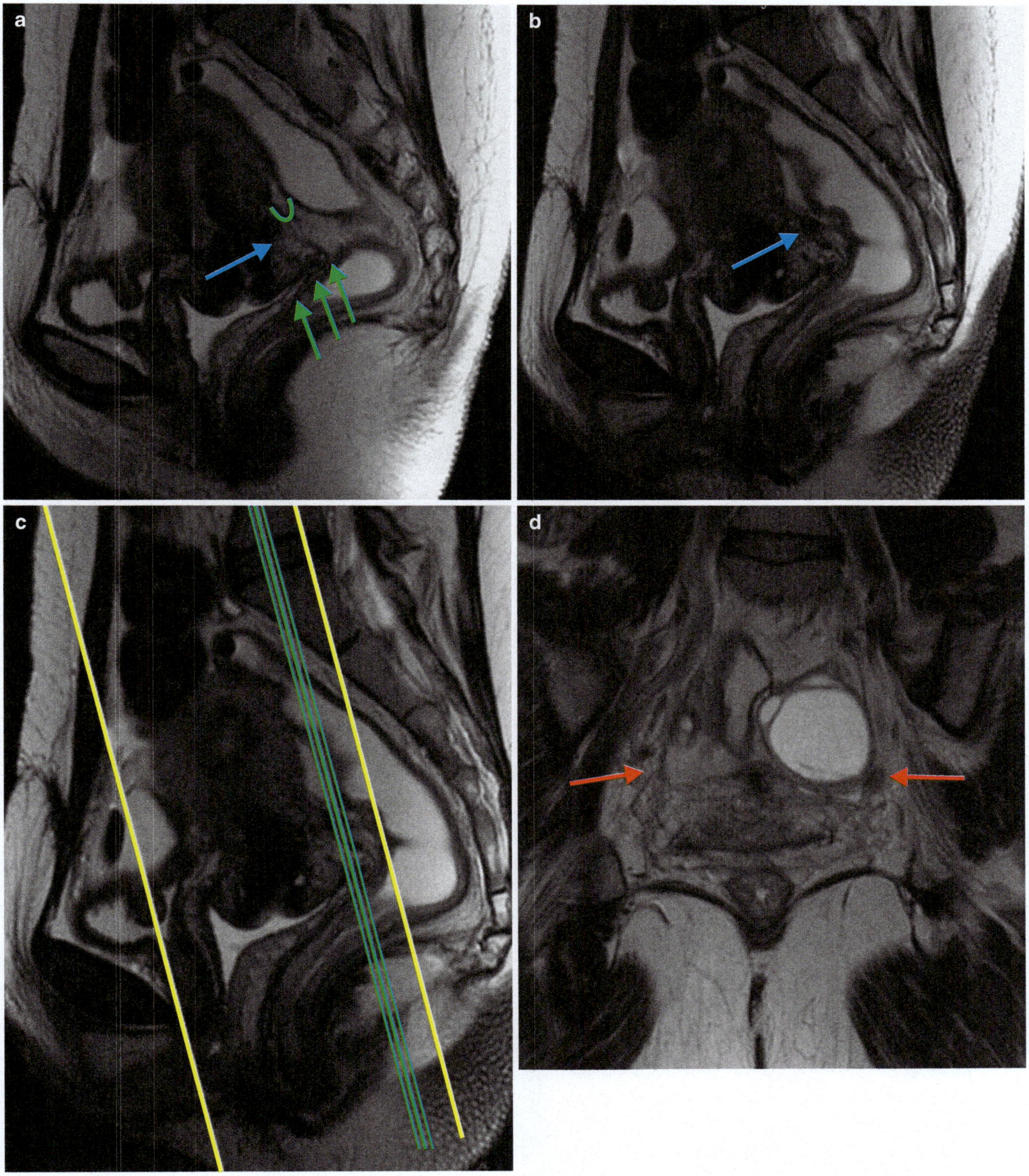

Fig. 4.60 Retrocervical region delimited in the cranial axis by the cul-de-sac (green line in **a**) and the upper portion of the rectovaginal septum (green arrows in **a** and ellipse in **i**), lateral (**c**–**h**) by the insertion of the uterosacral ligaments (red arrows) and anteroposterior by the cervix and the insertion of the vaginal fornix and rectum. Notice small retrocervical hypointense node (blue arrow in **b** and blue line in **e**, **h**). (**a**–**h**) T2-weighted sequence. (**a**–**c**, **f**) Sagittal. (**g**, **h**) Axial. (**i**) Laparoscopy showing the topography of the retrocervical region (blue ellipse)

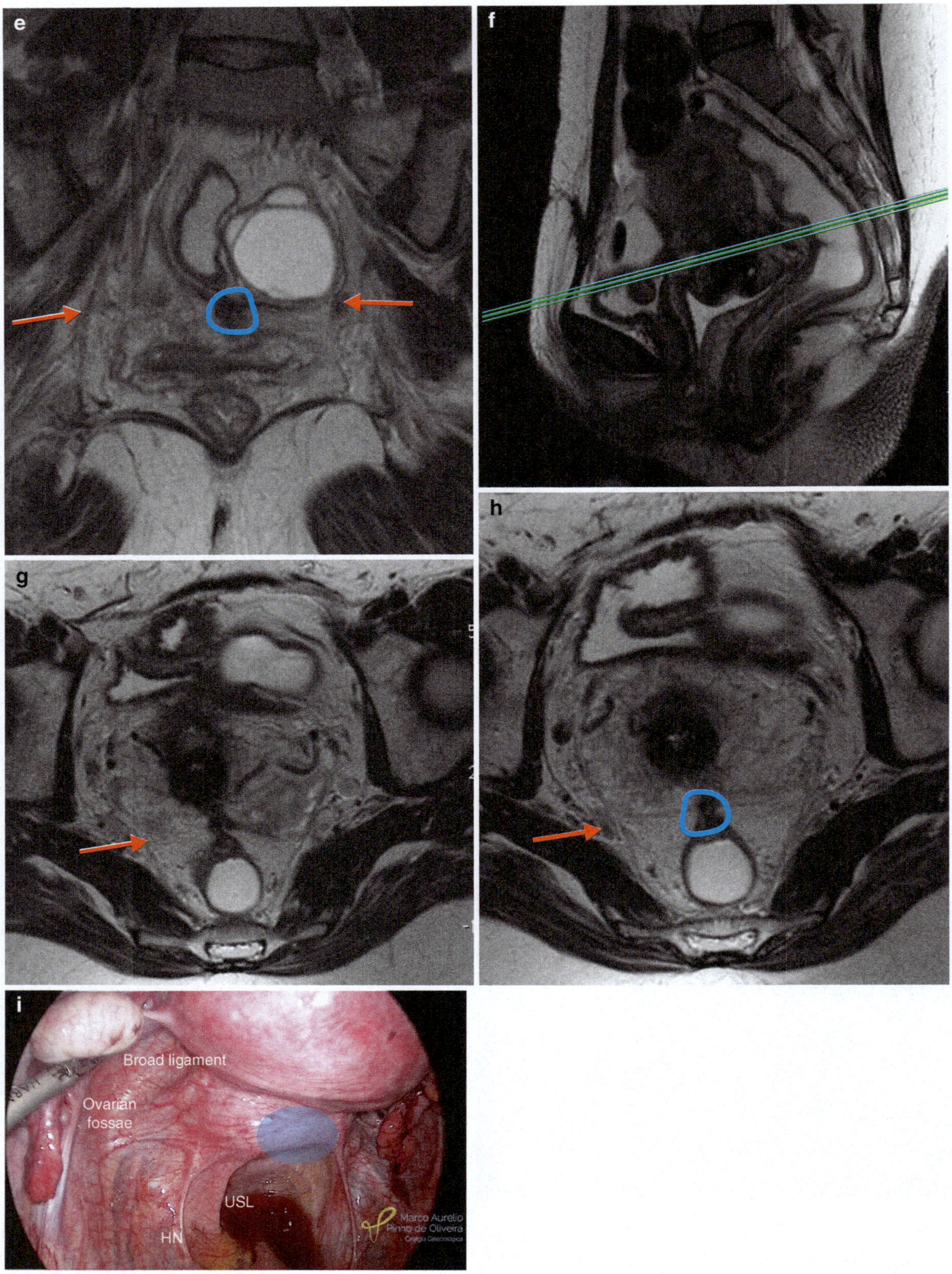

Fig. 4.60 (continued)

4.2.1.2 Most Common Aspects of the Endometriosis

The location is typically at the midline; as the lesion progresses, it extends in all directions, infiltrating adjacent structures and promoting adhesion, which may result in a frozen pelvis.

When there is a small retrocervical lesion, a well-prepared interpreter and a high-resolution examination may be required for the node to be identified with precision (Fig. 4.61) [30].

The retrocervical lesion has a typical extension pattern (Table 4.6):

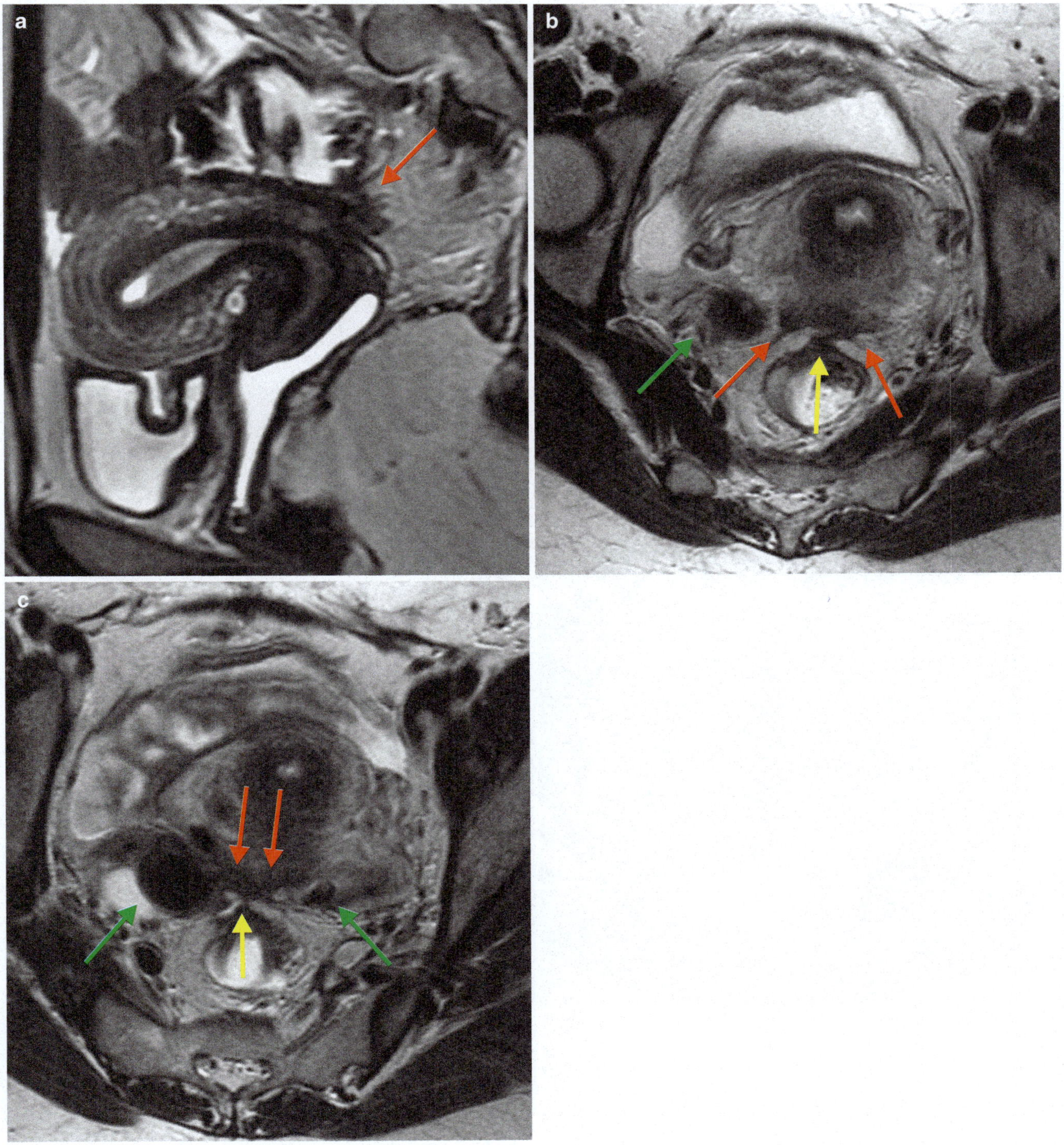

Fig. 4.61 The retrocervical lesion (red arrows), when small, may be presented as a discrete hypointense central node in T2, with no bleeding; as a consequence, for its detection, a well-trained interpreter and a high-resolution examination are required. (**a–c**) T2-weighted sequences. (**a**) Sagittal. (**b**, **c**) Coronal short axis. Notice medial and posterior deviations of ovaries with endometriomas (green arrows **b** and **c**) and discrete and superficial rectal engagement (yellow arrows)

Table 4.6 Retrocervical lesion extension pattern

• Lateral to the uterosacral ligament
• Inferior and anterior to the posterior vaginal fornix
• Inferior to the retovaginal space
• Superior, covering the uterine serosa
• Anterior to the uterus posterior myometrial wall
• Posterior to the rectal wall

- Lateral to the uterosacral ligaments, being able to compromise the parametrium (lateral compartment) and thus the uterine artery and the ureter, close to the hypogastric nerve (Fig. 4.62)
- Inferior and anterior to the posterior vaginal fornix, sometimes reaching the vaginal mucosa, obliterating the vaginal fornix (Fig. 4.63)

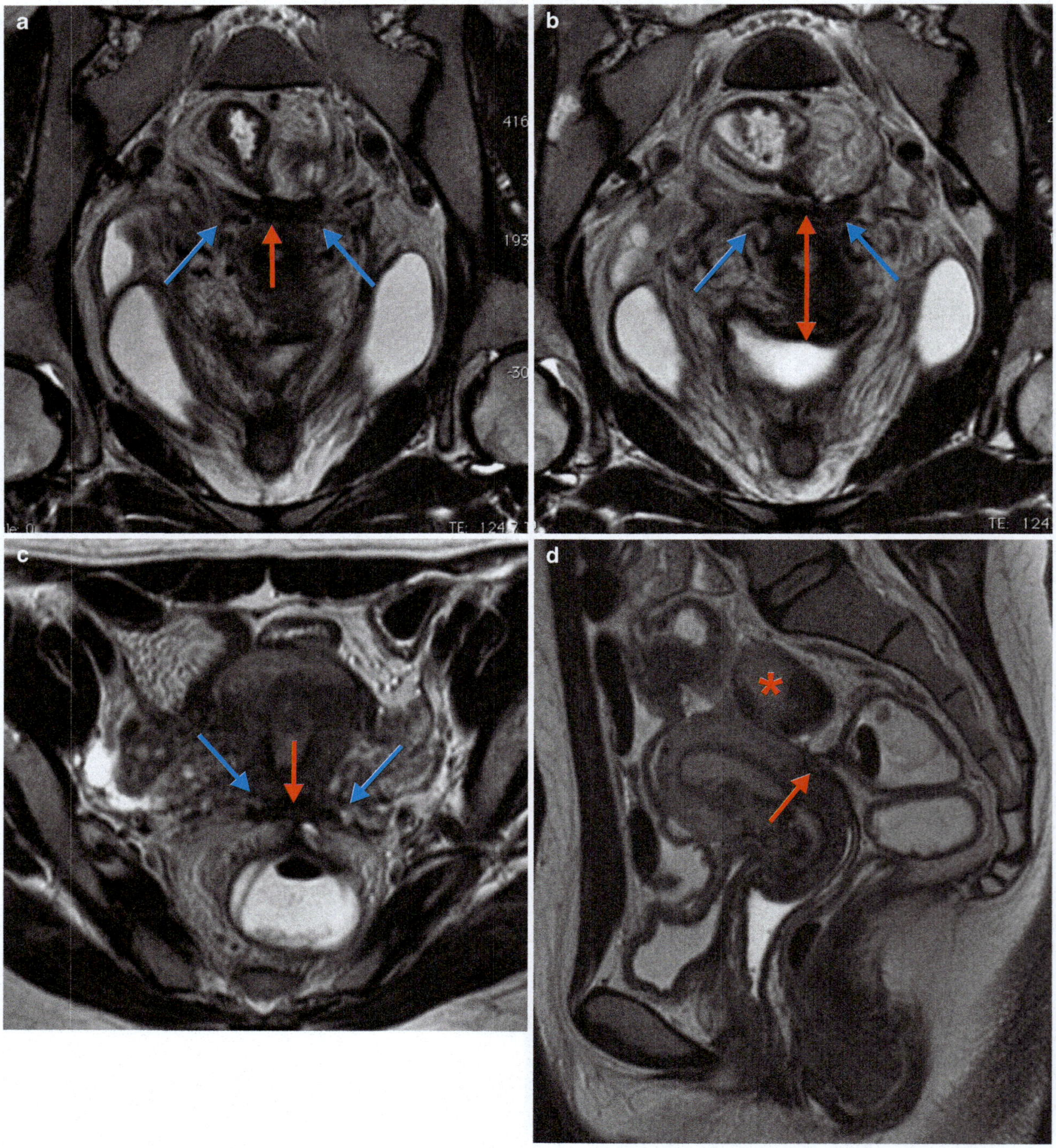

Fig. 4.62 Retrocervical lesion (red arrows **a**–**e**) with a lateral extension to the uterosacral ligaments (blue arrows **a**–**c**). Notice endometrioma in the right ovary (* **d**, **e**), medially deflected and retrouterine (sagittal). (**a**–**d**) T2-weighted sequences. (**e**) T1-weighted sequence. (**a**, **b**) Coronal short axis. (**c**) Axial. (**d**, **e**) Sagittal. (**f**) Laparoscopy demonstrating the lesion (black arrows), obliteration of the cul-de-sac with adnexal deviation, and peritoneal decidual reaction (green arrows)

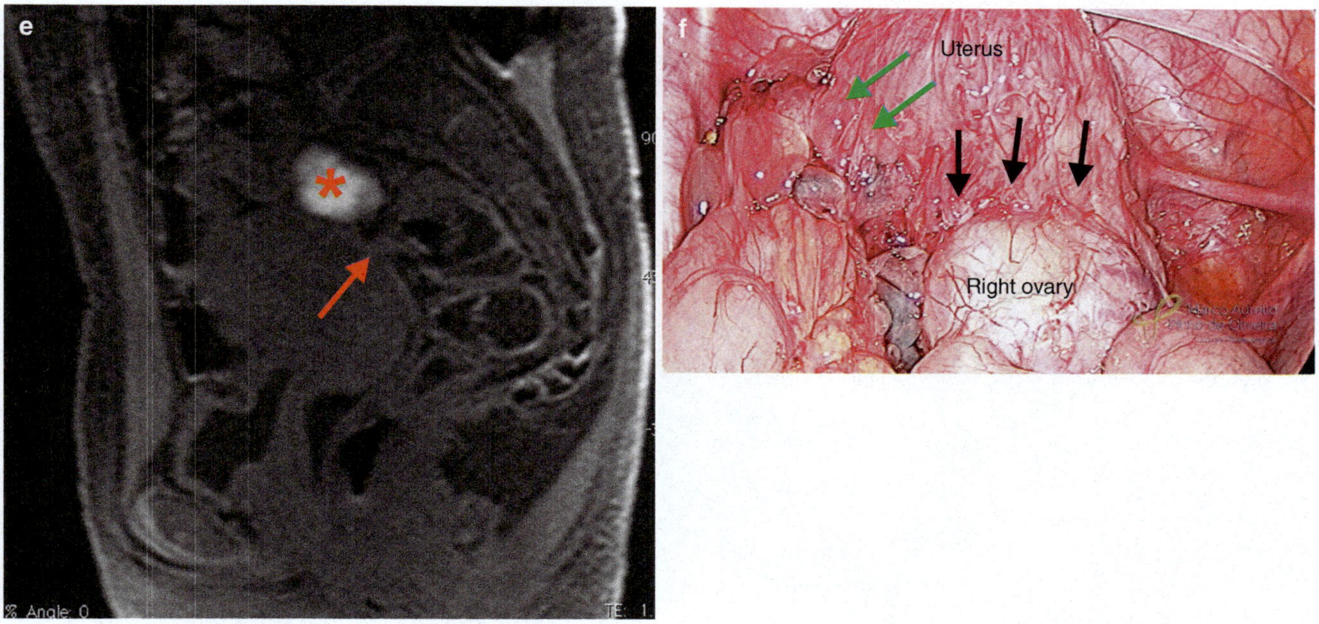

Fig. 4.62 (continued)

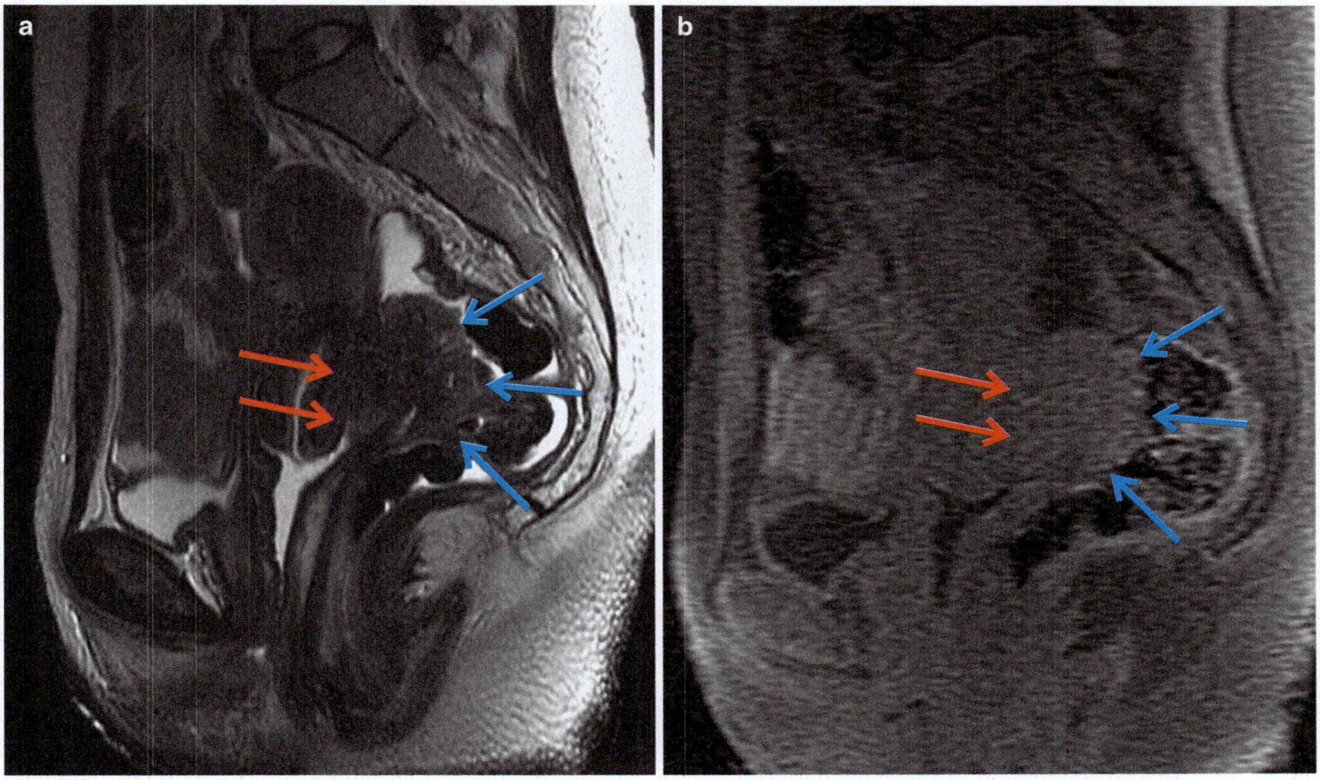

Fig. 4.63 (**a**, **b**) Inferior and anterior extension to the posterior vaginal fornix, obliterating the vaginal fornix (red arrows **a**–**d**). Notice further extension to rectal segments, obliterating the cul-de-sac and penetrating the intestinal wall (blue arrows **a**–**d**) and bilateral involvement of ligaments (green arrows in **c**, **d**). Lesion with predominance of fibrosis, hypointense in the T2-weighted sequences (**a**, **c**) and with an intermediate signal in T1 (**b**). (**a**, **b**) Sagittal. (**c**, **d**) Axial. (**e**, **f**) Laparoscopy of the beginning of the procedure (**e**) and after resection of the vaginal lesion (**f**)

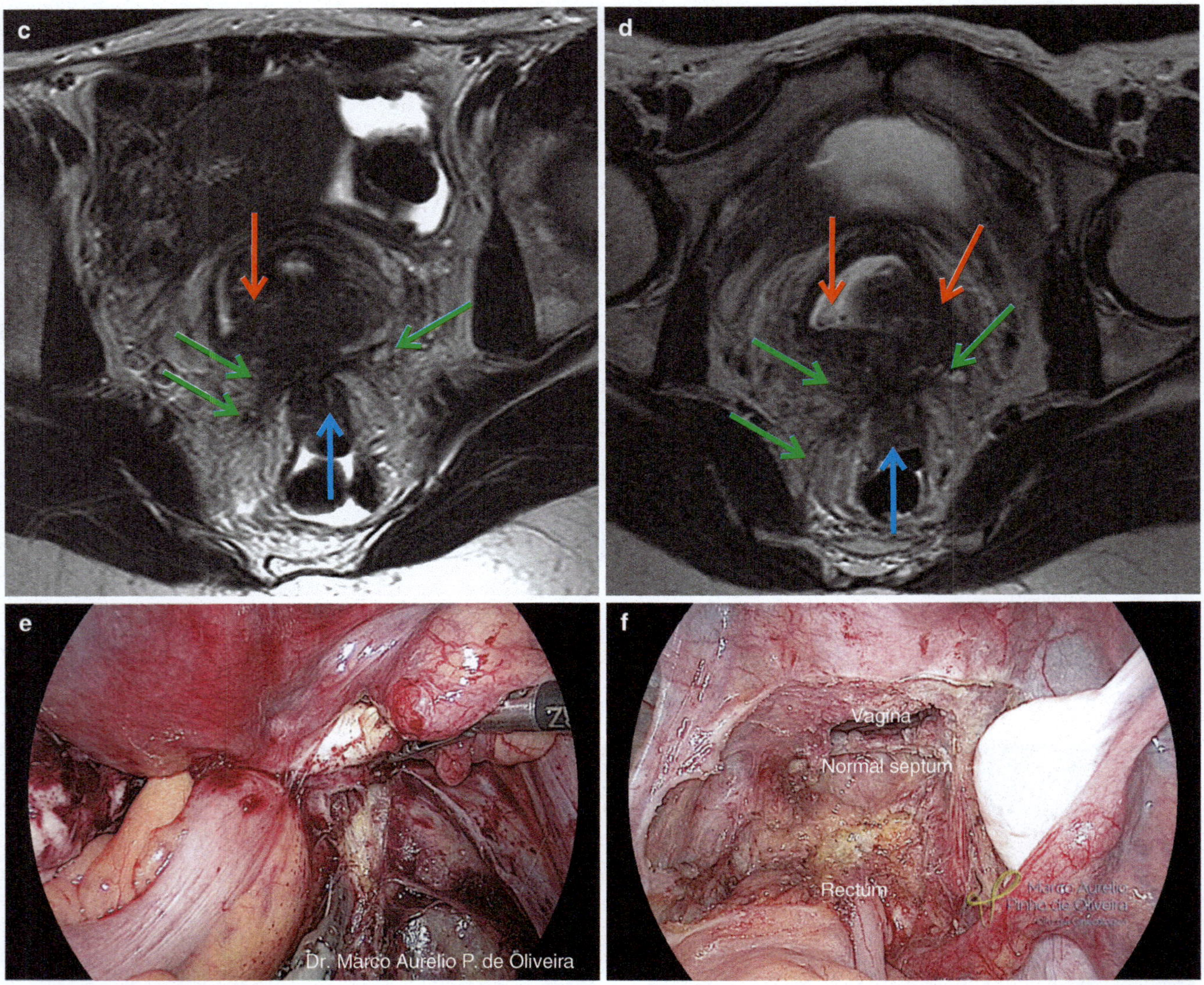

Fig. 4.63 (continued)

- Inferior to the rectovaginal space
- Superior, covering the posterior uterine serosa as a plaque-like lesion, from the fundus to the retrocervical region (Fig. 4.64)
- Anterior into the myometrium and being able to reach the uterine cavity (Fig. 4.65)
- Posterior to the rectal wall, obliterating the cul-de-sac and penetrating the intestinal wall, usually sparing the mucosa (Fig. 4.66)

A physical examination alone may be insufficient to assess the extent of infiltration of the endometriosis in this topography [31].

The pattern of the extent of the retrocervical lesion can be asymmetrical, with a predominance of the involvement of one organ. For example, the intestinal (in the rectum and sigmoide) or myometrial component (from the fundus to the cervix) can be more prominent than the retrocervical lesion (Fig. 4.67).

When the lesion is predominantly located in the torus uterinus, it promotes an asymmetric adherence, with ipsilateral uterine flexion, as well as rectal retraction. Likewise, when there is significant myometrial penetration, it produces an accentuated retroflexion of the uterus (Fig. 4.68) [26].

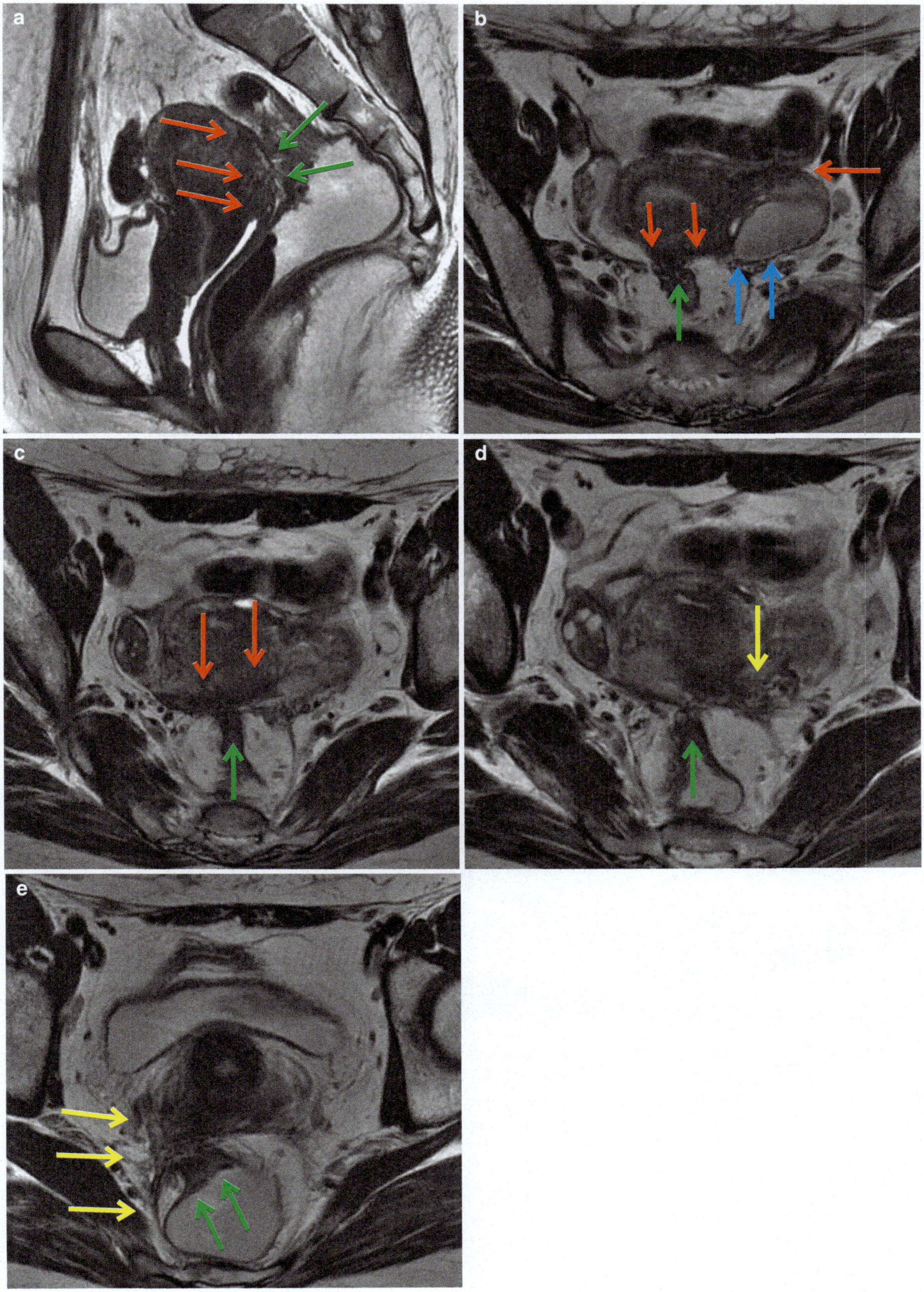

Fig. 4.64 Superior extension, covering the posterior uterine serosa, from the fundus to the retrocervical region (red arrows **a**–**c**) with a view of the mantle, obliterating the cul-de-sac (red arrow in **a**) and promoting important adherence with the adnexa (blue arrow in **b**) rectosigmoid (green arrows **a**–**e**) and vagina, superiorly retracted (**a**). Also, note bilateral ligament and right parametrial extension (yellow arrows **d** and **e**). T2-weighted sequences. (**a**) Sagittal. (**b**–**e**) Axial

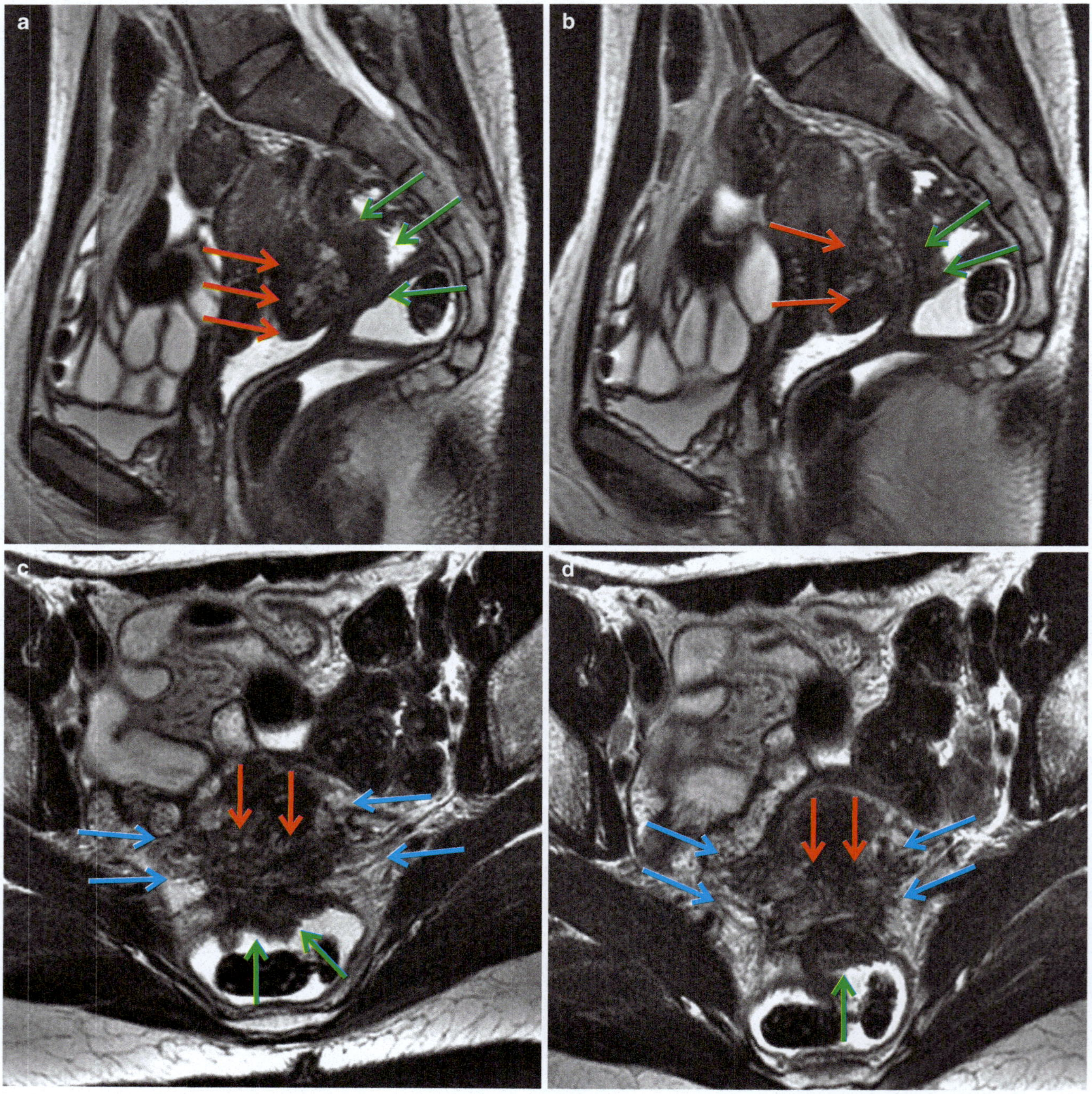

Fig. 4.65 Anterior extension to the myometrium of the isthmus and cervix, intravaginal and supravaginal, without reaching the uterine cavity (red arrows **a–d**). Notice extensive parametrium and bilateral ligament involvement (blue arrow **c**, **d**) and rectal involvement (green arrow **a–d**). (**a–d**) T2-weighted sequences. (**a**, **b**) Sagittal. (**c**, **d**) Axial

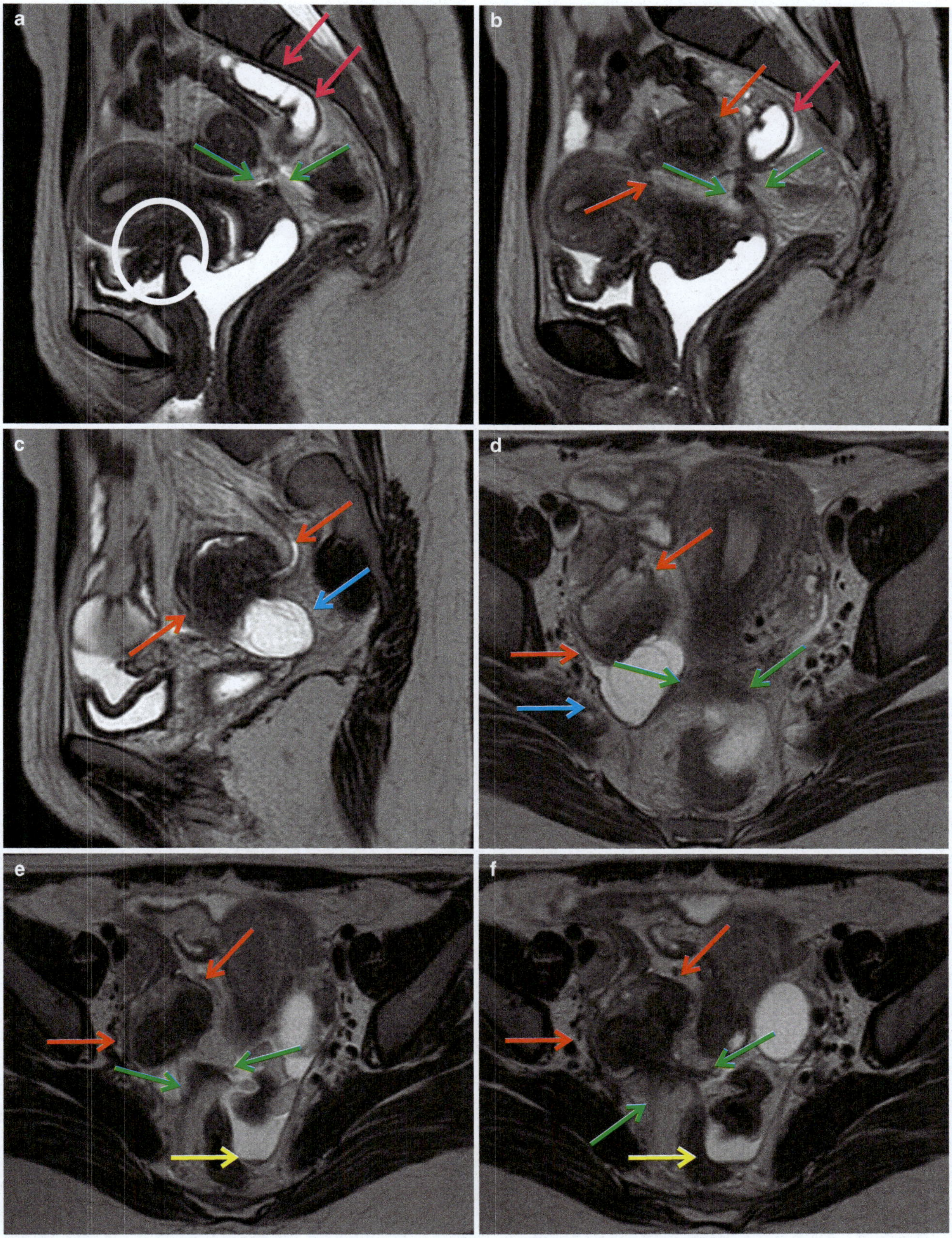

Fig. 4.66 Asymmetric posterior extension of retrocervical lesion (green arrows) to the cecum, which by anatomical variation insinuates itself in the pelvis (purple arrows **k**, **l**), penetrating into the mucosa, causing reduction of lumen (red arrows) and distension of the appendix (pink arrows), besides ligamentous involvement and pseudocyst formation (blue arrow). Notice liquid with hematic level in the cul-de-sac caused by peritoneal endometriosis (yellow arrow) and small deep endometriosis in the anterior compartment (white circle **a**). (**a**, **b**) MRI enterography showing the extension from the cecum to the pelvis (purple arrow **k**, **l**). T2-weighted sequences. (**a**–**c**) Sagittal. (**d**–**l**) Axial. (**h**–**l**) Coronal

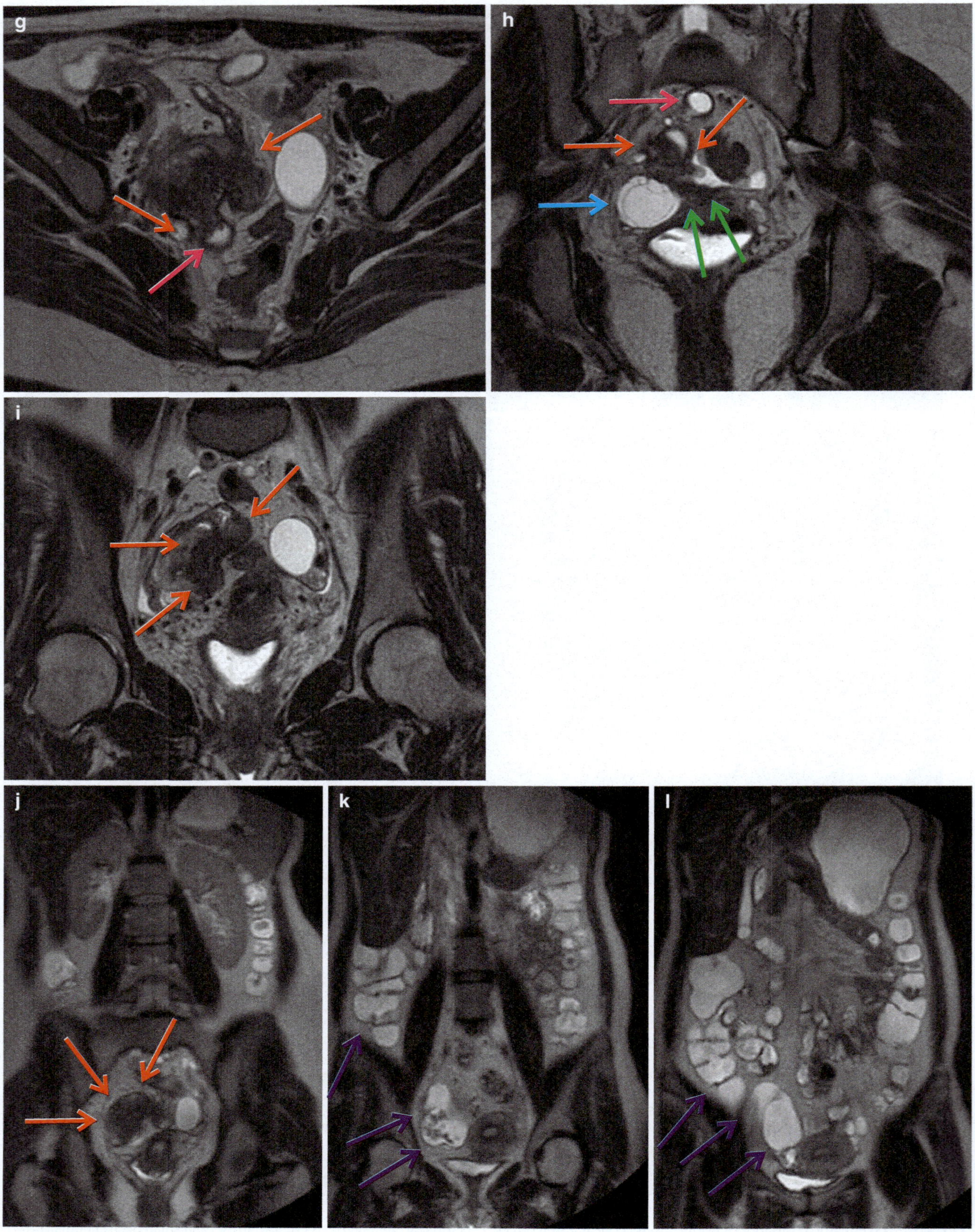

Fig. 4.66 (continued)

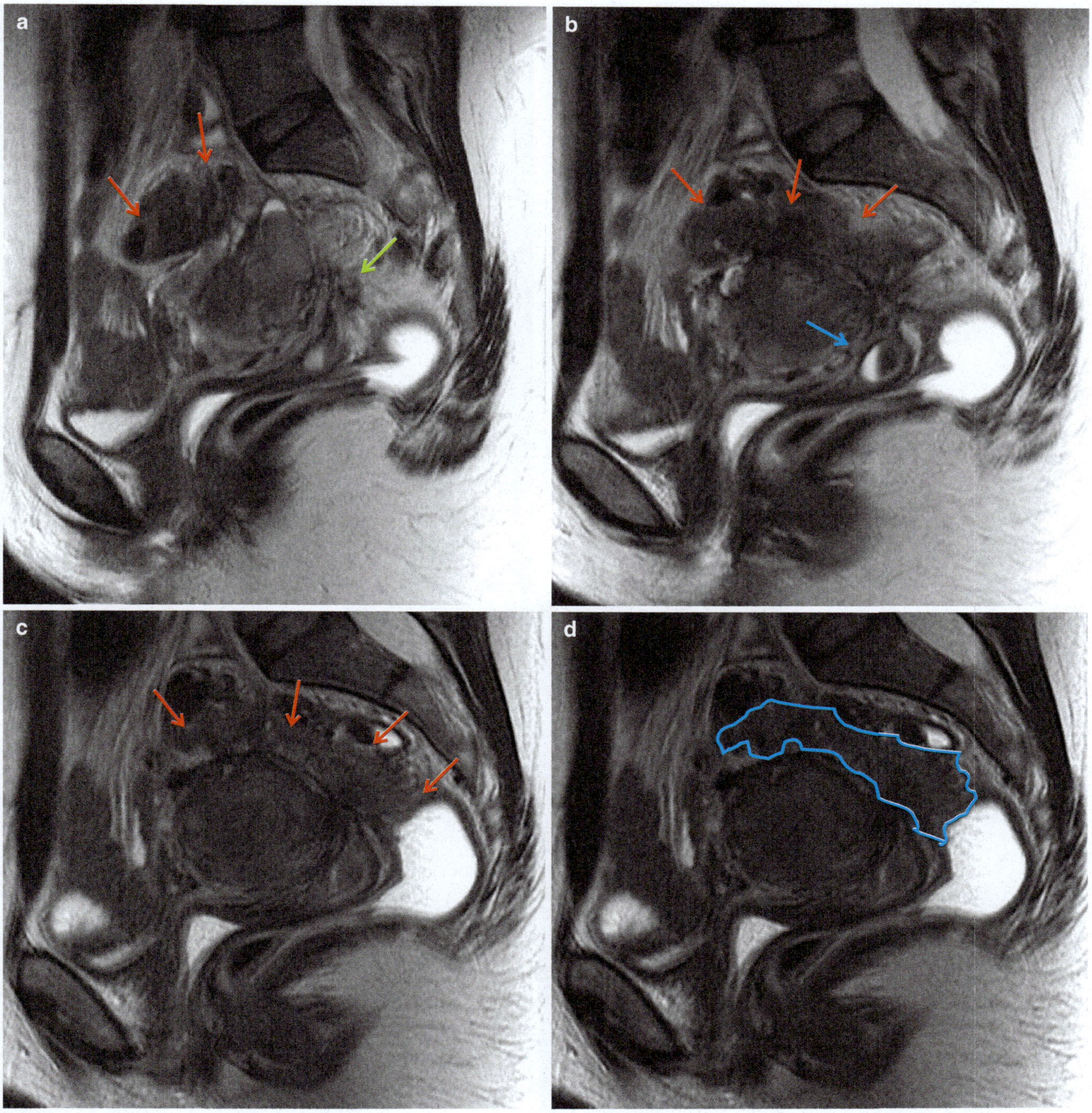

Fig. 4.67 Involvement with intestinal predominance (extensive in the rectum and sigmoid—red arrows and blue trace), asymmetrical, with the lesion epicenter in the retrocervical region, determining loop stenosis with a length of 15 cm. Notice ligament (green arrow in **a**) and vaginal extension (blue arrows) in addition to endometriomas and left hematosalpinx (yellow arrows). (**a–e**, **g**, **h**) T2-weighted sequences. (**f**) T1-weighted sequence. (**a–f**) Sagittal. (**l–h**) Coronal long axis. (**i**) Laparoscopy demonstrating extensive posterior adherence. (**j**) Surgical specimen from segmental resection. (**k**) Microscopy (40×) showing focus of endometriosis in the intestinal musculature

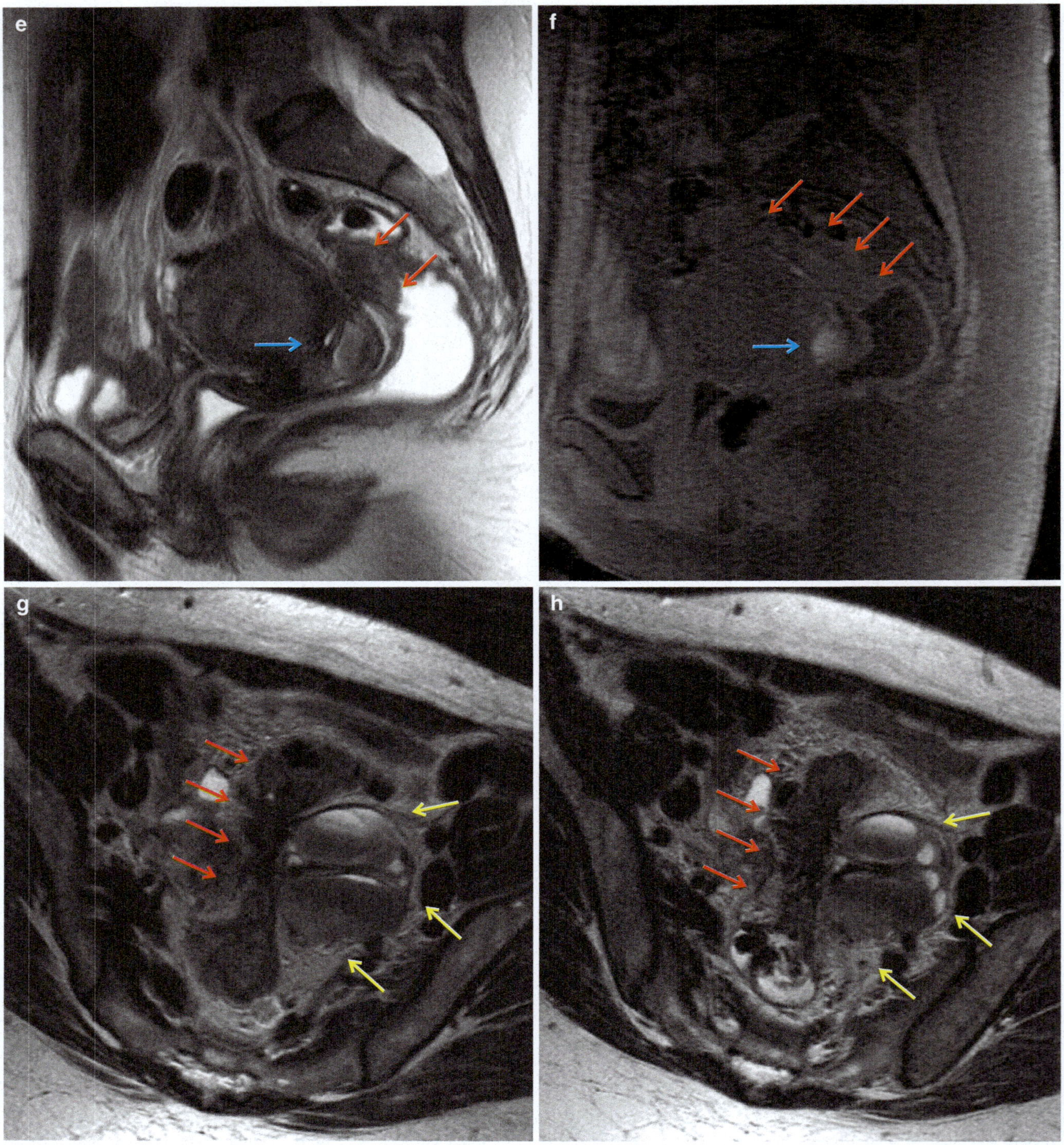

Fig. 4.67 (continued)

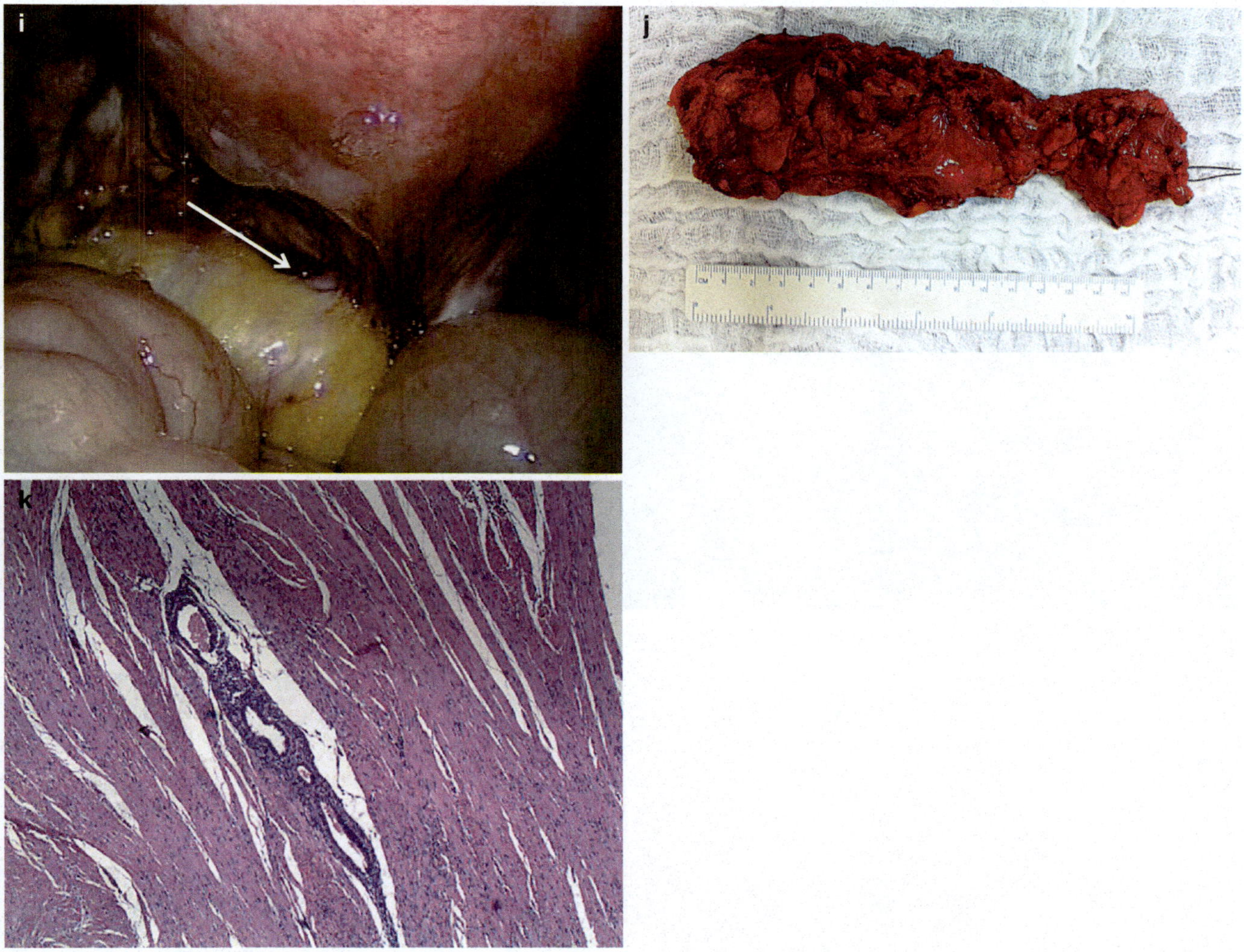

Fig. 4.67 (continued)

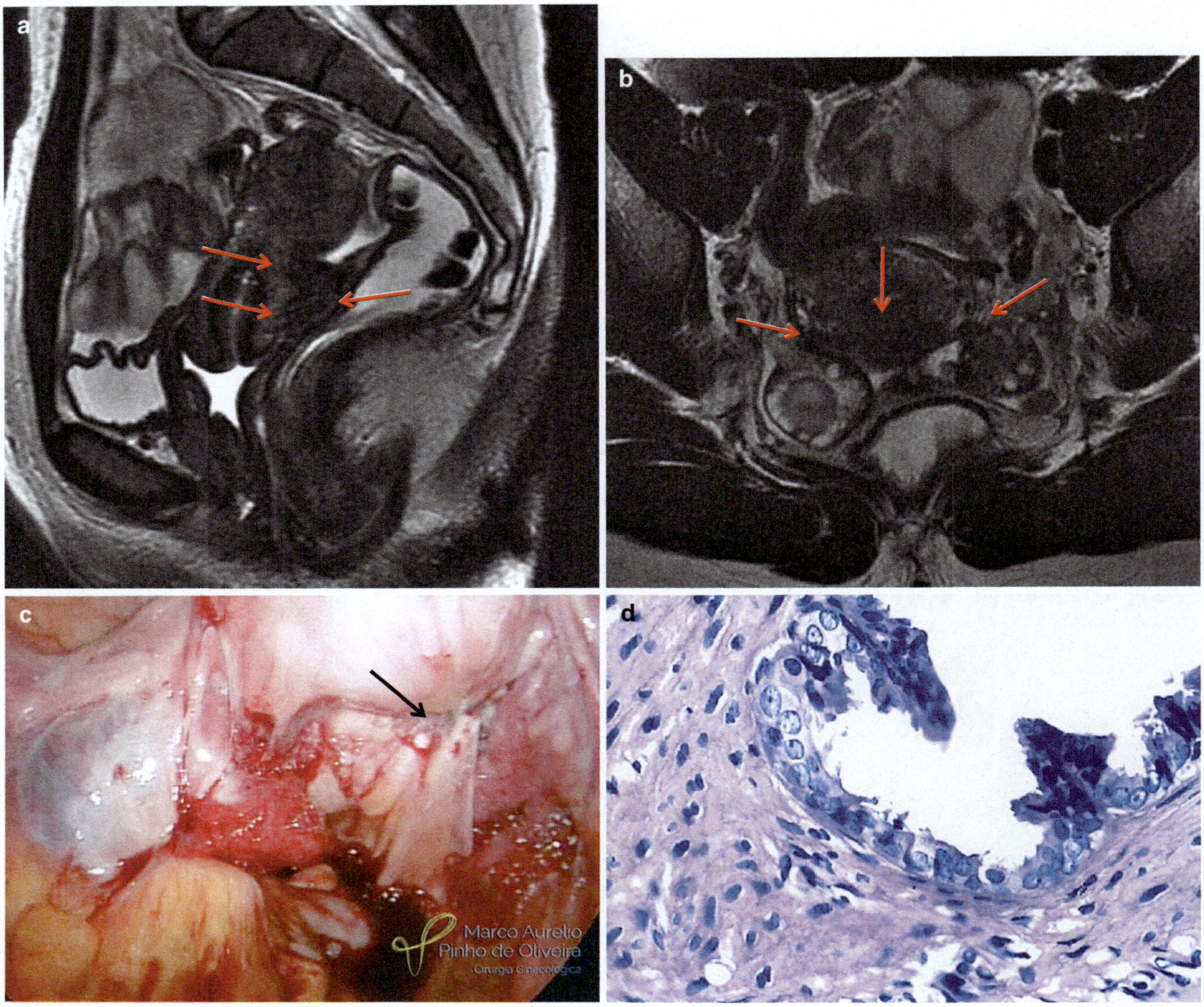

Fig. 4.68 Lesion with myometrial penetration (arrows) determining uterine retroversion and retroflexion (**a**) and posterior and medial deviation of the adnexa (**b**). (**a**, **b**) T2-weighted sequences. (**a**) Sagittal. (**b**) Coronal short axis. (**c**) Laparoscopy identifies retrocervical nodule, involving posterior myometrium. (**d**) Microscopy identifies endometriotic focus with compact cytogenic stroma

4.2.1.3 Clinical Symptoms

Symptoms may vary according to the extent of the retrocervical lesion, and patients may present a progressive dysmenorrhea, acyclic pelvic pain, dyspareunia, and intestinal disorders (dyschezia, tenesmus, diarrhea, and proctorragia), especially during menstrual periods [10].

4.2.1.4 MRI and Laparoscopic Findings

The lesions may have different morphologies in this region. The most common aspect is an irregular node with indistinct margins (Fig. 4.69).

However, the morphology can be plaque-like when an upper myometrium extension covers the posterior uterine wall (Fig. 4.70) [26].

These lesions are typically mostly composed of fibrous tissue and therefore are markedly hypointense in the T2-weighted sequence, with an intermediate signal in the TW1, and may be enhanced after the administration of gadolinium (Fig. 4.71).

The endometrial glandular ectopic component can be identified in the T2-weighted image as a hyperintense signal foci and, less commonly, hemorrhage as a hyperintense signal foci in the T1-weighted sequence (Fig. 4.72) [30, 31].

The underestimation of the extent of the retrocervical lesion can be avoided by the interpreter, by carefully analyzing the high-resolution images in the short-axis coronal plane (Fig. 4.73).

Furthermore, small lesions may go unnoticed in the sagittal plane, whereas the oblique coronal plane (short axis) is the best plane for identification (Fig. 4.61).

Another difficulty for correct interpretation in the retrocervical region is when the uterus finds itself in a retroflexed position. A small lesion may be missed, as well as uterosacral ligaments and the vaginal fornix possibly being misinterpreted as abnormal. This should be referred to the physician, to be clinically correlated. In these cases, it is important to try to identify bleeding foci and assess the posterior vaginal fornix in the sagittal contrast-enhanced study. In our experience, homogeneous gadolinium enhancement represents a normal vaginal wall (Fig. 4.74).

The laparoscopic appearance of a retrocervical lesion is easily recognized by the surgeon; however, it can be underestimated at the beginning of the procedure, especially when there is adherence and a frozen pelvis, with the associated distortion of the anatomy (Fig. 4.75) [26].

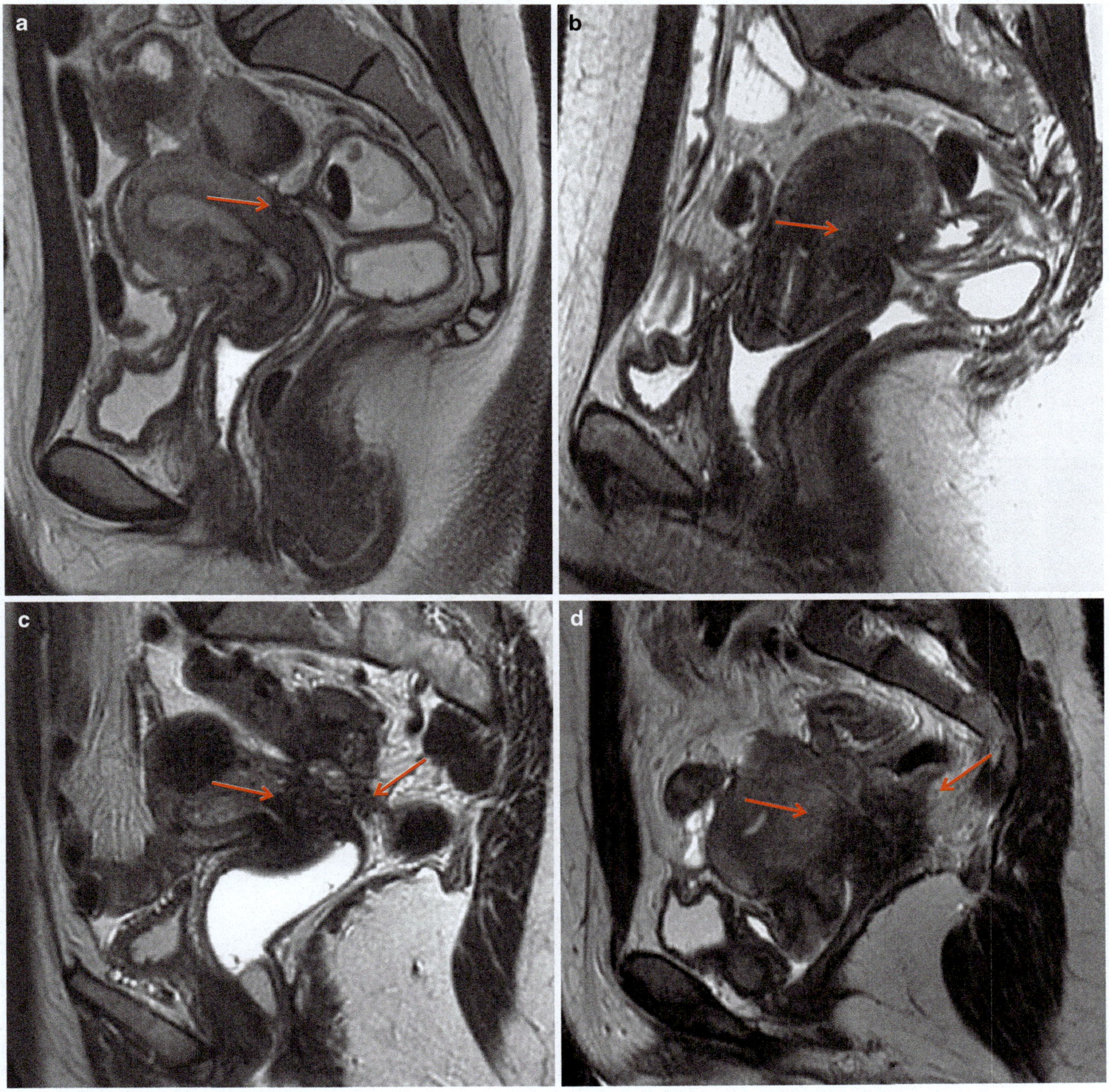

Fig. 4.69 Varied morphology of the lesion (arrow). Small node (**a**), slightly irregular nodules (**b**), poorly defined (**c**), and infiltrative mass (**d**). (**a–d**) T2-weighted sequences. Sagittal

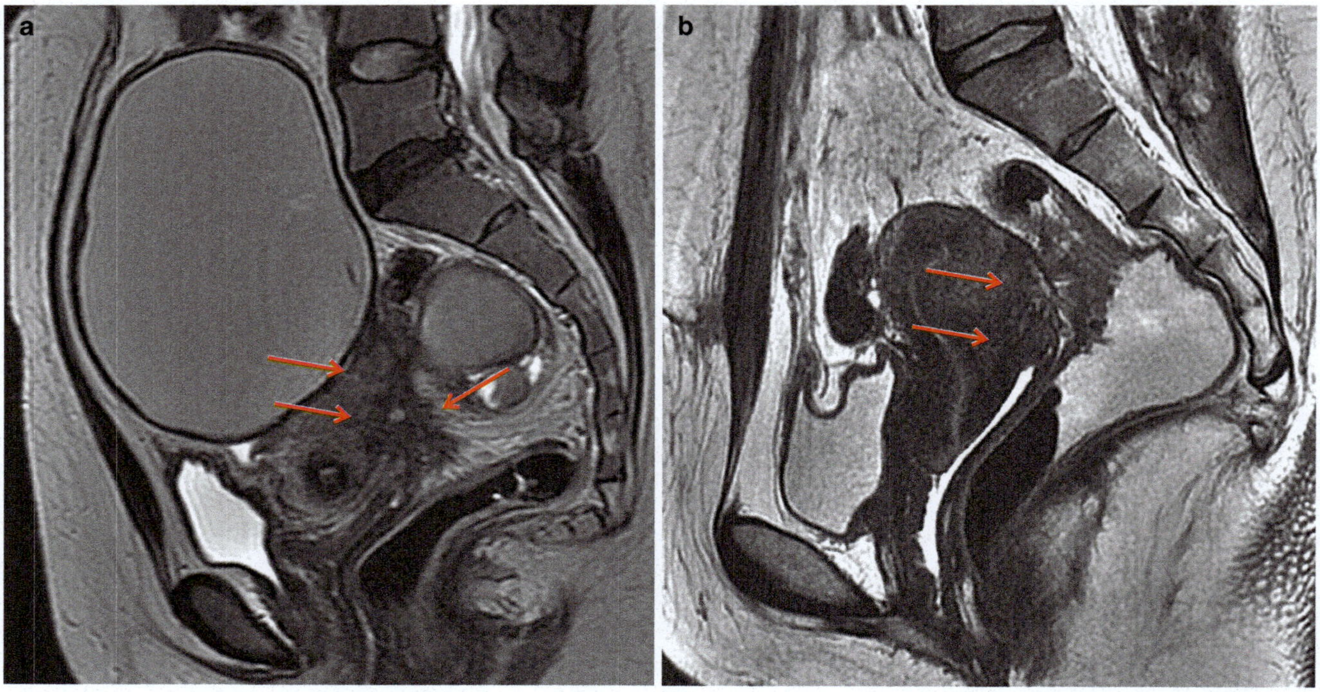

Fig. 4.70 Morphology of the mantle with superior extension covering the posterior uterine wall (arrows). (**a**, **b**) T2-weighted sequences. Sagittal

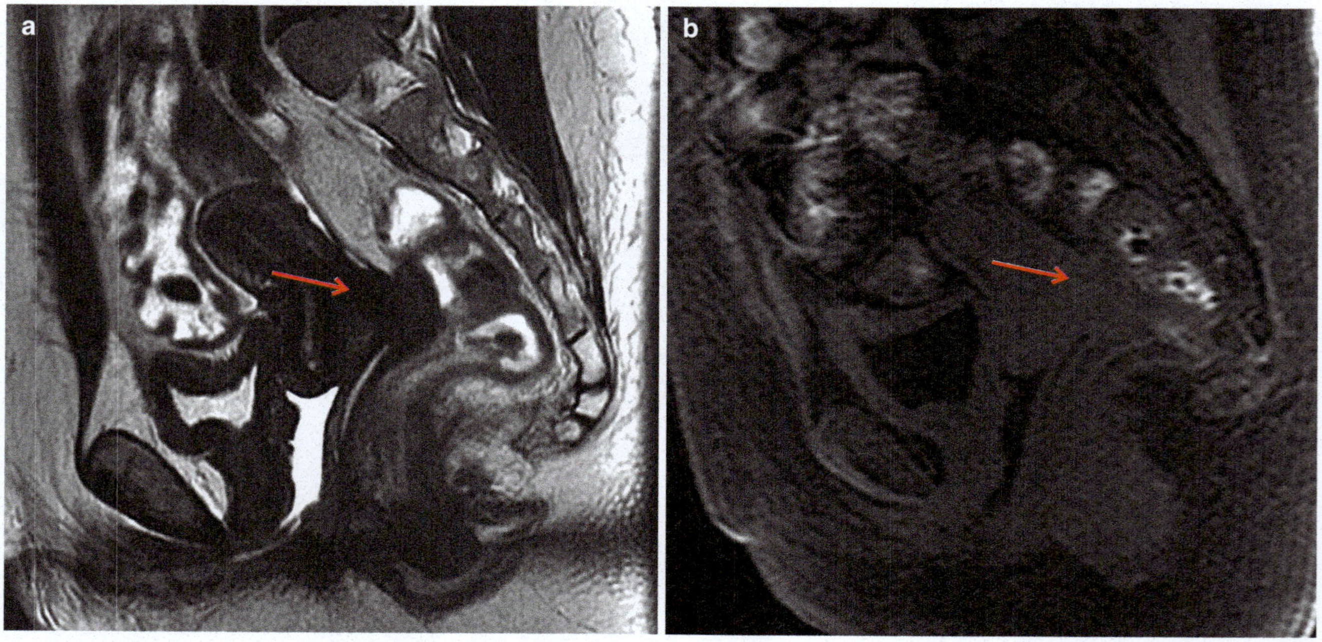

Fig. 4.71 Lesion with predominance of fibrous tissue markedly hypointense in T2-weighted sequences (arrows in **a**, **c**), with intermediate signal in T1 (arrow **b**) and discrete gadolinium enhancement (arrows in **d**). (**a**, **b**) Sagittal. (**c**, **d**) Axial. (**e**) Microscopy demonstrating endometrial focus with a little glandular component and cytogenic stroma with marked lymphocytic infiltration (100×)

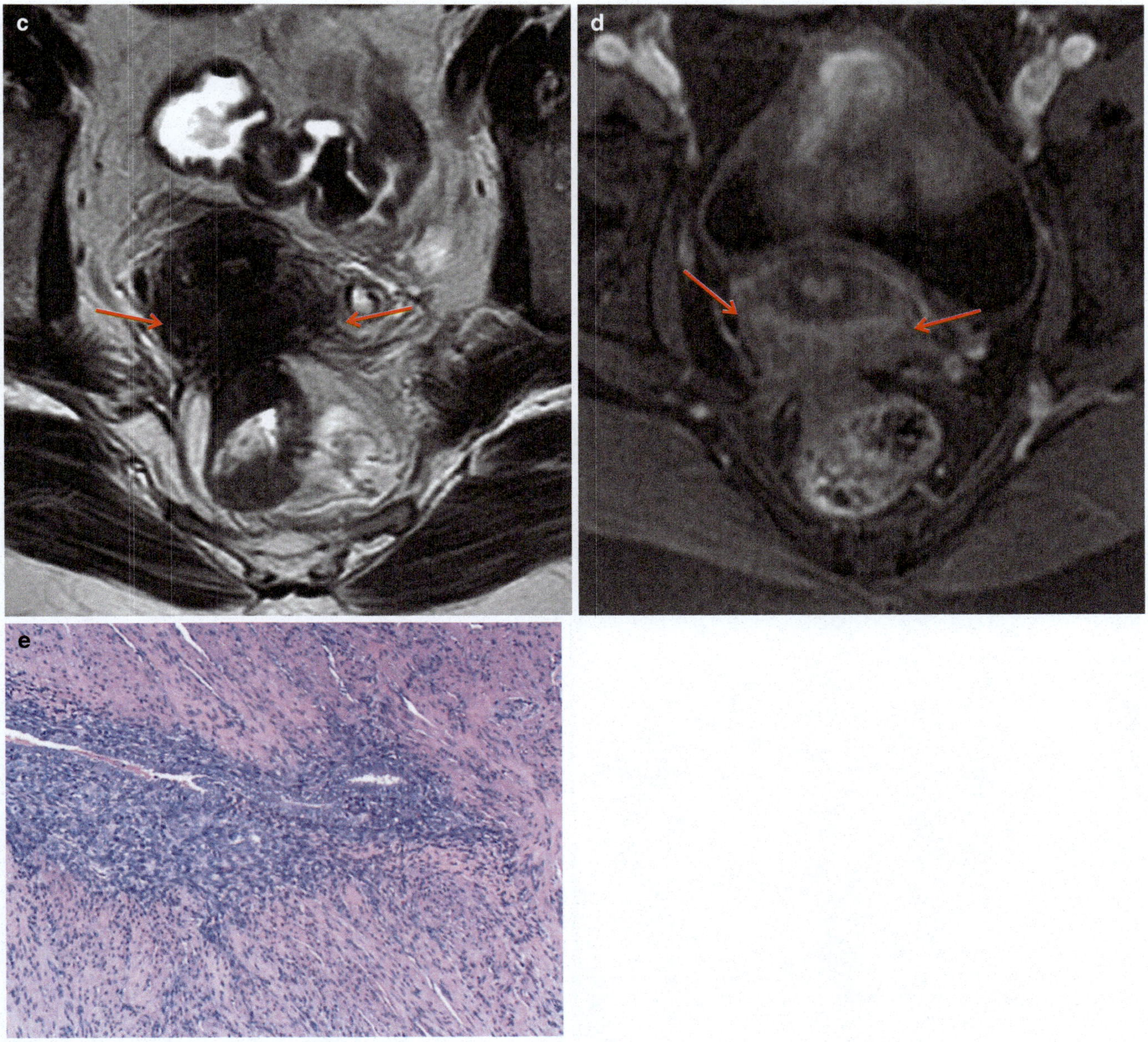

Fig. 4.71 (continued)

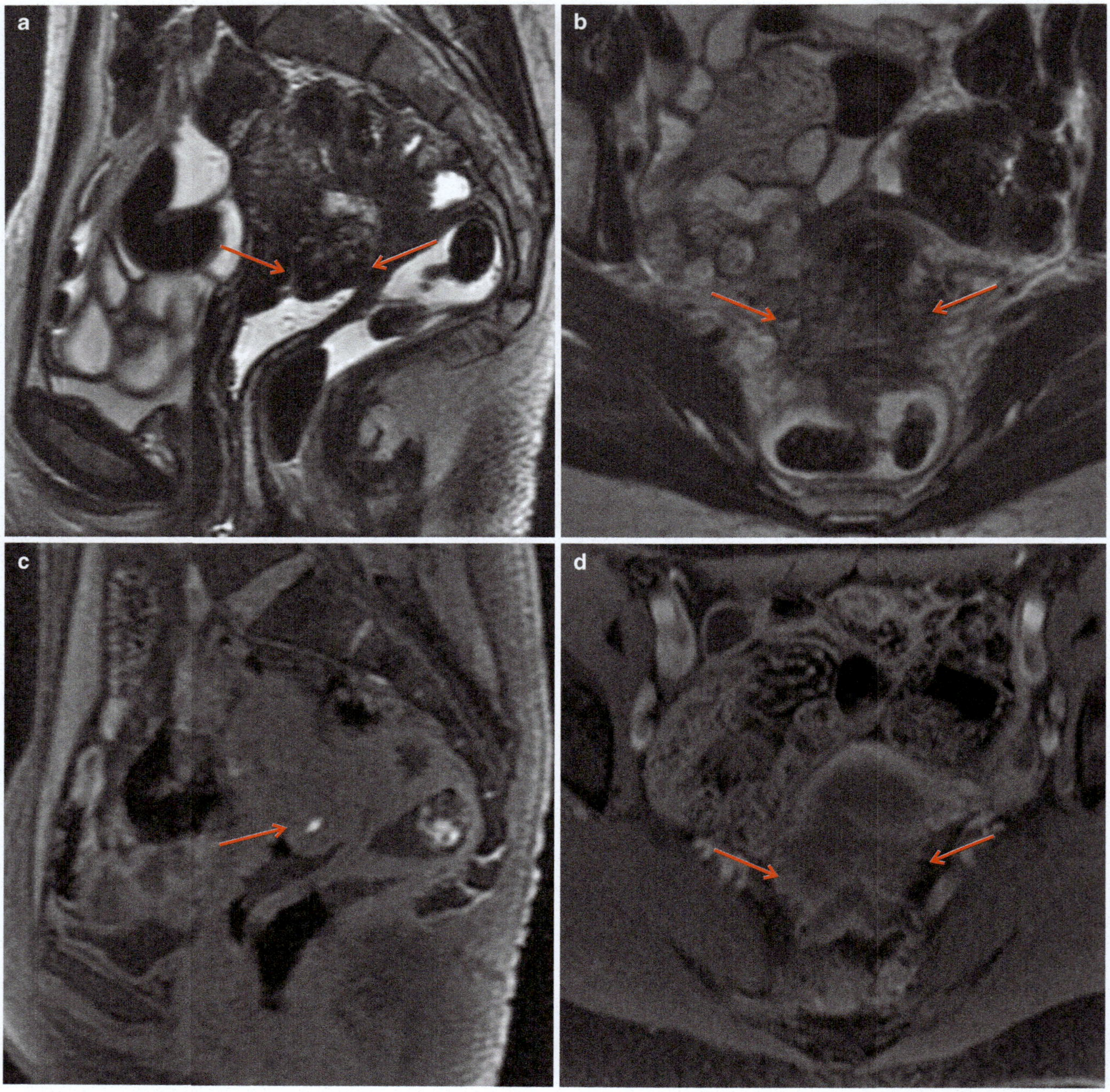

Fig. 4.72 Lesion with endometrial glandular ectopic component, being discreet in Case 1 (**a–d**) and prominent in Case 2 (**e–h**). As in Fig. 4.106 (**a–e**) and Fig. 4.108 (**e–h**). Multiple hypersignal foci in the T2 (**a**, **b**, **f**, **h**) and T1-weighted sequences, bleeding (**c–e**, **h**), and with gadolinium enhancement (**d**). (**a**, **c**) Sagittal. (**b**, **d**, **e**, **h**) Axial. (**i**) Microscopy showing endometrial glands and cysts

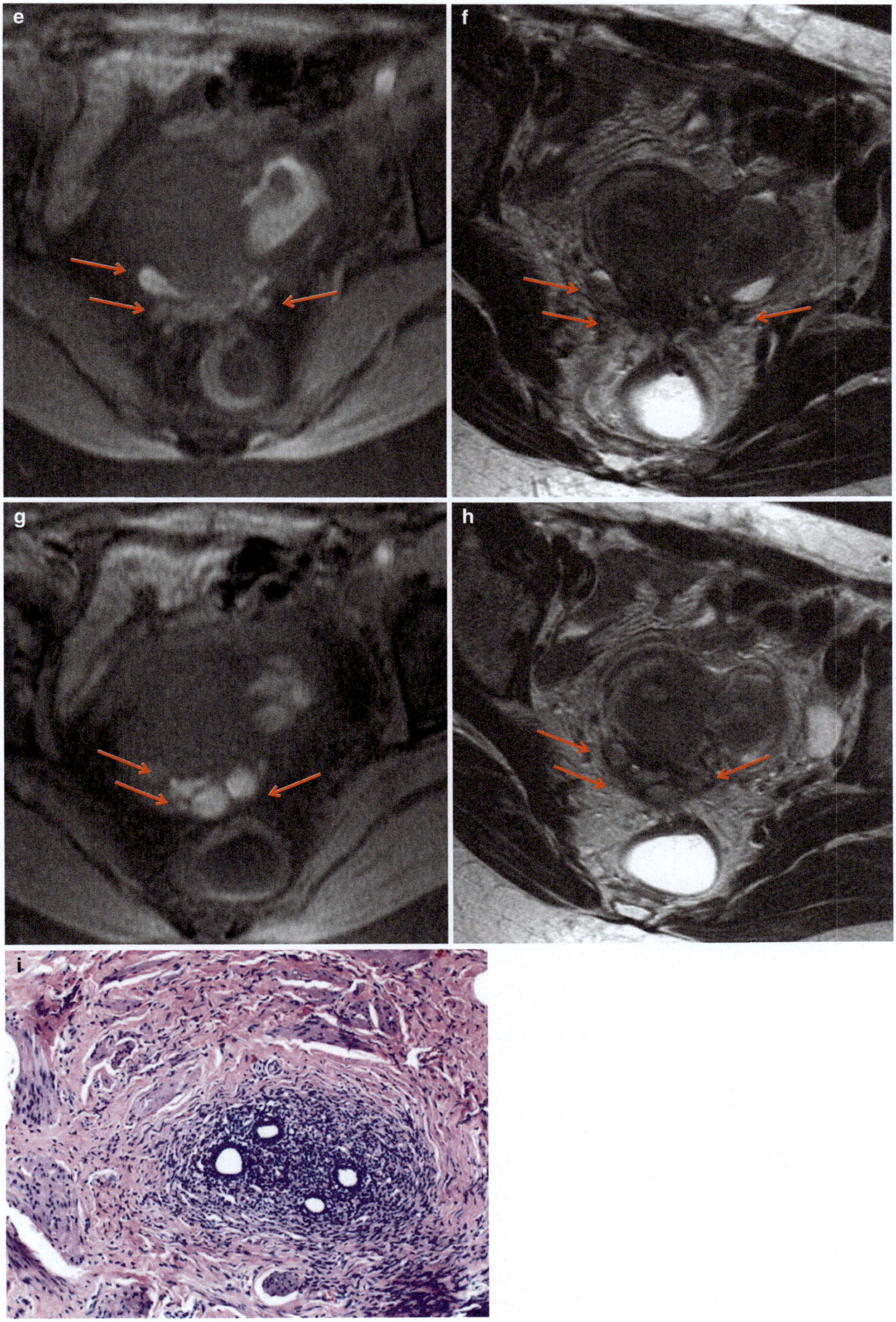

Fig. 4.72 (continued)

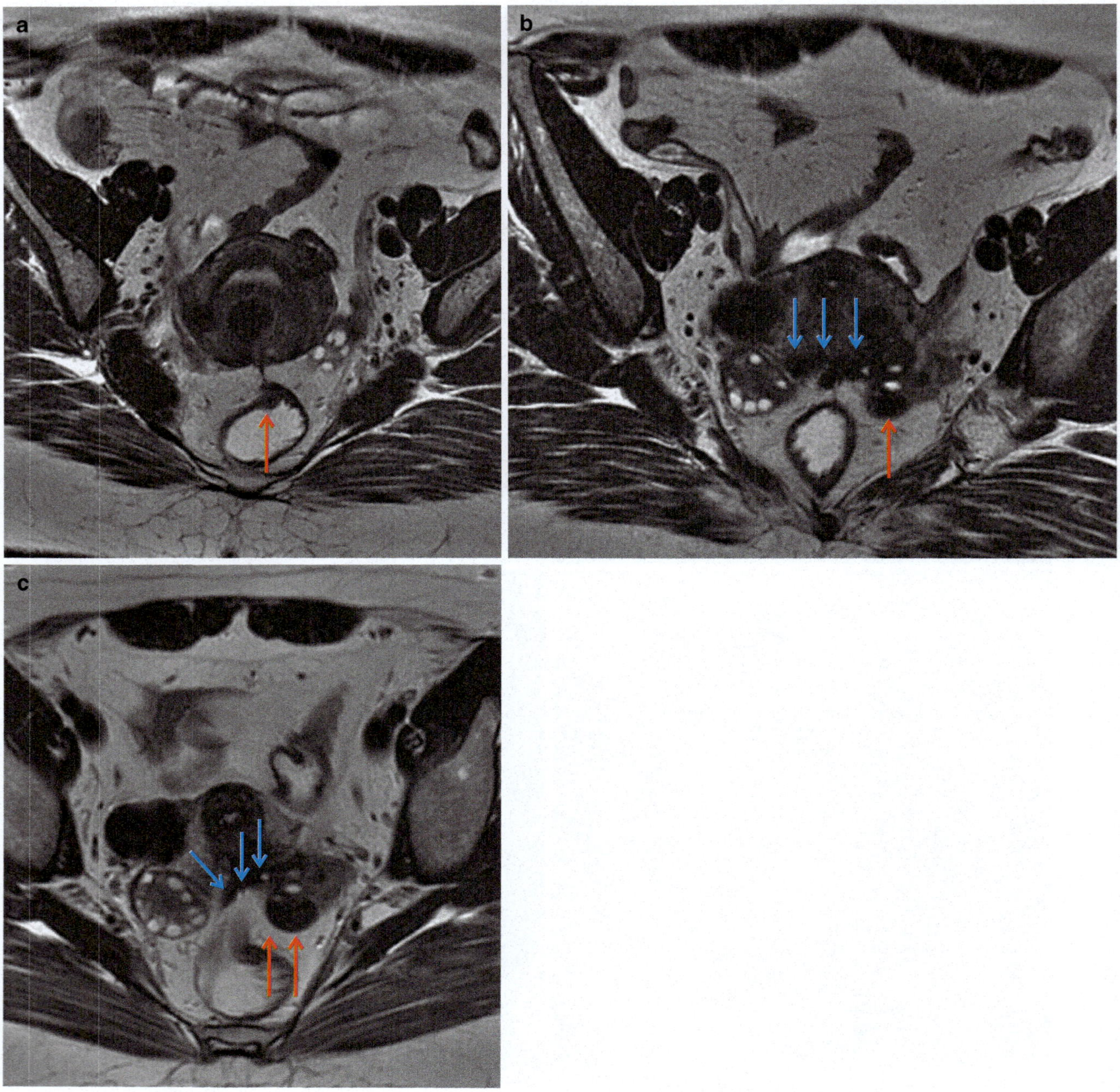

Fig. 4.73 Lesion extension toward the uterosacral ligaments promoting adherence and posteriorly deviating adnexa, larger on the left (blue arrows). Note proper assessment of the extent of the lesion in the short-axis coronal plane. Endometrioma in the left ovary (arrows **b**, **c**) and superficial involvement in the upper rectum (arrow **a**). (**a**–**c**) T2-weighted sequences. Axial

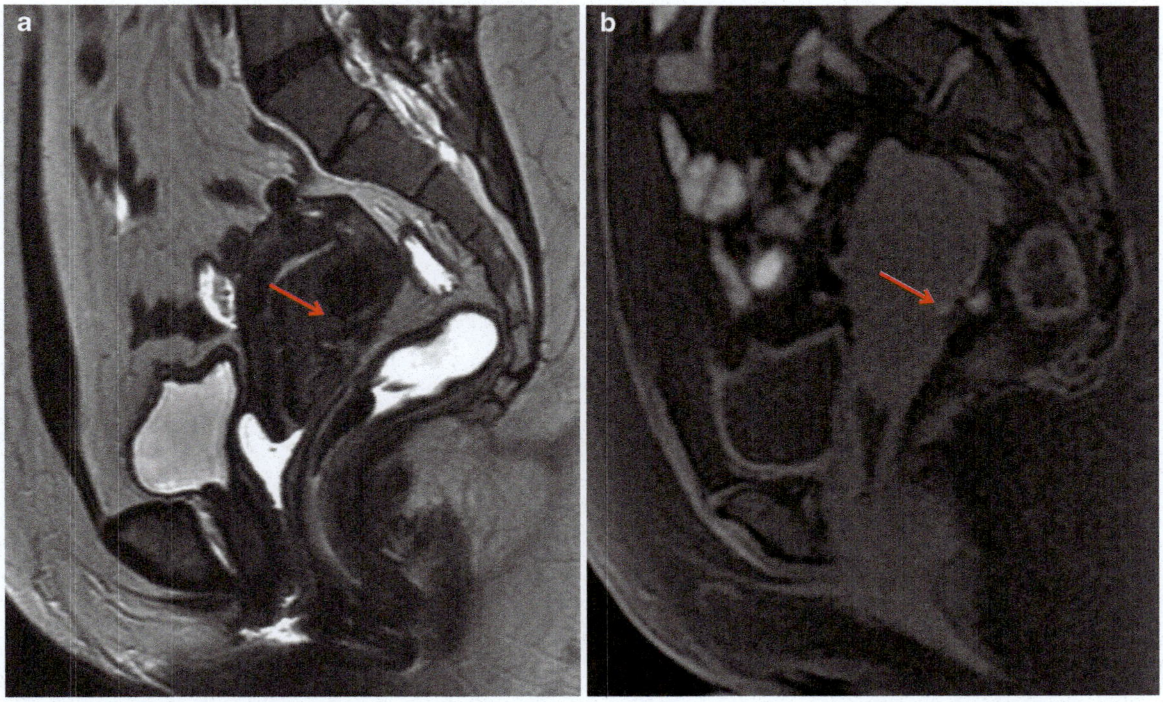

Fig. 4.74 Uterus in retroversion and retroflexion, making identification of the lesion in the retrocervical region difficult. Discreet blurring in the fatty planes in T2-weighted sequence in the sagittal plane (arrow **a**). Observe the images in the oblique coronal plane in T2-weighted sequence (as in Fig. 4.114) and bleeding in the T1-weighted sequence with fat suppression (arrow **b**). (**a**, **b**) Sagittal

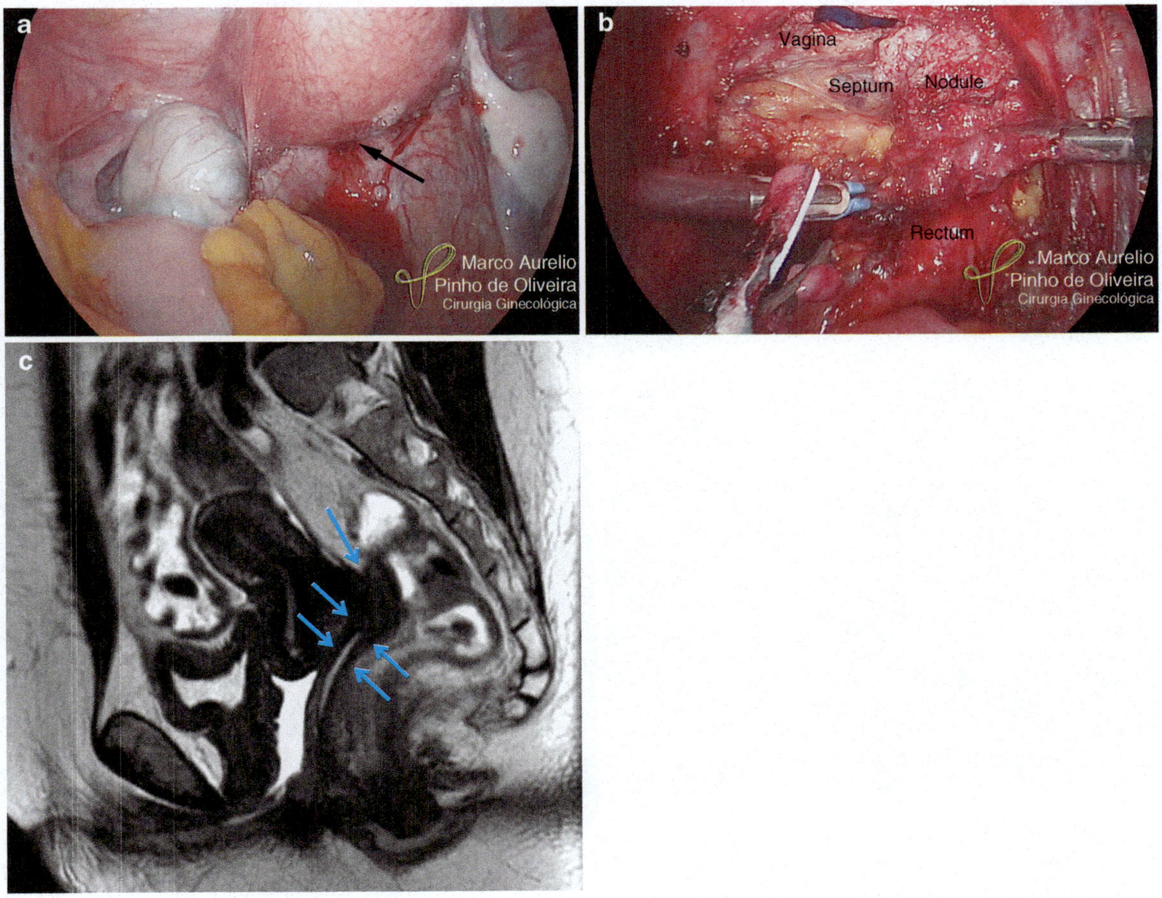

Fig. 4.75 (**a**) Retrocervical lesion. Low retrocervical nodule with inferior extension of the septum. (**b**) Nodule being resected, infiltrating the rectovaginal septum and vagina. (**c**) Lesion in the sagittal plane. Note the lower extension well identified by the method (arrows)

4.2.1.5 Comments on the Treatment

Surgical treatment includes the removal of the retrocervical lesion and the infiltrative component in adjacent structures. However, in relation to the myometrium, the preservation of an endometriotic component in the cervix may be considered in patients who wish to become pregnant (Fig. 4.76) [9].

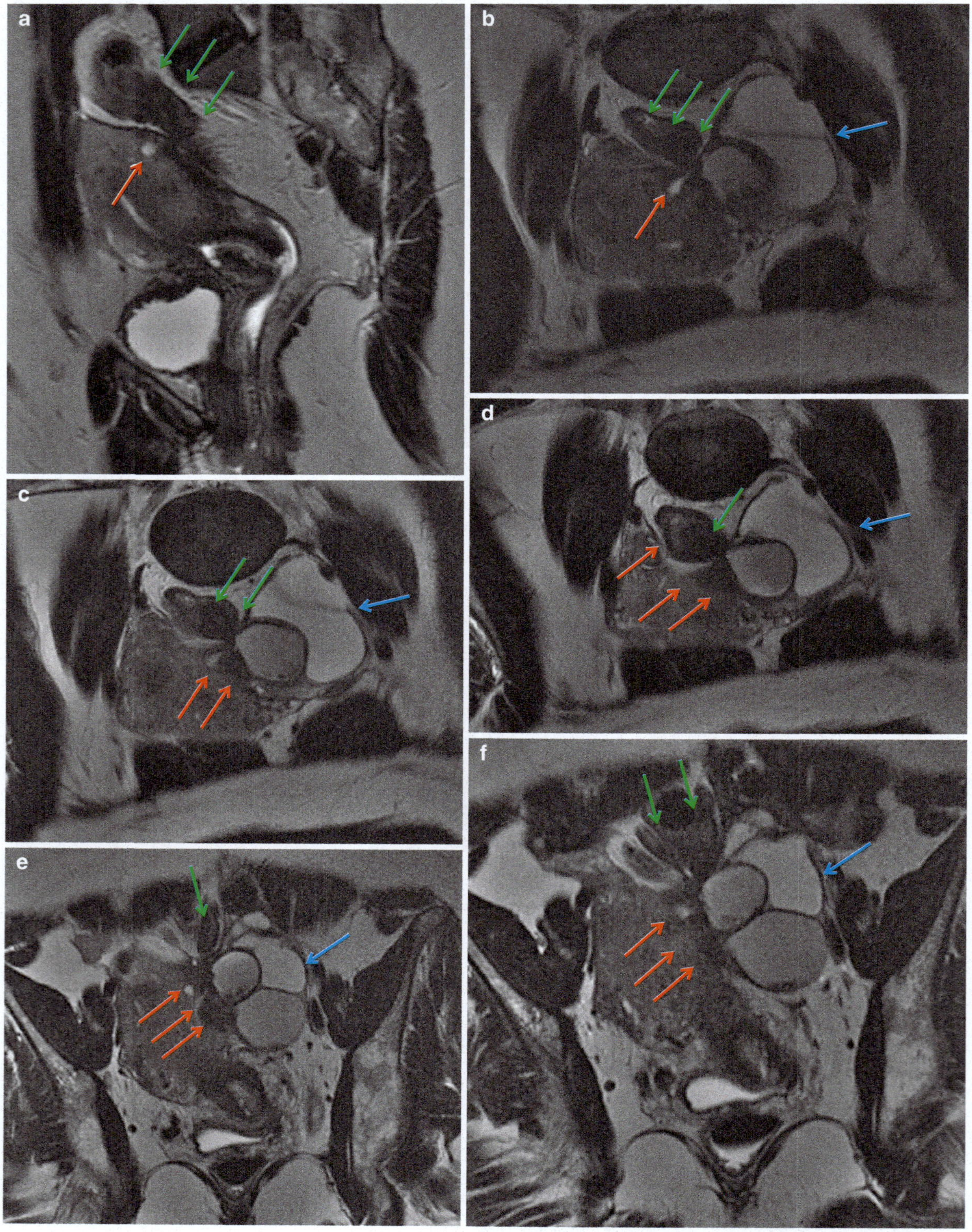

Fig. 4.76 Importance of MRI in identifying myometrial component that must also be removed during the surgical treatment of retrocervical lesion. In this case, although small, there is an important glandular component which can cause recurrence of the (red arrows). (**a–h**) T2-weighted sequences. (**a**) Sagittal. (**b–d**) Coronal short axis. (**e–h**) Coronal long axis. Notice extensive involvement associated to the sigmoid, reducing the loop lumen, extending itself near the descending colon (green arrows). Note adherence with the left attachment with hydrosalpinx and endometrioma (blue arrows **b–h**)

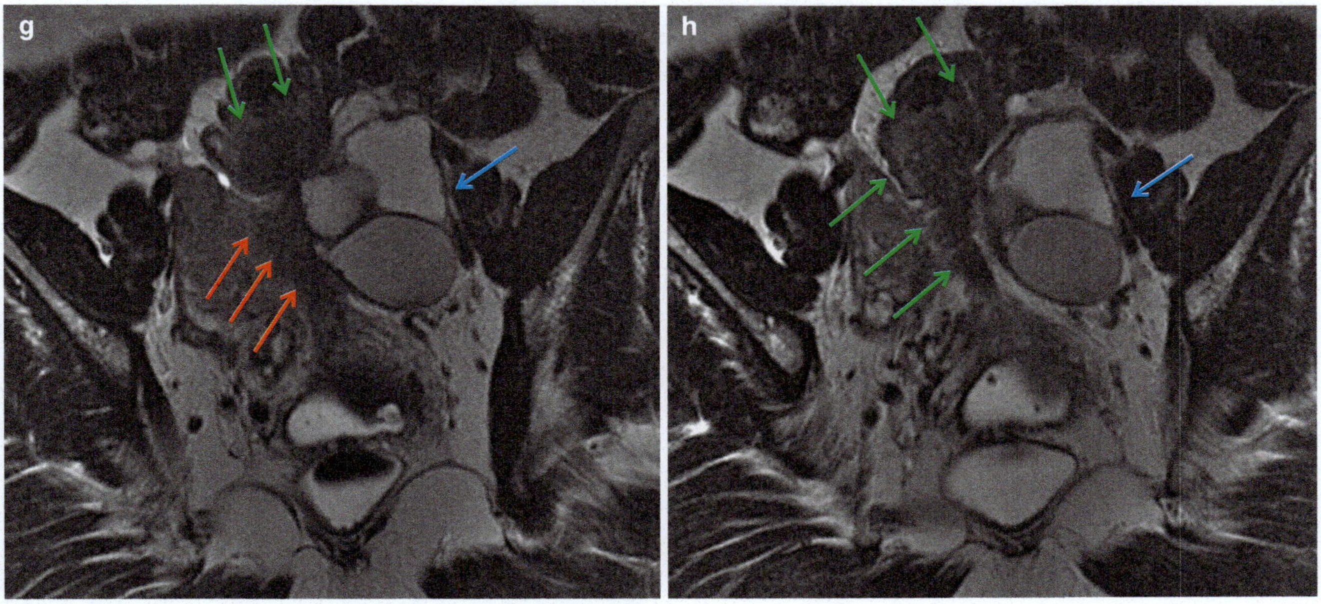

Fig. 4.76 (continued)

4.2.2 Rectovaginal Space

4.2.2.1 Anatomy

The rectovaginal space between the posterior vaginal and anterior rectum walls is filled by a connective tissue and superiorly suspended by the cardinal and uterosacral ligaments, laterally by the tendinous arch, and distally connected to the perineal body. It is bound anteriorly by the rectovaginal septum. This space allows the posterior vaginal wall and the anterior rectal wall, which have functional independence, to slide over each other, with considerable mobility [32, 33].

The rectovaginal space is well characterized in MRI images, especially in the sagittal and axial planes on T2-weighted sequences. It can range from a thin hypointense space to a large hyperintense space, according to the amount of fatty tissue (Fig. 4.77).

The length of the rectovaginal space depends on the cul-de-sac's depth. When the cul-de-sac is deep, running posteriorly to the upper third of the vagina, this space may be shorter (Fig. 4.78) [10].

4.2.2.2 Most Common Aspects of the Endometriosis

Endometriosis of the rectovaginal space was reported by Sampson at the beginning of the last century. However, the prevalence is lower, when compared with other sites affected by deep endometriosis [34, 35].

When present, it constitutes a severe presentation of deep endometriosis, affecting the lower vagina and rectum, as well as the inferior hypogastric nerves and the ureter, resulting in greater surgery complexity and increased complications, such as rectovaginal fistula [36].

4.2.2.3 Clinical Symptoms

The clinical symptoms are similar to those observed in the retrocervical region, such as cyclical or permanent pain, deep dyspareunia, and dyschezia, and hematochezia, when there is associated rectal involvement [9, 37].

The bimanual gynecological examination has a high specificity for the diagnosis of lesion in this topography, ranging from 96.3 to 99%, and it may reveal areas of fibrosis and nodular lesions, usually near the insertion of the uterosacral ligaments and the cul-de-sac [38, 39].

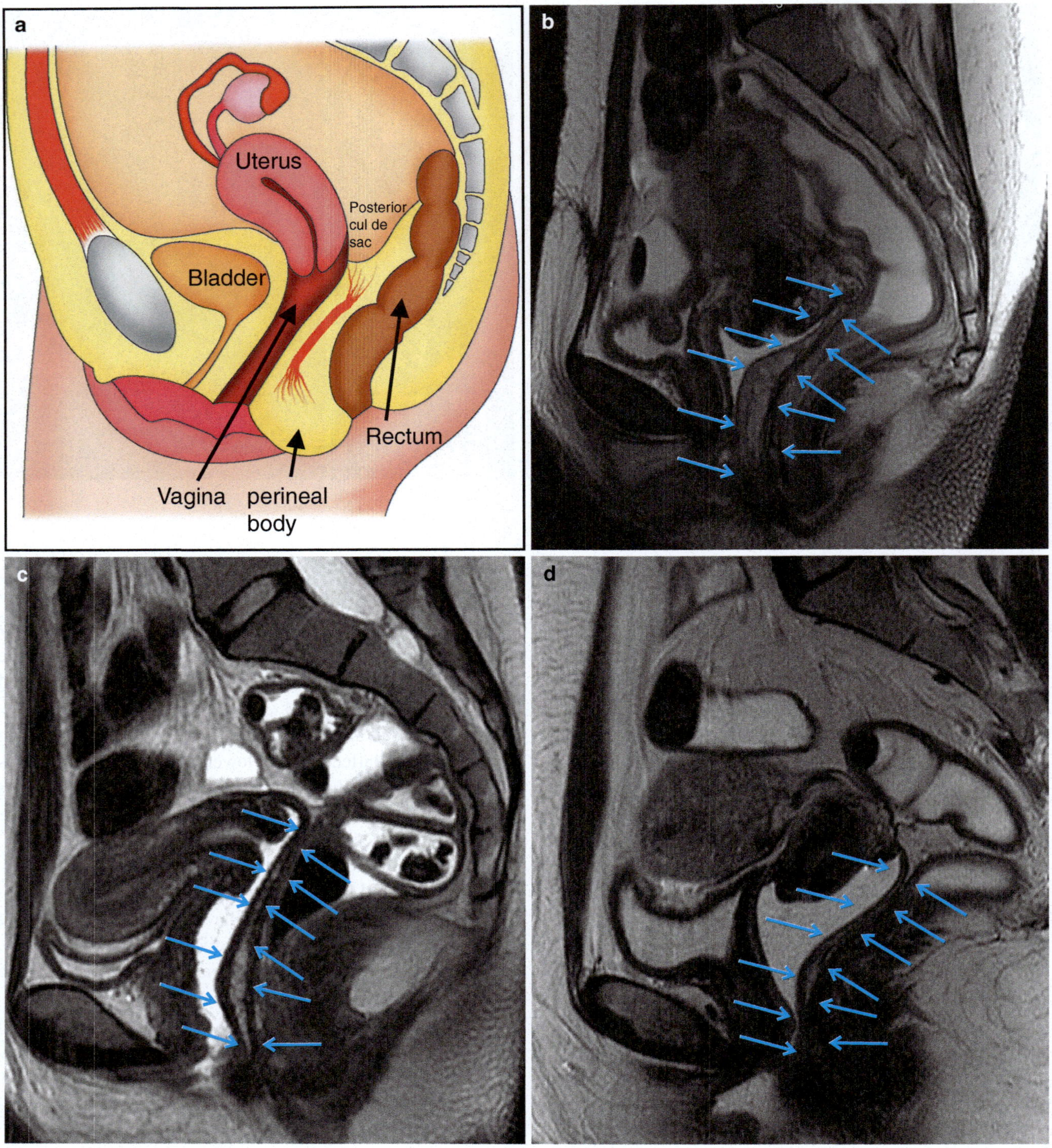

Fig. 4.77 Rectovaginal septum. Extraperitoneal space extending from the retrocervical region to the perineal body between the posterior wall of the vagina and the anterior rectum and anus (in diagram **a** and **b–d** arrow). Notice that the volume of the space is directly related to the amount of fatty tissue in the patient (**b**, larger; **d**, smaller). The greater the amount of fat tissue, the more hyperintense the signal it presents (arrows). (**a**) Diagram. (**b–d**) T2-weighted sequences. Sagittal

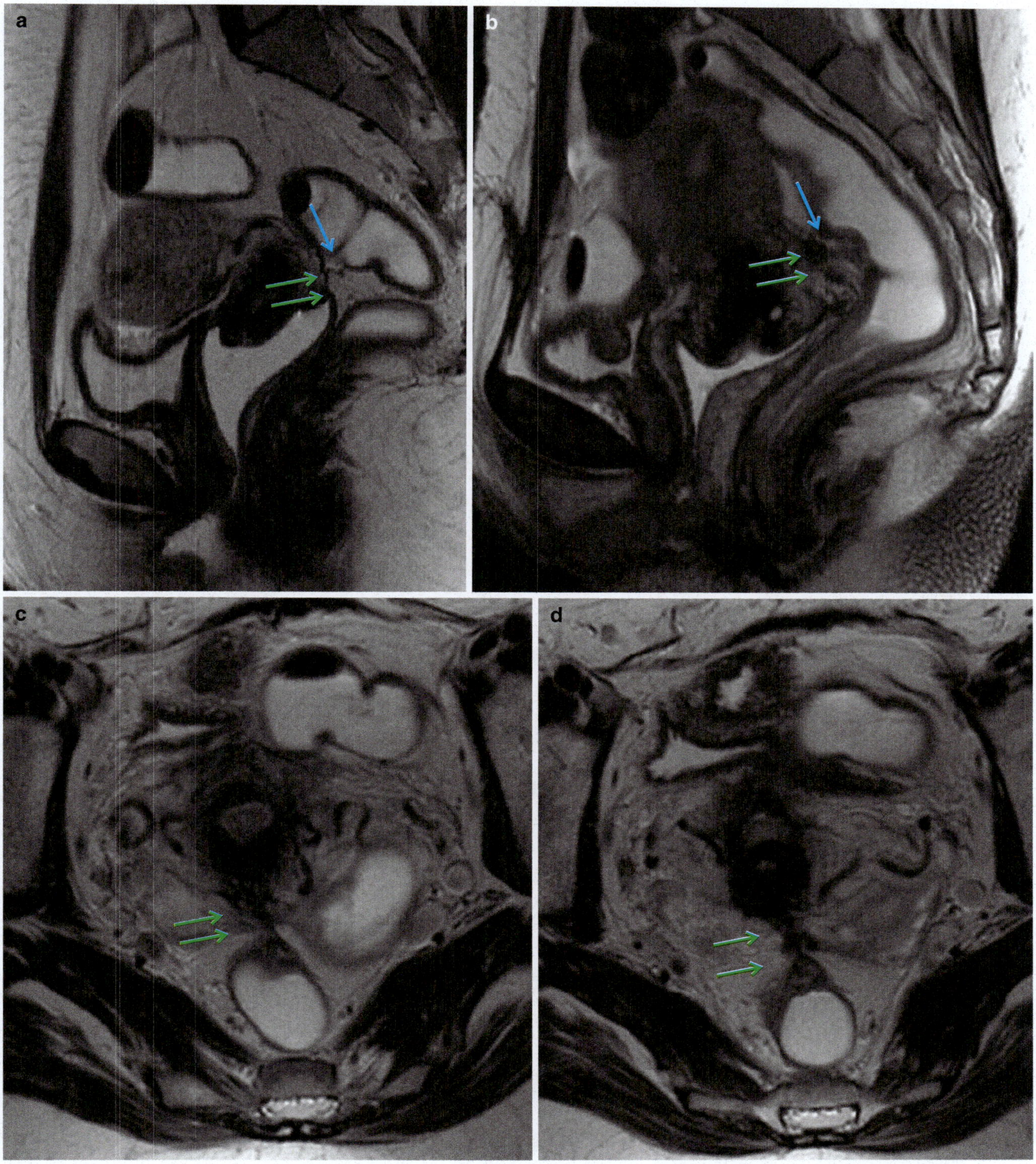

Fig. 4.78 Variations in depth of the posterior cul-de-sac modify the extent of the retrocervical region and the rectovaginal septum. (**a**, **e**) Normal exams in different patients. In (**a**), the depth of the posterior cul-de-sac (blue arrow) is less, and therefore there is a greater extent of the retrocervical region (green arrows). In (**e**), the depth is grater (blue arrow), with a smaller longitudinal extent of the retrocervical region (green arrow). Patients with greater depth will have an increased chance of developing early disease in the septum. Case 1 with less depth (**b–d**) compared to Case 2 (**m–h**). In Case 1, the initial retrocervical lesion is in the cervical plane and the vaginal fornix (green arrows in the sagittal and short axis), and in Case 2, it begins at the septum in the plane of the upper third of the vagina (green arrow in the sagittal and axial with bleeding focus in **f**). (**a–g**) T2-weighted sequences. (**h**) T1-weighted with fat suppression. (**a**, **b**, **e**, **f**, **h**) Sagittal. (**c**, **d**, **g**) Coronal short axis

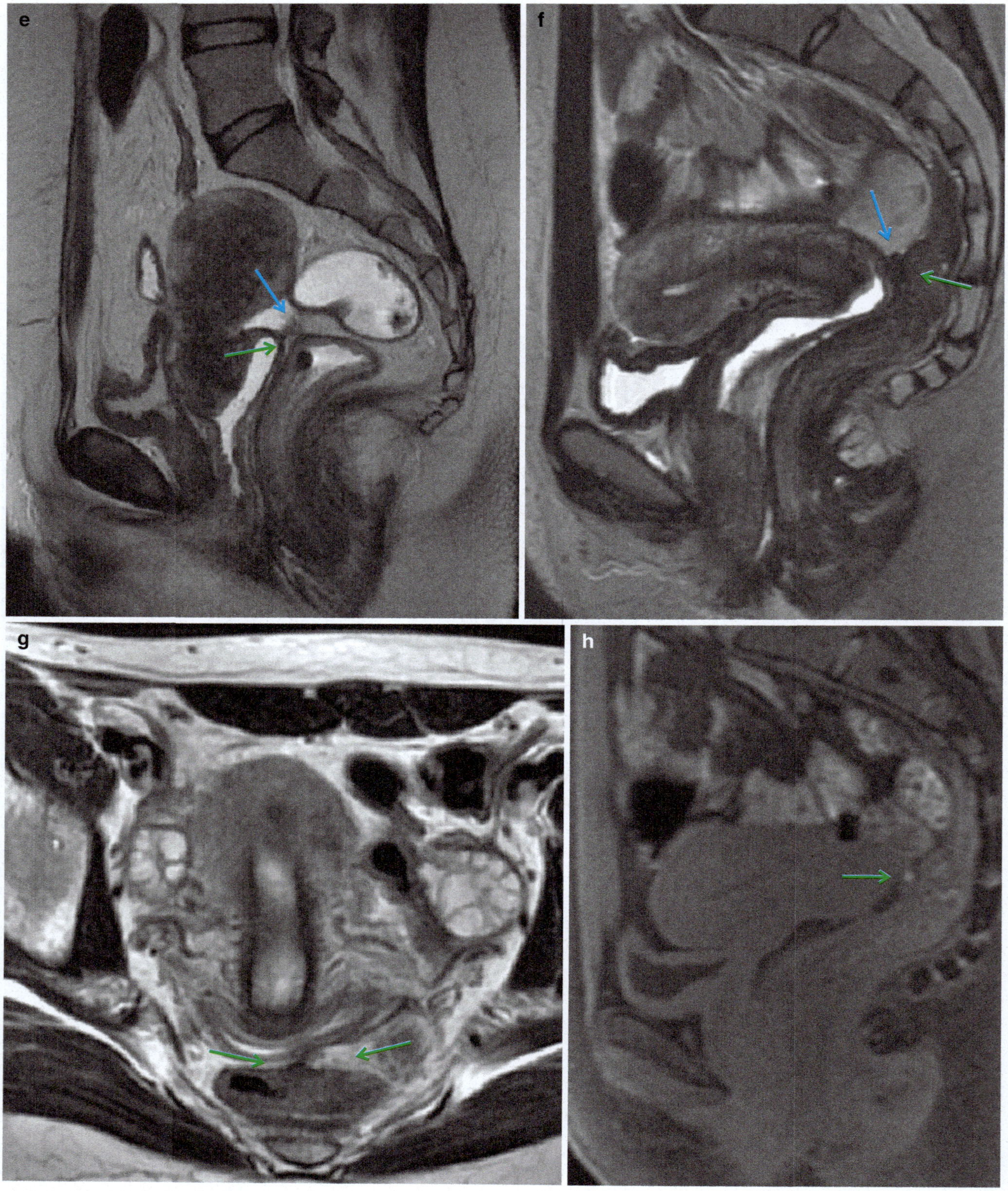

Fig. 4.78 (continued)

4.2.2.4 MRI and Laparoscopic Findings

Lesions may obliterate the rectovaginal space and the cul-de-sac and determine adhesion between the cervix, the vagina, and the rectum (Fig. 4.79).

There may be extension to the paracolpos and the parametrium (lateral compartment); therefore the relationship with the uterine arteries, ureters, and inferior hypogastric nerves should be described (Fig. 4.80).

Moreover, there is a greater possibility of involvement of the levator ani muscle, and it should be reported in the radiologist report (Fig. 4.81).

The lesion signal intensity usually reflects the predominance of fibrous tissue, with hypointense lesions in the T2-weighted sequences and intermediate signal intensity in the T1-weighted sequences (Fig. 4.82).

However, some lesions may present an abundant glandular component. In these cases, ectopic endometrial foci exhibit hyperintense signal on T1-weighted images with fat saturation (reflecting the hematic content), with variable signal intensity on T2-weighted images, mostly hyperintense (Fig. 4.83) [30, 31].

At laparoscopy, the "tip of the iceberg" is observed at the beginning of the procedure, since most of the subperitoneal and deep nodule is hidden in the extraperitoneal space. Therefore, these lesions are often more palpable than visible, and MRI may guide the surgical planning (Fig. 4.84) [36].

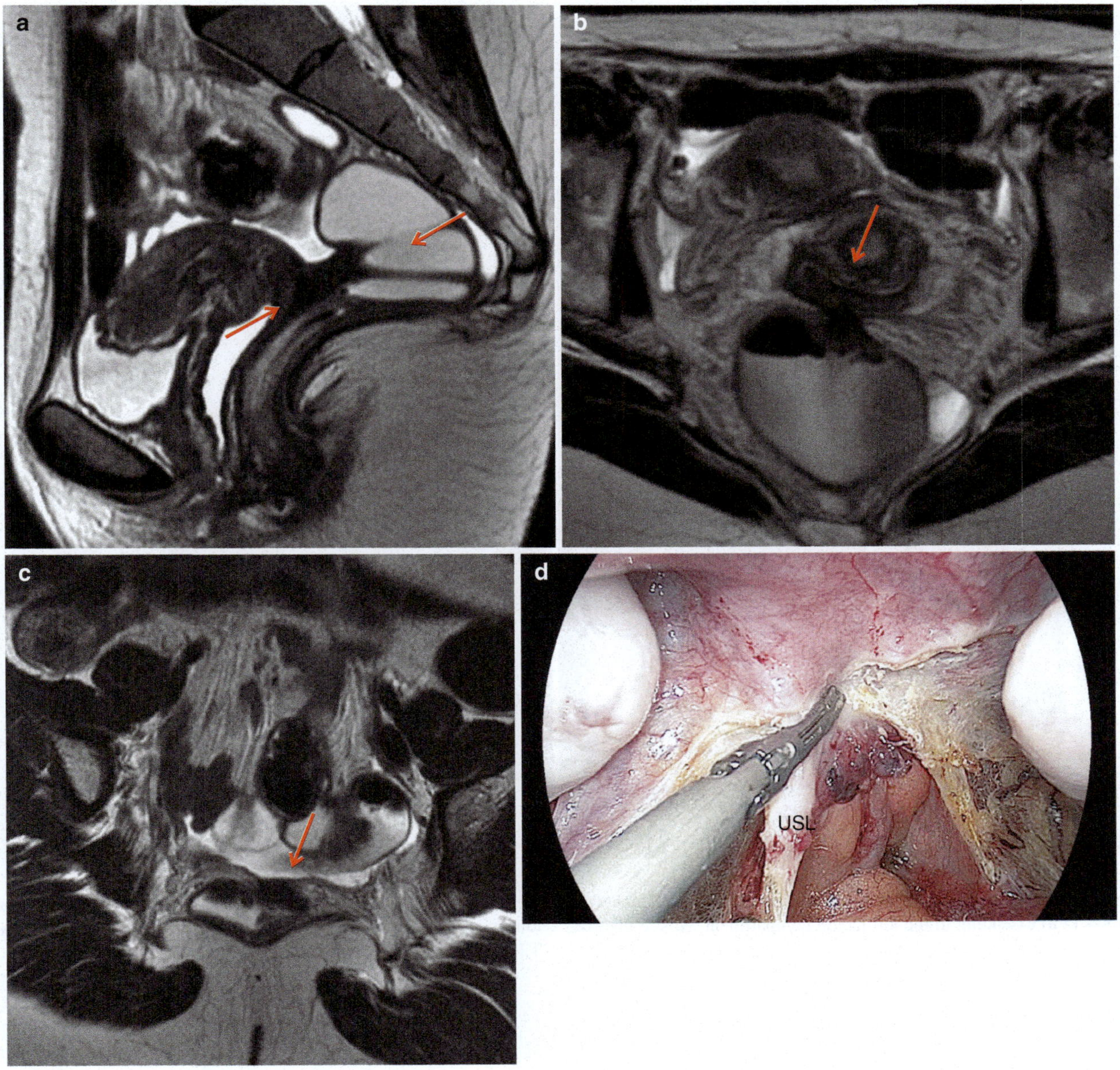

Fig. 4.79 Lesion obliterates the rectovaginal septum and the posterior cul-de-sac and determines adhesion between the vagina and rectum (arrows) with intestinal deep penetration. T2-weighted sequences. (**a**) Sagittal. (**b**) Axial. (**c**) Oblique coronal. (**d**) Laparoscopy (start of the procedure) identifies the tip of the lesion (arrow). (**e**) Microscopy of the lesion demonstrating the endometrial glandular structure between the muscle tissue

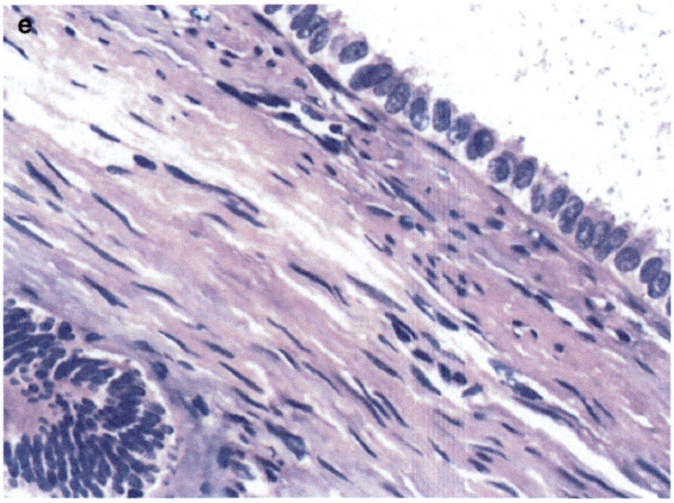

Fig. 4.79 (cotinued)

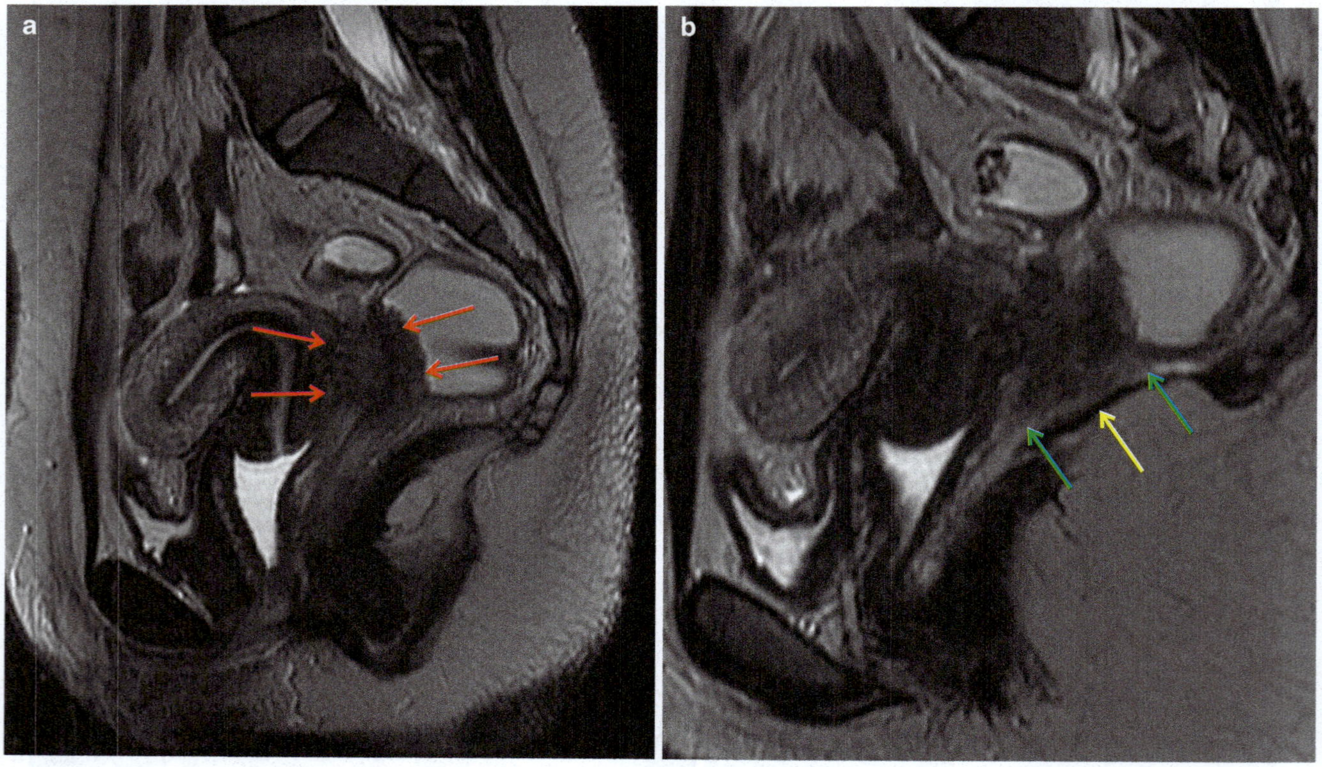

Fig. 4.80 Nodule in rectovaginal septum with rectal involvement (red arrows in **a**) extending to the left lateral compartment. Notice involvement of the lower hypogastric nerve (green arrows **b–d**). Compare it to the right side, without any involvement (blue arrow in **d**). The lesion touches the iliococcygeus muscle (yellow arrows **b–d**). (**a–d**) T2-weighted sequences. (**a**, **b**) Sagittal. (**c**, **d**) Coronal short axis

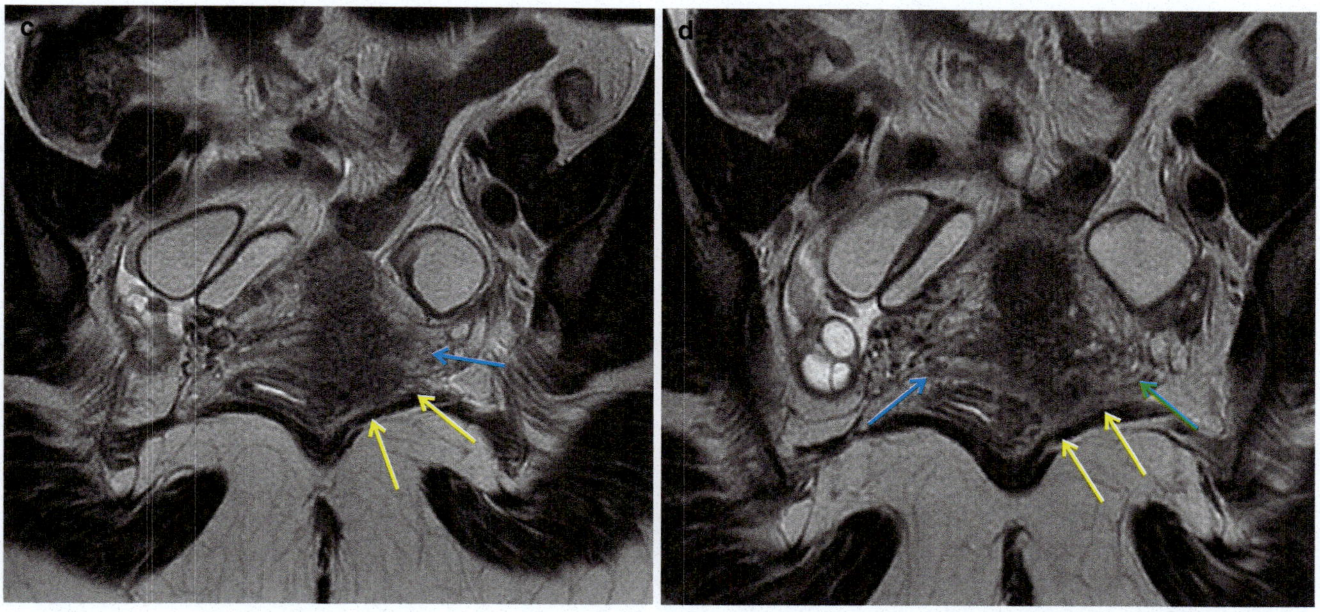

Fig. 4.80 (continued)

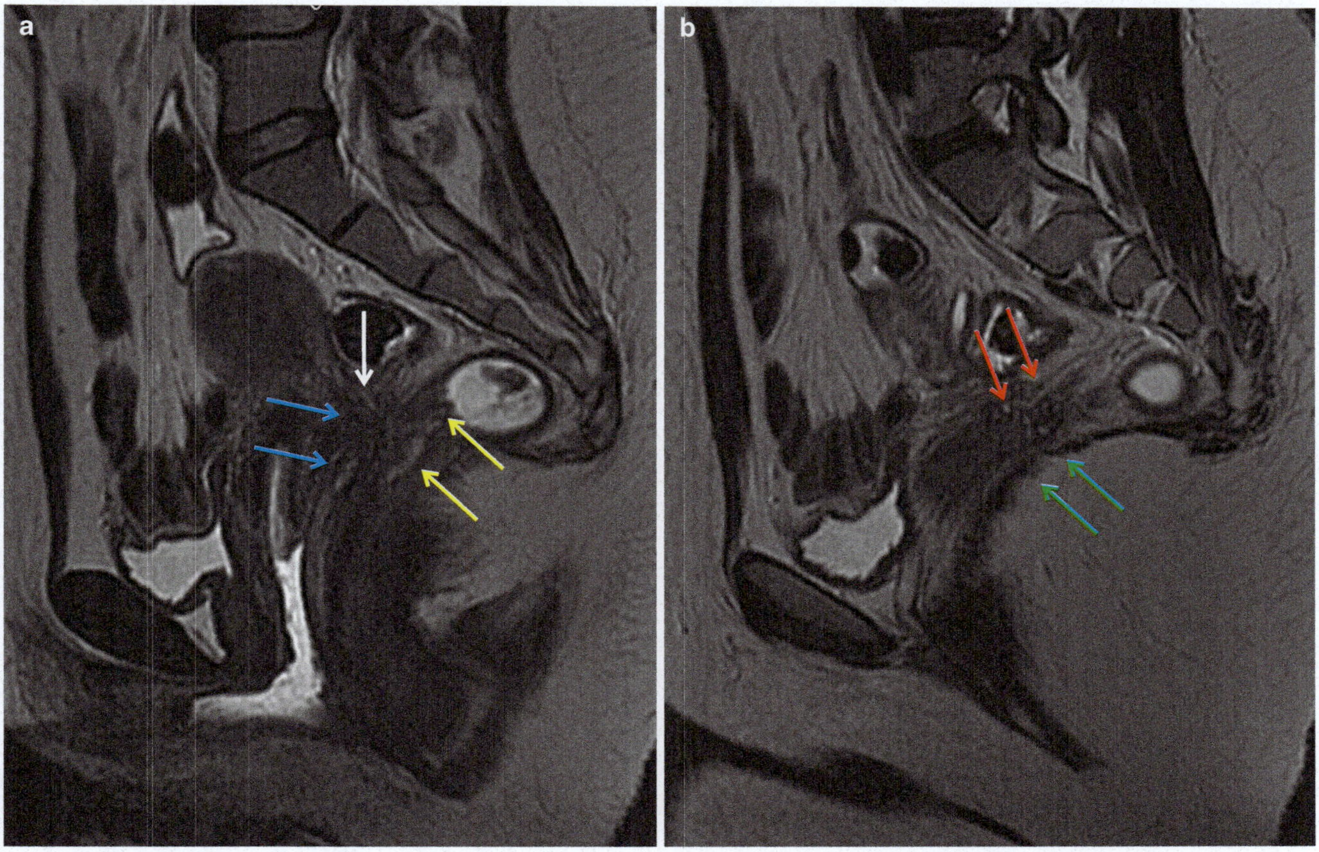

Fig. 4.81 Nodule of the rectovaginal septum (blue arrows) with involvement of the levator ani muscle (bilateral iliococcygeal) (green arrows in **b**, **f**). Extensive infiltrative lesion, following the muscle, with a predominance of fibrosis and well identified in the sagittal (**a**, **b**) (arrows) and axial planes (**c**–**f**) in T2-weighted sequences, and no bleeding in T1-weighted sequence with fat suppression, in the axial plane (**e**). Notice obliteration of the cul-de-sac (white arrow in **a**), rectal (yellow arrow A, **c**–**f**), and vaginal extension (**a**, **e**, **c**) and extension to the paracolpos, comprising the hypogastric nerve (red arrows)

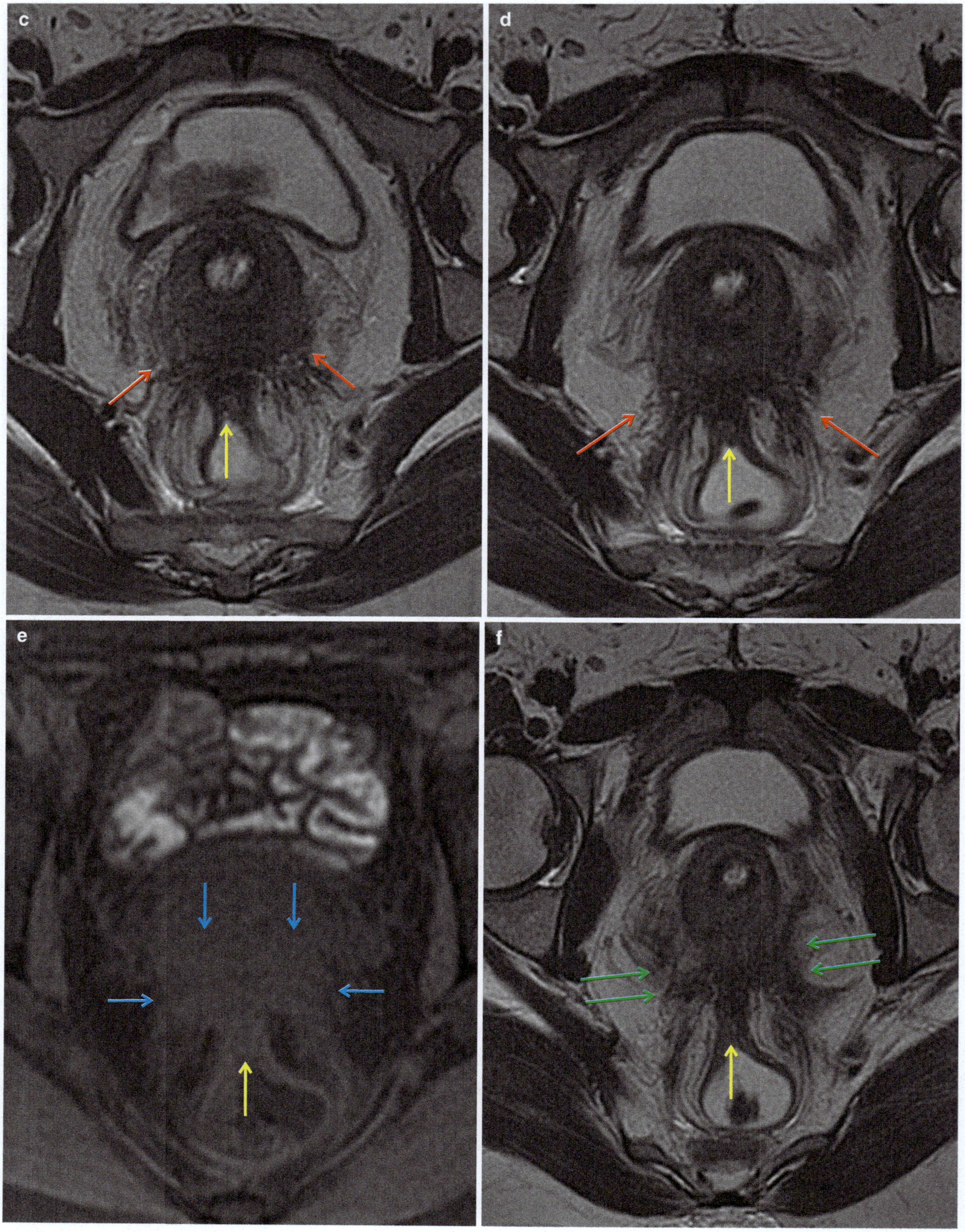

Fig. 4.81 (continued)

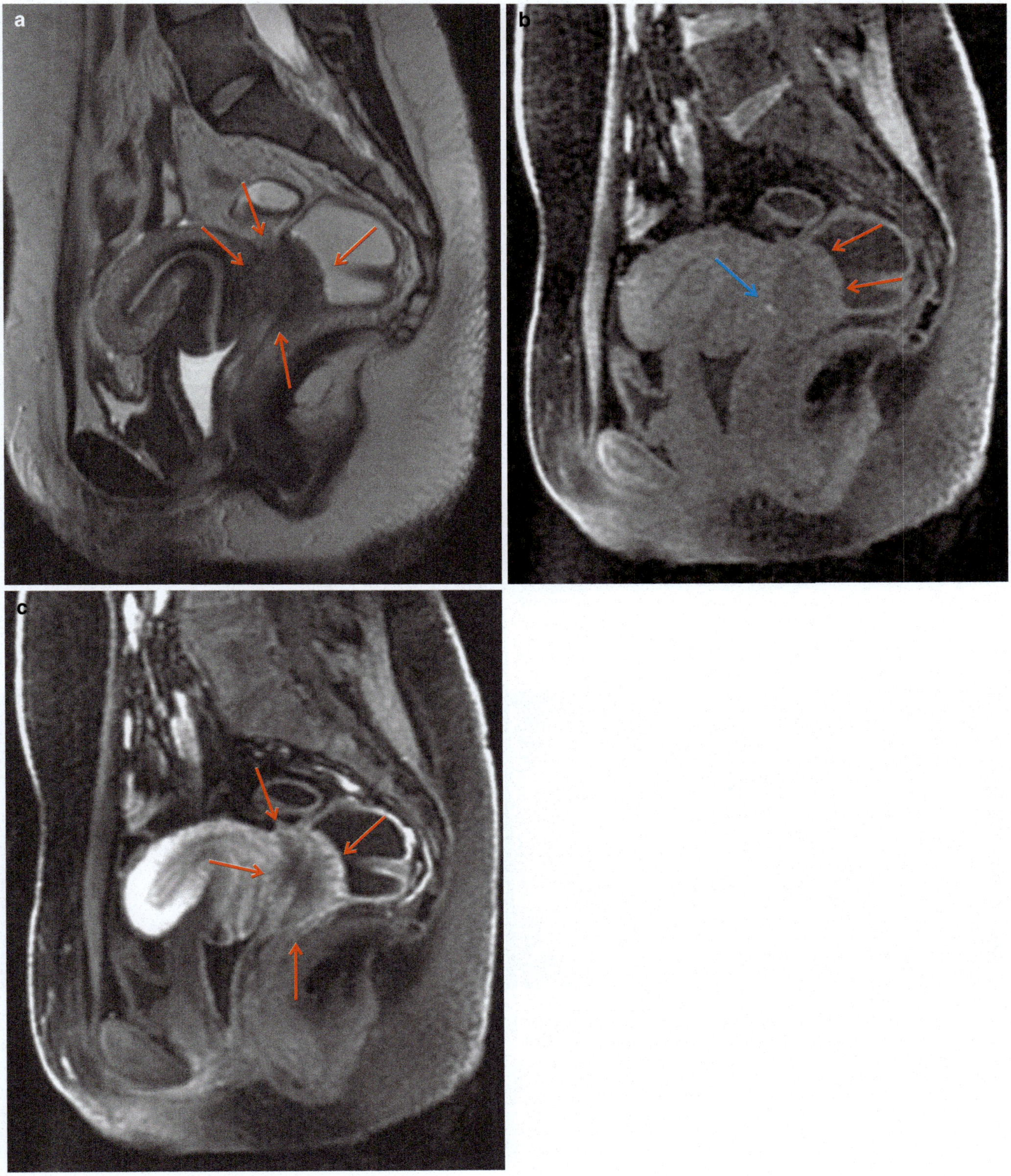

Fig. 4.82 Lesion in the rectovaginal and retrocervical septum (red arrows) with a predominance of fibrous tissue, hypointense in T2-weighted sequences (arrow in **a**), with intermediate signal in T1 (**b**), and with gadolinium enhancement (**c**), especially the intestinal part (arrow in **c**). Notice only one bleeding focus (arrow in **b**). (**a**–**c**) Sagittal

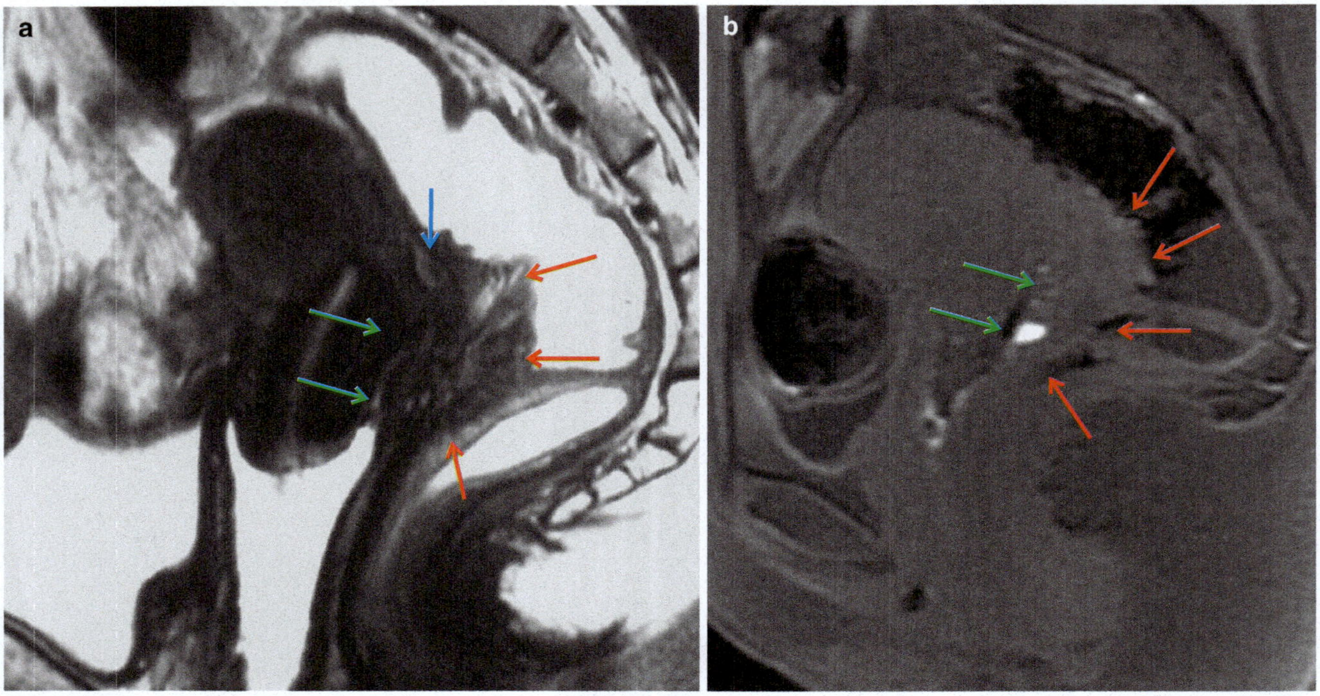

Fig. 4.83 Extensive lesion in the rectovaginal septum with posterior vaginal involvement, obliterating the vaginal fornix (green arrows), and the posterior cul-de-sac (blue arrow), in addition to deep rectal involvement (red arrows). Note the ectopic endometrial tissue with hyperintense signal in T2-weighted images (**a**) and T1 with fat saturation (**b**), reflecting the hematic content (arrows in **b**). (**a**, **b**) Sagittal

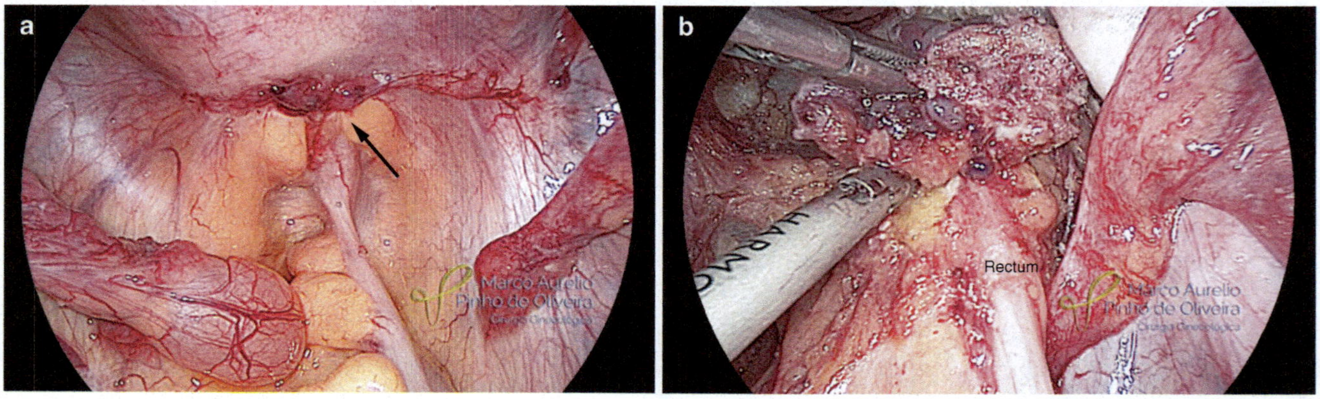

Fig. 4.84 In the initial laparoscopic view (**a**) the lesion seems small (arrow **a**), the largest part being deep in the rectovaginal septum (**c**–**f**), penetrating the lower rectum (blue arrows) and the vagina (red arrows). Notice the predominance of fibrous tissue, hypointense in T2 (**c**, **e**, **f**, intermediate in T1 with bleeding focus (arrow in **d**). (**a**, **b**) Laparoscopy. (**a**) Beginning of the procedure. (**b**) Removing the lesion (**g**) Microscopy of intestinal component. Rectum with endometriosis and decidual reaction. On the right, notice rectal mucosa (400×)

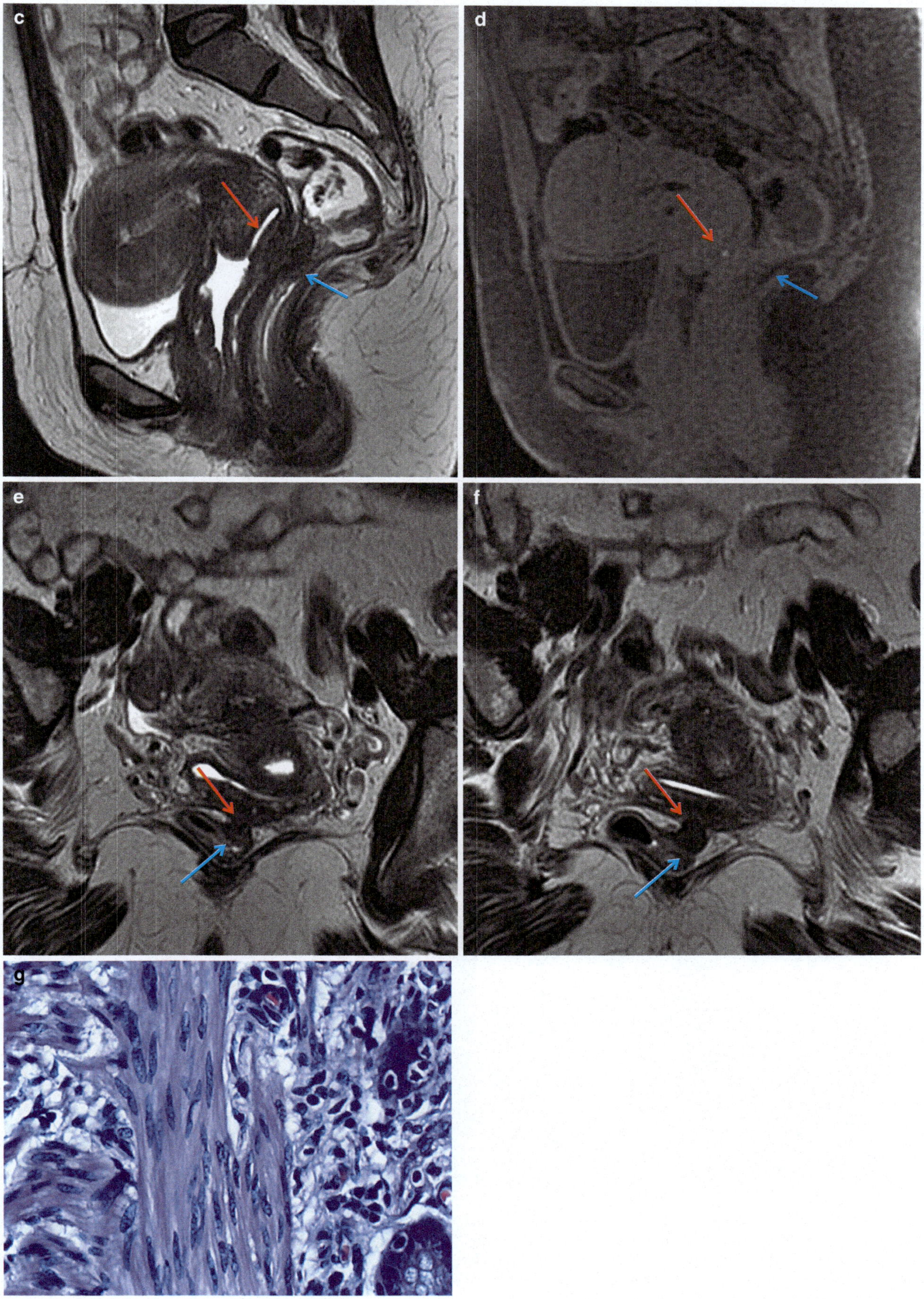

Fig. 4.84 (continued)

4.2.2.5 Comments on the Treatment

The treatment for rectovaginal space endometriosis lesions is surgery. The surgical planning will be influenced by the rectal and vaginal involvement and the obliteration of the cul-de-sac [39, 40].

After conducting ureterolysis and neurolysis, the uterosacral ligaments and posterior vaginal lesions are resected. Colpectomy and excision of the rectum wall may be required (Fig. 4.85).

Mid-to-lower rectum lesions increase surgical complexity and may require an expert surgeon. Even in experienced hands, a rectovaginal fistula can occur, and sometimes a protective ileostomy may be necessary. The MRI information helps the patient to understand the risk of the surgery and the chance of complications (Fig. 4.86) [9, 39].

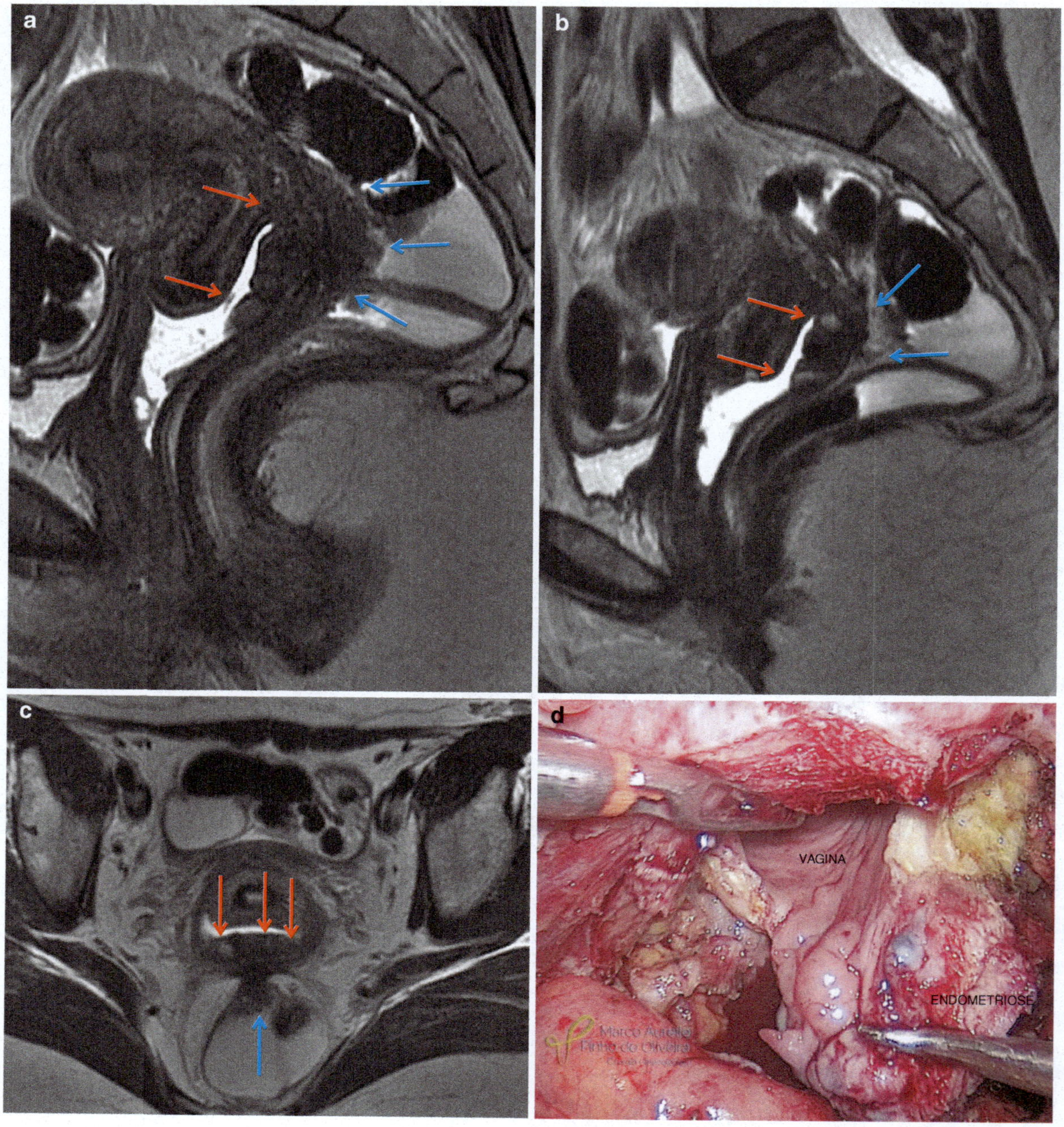

Fig. 4.85 Extensive lesion of the rectovaginal septum, with a vaginal component, obliterating the prominent cul-de-sac (red arrows) and rectum (to the lower segment—blue arrows). T2-weighted sequence. (**a**, **b**) Sagittal. (**c**) Axial. (**d**) Laparoscopy. After conducting ureterolysis and neurolysis, observe the resection of the posterior vaginal wall lesion. (**e**, **f**) Vaginal endometriotic node microscopy. (**e**) Magnification 400×. The cytogenic stroma is myxoid, probably due to iatrogenic action (decidual) and with hemosiderin inside the gland. (**f**) Image with a smaller enlargement of 40×

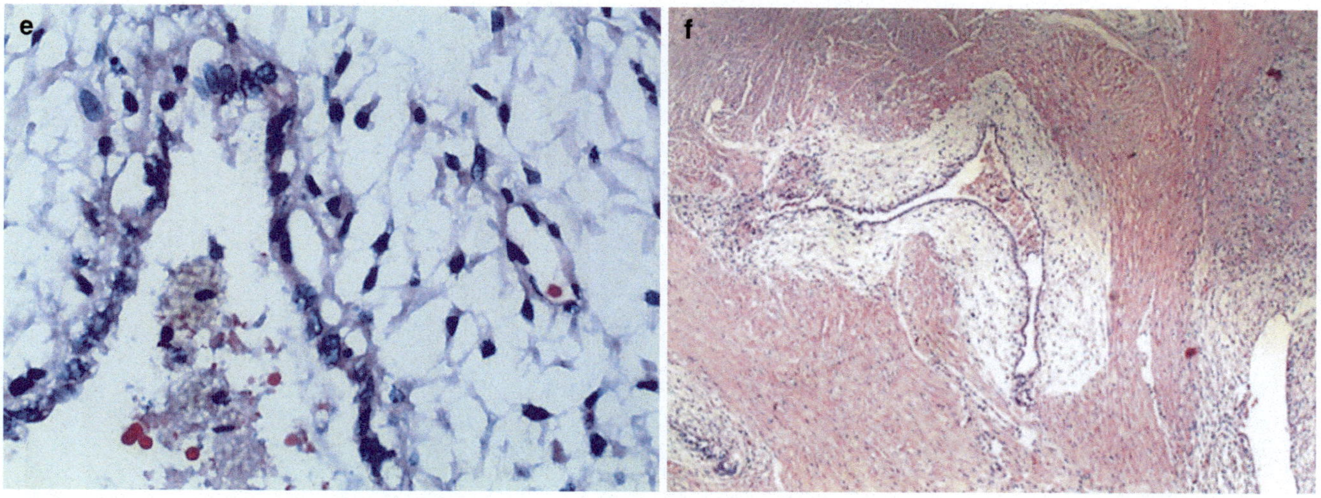

Fig. 4.85 (continued)

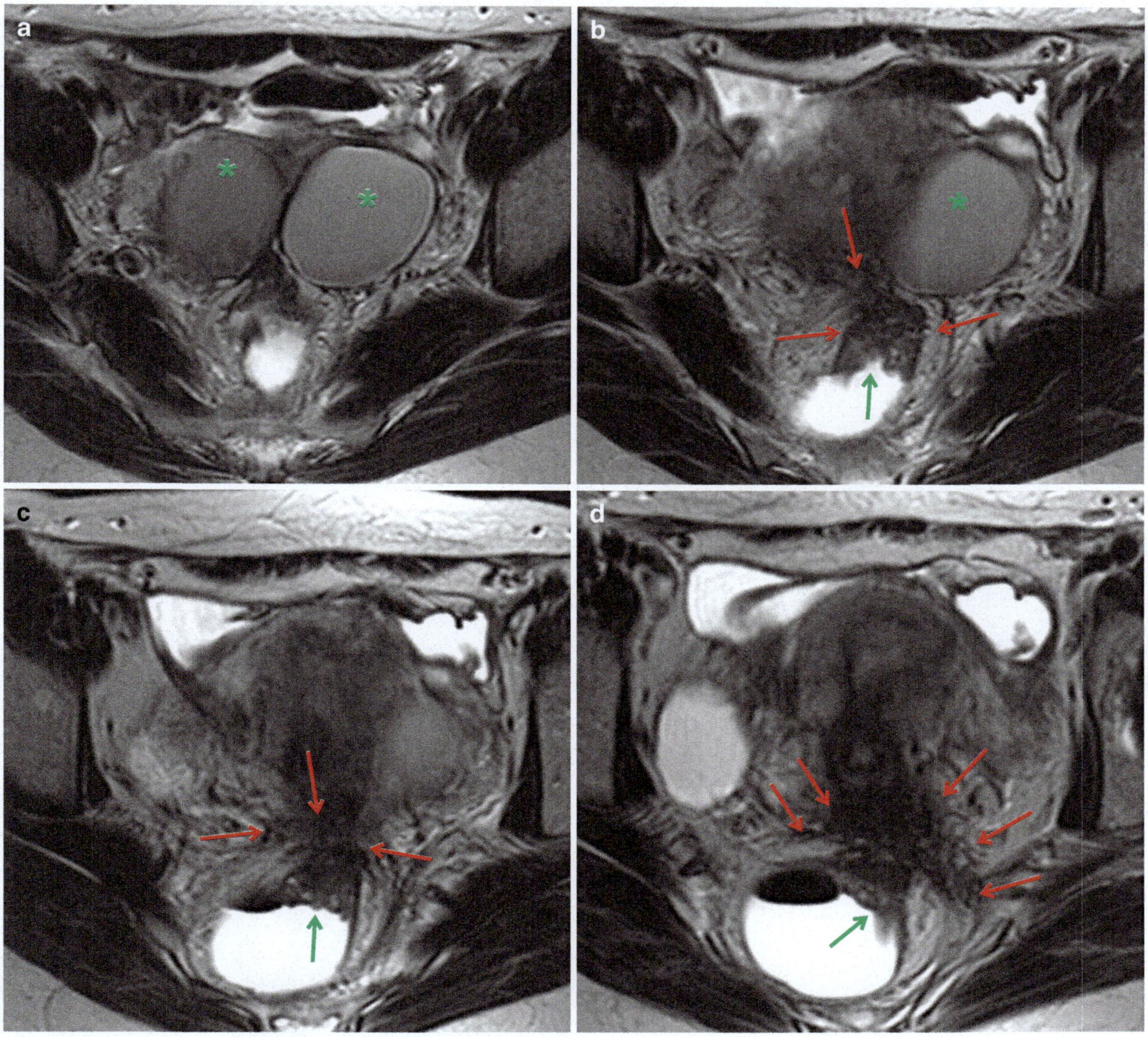

Fig. 4.86 (**a–g**) Extensive retrocervical and rectovaginal septum lesion (red arrows), with ligamentous commitment to the left, with involvement of the parametrium and pelvic floor (blue arrow) and the distal sigmoid and rectum (green arrows). Notice right bladder endometriosis (green arrow in **e**) and bilateral endometriomas (*). (**h**, **i**) Protective ileostomy in the right iliac fossa and discreet rectovaginal fistula (green arrow **i**). (**a–i**) T2-weighted sequences. (**a–e**) Coronal long axis. (**f**, **g**) Sagittal. (**h**, **i**) Axial

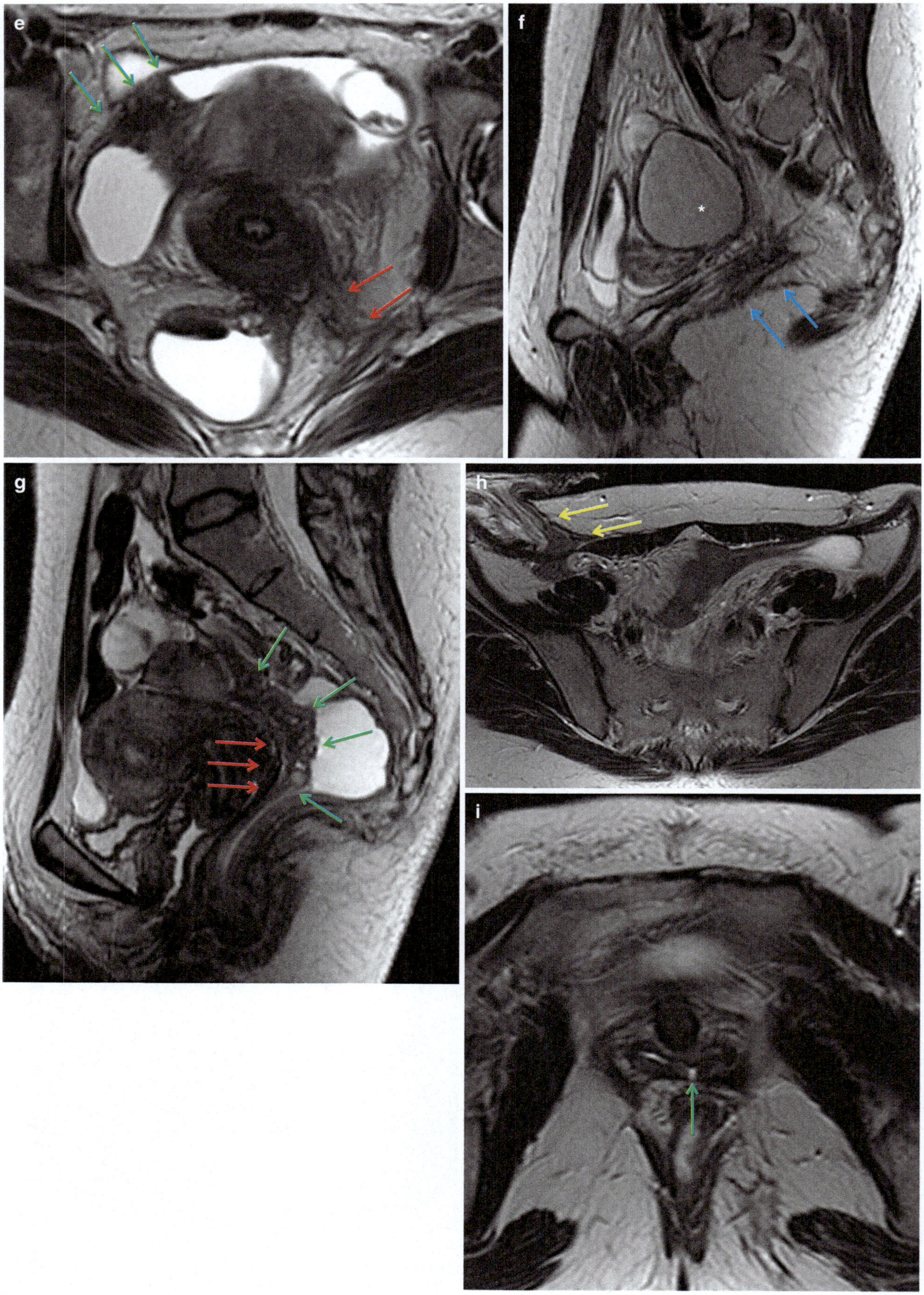

Fig. 4.86 (continued

4.2.3 Uterosacral Ligaments

4.2.3.1 Anatomy

The uterosacral ligaments are components of the pelvic fascia, an extraperitoneal structure of the pelvic floor, and form the pericervical ring. In conjunction with the cardinal ligaments, they support the uterine cervix and the vagina. The ligaments connect the cervix and the vagina to the sacrum, usually at the fourth vertebra level, and fuse with the presacral fascia, forming the lateral boundary of the posterior cul-de-sac (Fig. 4.87) [32].

Histologically, this ligament is a well-defined dense structure, comprising collagen, fatty and fibrous tissue, and rare smooth muscle fibers, interspersed with arteries, veins, and nerves for the cervix and the superior vagina [41].

In the MR images, the uterosacral ligament should be well-defined and slightly hypointense in the T2-weighted sequence, with an intermediate signal in the T1, without any bleeding (Fig. 4.88).

It is about 12–14 cm in length, and its thickness may vary during its path from the pericervical region to the

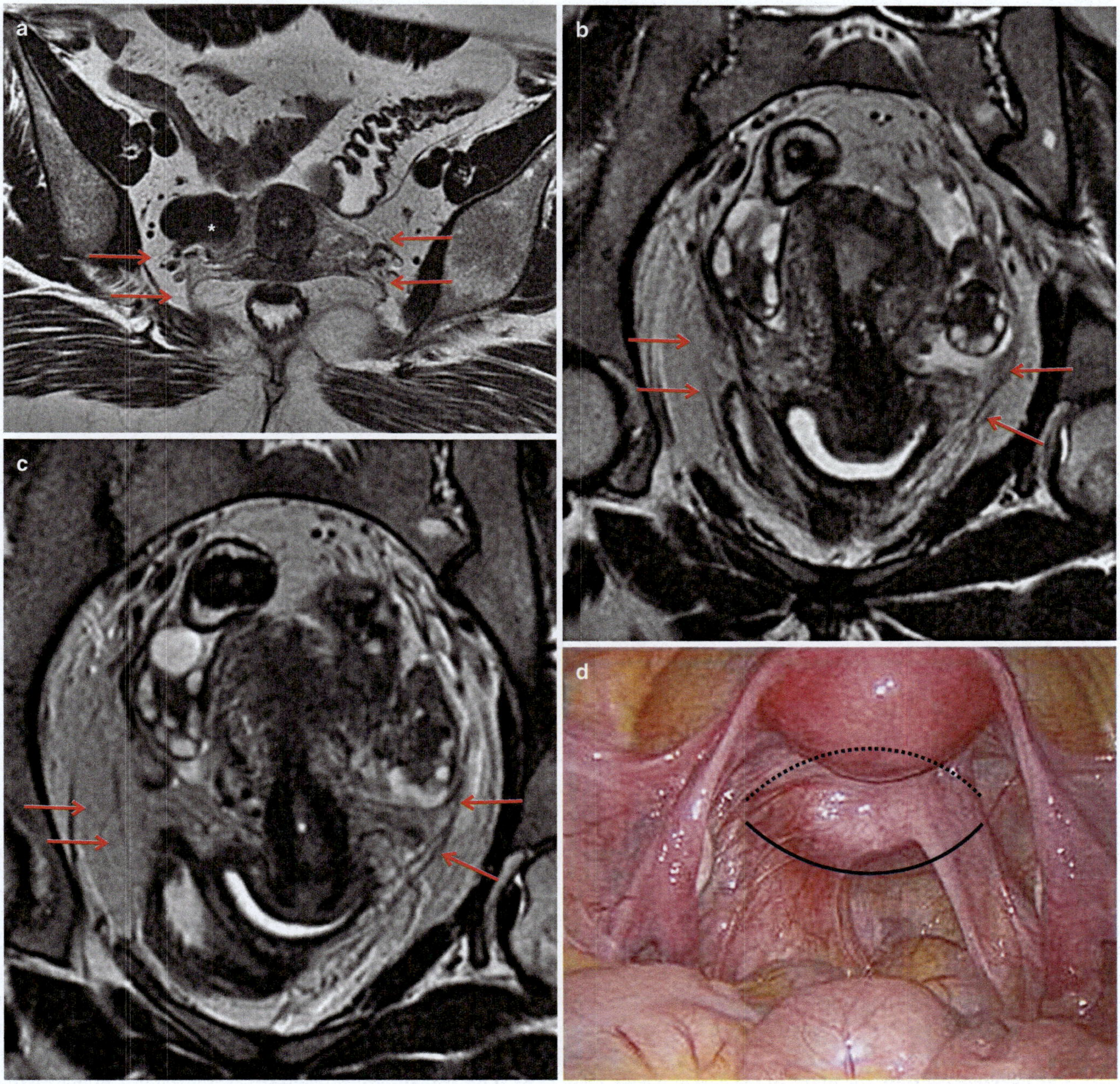

Fig. 4.87 Pericervical ring. The uterosacral ligaments together with the cardinal ligaments arise from the cervix and the upper vagina (arrows **a**–**c**). The ligaments connect the cervix and vagina to the sacrum and form the lateral boundary of the posterior cul-de-sac (**d**). (**a**, **c**) T2-weighted sequences. (**a**) Coronal, short axis. Note ligamentous leiomyoma to the right (*). (**b**, **c**) Coronal long axis. (**d**) Laparoscopy showing the region of the pericervical ring within the ellipse

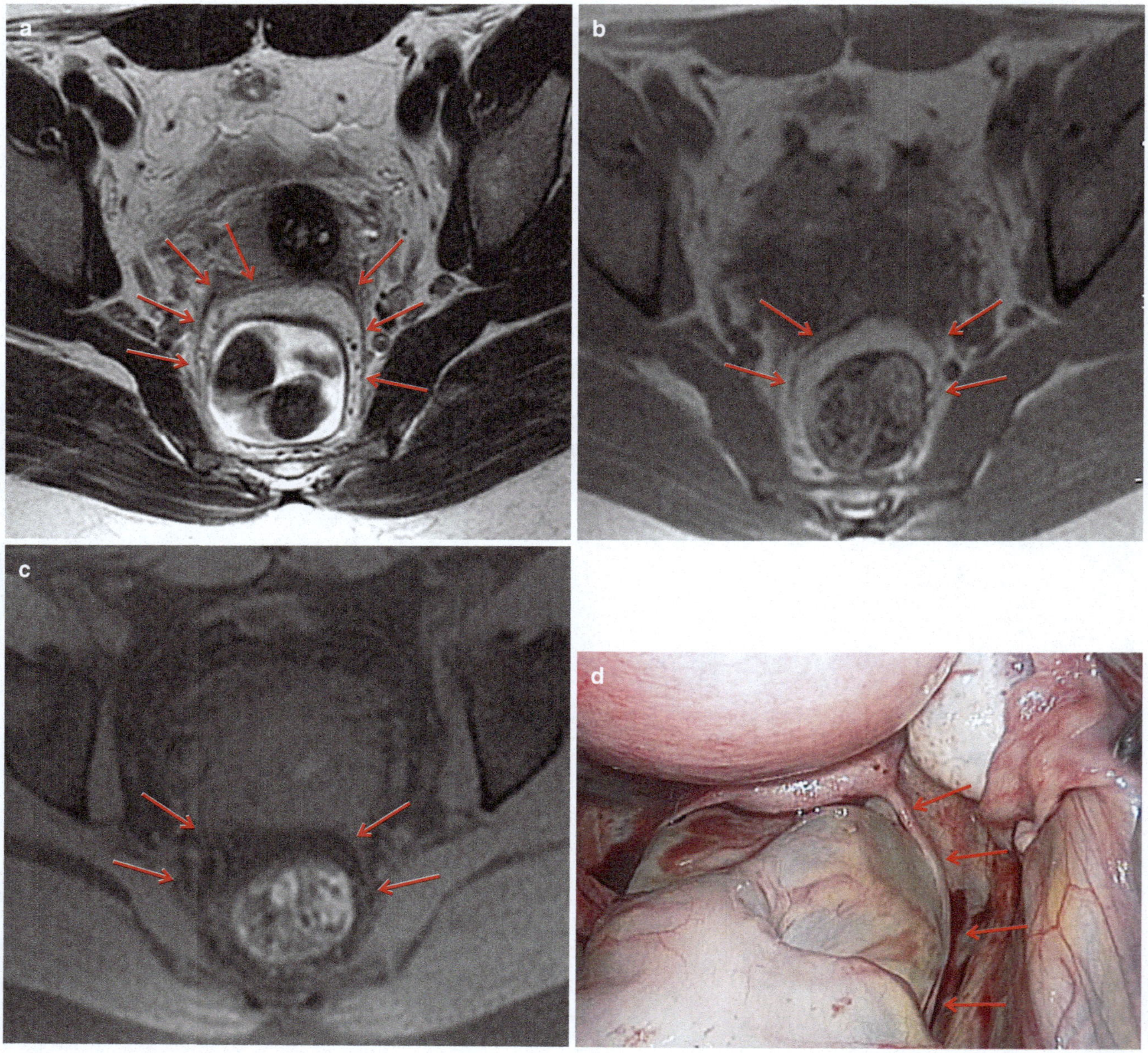

Fig. 4.88 (**a**) Normal uterosacral ligament (arrows) must be well-defined, slightly hypointense in T2-weighted sequence (**a**) with an intermediate signal in T1 (**b**), with no bleeding in the T1-weighted sequence with fat suppression (**c**). (**a**–**c**) Axial. (**d**) Laparoscopy showing normal right uterosacral ligament

sacrum, getting thinner as the sacrum is approached. We consider 4 mm as the maximum normal thickness in MRI (Fig. 4.87) [41].

The understanding of anatomy is the most important factor for the identification of this ligament by MRI, in addition to the high spatial resolution on T2-weighted images. The ligament has a complex path, and for didactic purposes, we separate it into three parts:

(a) **The cervical section**: the plane of the cervical ring, also called the *torus uterinus*, involves the cervix and the vaginal vault, being predominantly a posterior insertion, with some anterior fibers that merge and adhere to the cardinal ligament (Fig. 4.89). The uterosacral ligament interfaces anteriorly with the parametrium and posteriorly with the mesorectum and the cul-de-sac, containing branches of the hypogastric plexus (Fig. 4.89). The cervical pathway is lateral-horizontal in relation to the cervix and vagina. This is the thickest section of the ligament, ranging from 5 to 20 mm in cadaver studies under tension and 20–30 mm in width (Fig. 4.89) [41].
(b) **The intermediate section**: in the lateral plane of the posterior cul-de-sac, with oblique, lateral, and posterior directions, contacting the mesorectal fascia and mesorectum, with proximity to the piriformis muscle,

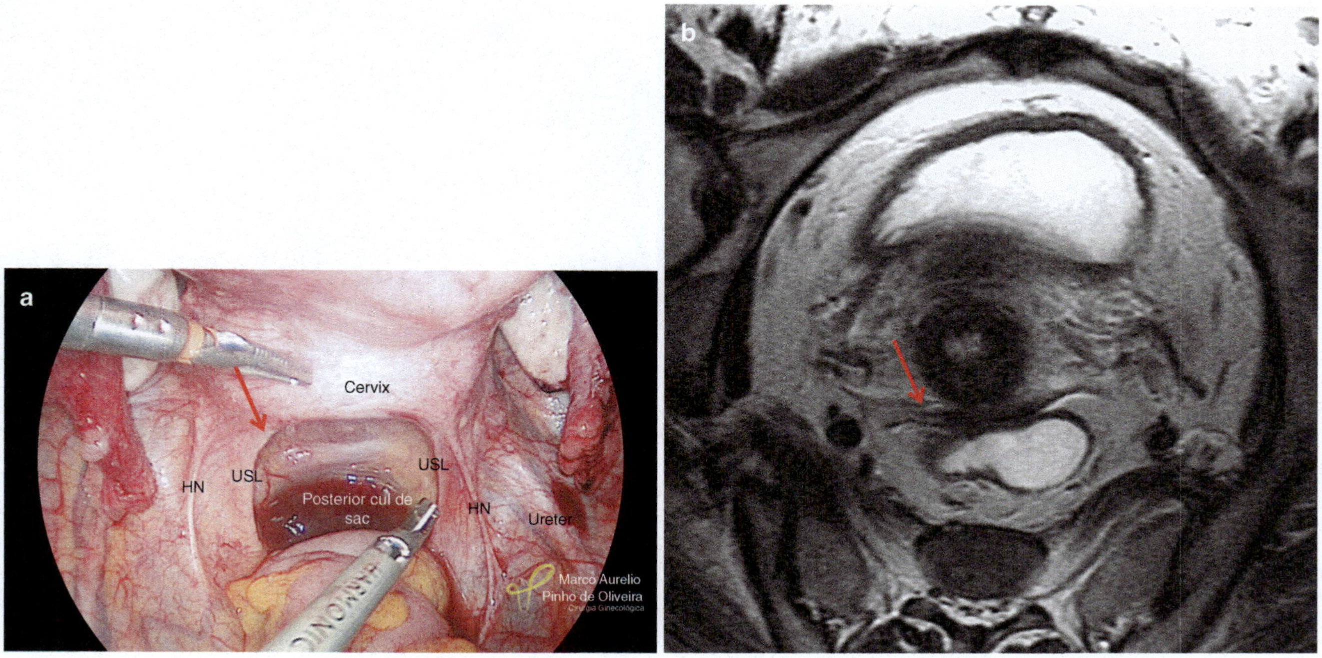

Fig. 4.89 Cervical segment. The cervical path is lateral and horizontal to the cervix and vagina. It is the thickest portion of the ligament, measuring up to 4 mm when normal (arrowheads). (**a**) Laparoscopy. (**b**) T2-weighted Sequence. Coronal short axis

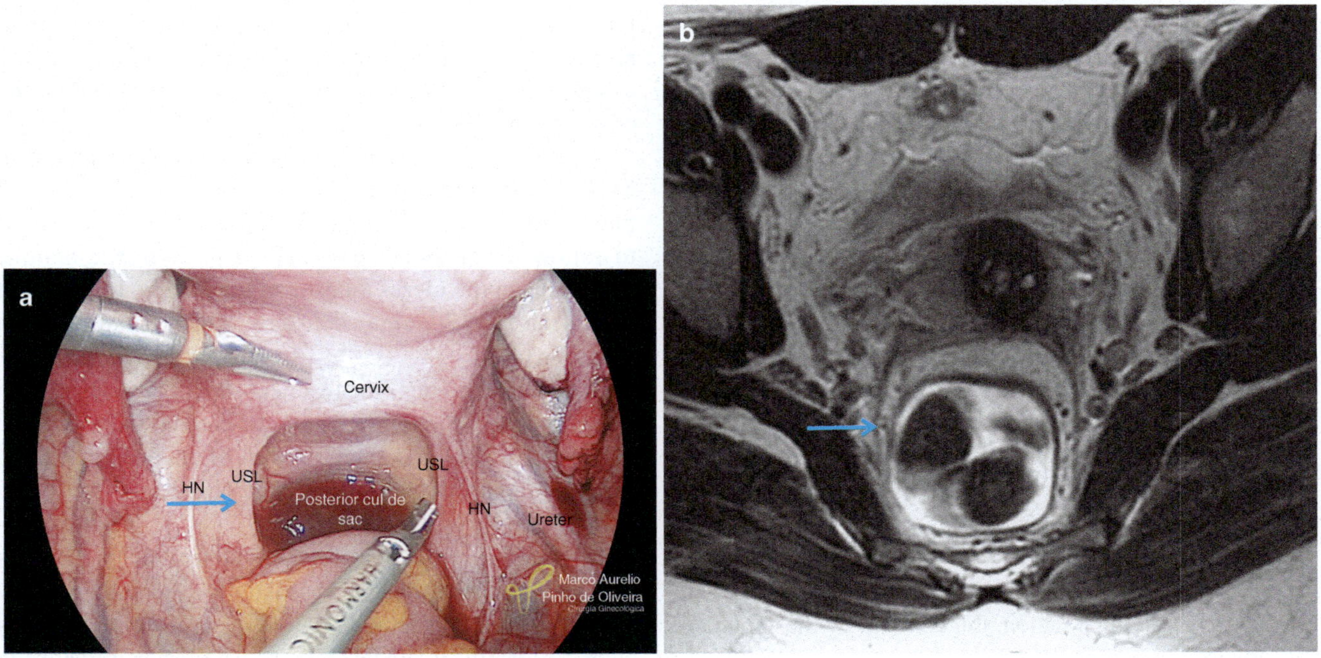

Fig. 4.90 Intermediate segment (arrows). Side view of the posterior cul-de-sac, with oblique, lateral, and posterior direction contacting the mesorectal fascia and mesorectum near the piriformis muscle and sacral plexus. (**a**) Laparoscopy. (**b**) T2-weighted Sequence. Axial

sciatic nerve, and sacral plexus. It is 5 cm long (Fig. 4.90).

(c) **The sacral section**: in the plane of the sacral insertion, with oblique, posterior, and superior direction, adhered to the presacral fascia and closely related to the emerging sacral roots (Fig. 4.91).

The insertion in the pelvic fascia has two subdivisions: (a) vertical sacrococcygeal articulation, S3, and (b) transversal to the sacral foramen, the sacroiliac joint, attached to the fascia covering the piriformis and the levator ani muscles. It is the thinnest section of the ligament (<0.5 mm) [41].

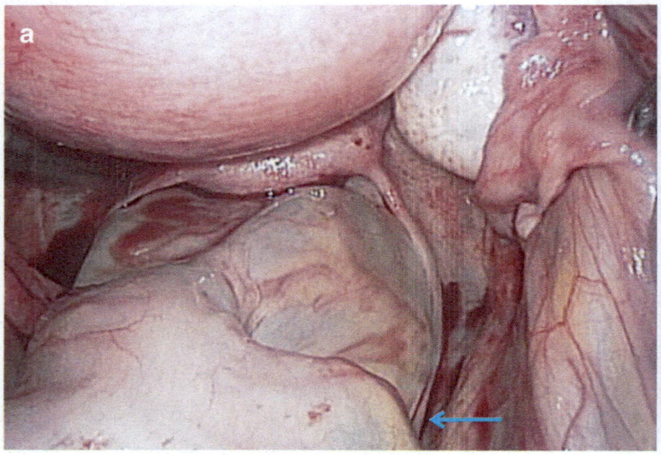

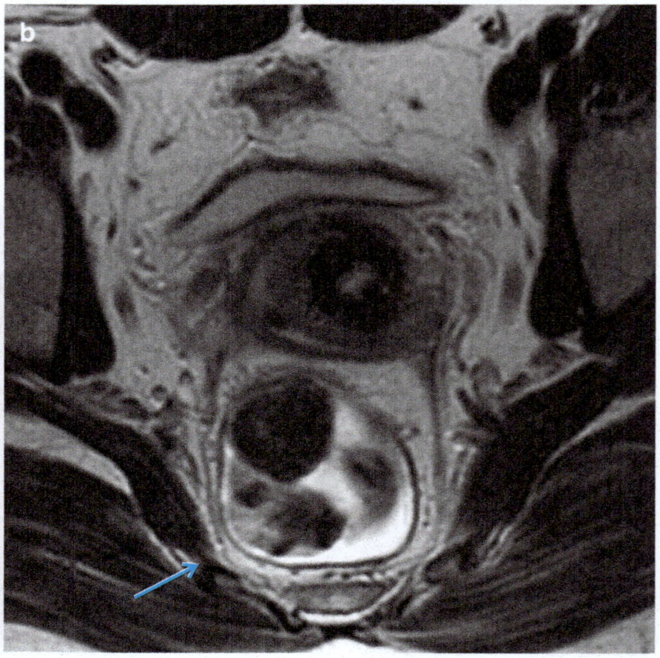

Fig. 4.91 Sacral portion. In the sacral insertion plane, the ligament has an oblique, posterior, and superior direction, adhered to the presacral fascia and closely related to the emerging sacral roots (arrows). (**a**) Laparoscopy. (**b**) T2-weighted sequence. Axial

4.2.3.2 Most Common Aspects of Endometriosis

These ligaments are very important because they are the most frequent site of deep endometriosis. Bazot identified uterosacral lesions in 80% of the patients studied [42, 43].

According to Chapron, the frequency of involvement is asymmetrical, with a predominance of the left side, probably due to peritoneal flow theory. However, other authors did not have the same experience, observing bilateral ligament symmetrical involvement, associated with medial posterior, retrocervical, or rectovaginal septum lesions [5, 34].

4.2.3.3 Clinical Symptoms

The majority of the lesions are symptomatic, and the patients affected present deep, progressive dyspareunia, typical of the involvement of this ligament [26].

When the extension of the lesion reaches the sacral section of the ligament, the patient may report lumbar pain with spread to the inguinal region, thigh or leg, by the simultaneous involvement of nerve fibers.

Implants can be noticed on physical examination, with thickening and pain on examination in the mobilization of uterosacral ligaments.

4.2.3.4 MRI and Laparoscopic Findings

Understanding the anatomy and pattern of endometriosis involvement in this ligament is one of the major challenges for the radiologist. This understanding coupled with high-resolution T2-weighted images directed at the ligament is essential for the characterization of the normal aspect and endometriosis lesion.

To improve the identification and characterization in MRI, we suggest the images are acquired in the axial plane with an angulation of 25° (anteroinferior direction) to follow the ligament path and to perform the oblique sequences of the uterus (short and long axes), high spatial resolution on T2-weighted image, with a smaller depth (3–4 mm) [44].

The identification of the ligament should be performed in all planes, the best in order being the coronal short axis, the oblique axis, and the sagittal. Because of their complex pathway, the authors define any ligament changes in two planes as suspicious (Fig. 4.92).

Another factor that may hinder ligament identification is inadequate preparation and its proximity to loops, especially with the redundant sigmoid. The use of several cutting planes helps to identify it. Bazot described a greater difficulty in characterizing the left uterosacral because of its relation with the sigmoid [8].

In addition, uterine retroversion, multiple endometriomas, and the pelvis may make it difficult to identify and detect uterosacral lesions (Fig. 4.93) [45].

The criteria for lesions of the uterosacral ligament in MRI are (Table 4.7):

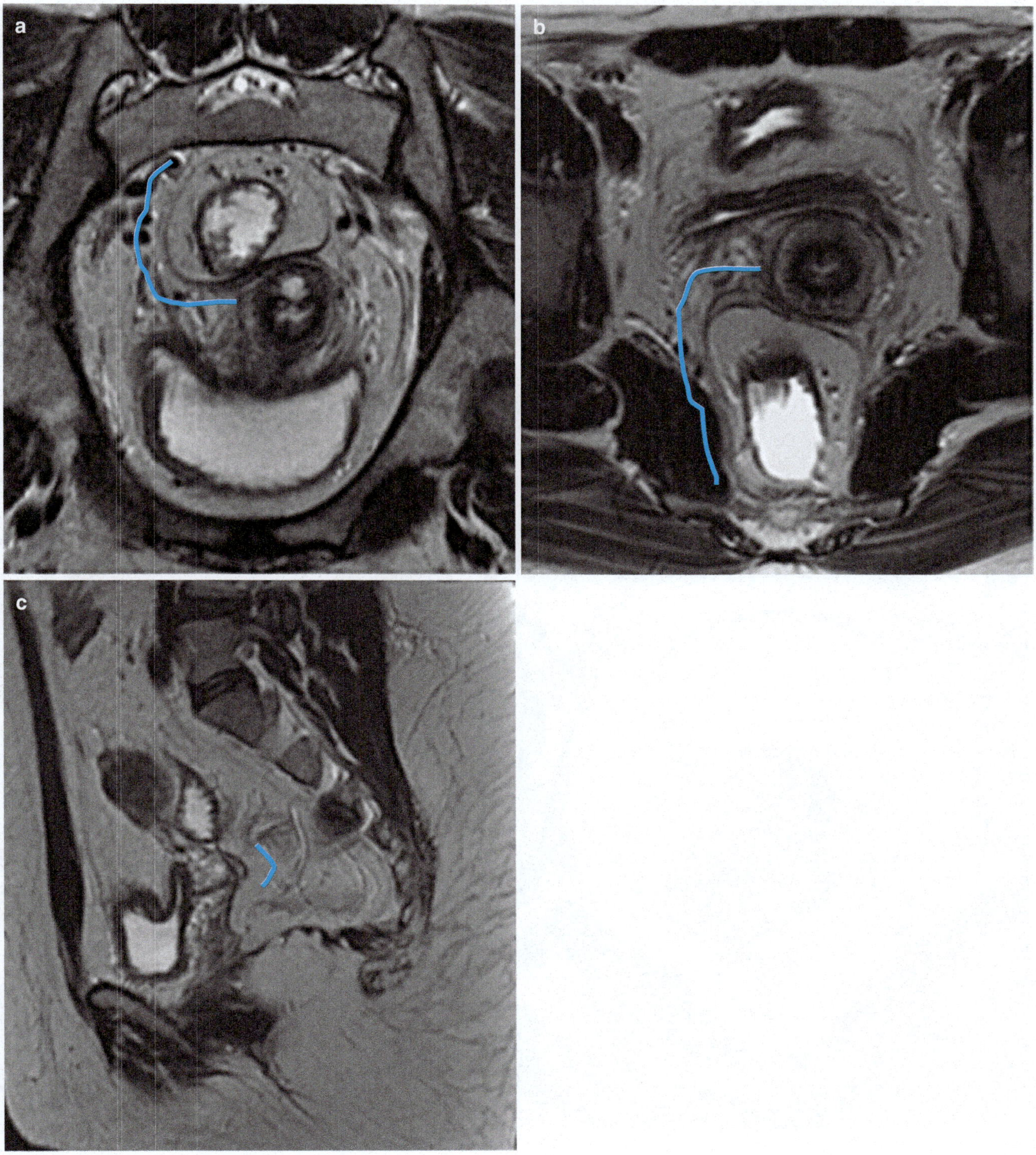

Fig. 4.92 Because of the multiple adjacent structures and its oblique direction, the identification of the uterosacral ligament should be performed in the coronal short axis (**a**), oblique axial (**b**), and sagittal (**c**) (parallel to the path). T2-weighted sequences

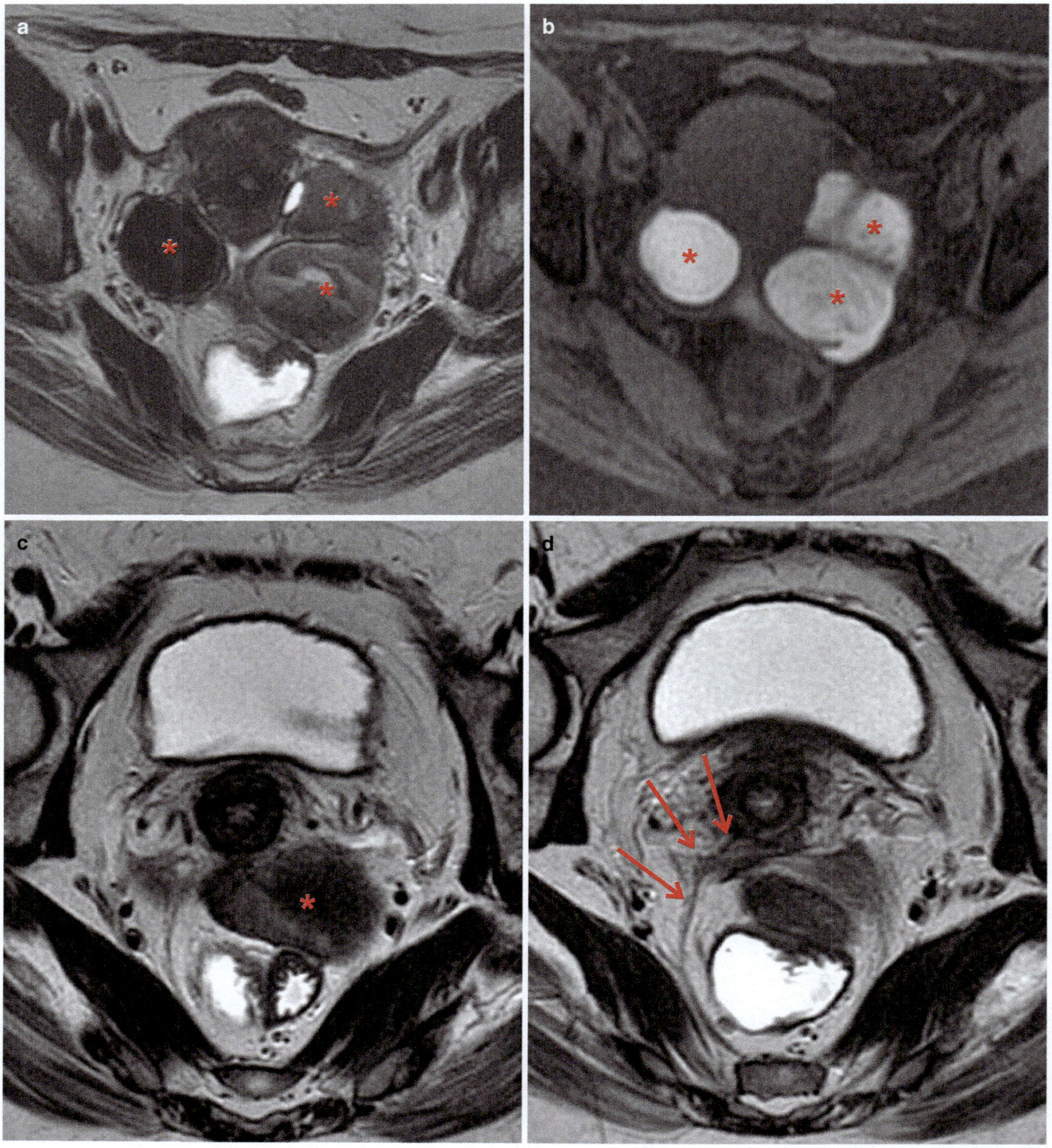

Fig. 4.93 (**a**, **b**) Bilateral endometriomas (*) difficult to identify the lesion in the right uterosacral ligament (arrows). Seek to identify in all planes (arrows **d**–**g**). (**a**, **c**–**g**) T2-weighted sequences. (**b**) T1 weighted. (**a**–**d**) Oblique axial. (**e**) Sagittal. (**f**, **g**) Coronal short axis. (**h**–**k**) Laparoscopy with resection of the capsule of the endometrioma (**h**) and uterosacral ligament (**i**). Lesion and resection of the ovarian fossa (**k**). (**l**) Ligament microscopy (100×) showing endometriotic cysts and extensive pericystic infiltration

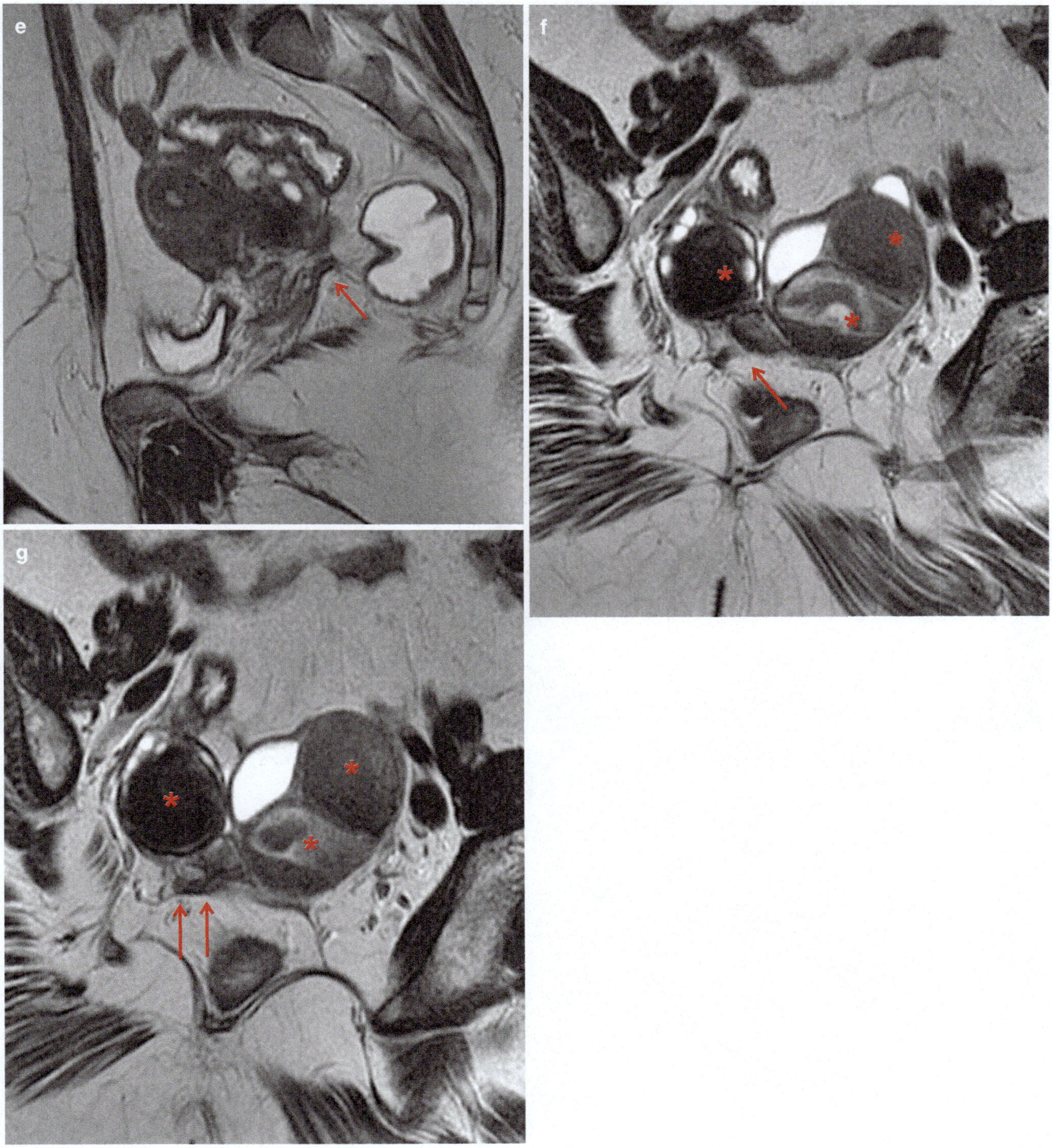

Fig. 4.93 (continued)

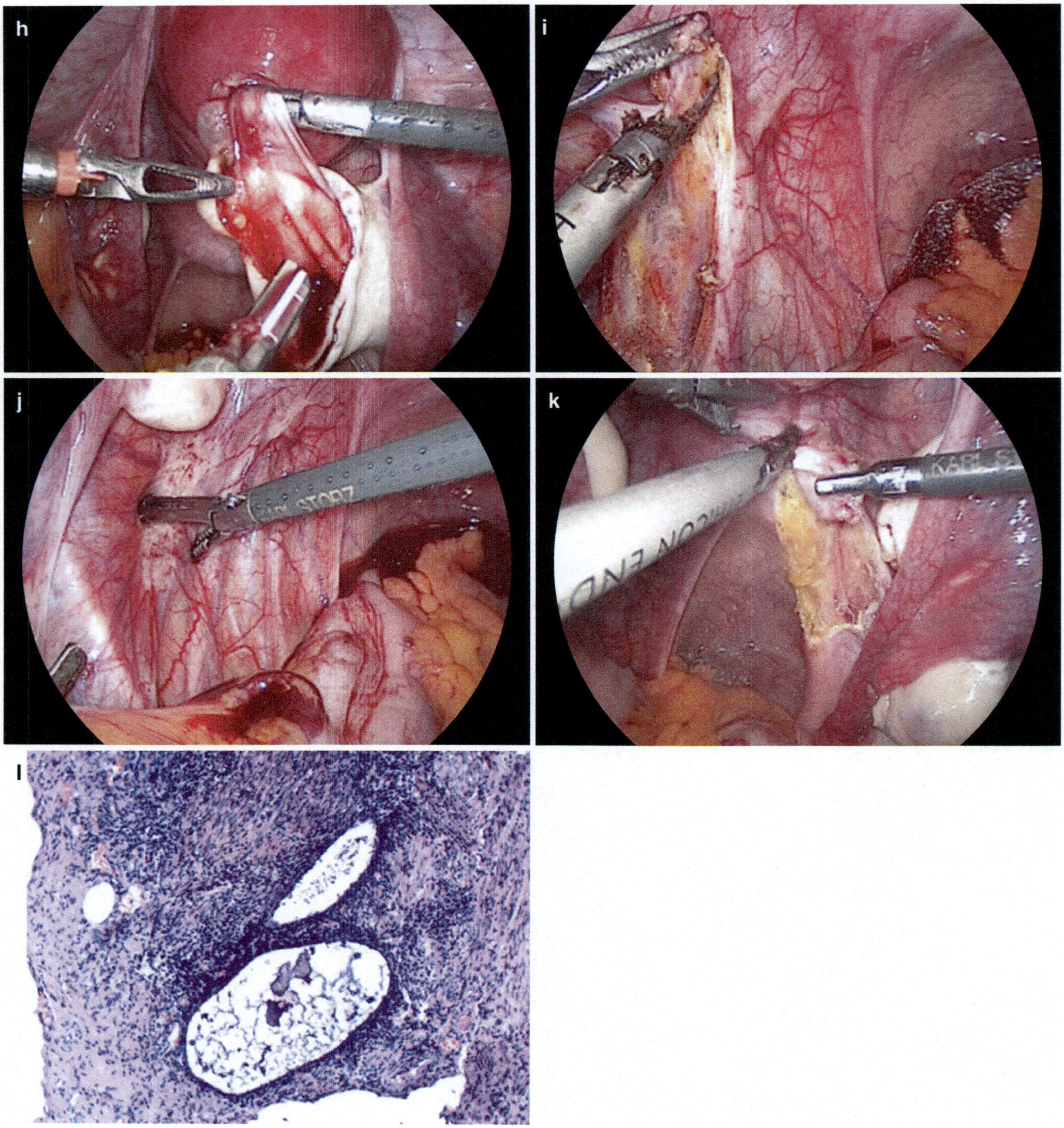

Fig. 4.93 (continued)

Table 4.7 Criteria for uterosacral ligament lesion

Ligament thickening > or equal to 5 mm
Signal modification
Nodule and mass

1. **Thickening**: defined as a thickness equal to or greater than 5 mm. Usually it is accompanied by contour irregularity and ligament retraction (Fig. 4.94). The retraction changes its position, to having a superior path, and adhere to the adnexa and the rectum and sigmoid, hindering their full identification (Fig. 4.95).

The most common involvement is of the cervical section; however, it may extend to the sacral section. When bilateral, we usually describe this form of impairment as the "mustache sign" (Fig. 4.96).

2. **Signal modification**: The ligament acquires a fairly hypointense signal on T2-weighted images, due to fibrosis, and when there is glandular tissue may vshow hyperintense foci on T2, and in the presence of bleeding, hyperintense on T1 (Fig. 4.97).

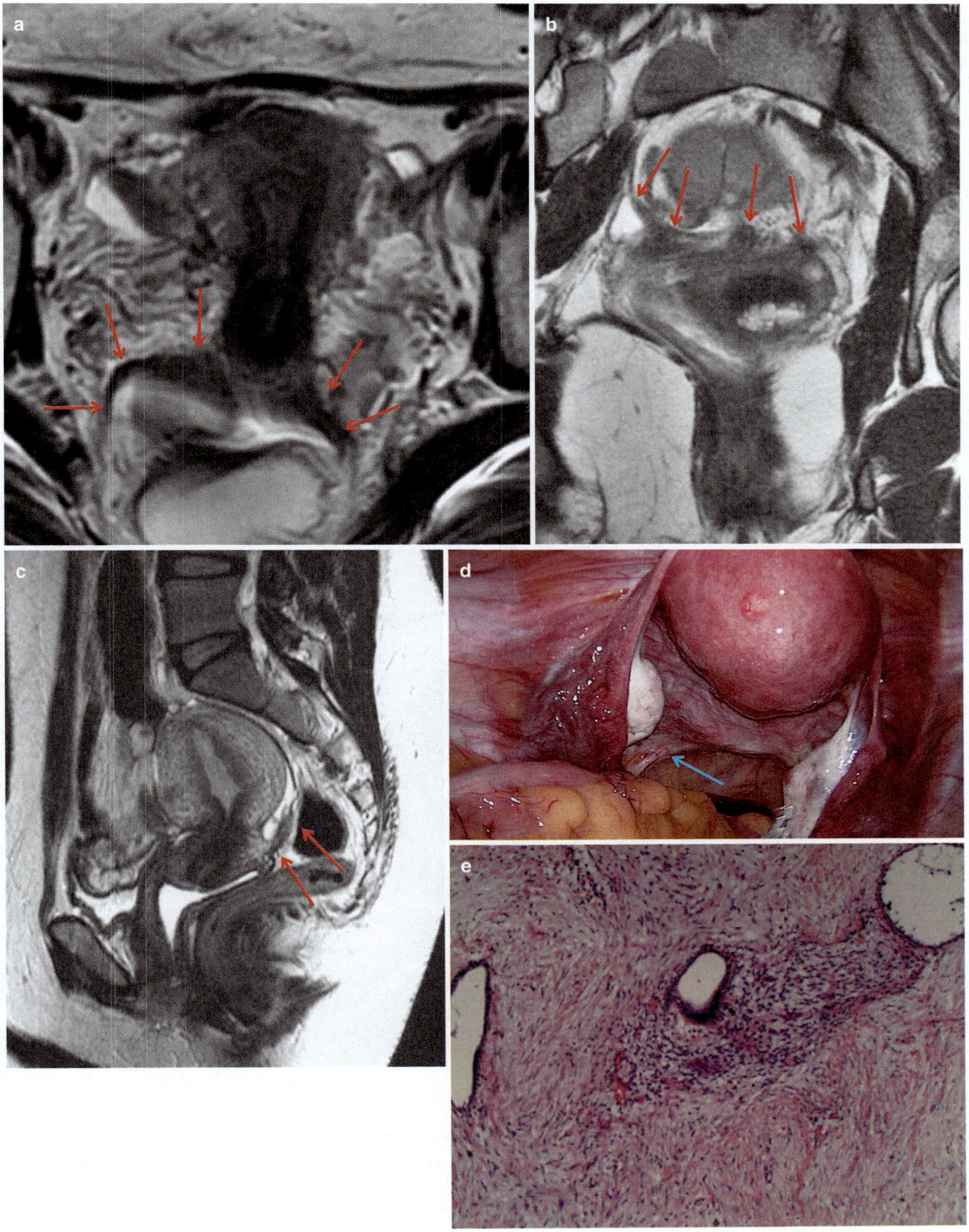

Fig. 4.94 Thickening (thickness greater than 5 mm) of the cervical and intermediate portions of the two uterosacrals (arrows) accompanied by contour irregularity and ligamentous retraction on the right (**b**, **c**). (**a**–**c**) T2-weighted sequences. (**a**) Coronal long axis. (**b**) Coronal. (**c**) Sagittal. (**d**) Laparoscopy. (**e**) Microscopy (100×). Endometriotic cysts and central lymphoplasmacytic infiltration

3. **Nodules and mass**: the endometriotic nodule can be prominent and form a lump or mass. When presented, the lesion goes beyond the ligament and compromises the adjacent structures, especially the mesorectum, rectum, sigmoid, vagina, and pelvic floor. The lesion is poorly delimited and infiltrative and exhibits the same signal characteristics as in ligament thickening (Fig. 4.98).

Because of the proximity to the ureter and the inferior hypogastric nerve, special care should be taken by the radiologist to identify the relationship of the lesion with these structures (Fig. 4.99).

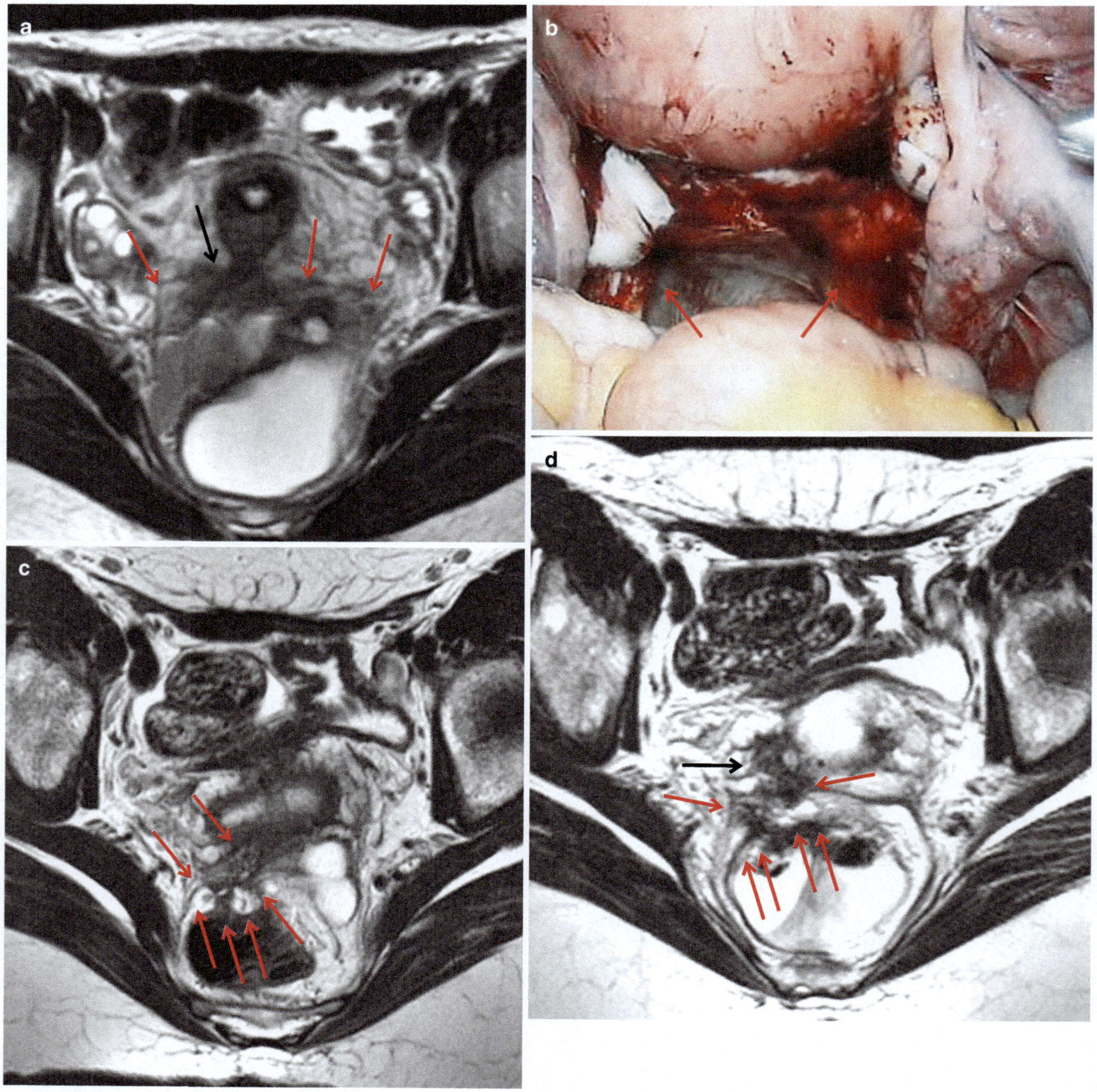

Fig. 4.95 (**a**, **b**) Case 1: Thickening and retraction of the ligaments, the left adhered to the adnexa and the rectum (red arrows). Note parametrial extension (black arrow). (**ec**) Case 2: Thickening, irregularity and retraction to the right, with mesorectal extension, adhered to the rectum. Observe additional lesion on the sigmoid (green arrow). (**a**, **e–c**) T2-weighted sequences. (**a**, **c**, **d**) Axial. (**e**) Sagittal. (**b**) Laparoscopy. Arrows showing bilateral ligament lesion and adherence with the adnexa

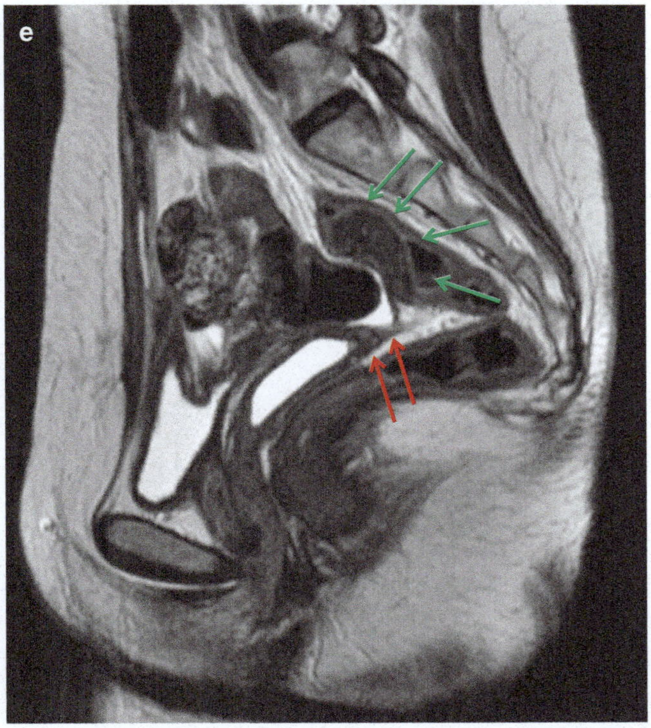

Fig. 4.95 (continued)

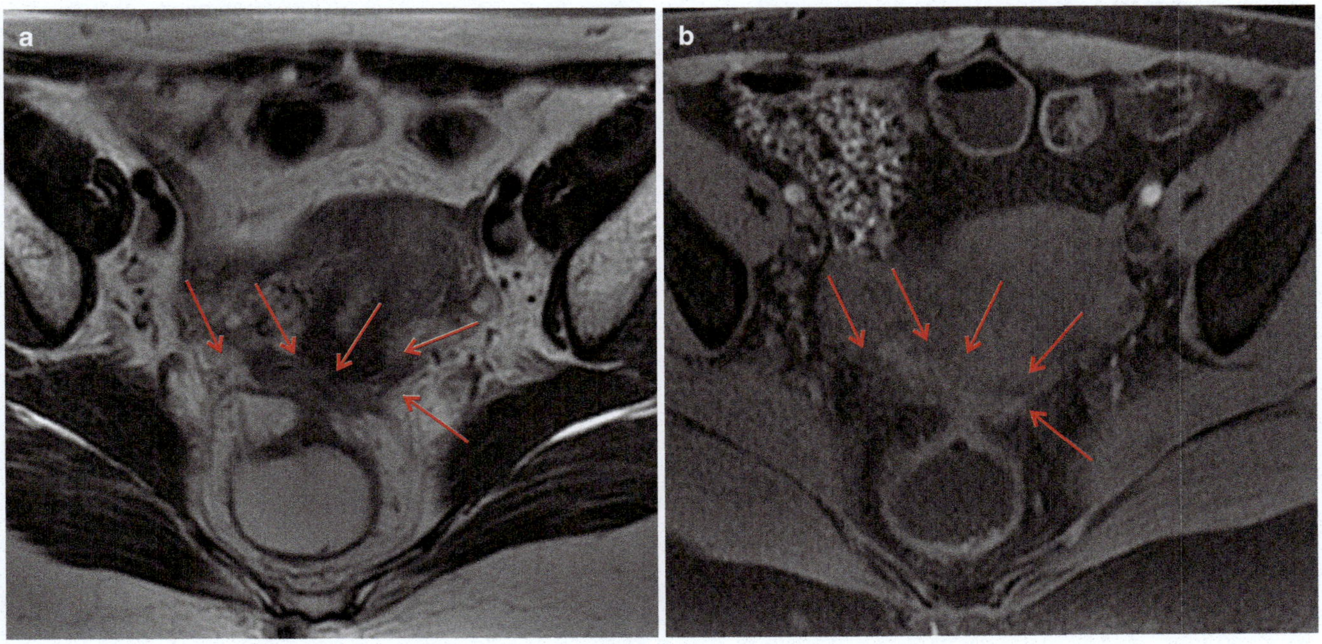

Fig. 4.96 Retrocervical lesion and bilateral thickening of the cervical portion (mustache sign - arrows in **a**, **b**, **k–o**). In Case 1 (**a–i**), adhesion is observed with right attachment and in Case 2 (**m–o**) with left attachment. Compromising the cervical and intermediate portions of the uterosacral ligaments. (**a**, **c**, **e**, **g**, **i**, **k–o**) T2-weighted sequences. (**b**, **d**, **f**, **h**, **j**) T1-weighted with fat suppression. (**a**, **b**) Axial. (**c–j**) Sagittal. (**k**, **l**, **n**, **o**) Coronal short axis. Note the discrete bleeding on the lesion in **b**, **d**, **f**, **h**. (**j**) Reference for localization of the lesion in (**k**, **l**). Note extension to the rectum in both cases and endometriomas in the right ovary in Case 1

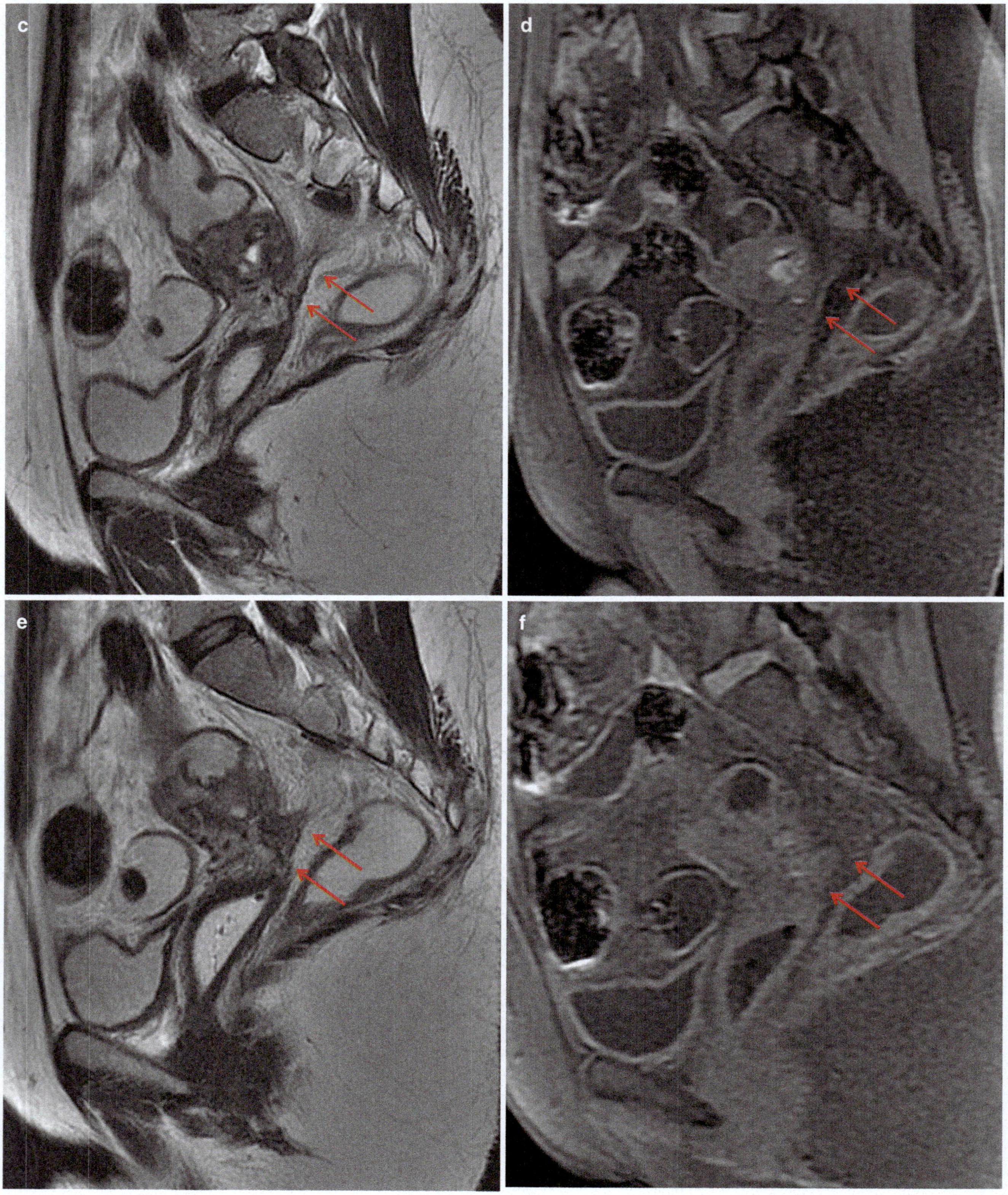

Fig. 4.96 (continued)

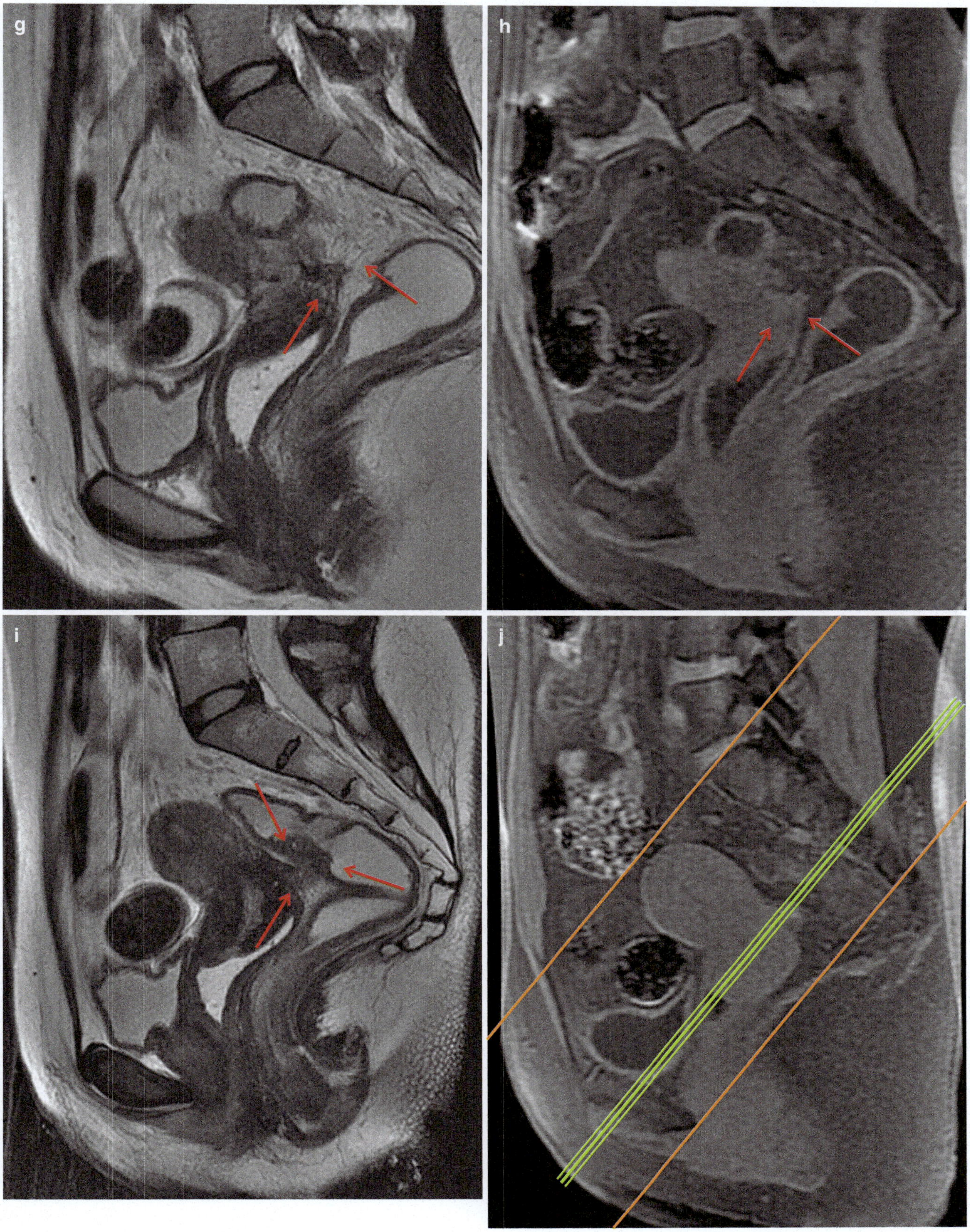

Fig. 4.96 (continued)

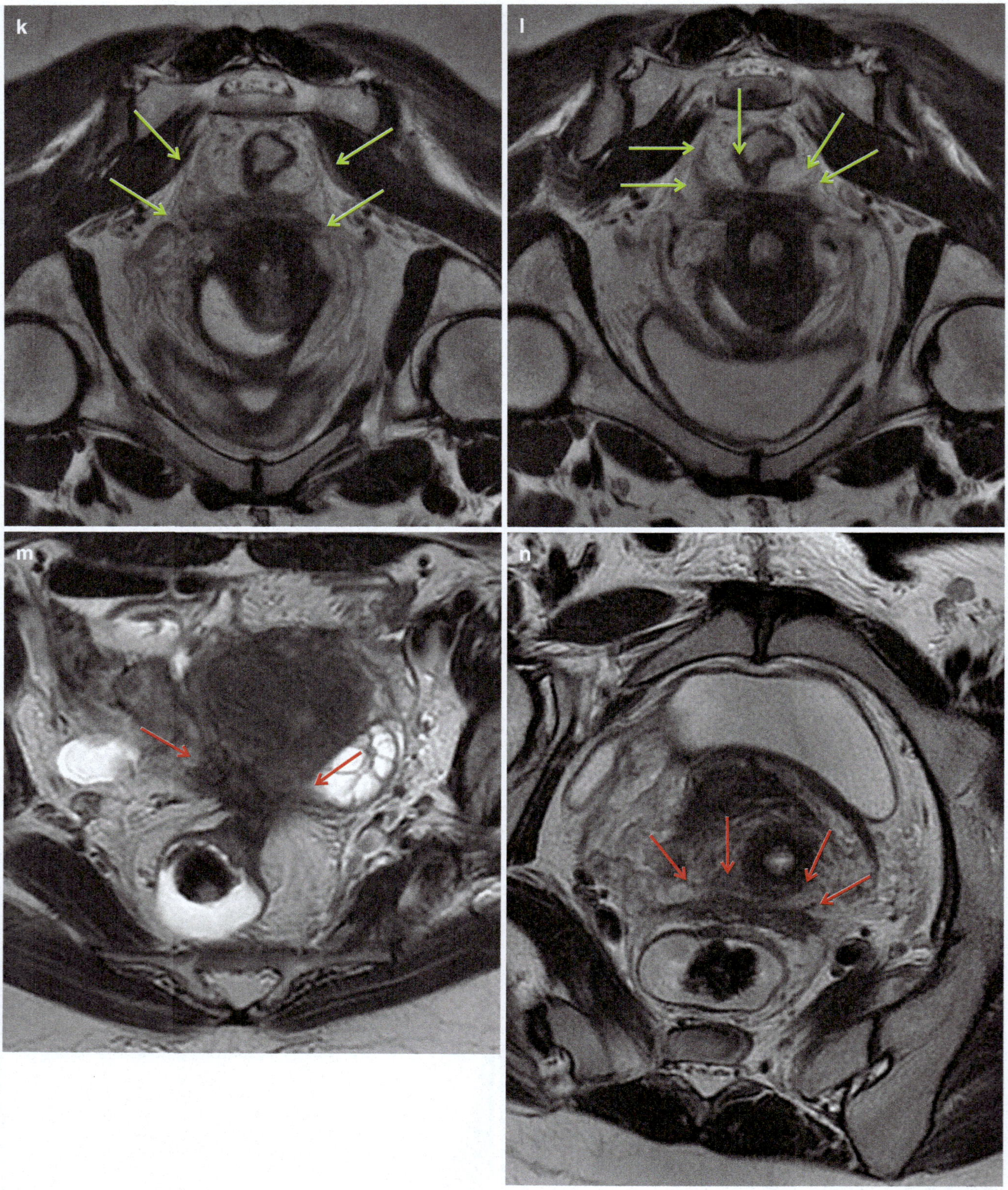

Fig. 4.96 (continued)

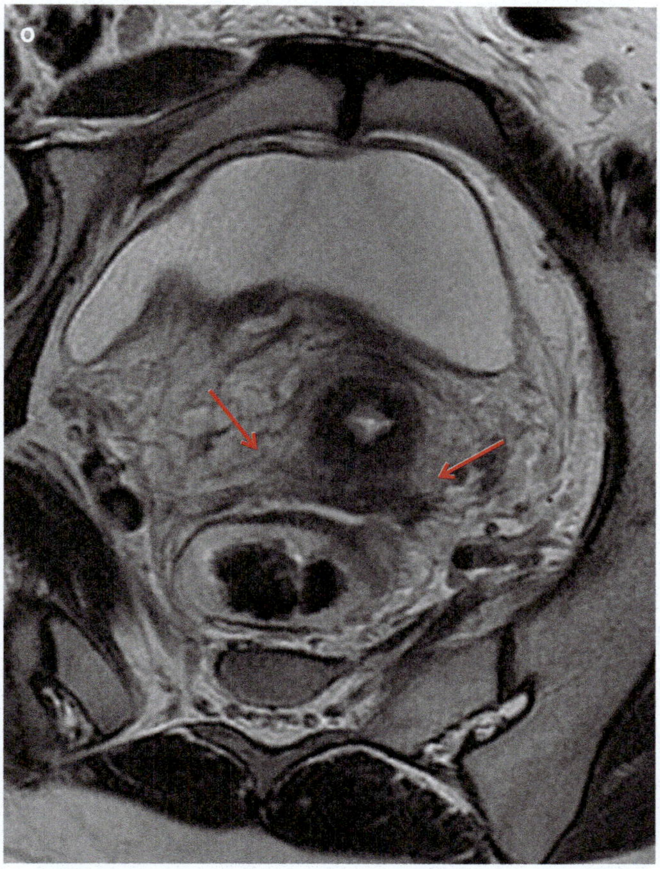

Fig. 4.96 (continued)

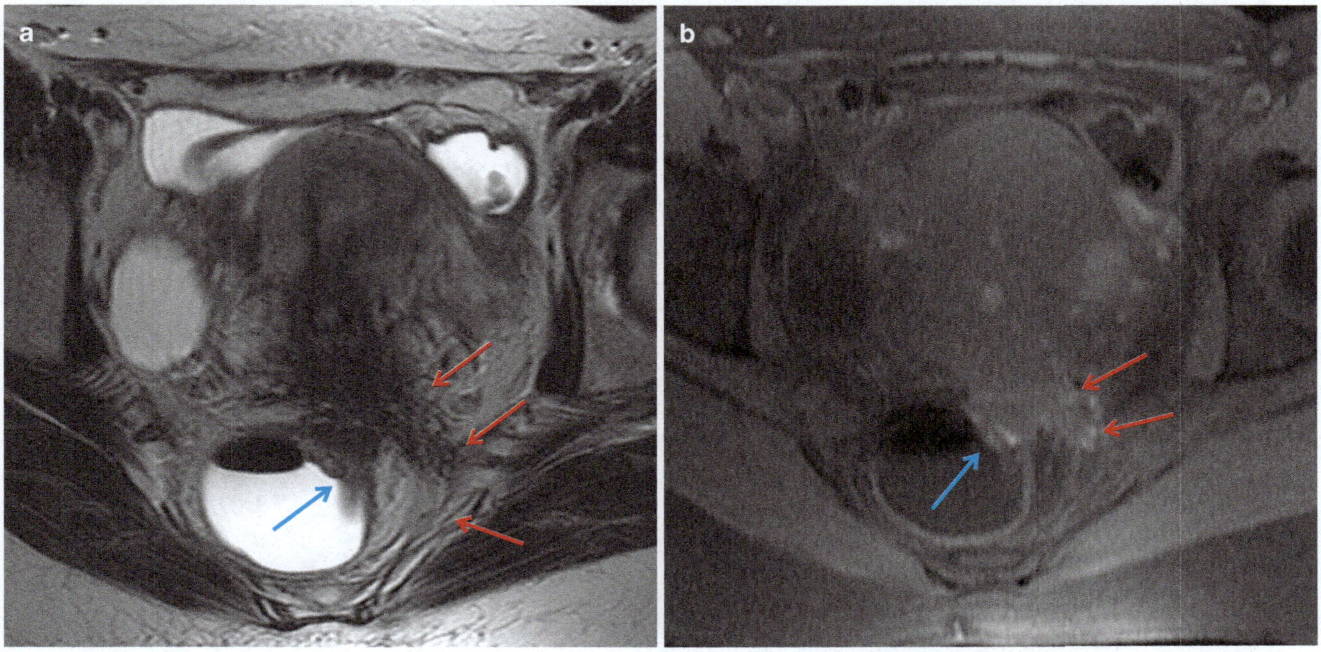

Fig. 4.97 Ligament lesion involving the entire caudal extension of the left uterosacral ligament (red arrows). Hepatic, heterogeneous, predominantly hypointense nodule in T2-weighted images (**a**, **c**, **e**), with hypertensive foci in T2 and T1 (**b**, **d**, **f**), indicating ectopic endometrial tissue with bleeding. The same as in case 1 in Fig. 4.127. Note associated bladder and rectal lesions (blue arrows). (**g**) Laparoscopy. Resection of thickened, irregular uterus ligament. (**h**) Microscopy. Endometrial cyst joined to fatty and fibrous tissue (40×)

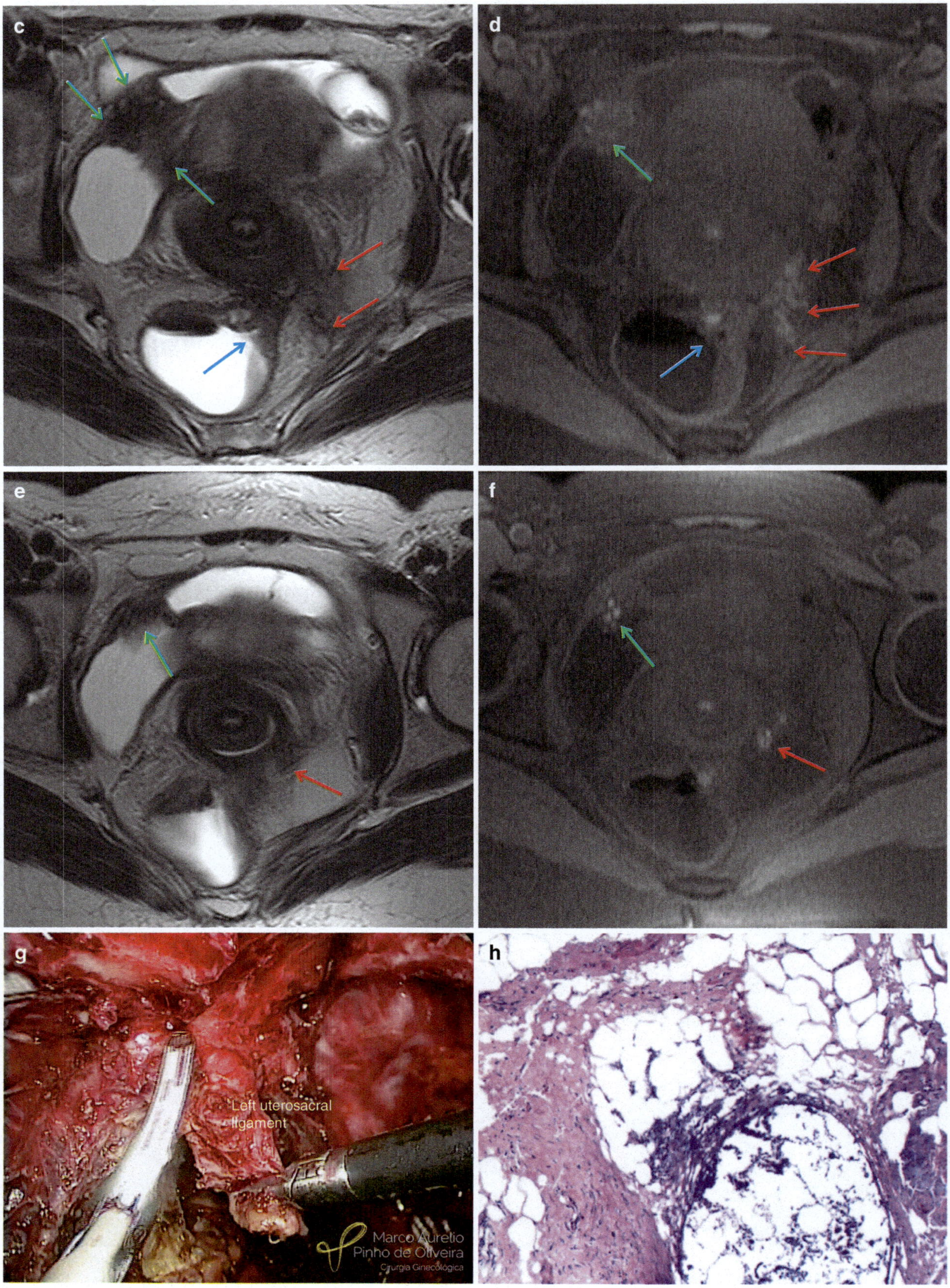

Fig. 4.97 (continued)

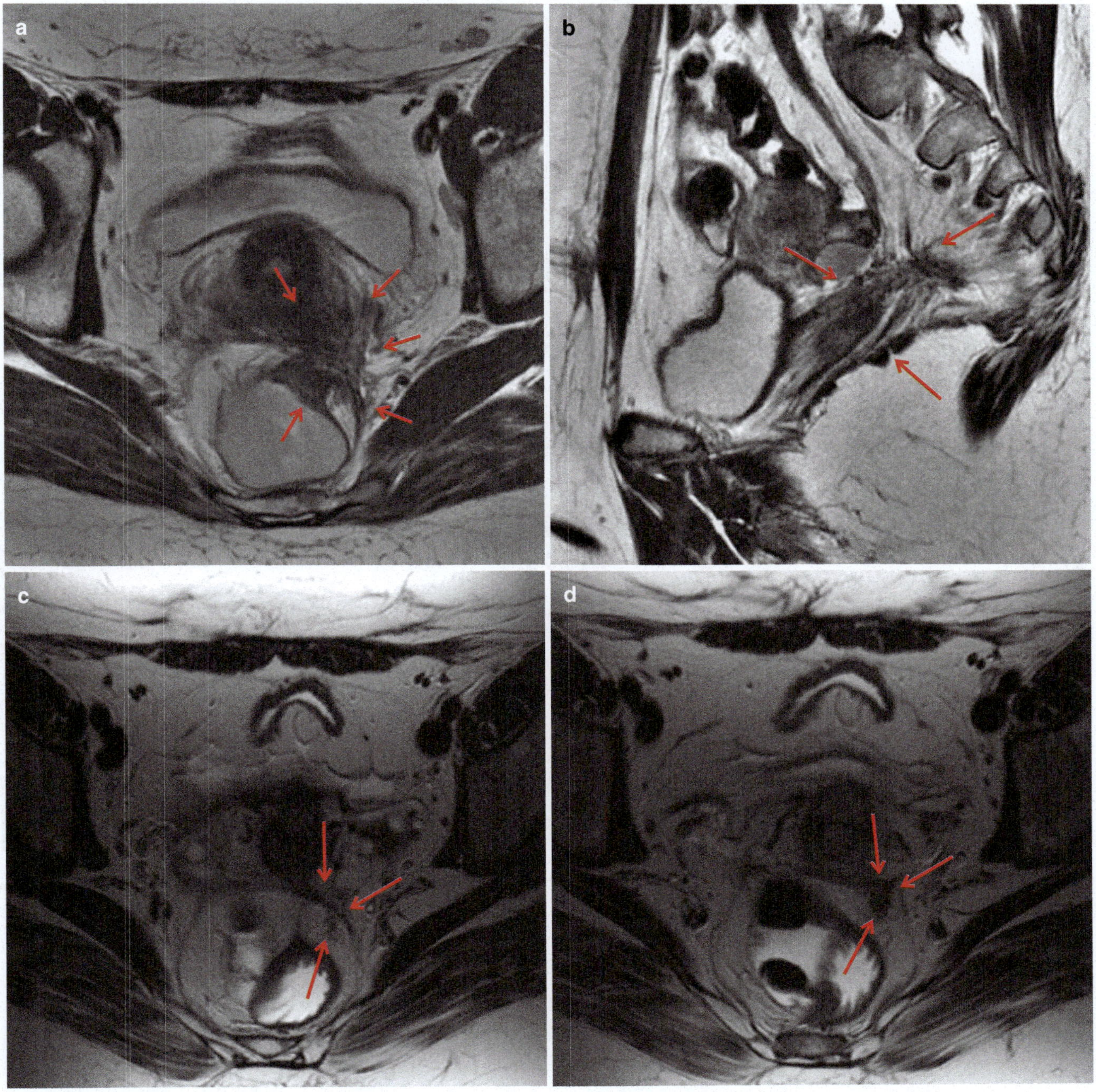

Fig. 4.98 Case 1: (**a**, **b**) Endometriotic nodule prominent on the right (red arrows), exceeding the edge of the ligament, compromising the mesorectum, rectum (lateral wall), vagina, and pelvic floor. The lesion is poorly delimited and infiltrative. Case 2 (**c**–**g**): Thickening and penetration in the mesorectum. (**a**–**e**) T2-weighted sequences. (**a**, **c**, **d**) Axial. (**b**, **e**) Sagittal. (**f**, **g**) Laparoscopy showing rectum and uterus sacrum. (**h**, **i**) Microscopy. (**h**) Endometriotic cyst containing red blood cells and histiocytic cells (100×). (**i**) Endometriotic glandular structure (400×)

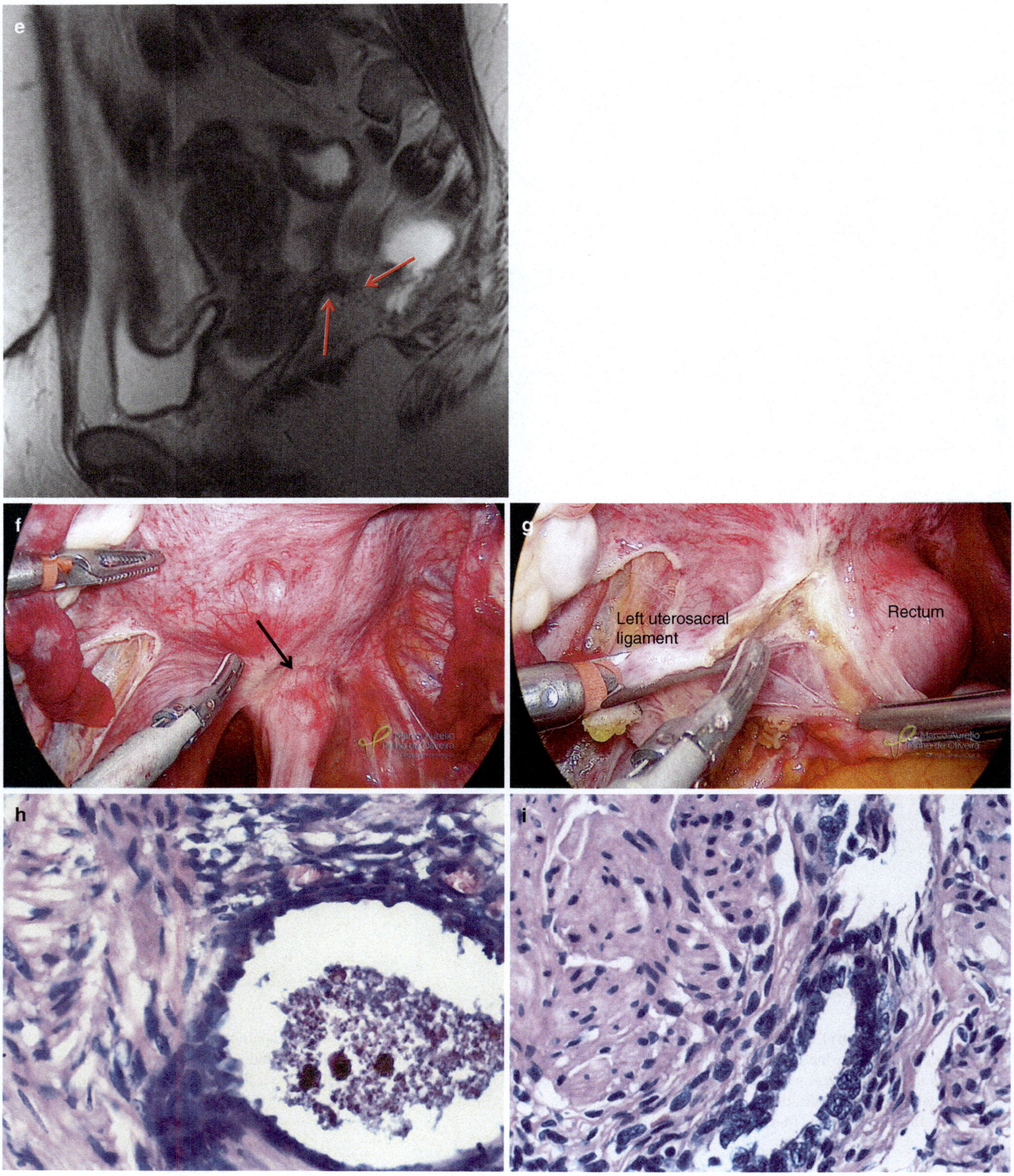

Fig. 4.98 (continued)

4.2.3.5 Treatment Comments

The sacral section of the uterosacrum contains nerve trunks of the upper hypogastric plexus, vulnerable to damage during a surgical procedure. In addition, there is proximity to the ureter, located anterior to the free edge of the ligament, about 2–3 cm from the cervical fixation (Fig. 4.99) [41].

Thus, in order to perform complete resection of the ligamentous lesion, the stages of neurolysis and ureterolysis and identification of the parietal spaces are very important (Fig. 4.100) [9].

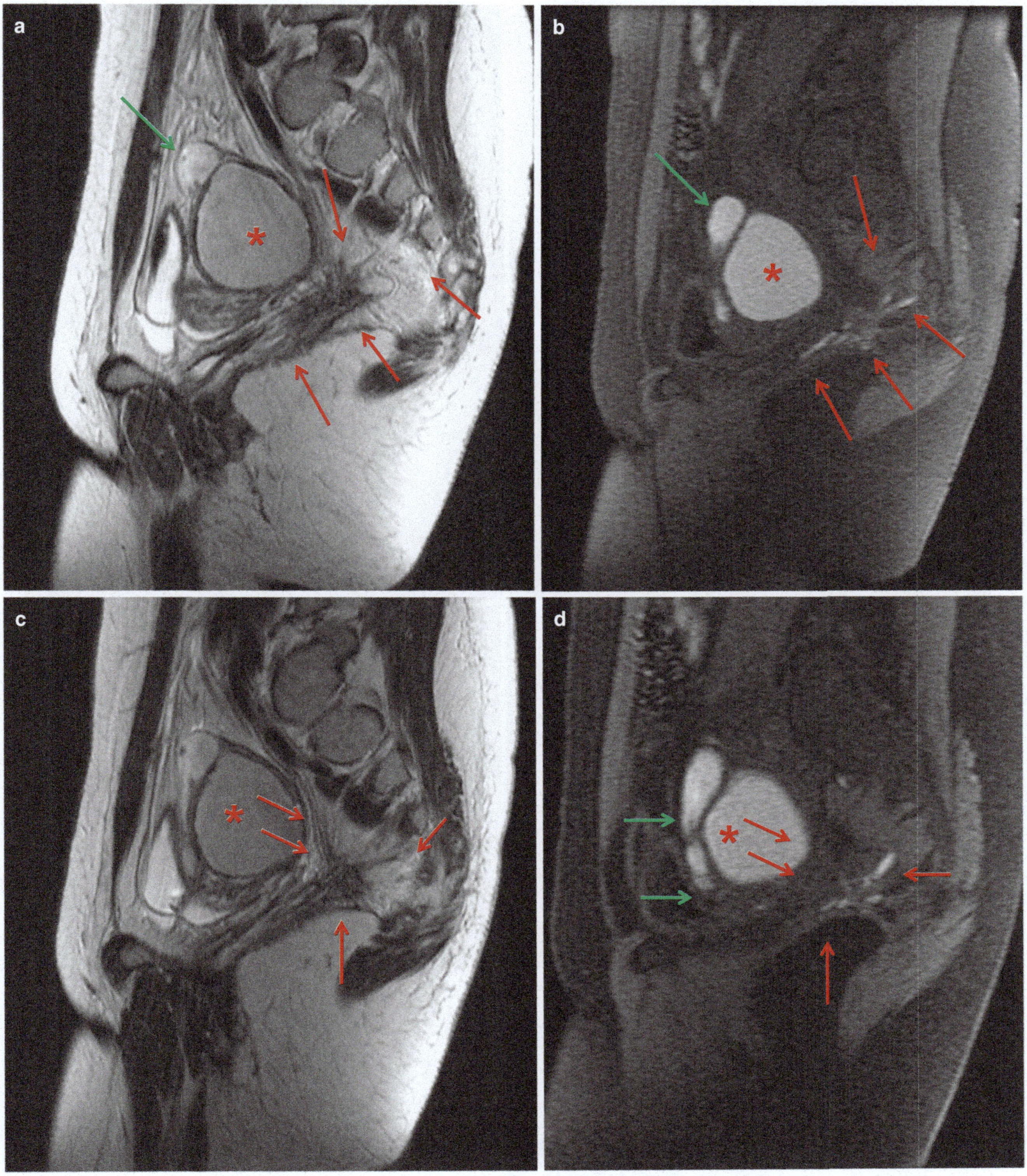

Fig. 4.99 Extensive lesion (red arrows **a**–**e**) with strong glandular component (bleeding clearly seen, **d**, **f**), penetrating the iliococcygeus muscle, involving the hypogastric nerve and subsequently penetrating the neural foramen. With proximity to the ureter and adherence with the adnexa, which presents endometrioma (*). Note hematosalpinx anterior to the endometrioma (green arrows). (**a**, **c**, **e**) T2-weighted sequences. (**b**, **d**, **f**) T1-weighted with fat suppression. (**a**–**f**) Sagittal. (**g**) Resection of the lesion. (**h**) Microscopy. Nodule with endometriosis and decidual reaction (400×)

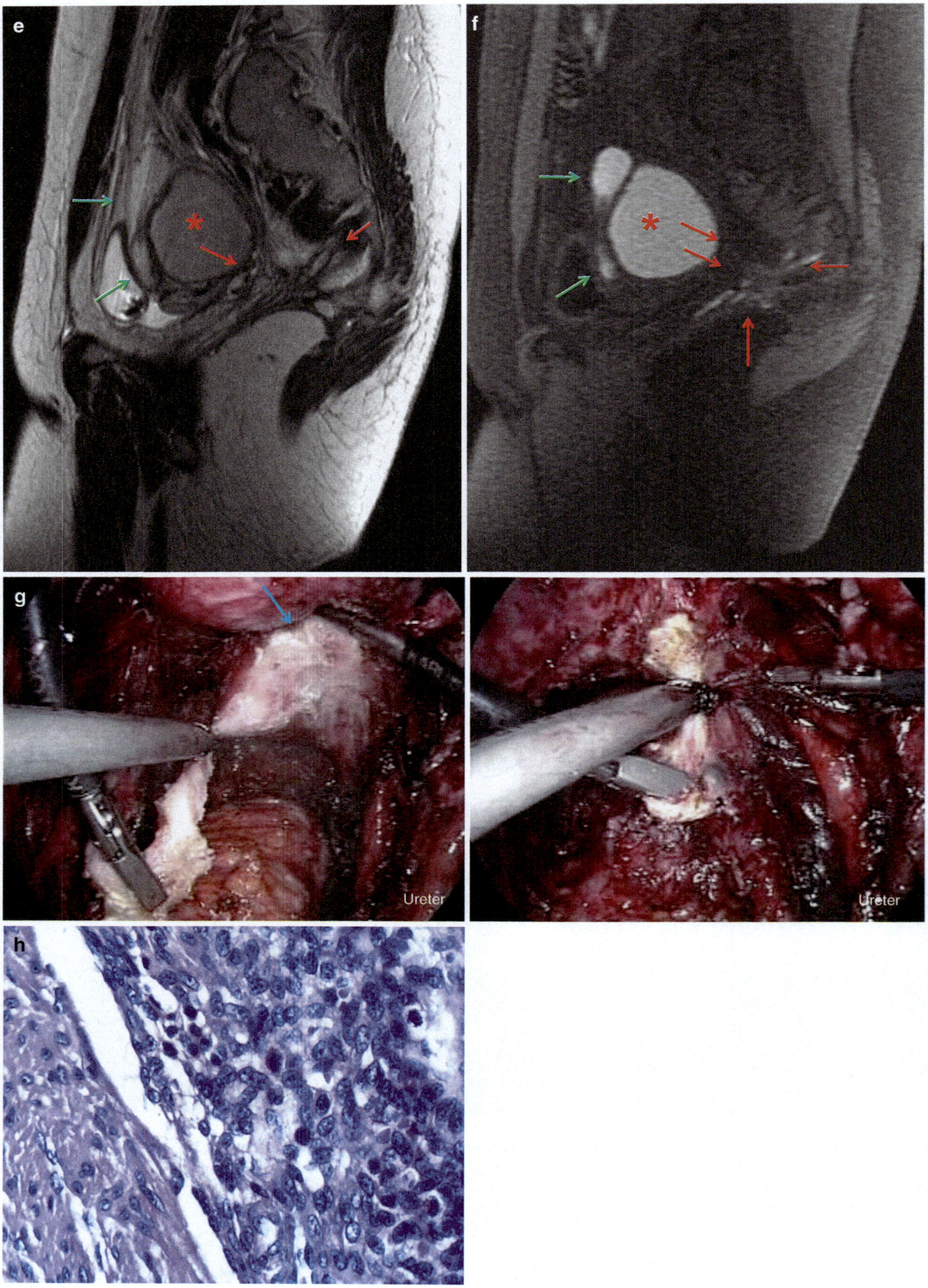

Fig. 4.99 (continued)

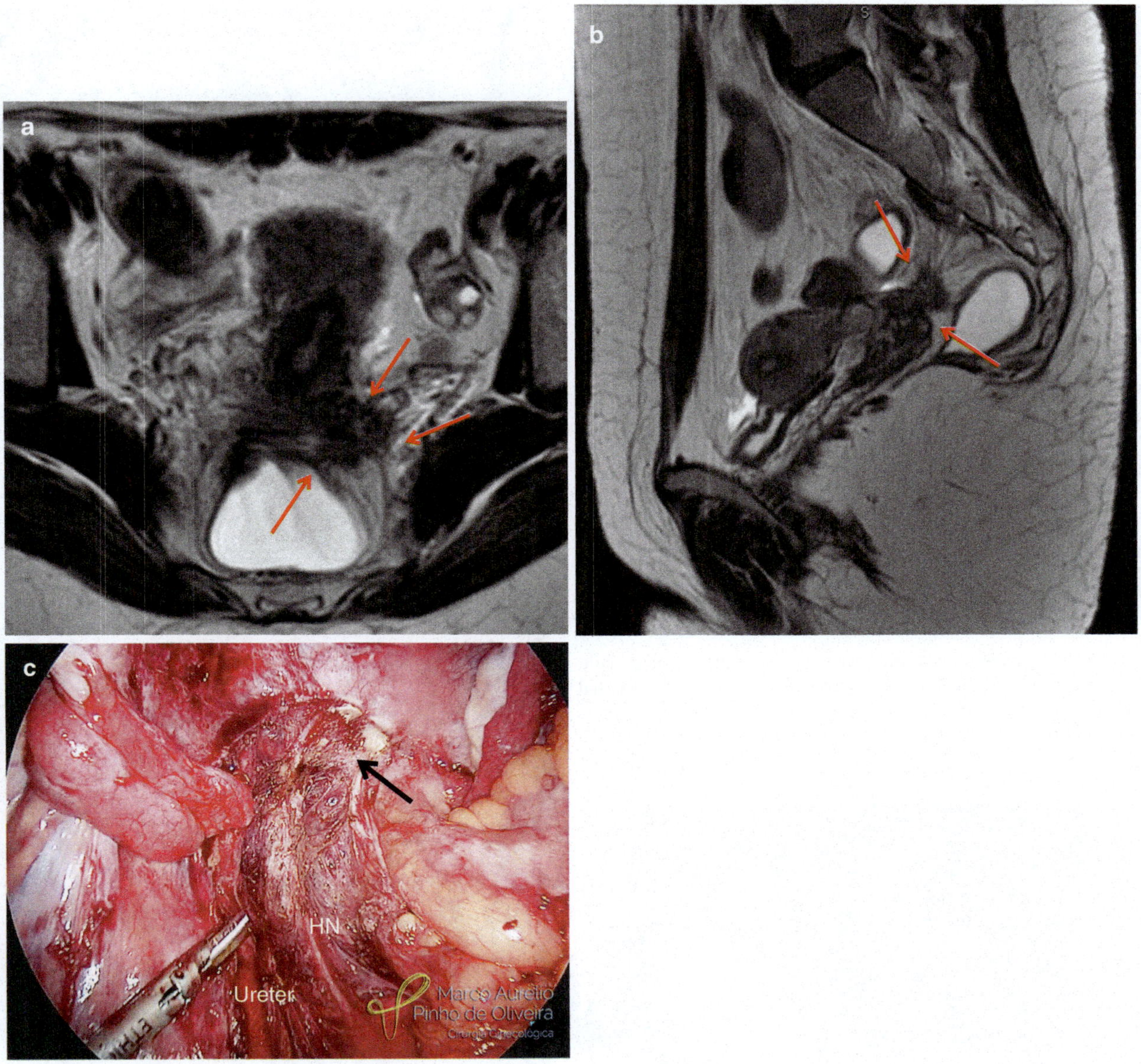

Fig. 4.100 (**a**, **b**) Extensive nodule in the left uterosacral ligament with rectal surface involvement. T2-weighted sequence, being (**a**) axial and (**b**) sagittal. (**c**) Laparoscopy. The arrow indicates the resected left uterosacral ligament. Note preservation of the hypogastric nerve (arrow)

4.2.4 Vagina (Posterior Vaginal Fornix) Anatomy

The upper vaginal section or the vaginal dome surrounds the intravaginal cervix, receiving the name the vaginal fornix. The posterior vaginal fornix is longer than the anterior one (Fig. 4.101).

The vaginal ring formed by the uterus and the cardinal ligaments surrounds the vaginal fornix.

The wall of the vagina consists of the mucosa, a muscular layer with longitudinal smooth fibers, and the adventitia, a layer of dense connective tissue, which connects the vagina to the adjacent structures. These layers can be identified in MRI, especially with the addition of vaginal gel (Fig. 4.102) [43, 46].

In addition to helping to define the vaginal wall, vaginal gel delineates the vaginal cul-de-sac, and the cervix, and allows a better analysis of the retrocervical region, the recto-vaginal septum, the posterior cul-de-sac, and the uterosacral ligaments (Fig. 4.103) [43].

In MRI, the vagina is well delimited, has a predominantly hypointense signal on the T2-weighted sequence and intermediate in T1 and intense enhancement by gadolinium, and has a thickness equal to or less than 3 mm (Fig. 4.102) [43].

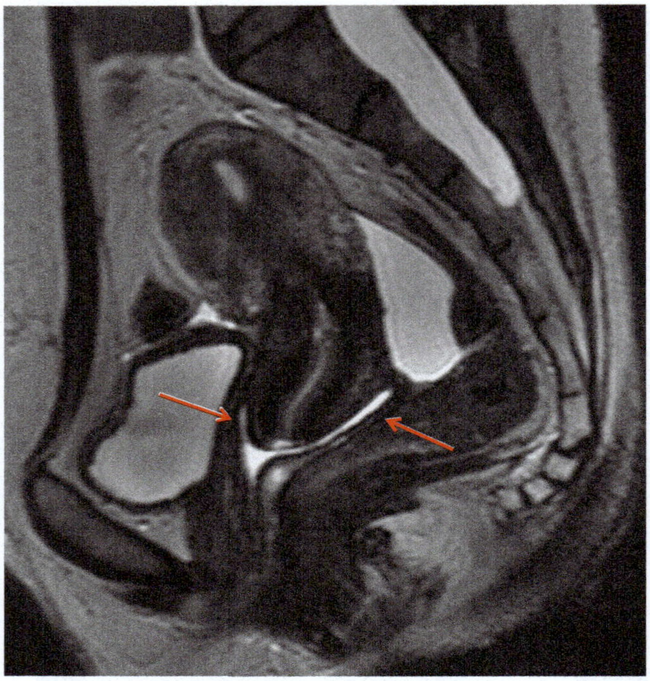

Fig. 4.101 The superior portion of the vagina, or the vaginal vault, surrounds the intravaginal cervix (arrows), known as the vaginal fornix

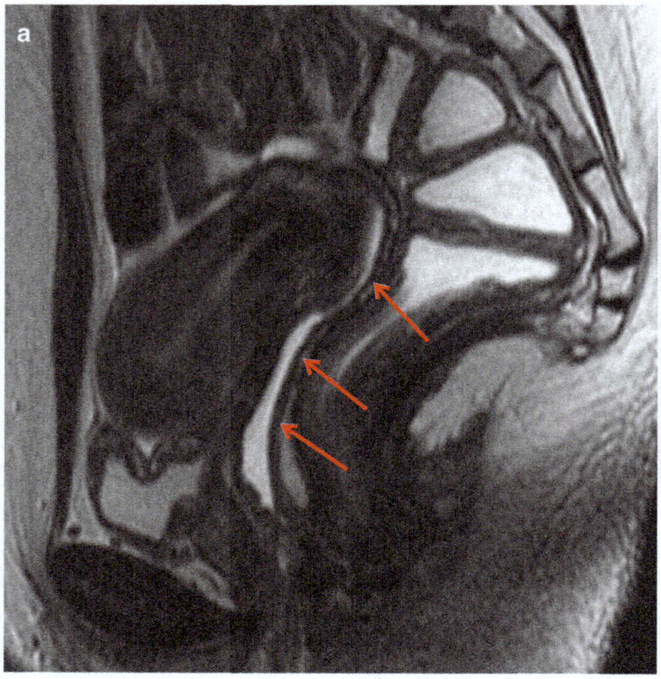

Fig. 4.102 The layers of the vaginal wall (arrows) can be identified in MRI with the addition of vaginal gel. The vaginal wall is well delimited (**a**–**c**), with a thickness of less than 3 mm, predominantly hypointense in the T2-weighted sequence (**a**, **b**) and intensely enhanced by gadolinium (**c**). (**a**–**c**) Sagittal

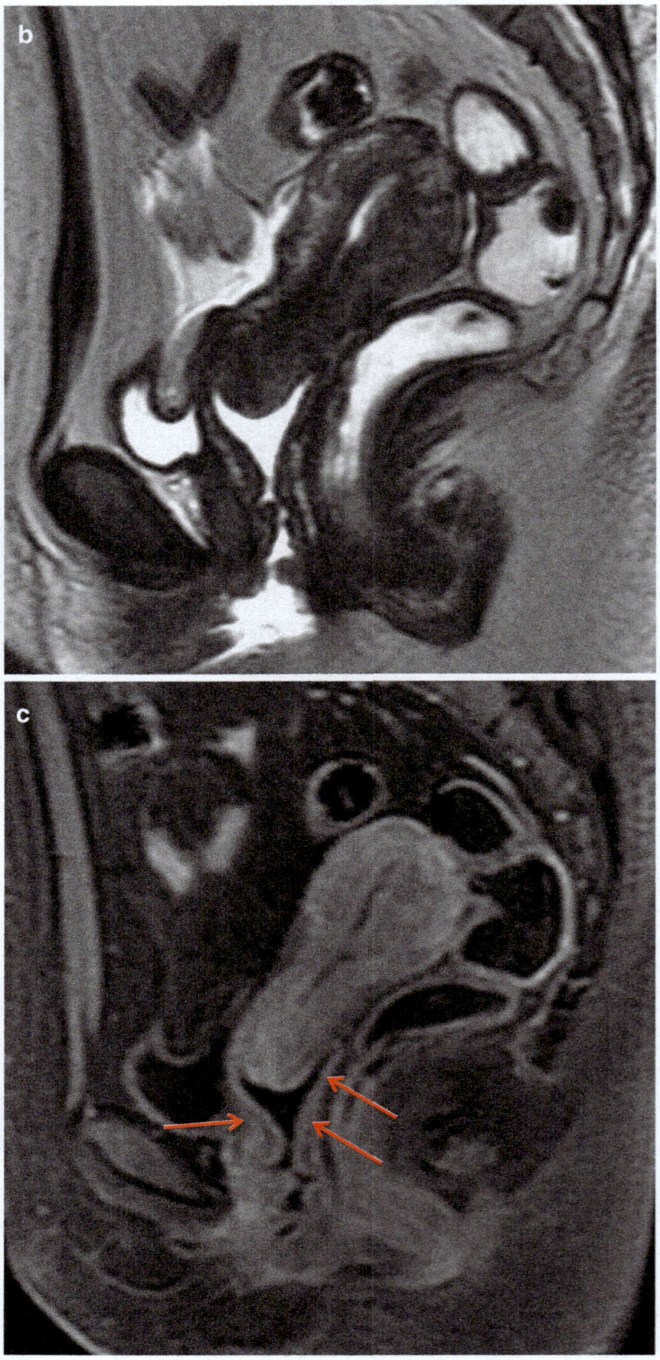

Fig. 4.102 (cotinued)

4.2.4.1 Common Aspects of Endometriosis

Infiltrative endometriosis is less prevalent in the vaginal wall, and when present, it is usually the extension of a lesion to another site of the pelvis, especially retrocervical. Vimerceti identified four vaginal lesions in 90 patients, and in all cases the dominant involvement was located in the posterior cul-de-sac (Fig. 4.104). However, isolated vaginal lesions can be demonstrated (Fig. 4.105) [26, 45].

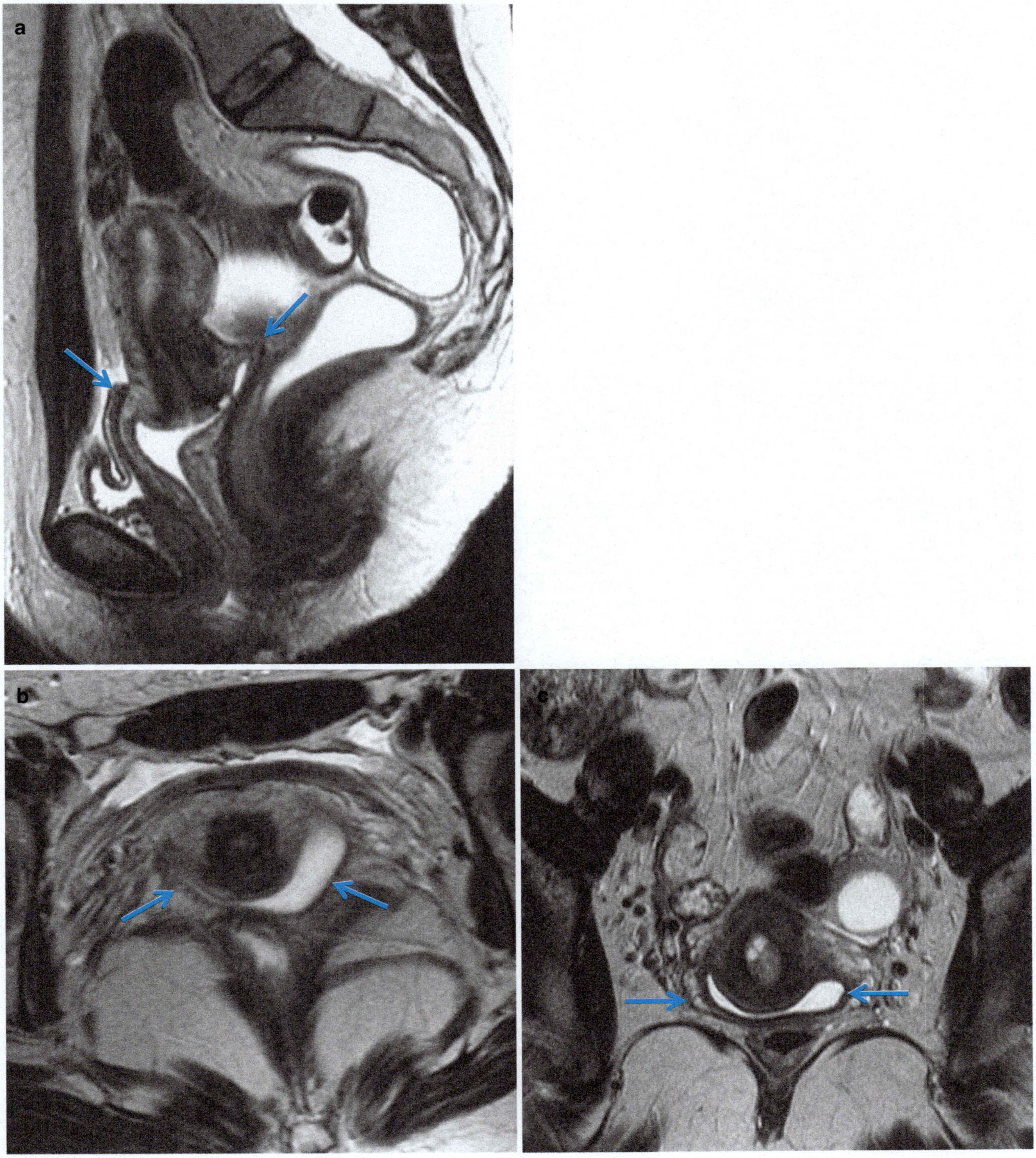

Fig. 4.103 The importance of vaginal gel. It delineates the posterior cul-de-sac and the cervix (**a**–**c** arrows). T2-weighted sequences. (**a**) Sagittal. (**b**) Oblique axial. (**c**) Coronal short axis

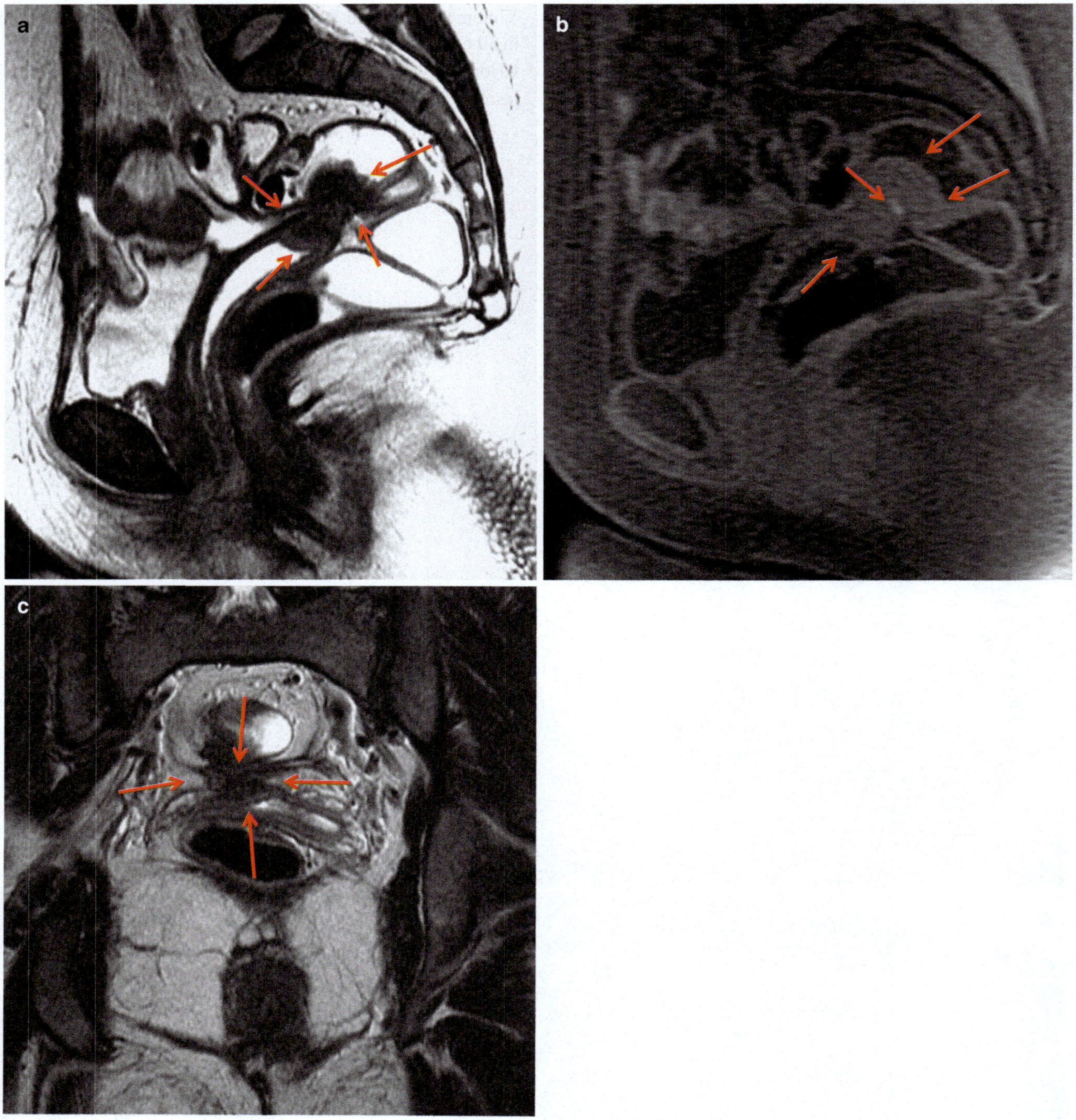

Fig. 4.104 Vaginal and rectovaginal septum nodule, causing obliteration of the posterior cul-de-sac and rectal involvement (arrows). Nodule with predominance of fibrosis (hypointense in T2- [**a**, **c**] and with a discrete focus of central bleeding [**b**]). After three surgeries and under hormonal block, maintaining vaginal bleeding. (**a**, **c**) T2-weighted sequences. (**b**) T1-weighted sequences. (**a**, **b**) Sagittal. (**c**) Coronal short axis

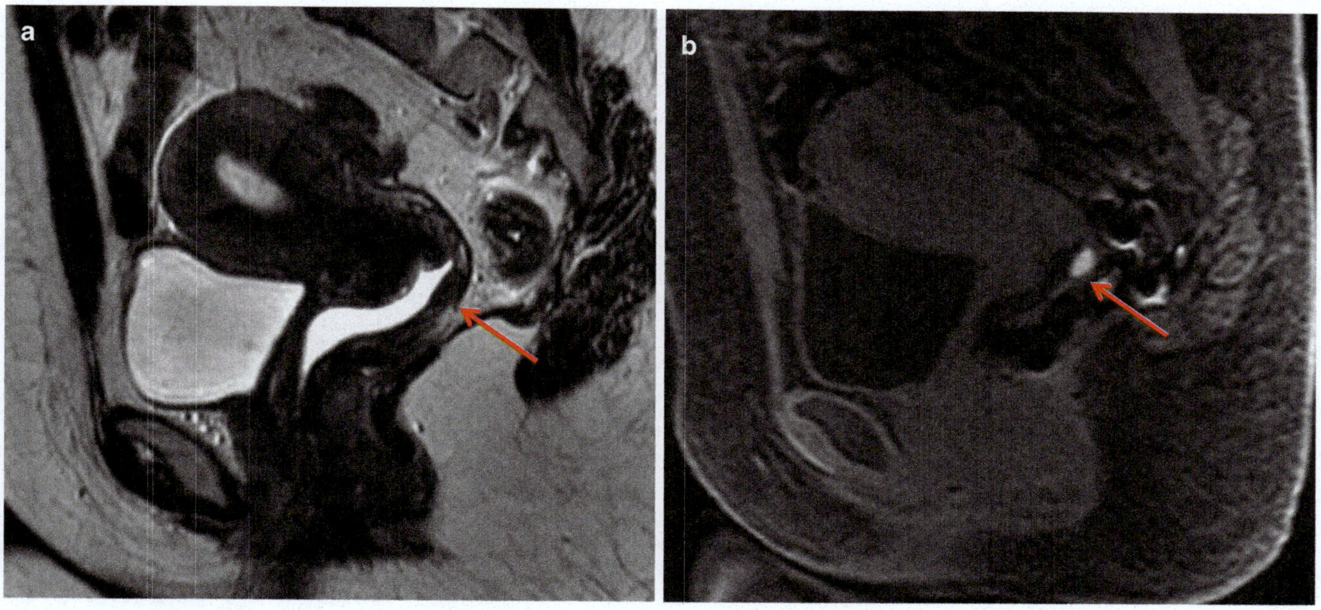

Fig. 4.105 Isolated vaginal lesion (arrow). Small vaginal nodule in upper and posterior thirds, hypointense in T2-weighted sequence (**a**) and hyperintense in T1-weighted sequence (**b**), due to bleeding. (**a**, **b**) Sagittal

4.2.4.2 Clinical Symptoms

Vaginal endometriosis may be an incidental finding in asymptomatic patients; however, more frequently, patients present dysmenorrhea and dyspareunia [26].

Gynecological examination, touch or specular exam, has a high specificity (87–100%), with identification of a bluish, hardened painful lesion [9].

4.2.4.3 MRI and Laparoscopic Findings

The appearance of the image varies according to the size and extent of the lesion. Thickening of the posterior vaginal wall, no nodule formation, small nodules, and large infiltrating nodules, with involvement of the vaginal inner layer and obliteration of the vaginal cul-de-sac, can be observed (Figs. 4.106 and 4.107).

Larger lesions usually have their epicenter in the recto-vaginal septum or retrocervical region and have vaginal extension.

Infiltrative endometriosis nodules demonstrate low signal on the T2-weighted sequences, due to the predominance of fibrous tissue, which may hamper their identification due to the vaginal wall having similar signal characteristics (Fig. 4.108).

However, the presence of hyperintense cystic areas on T2-weighted (endothelial ectopic glands) or hypersignal foci on T1-weighted sequences with fat saturation, reflecting bleeding, help to identify small lesions (Fig. 4.109) [26].

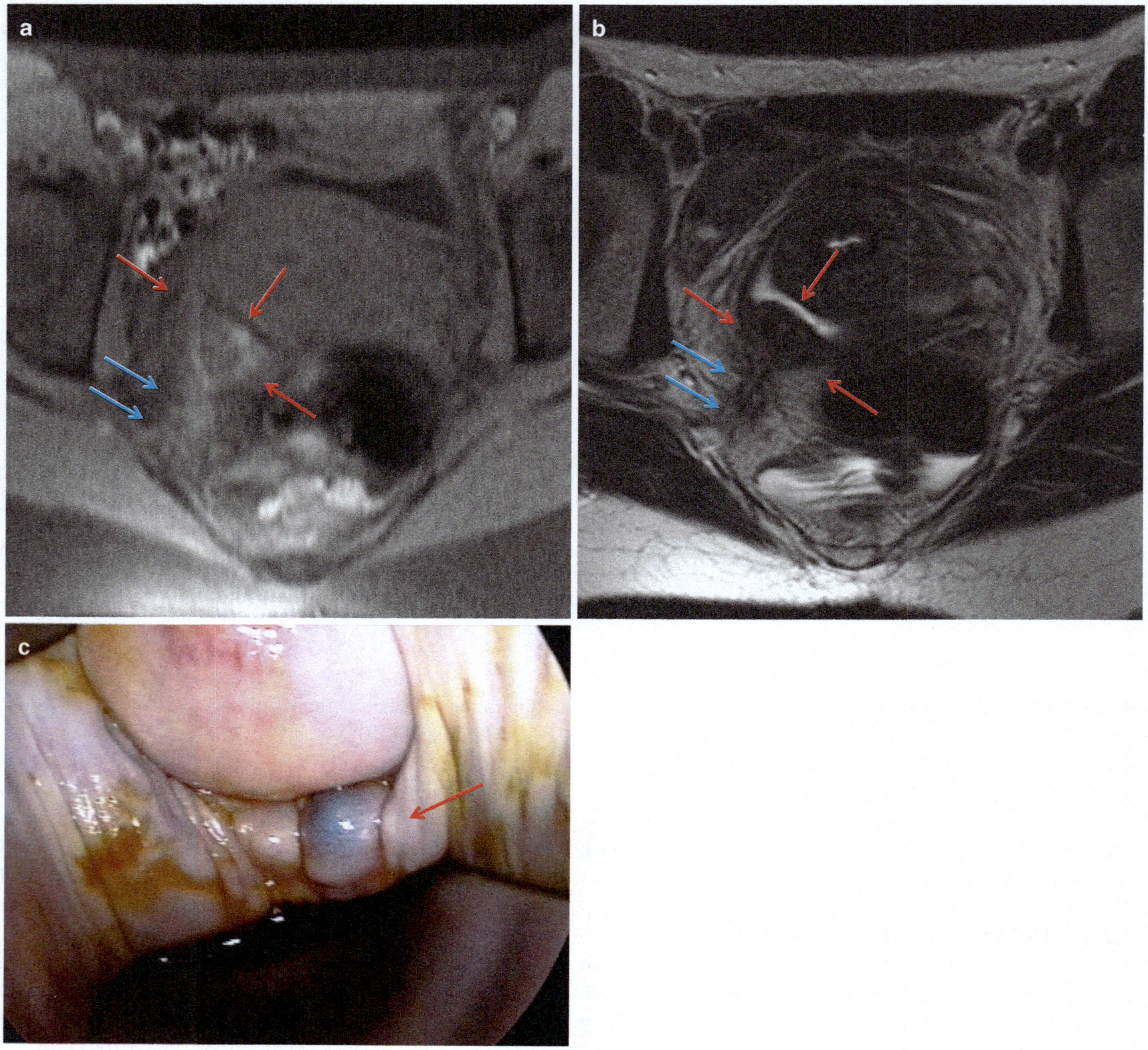

Fig. 4.106 Thickening of the right posterior vaginal wall, forming infiltrative nodules (red arrows), with compromised vaginal inner layer and obliteration of the posterior cul-de-sac, and extension to the utero-sacral ligament and mesorectum (blue arrow). Note hypersignal in T1 (**a**) and hyposignal in T2-weighted sequences (**b**). (**a**, **b**) Axial. (**c**) View of bluish vaginal nodule in the posterior cul-de-sac

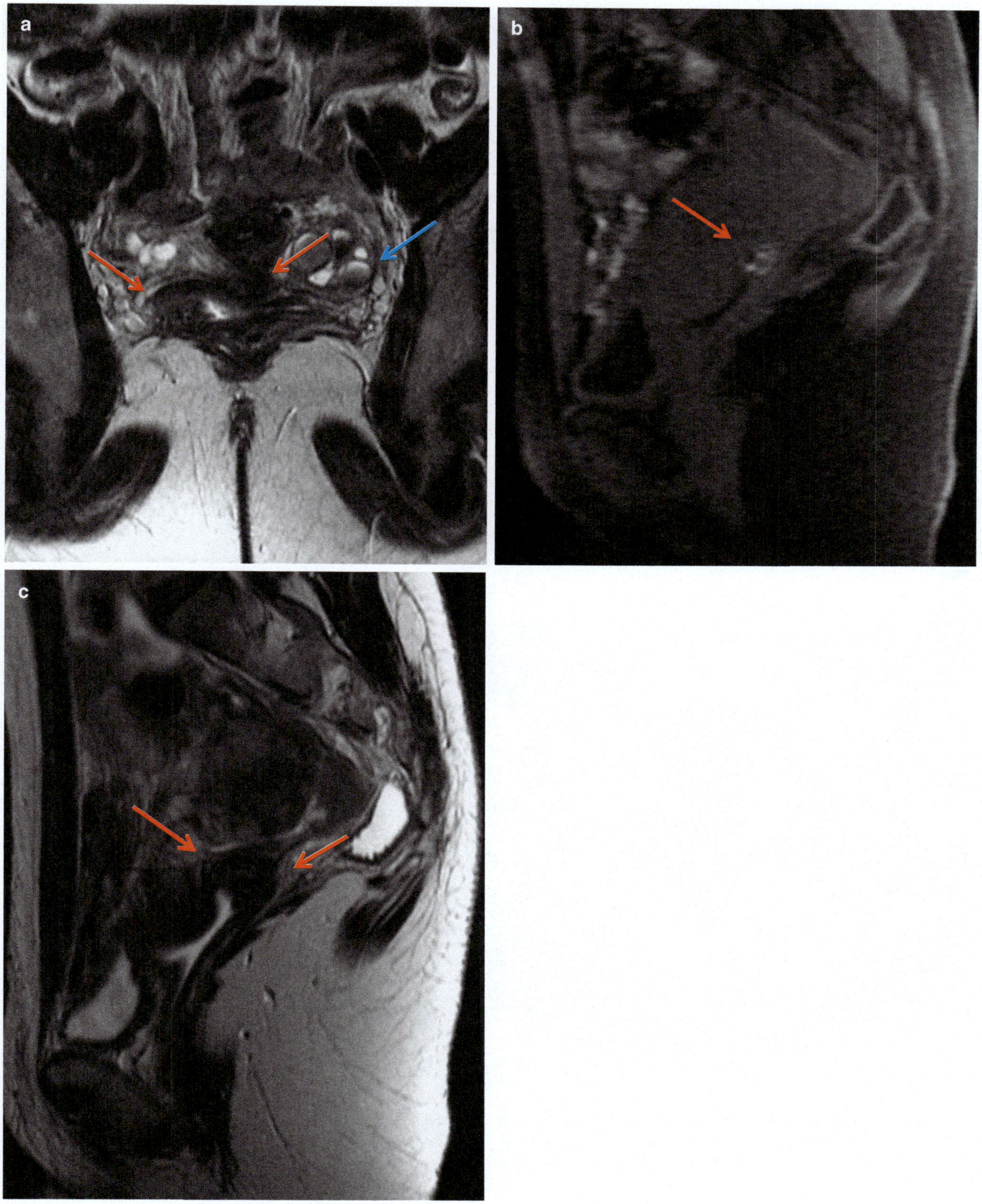

Fig. 4.107 Thickening of the right posterior vaginal wall by infiltrative lesion (arrows), with compromised vaginal inner layer, hypointense in T2-weighted sequences (**a**, **c**) and hyperintense in T1 (**b**), obliterating the vaginal fornix. Note multiple endometriomas in the left ovary (blue arrow in **a**). (**a**) Short axis. (**b**, **c**) Sagittal

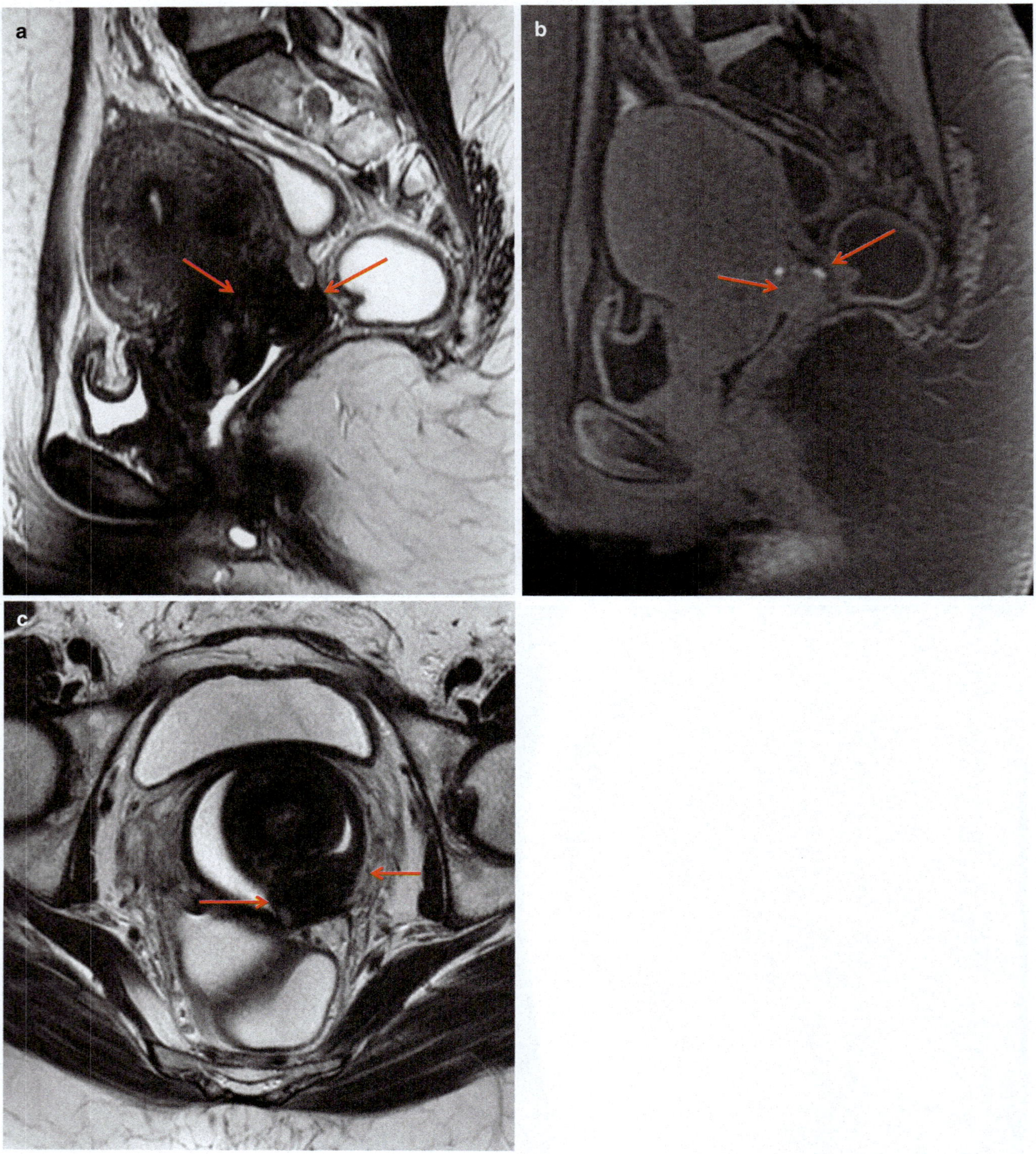

Fig. 4.108 Vaginal nodule in the upper third and left posterior, partly obliterating the fornix, hypointense in T2-weighted sequences (**a**, **c**), with predominance of fibrous tissue. Note discrete bleeding foci in the T1-weighted sequence (**b**) that help identify the lesion. (**a**, **b**) Sagittal. (**c**) Coronal short axis

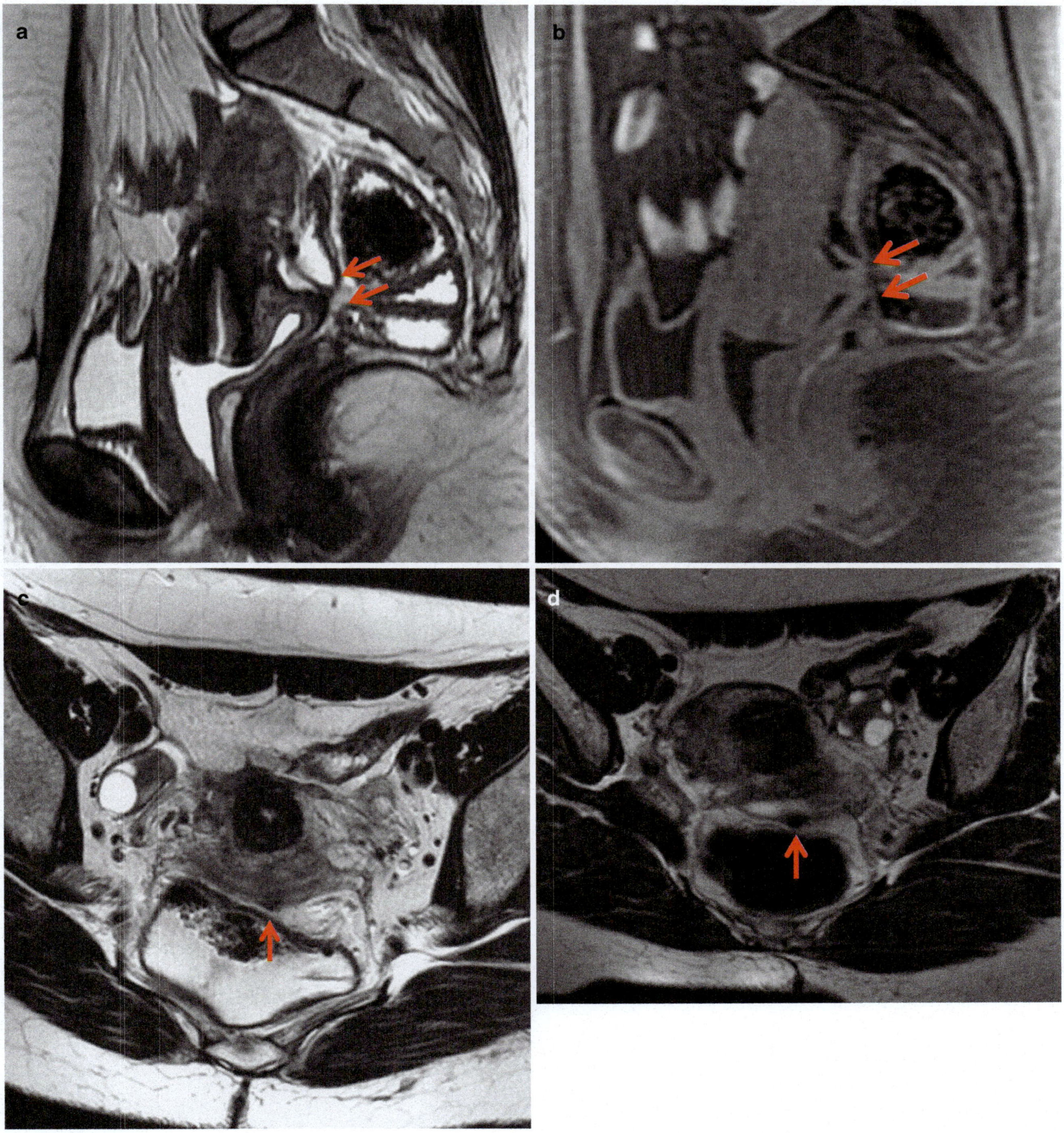

Fig. 4.109 Isolated vaginal lesion (arrows), small, difficult to identify in the T2-weighted sequence (**a**, **c**, **d**), hypointense, and without expression in the T1-weighted sequence with fat saturation (**b**) (arrows). (**d–f**) Same patient 1 year later, maintaining dyspareunia, with slight prominence of the lesion. Note well-delimited nodule in the short-axis coronal plane (**c**, **d**)

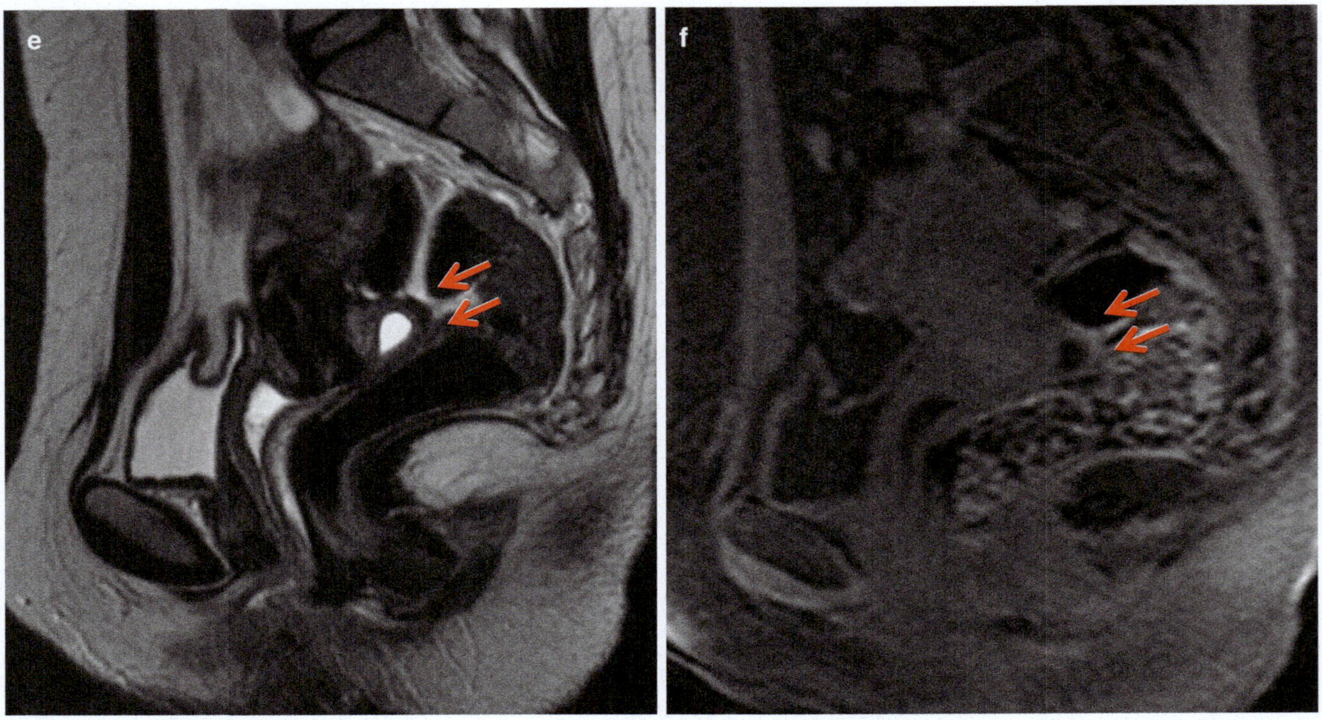

Fig. 4.109 (continued)

4.2.4.4 Treatment Comments

The surgical treatment requires colpotomy or posterior colpectomy. This procedure, when performed in conjunction with lower rectal resection, may carry a risk of developing a postoperative rectovaginal fistula (Fig. 4.110) [26].

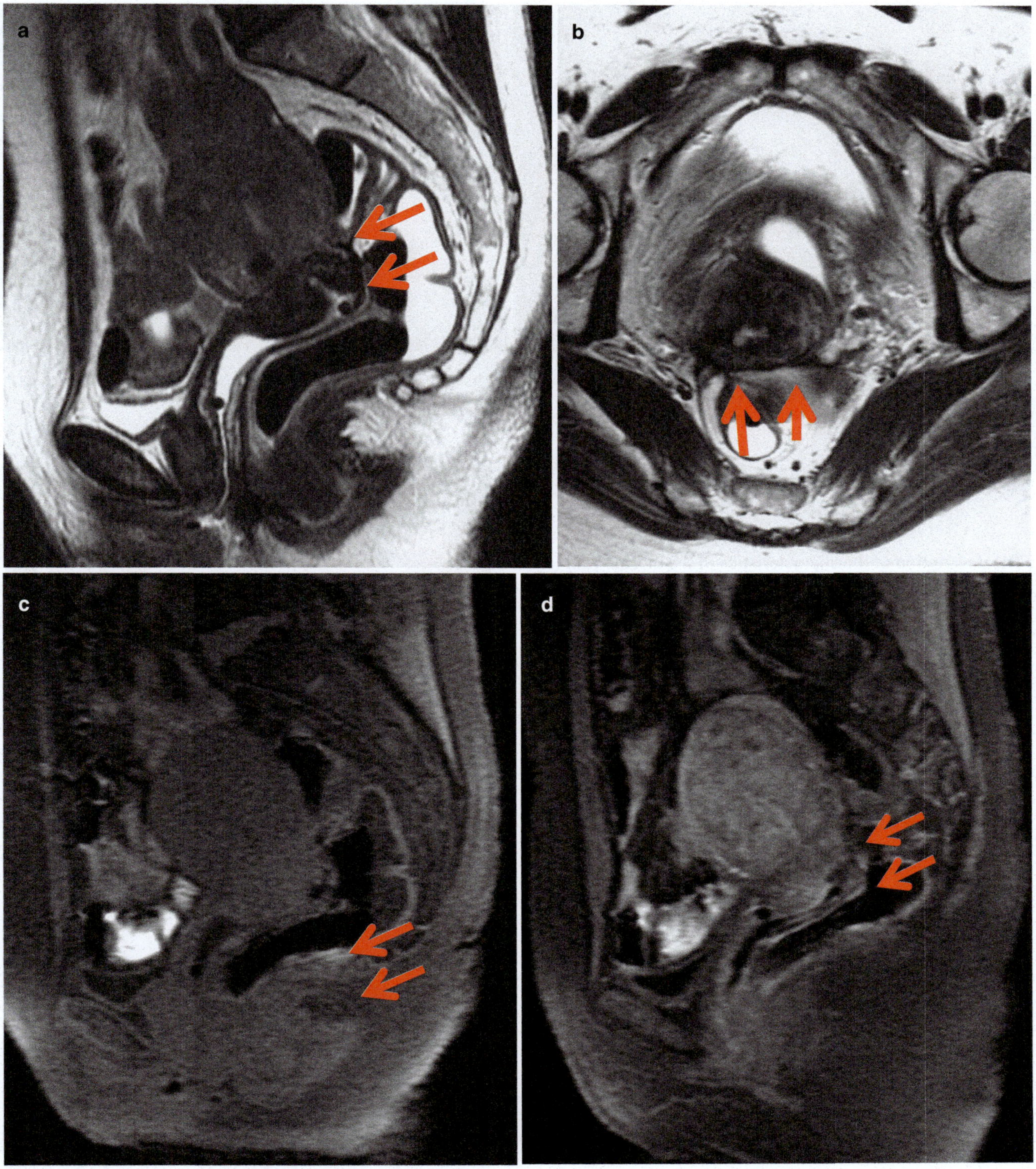

Fig. 4.110 Postsurgical findings of posterior colpectomy. Focal tapering, signal modification to markedly hypointense in T2 (**a**, **b**), and susceptibility artifacts seen on the T1-weighted sequence (**c**, **d**) with focal hypercaptation (**d**). (**a**, **c**, **d**) Sagittal. (**b**) Axial. (**e**, **f**) Laparoscopy during colpectomy (arrow)

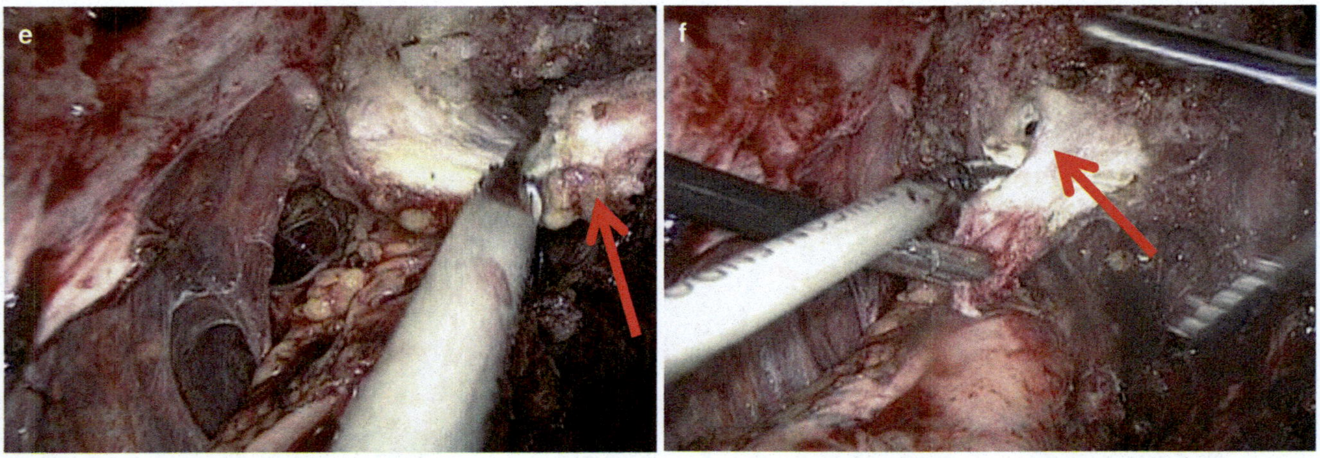

Fig. 4.110 (continued)

4.2.5 Myometrium Anatomy: Posterior Compartment

The description of the characteristics of the uterine wall (signal and zonal anatomy) is in the section on lesions of the myometrium in the anterior compartment, since it is similar.

The posterior face of the uterus is also covered by the visceral peritoneum and continues with the peritoneum of the anterior surface of the rectum, forming inferiorly the posterior cul-de-sac. Inferiorly, the peritoneum covers the supravaginal cervix and the upper part of the vagina (Fig. 4.111) [9].

The cervix differs from the rest of the uterus in its histological structure, presenting few smooth muscle fibers and a greater amount of connective tissue. In this way, the zonal anatomy is different from the rest of the uterus in MRI and presents four distinct zones on the T2-weighted sequence: (a) a central segment or endocervical canal, covered by the mucosa, with longitudinal folds, called palmate folds; (b) the fibrous stroma, which involves the mucosa and presents a hypointense sign;(c) a continuous muscle layer with the outer myometrial layer of the uterine body and the serosa; and (d) hypointense (Fig. 4.112) [24, 39].

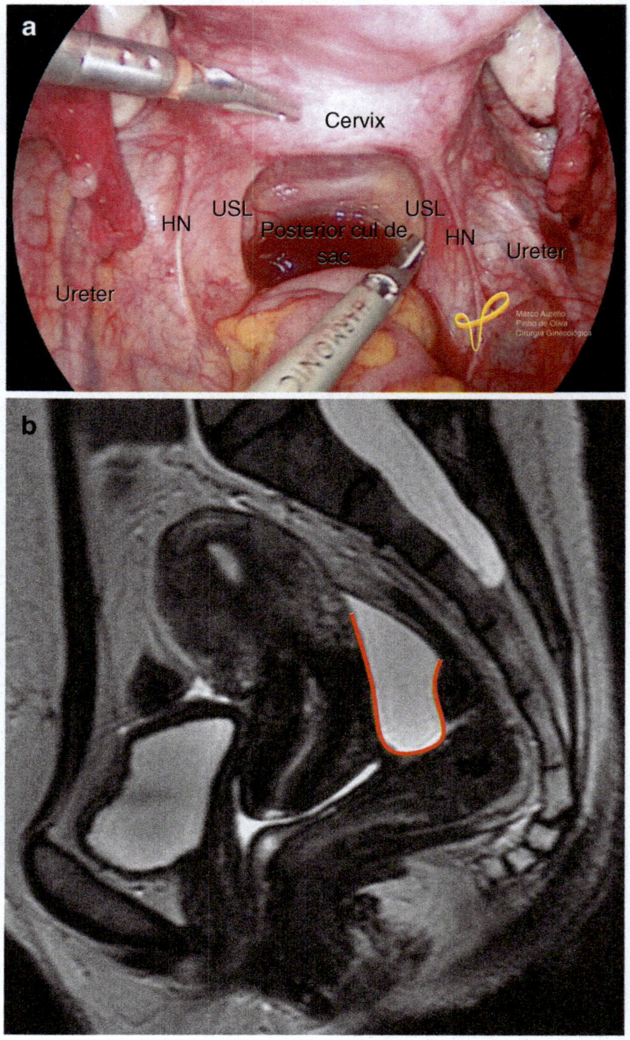

Fig. 4.111 The posterior face of the uterus is also covered by the visceral peritoneum and continues with the peritoneum of the anterior surface of the rectum, forming the posterior cul-de-sac (marked in [**b**]). Inferiorly the peritoneum covers the supravaginal cervix and the superior part of the vagina. (**a**) Laparoscopy. (**b**) T2-weighted sequence. Sagittal

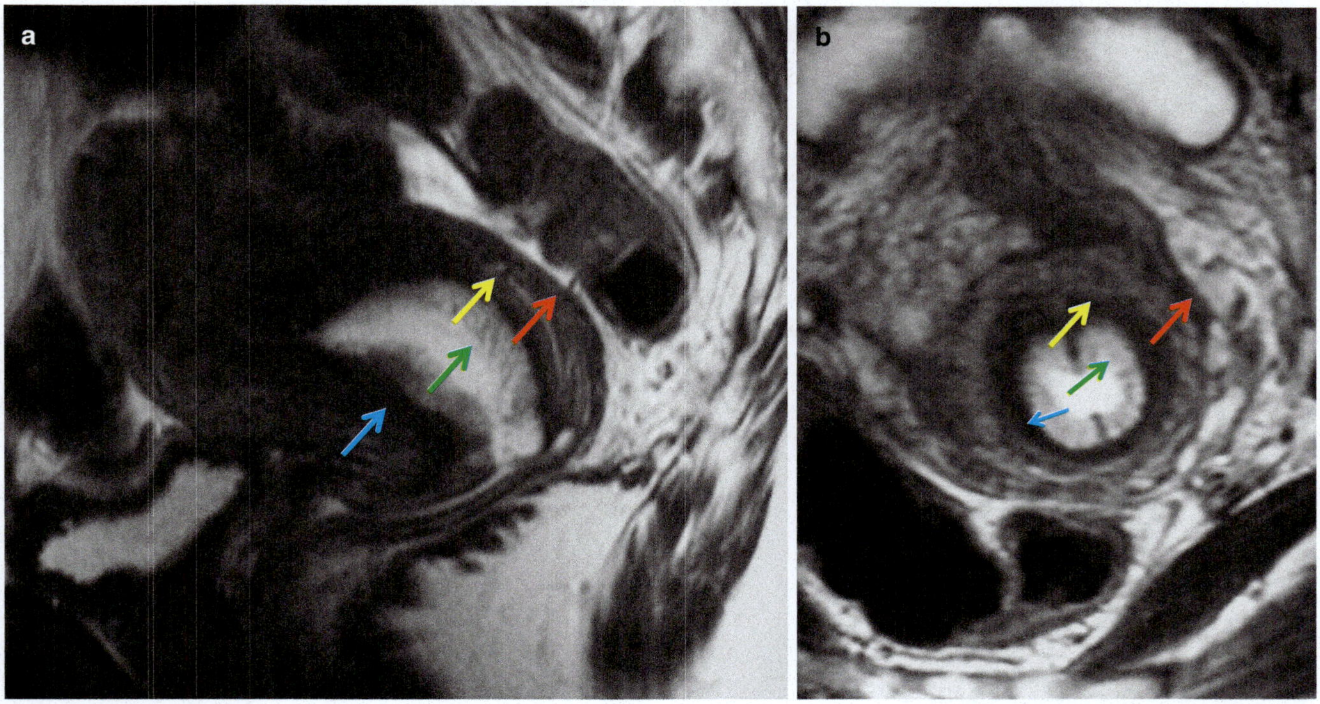

Fig. 4.112 Zonal anatomy of the cervix. Note central portion or endocervical canal, covered by the mucosa, with longitudinal folds called palmate folds (green arrows), fibrous stroma (blue arrows), which involve the mucosa and present hypointense signal, continuous muscular layer (yellow arrows), with the myometrial layer of the uterine body and serosa, hypointense (red arrows). (**a**, **b**) T2-weighted sequences. (**a**) Sagittal. (**b**) Coronal short shaft

4.2.5.1 Most Common Aspects of Endometriosis

Myometrial involvement of endometriosis in the posterior compartment was better identified and graded with the use of MRI. The incidence of this type of lesion in posterior deep endometriosis is still little known; however, it is very important for surgical planning, for avoiding relapse, and for the obstetric prognosis of the patient, if there is a need for myomectomy or hysterectomy for complete resection of the lesion.

The degree of myometrial penetration may vary, and may be discrete or prominent, sometimes being the main aspect of the lesion, coming close to the uterine cavity (Fig. 4.113).

This type of involvement can be observed in patients who underwent complete resection of deep endometriotic lesions in other sites and who presented with uterine disease (Fig. 4.114).

The process is different from adenomyosis. In myometrial endometriosis the onset of myometrial involvement is peripheral, with penetration from the visceral peritoneum and external myometrial layers. However, histologically, they resemble endometrial glands and stroma between the muscle bundles of the myometrium. In rare cases, there is only stroma (Fig. 4.115).

In most cases, the glands present the aspect of the proliferative phase and respond little to cyclic stimuli, with a low incidence of bleeding (Fig. 4.115).

The muscle fibers around the adenomyosis focus are hypertrophic and hyperplastic, contributing to wall thickening and uterine volumetric enlargement (Fig. 4.116).

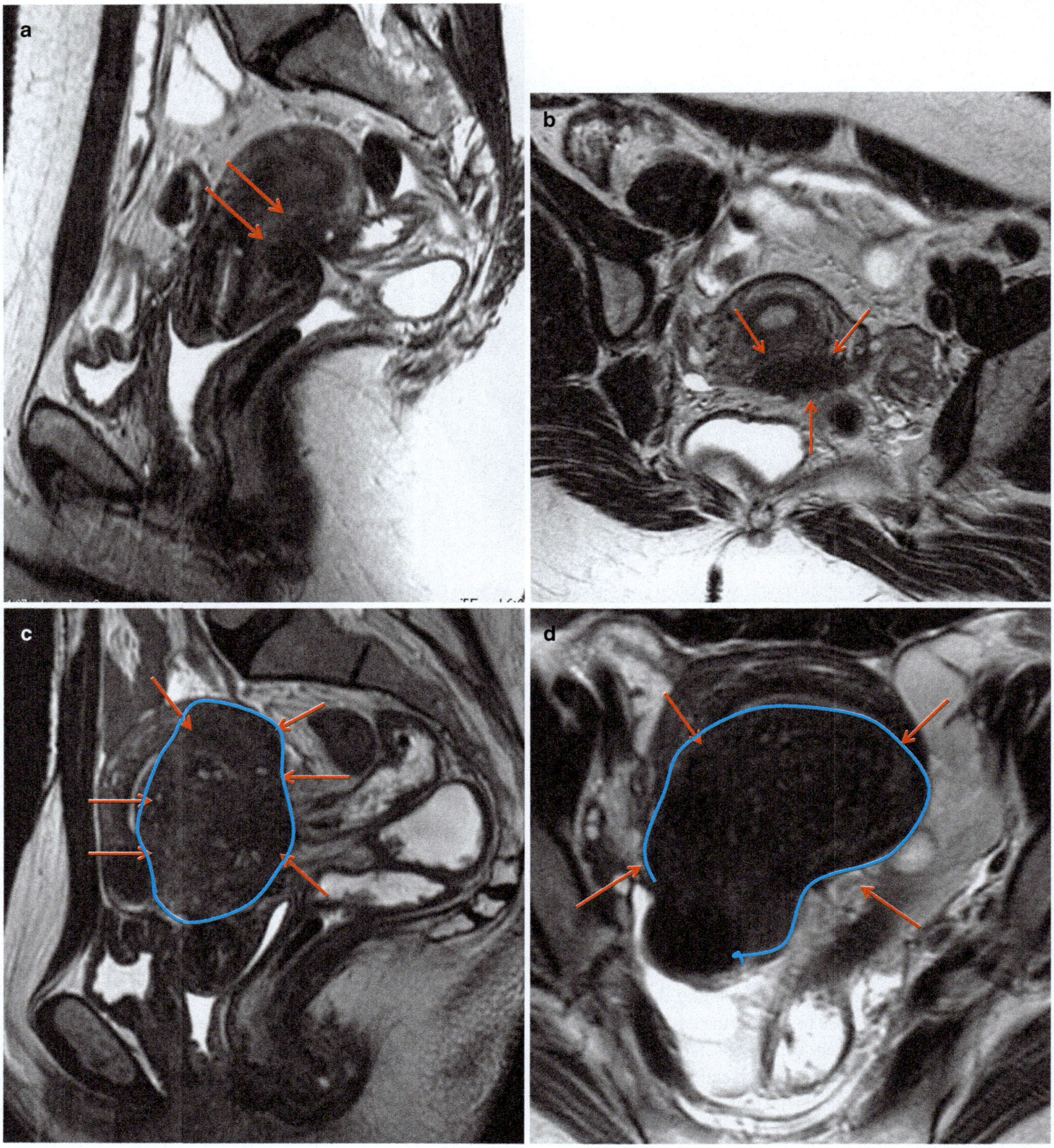

Fig. 4.113 Variation of the degree of myometrial penetration. Case 1: (**a**, **b**) Small lesion in the isthmus and cervix (arrows). Case 2: (**c**, **d**) Significant lesion in the entire posterior wall (blue arrows and line). (**a**, **d**) T2-weighted sequences. (**a**, **c**) Sagittal. (**b**) Coronal short axis. (**d**) Axial

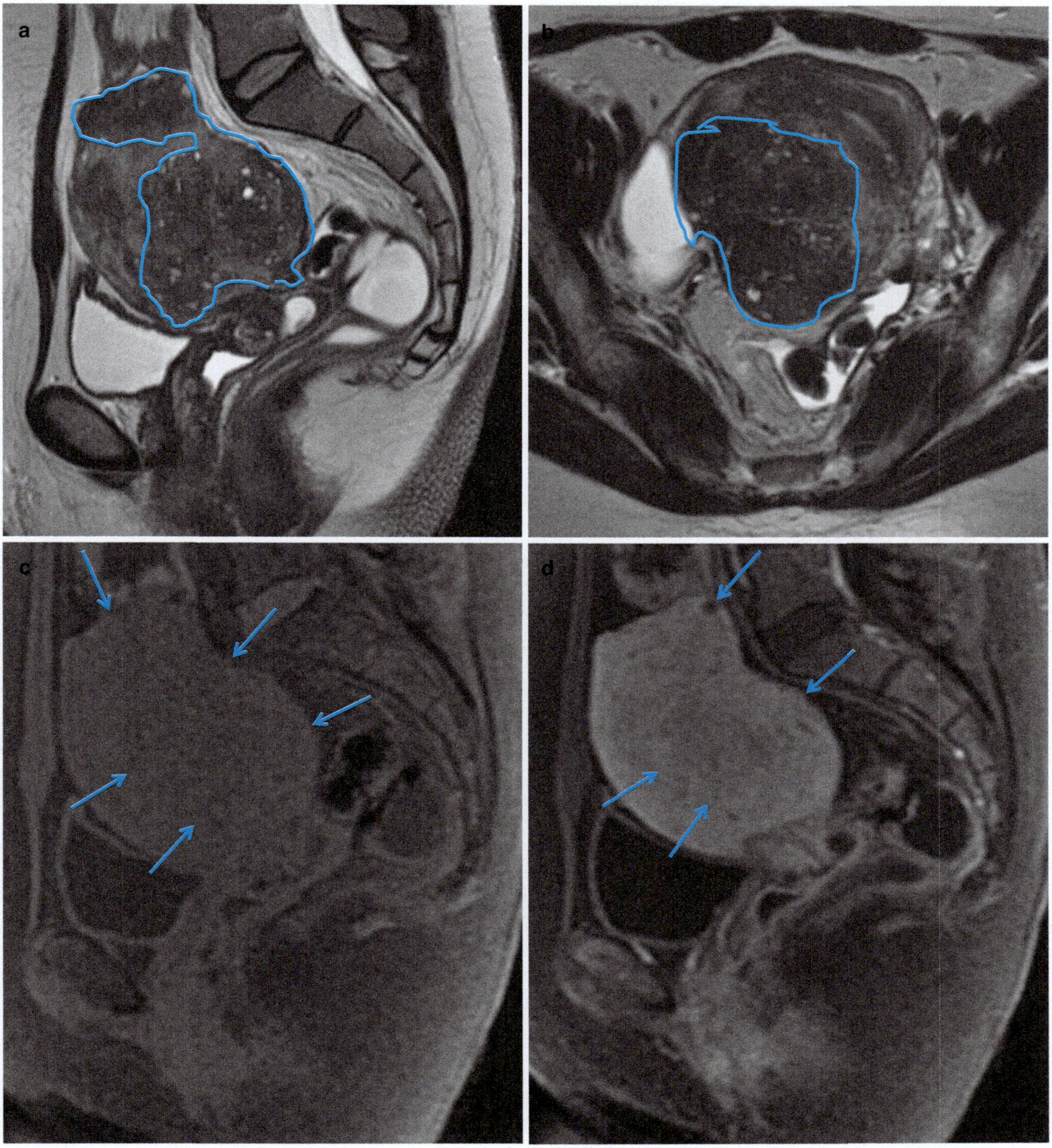

Fig. 4.114 Extensive myometrial lesion (blue lines in **a**, **b** and arrows in **c**, **d**) ill-defined, predominantly hypointense, with hyperintense foci in T2-weighted sequences (**a**, **b**) and intermediate signal on T1 (**c**), with nonhomogeneous enhancement (**d**). Note multiple foci of hypertensive ectopic endometrial glands and cysts in T2. Same case as Fig. 4.160, with progression of myometrial involvement in the fornix. (**a**, **c**, **d**) Sagittal. (**b**) Axial

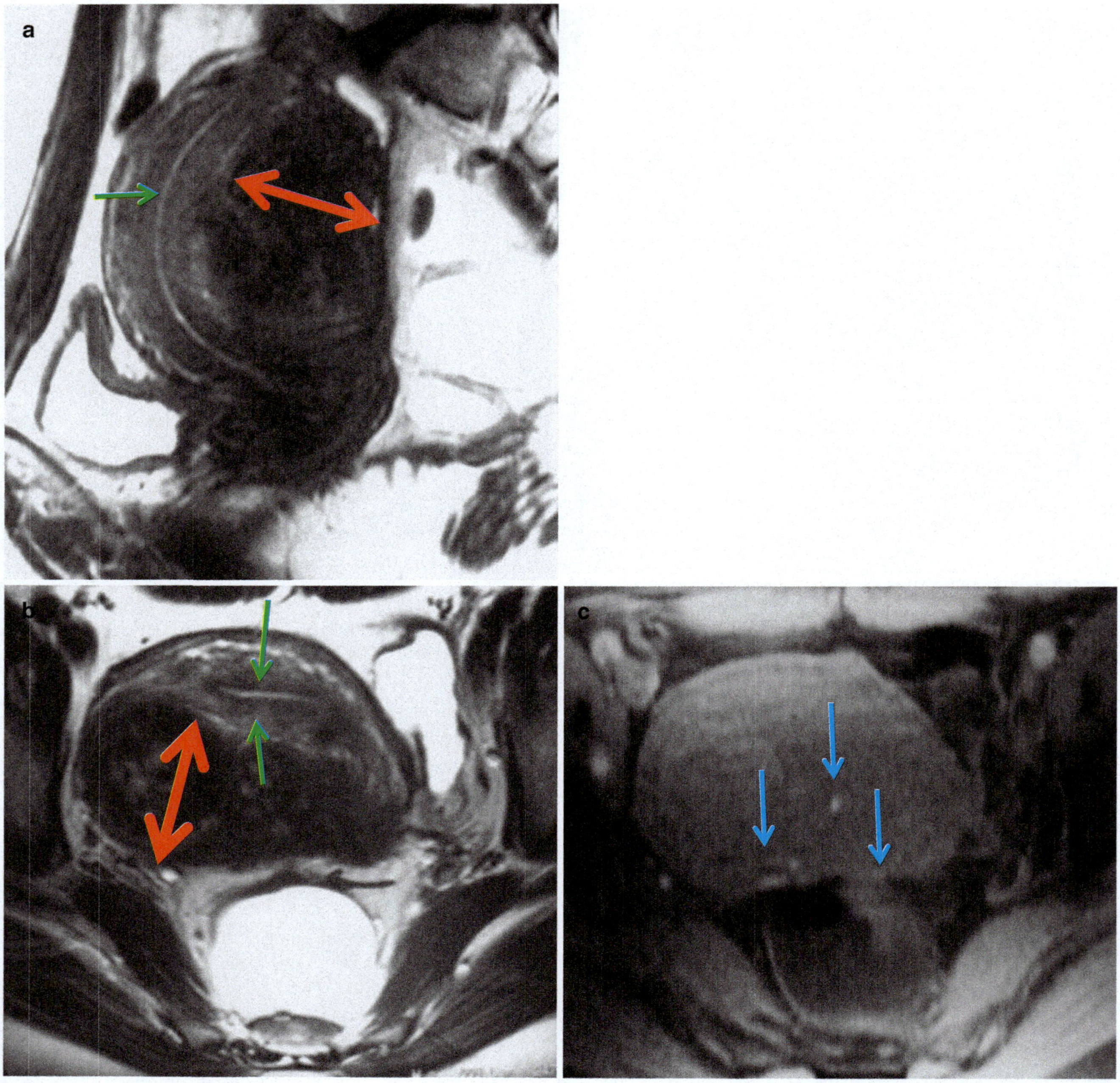

Fig. 4.115 In myometrial endometriosis the onset of the involvement is peripheral, with penetration from the visceral peritoneum and external layers (double arrows in **a**, **b**). Note normal junction zone (green arrows). (**a**, **b**) T2-weighted sequences. (**c**) T1-weighted fat suppression demonstrating scattered bleeding foci in the myometrium and retrouterine (blue arrows). (**a**) Sagittal. (**b**, **c**) Axial

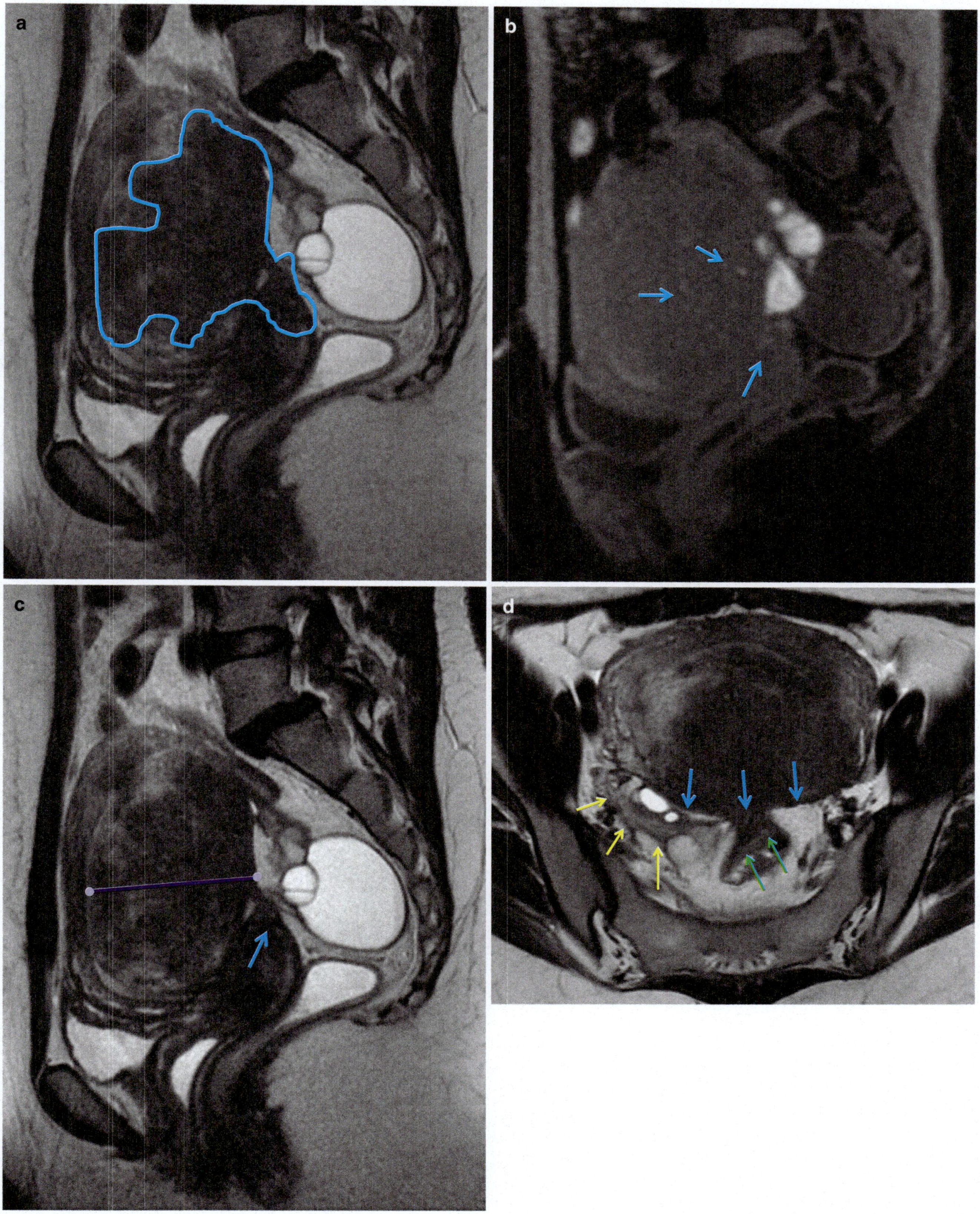

Fig. 4.116 Globular uterus, extended and asymmetric due to the penetration of endometriosis in the posterior wall, from fundus to the cervix (marked) to the uterine cavity ([**c**]—depth of 5.9 cm) with hypointense signal on T2 (**a**, **c**, **d**, **g**) and discrete bleeding foci (**b**). Note retrocervical endometriosis with superior extension (blue arrows **c**, **d**, **f**), rectal penetration (green arrows in **c**, **d**), and adnexal deviation with endometrioma and right hematosalpinx (yellow arrows in **d**, **e**)

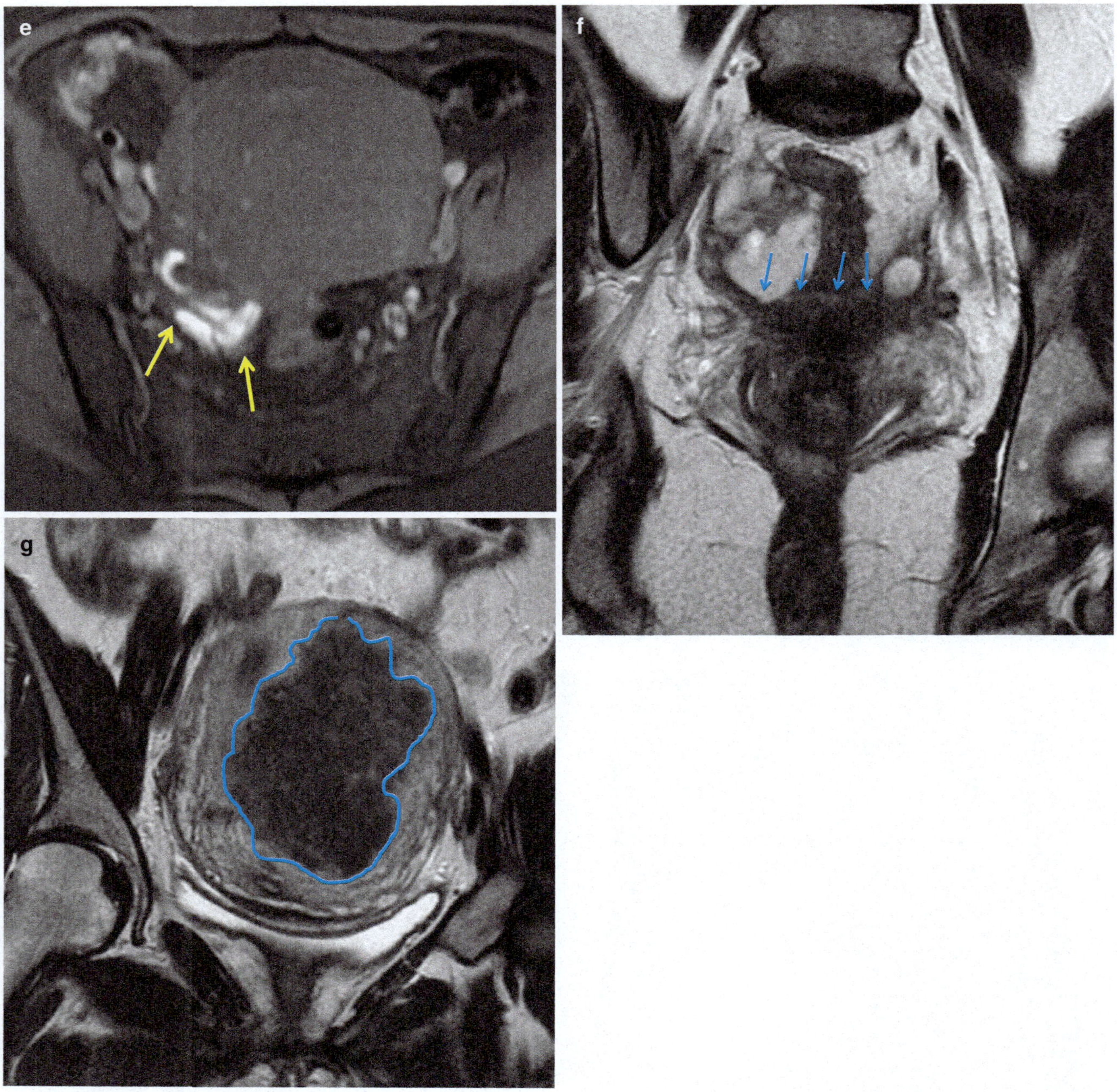

Fig. 4.116 (continued)

4.2.5.2 Clinical Symptoms

Symptoms of myometrial involvement are poorly specific, but patients may report dysmenorrhea and abnormal uterine bleeding.

4.2.5.3 MRI and Laparoscopic Findings

The MRI morphology of posterior myometrial involvement differs somewhat from that of the anterior compartment. It can be isolated and smaller in the cervix with extension of the retrocervical or rectovaginal lesion, producing signal modification in the myometrium or cervical stroma. The evaluation of the degree of penetration can be made more difficult, because the cervical wall has a hypointense signal on T2, and also by the deep lesion predominant in the myometrium. When there is a glandular component, this analysis is easier (Fig. 4.117).

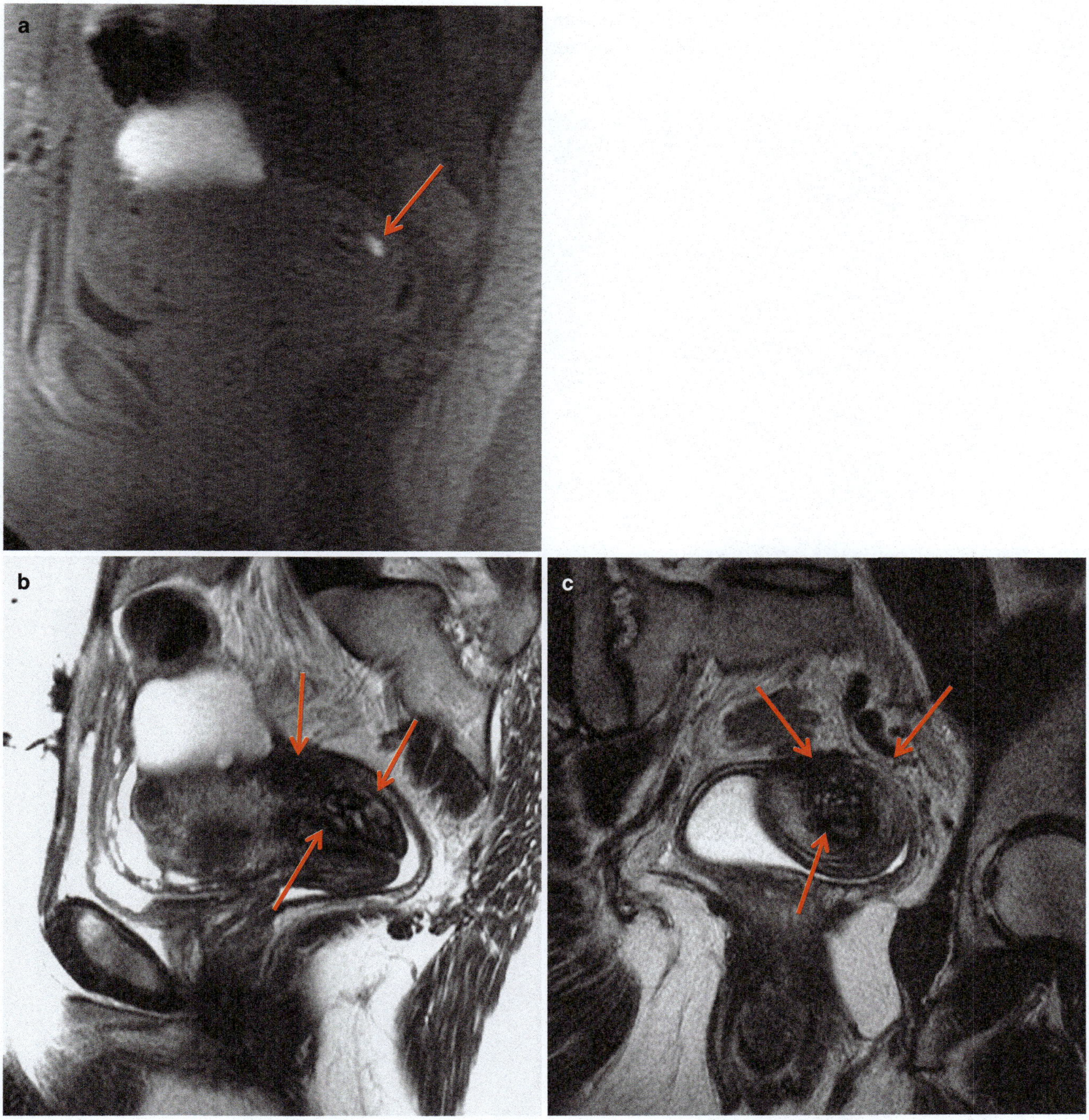

Fig. 4.117 Penetration in the cervix causing signal modification in the myometrium and cervical stroma. The evaluation of the degree of penetration was facilitated by the strong glandular component (hyperintense multiple foci on T2 and T1—arrows). (**b**, **c**) T2-weighted sequences. (**a**) T1 weighted with fat suppression. (**a**, **b**) Sagittal (**c**) Coronal short axis

On the other hand, the posterior compartment lesion, especially those with mantle morphology, following the uterine surface, may have prominent myometrial penetration, greater than the epicenter of the lesion, penetrating the entire posterior wall (Fig. 4.118).

Extensive myometrial lesions may even mimic adenomyosis, especially in patients under hormonal suppression, where there is a reduction in the signal intensity of the myometrium on the T2-weighted sequence, resulting in a loss of zonal anatomy, assuming a signal similar to that of the myometrial lesion. In addition, the two pathologies can coexist. In these patients, it is very important to compare examinations with those prior to the hormone therapy (Fig. 4.119) [26, 27].

The myometrial lesion is poorly delimited and shows a predominantly hypointense signal on the T2-weighted sequence and the T1-weighted sequence. T2 hyperintense foci can be observed, representing ectopic endometrial glands and cysts as well as bleeding foci (Fig. 4.120).

The degree of myometrial involvement may be underestimated during laparoscopy and should be detailed in the MRI report. Thus, it is necessary to describe the degree of penetration of the endometriotic process, in addition to its distance from the uterine cavity (Table 4.9 and Fig. 4.121).

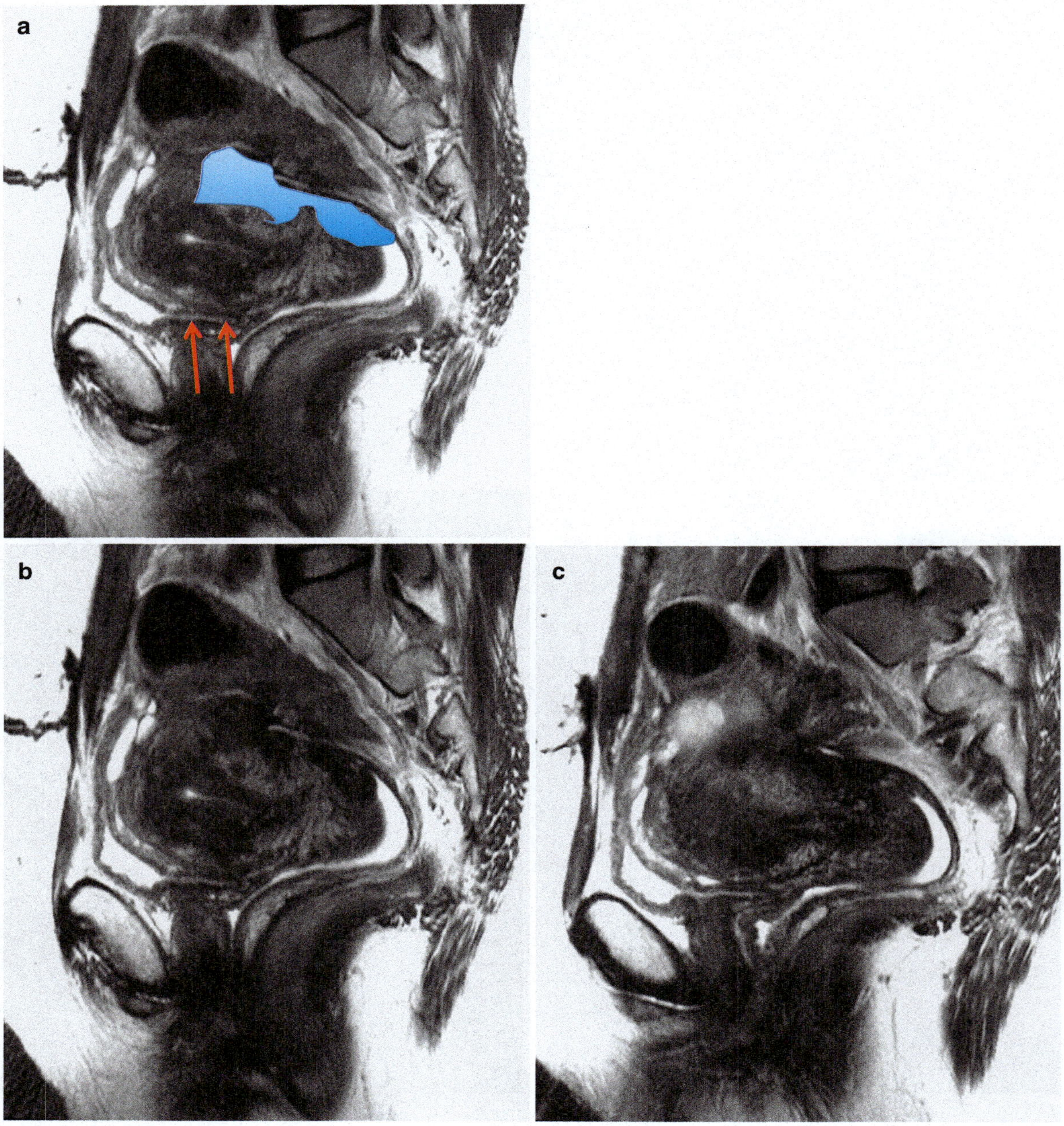

Fig. 4.118 Plaque-like morphology of the myometrial lesion ("blue highlighted area"), following the uterine surface, in correlation with retrocervical and retrouterine lesions, with sigmoid penetration. Note simultaneous anterior uterine adenomyosis (red arrows). (**a–c**) T2-weighted sequences. (**a**) Reference for (**b**, **c**). Sagittal

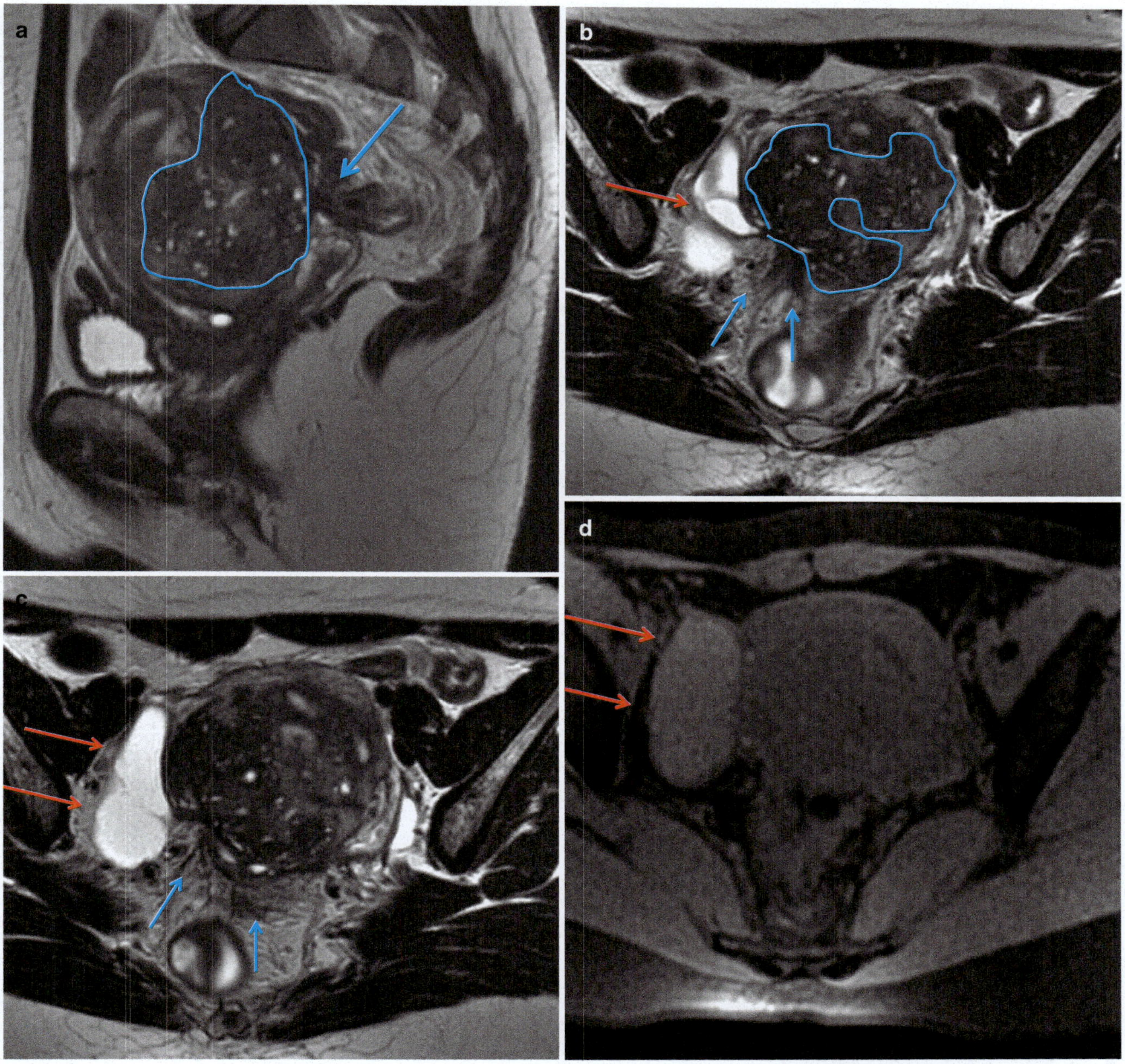

Fig. 4.119 Extensive myometrial lesion mimicking adenomyosis, globular and asymmetrical aspect of the uterus, thickening of the posterior wall, and extension until near the uterine cavity (marked in blue). Note a small retrocervical lesion, rectal and on right uterosacral ligament lesion (blue arrows), causing tubal adhesion and dilation (red arrows). (**a–c**) T2-weighted sequences. (**d**) T1-weighted. (**a**) Sagittal. (**b–d**) Axial

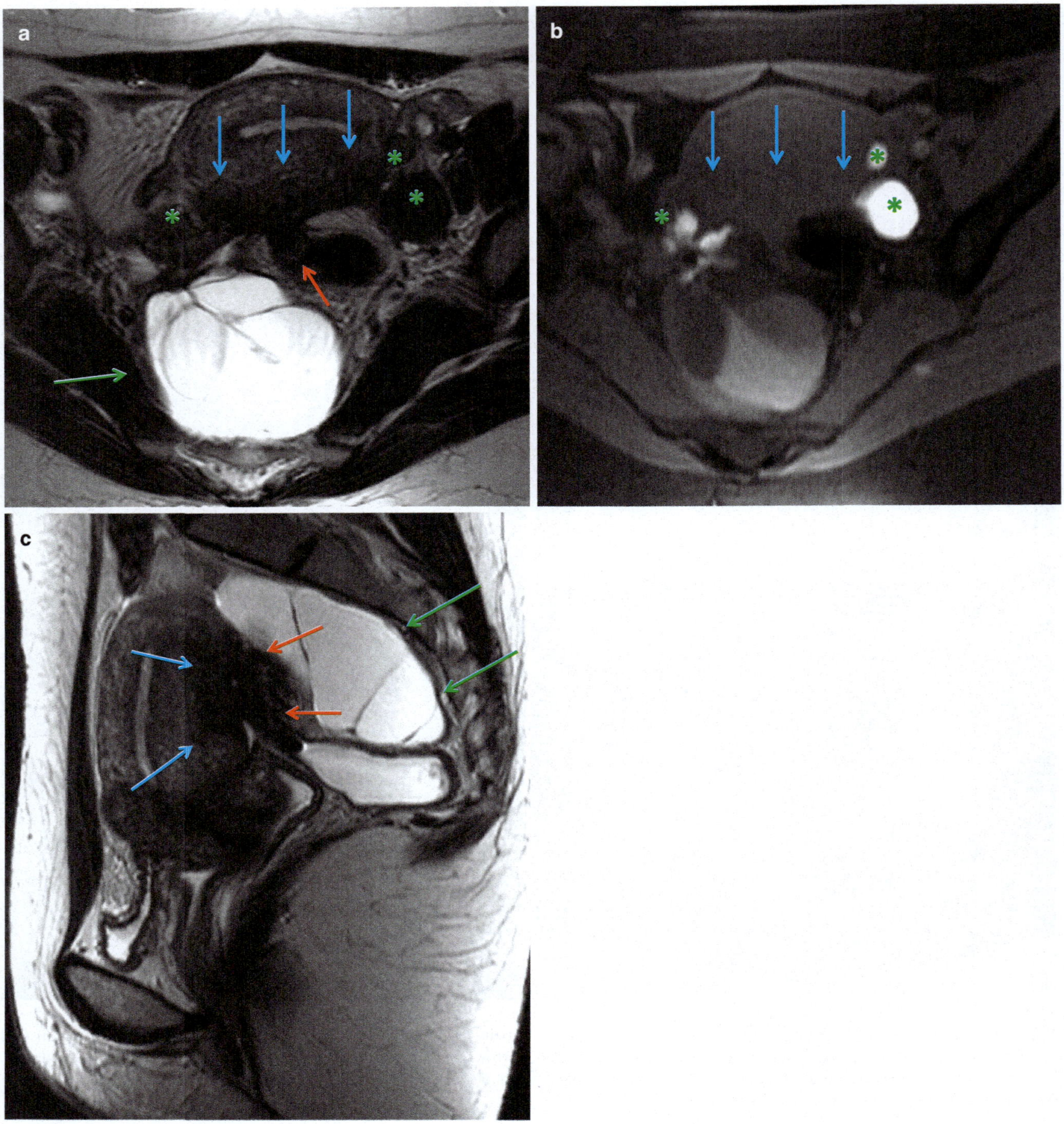

Fig. 4.120 Poorly defined myometrial lesion, predominantly hypointense with discrete hypersignal foci (glands and ectopic endometrial cysts) on T2-weighted sequences ([**a**, **c**] blue arrows) and with an intermediary signal on T1 (**b**), without bleeding. Note retrouterine endometriosis with deep penetration in the sigmoid (red arrows), uterosacral and broad ligaments on the right, adnexal adherence and posterior pseudocyst (green arrows), as well as bilateral endometriomas (*). (**a**, **b**) Axial. (**c**) Sagittal

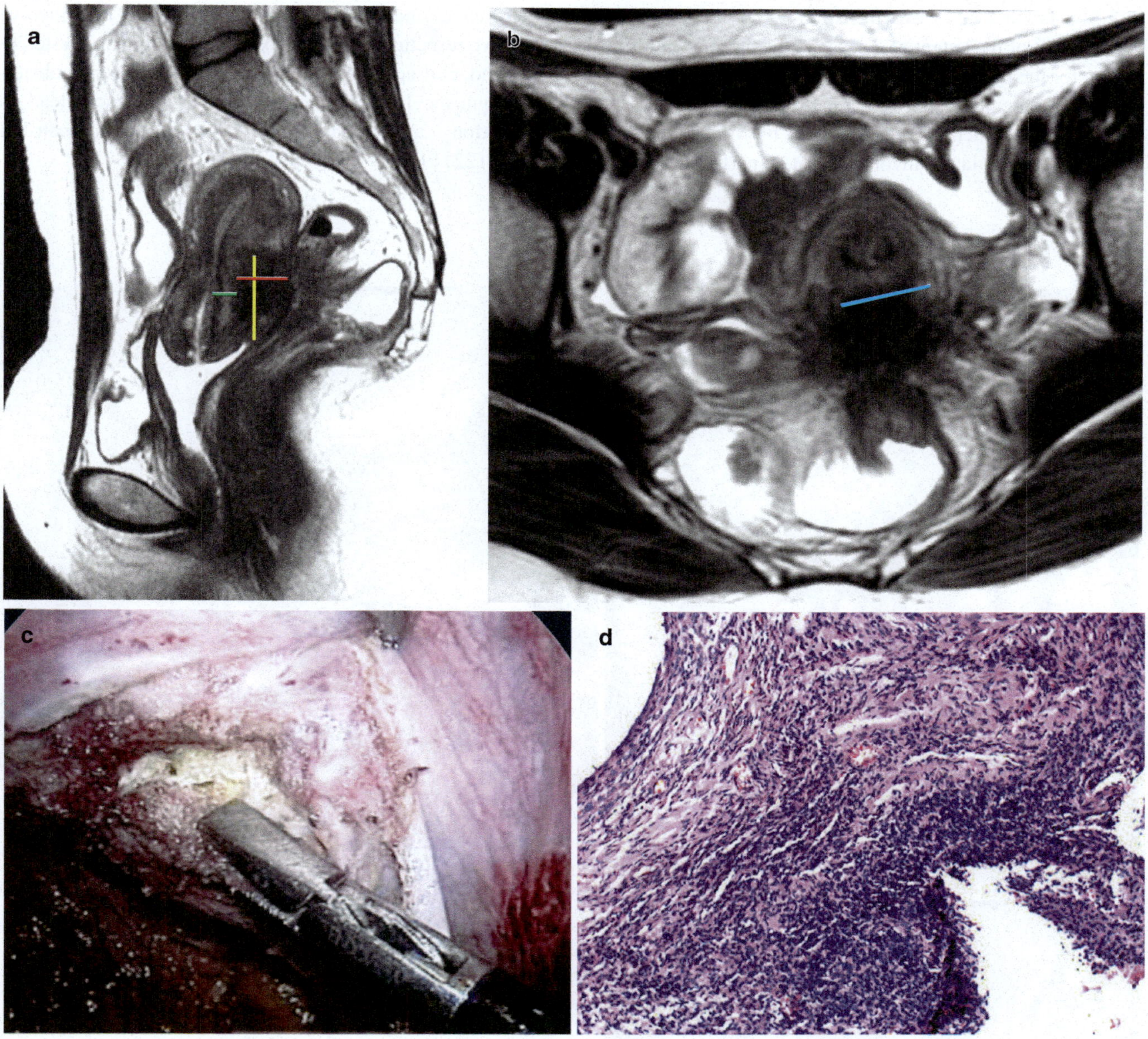

Fig. 4.121 Descriptive criteria. Lesion length in the longitudinal axis (yellow) and transverse axis (blue), the penetration of the endometriotic process in the myometrium (red), and the distance to the uterine cavity (green). (**a**, **b**) T2-weighted sequences. (**a**) Sagittal. (**b**) Axial. (**c**) Laparoscopic myometrial lesion resection. (**d**) Microscopy (100×). Fibrosis and lymphoplasmacytic infiltrate

4.2.5.4 Treatment Comments

Assessment of the extent of disease in the uterine wall is necessary for the proper planning of surgical excision, since successful treatment depends on radical surgical removal. Thus, if myometrial penetration is identified by MRI, resection of the uterine musculature involved must be performed [9].

However, when penetration is prominent, it may involve extensive resection of the cervix and, occasionally, hysterectomy and, consequently, modification of the patient's obstetric prognosis. In addition, cervical resection can lead to amputation and occlusion, causing hematometrium (Fig. 4.122) [9].

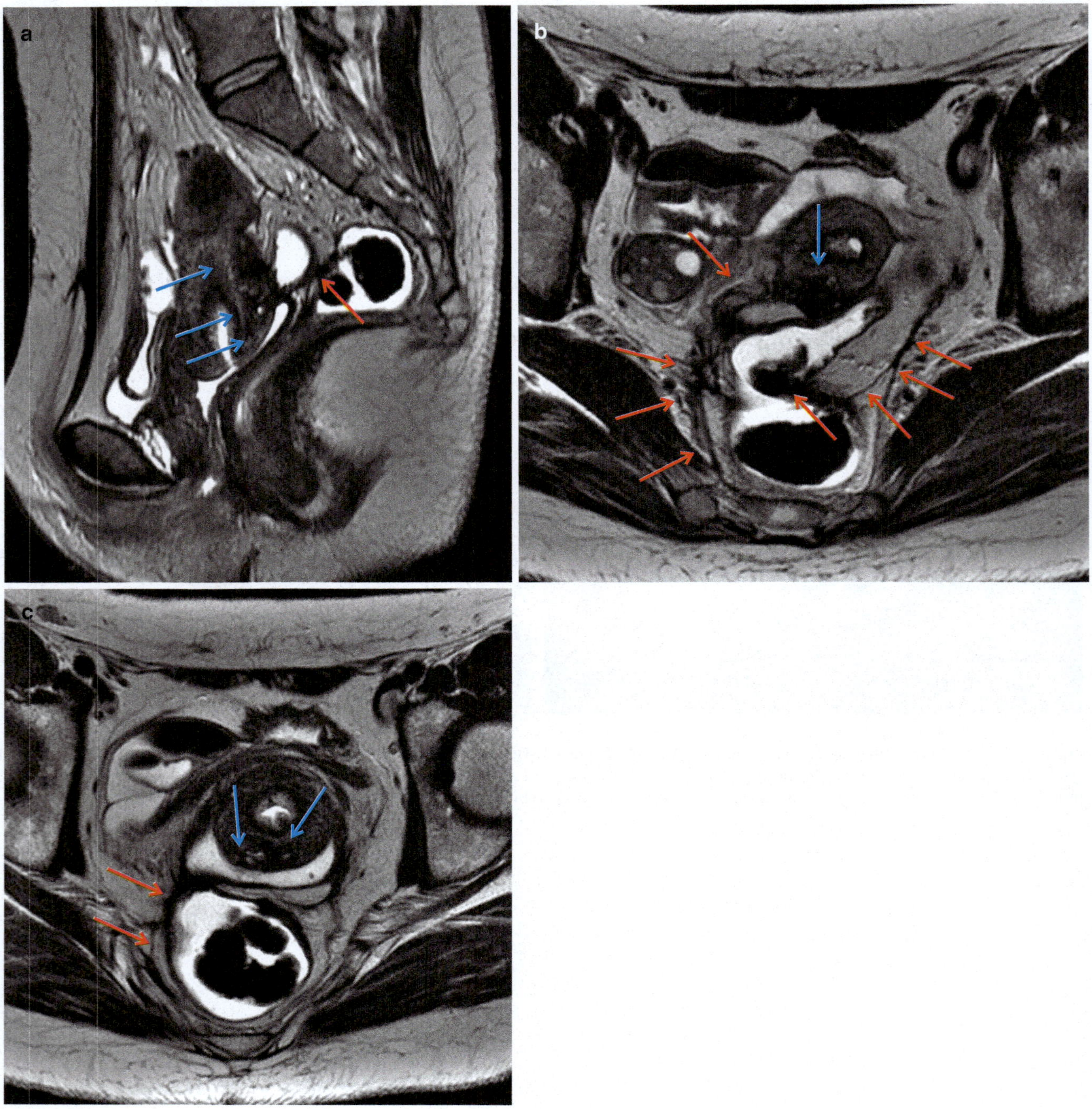

Fig. 4.122 Posterior compartment lesion. The cervical myometrial component (blue arrows) was not resected to avoid modifying the obstetric prognosis of the patient. Note postsurgical changes (red arrows) in retrocervical, ligamental, right parametrial, and perirectal with well-defined hypointense tissue on T2 weighted, in addition to colonic anastomosis. T2-weighted sequences. (**a**) Sagittal. (**b**, **c**) Axial

4.2.6 Rectum and Sigmoid

4.2.6.1 Anatomy

The rectum has intraperitoneal location, with the majority extraperitoneal. Only the anterior and lateral sections of the upper rectum and part of the middle are covered by a thin layer of visceral peritoneum to the peritoneal reflection, which in women is lower, 7.5–5 cm from the anal margin (Fig. 4.123) [47].

At its lower end, the rectum presents posterior indentation by the levator ani muscle, forming the anorectal junction (Fig. 4.123).

The rectum presents lateral curves, which correspond, in the intraluminal aspect, to the Houston or rectal valves. There are generally two to three valves, which aid in segmentation of the organ into upper, middle, and lower and in the identification of the junction with the sigmoid (Fig. 4.124).

According to Brown, MRI is accurate enough to describe the anatomy and pathologies of the rectal wall, anal sphincter, and mesorectum [48].

However, to do this, it is necessary to carry out the study with the appropriate sequence and the ideal coil, similar to that described in the protocol session. That is, T2-weighted sequence with high spatial resolution and an eight-channel coil, directed at obtaining sections perpendicular to the intestinal lesion.

In our experience, the use of a glycerin suppository also helps to characterize the majority of the rectal wall layers, by cleaning the lumen and its irritative effect on the wall, fostering the slight thickening of the mucosa and submucosa, and facilitating the distinction of the lesion and the analysis of the degree of penetration (Fig. 4.125).

Histologically, the rectal wall consists of three layers: the mucosa, the submucosa, and the muscularis propria, identified by MRI—(a) the mucosa, an internal hypointense thin line in continuity with the lumen; (b) the submucosa, which appears as a thicker band with a hyperintense signal; and (c) the muscularis propria with a hypointense signal (Fig. 4.125) [47].

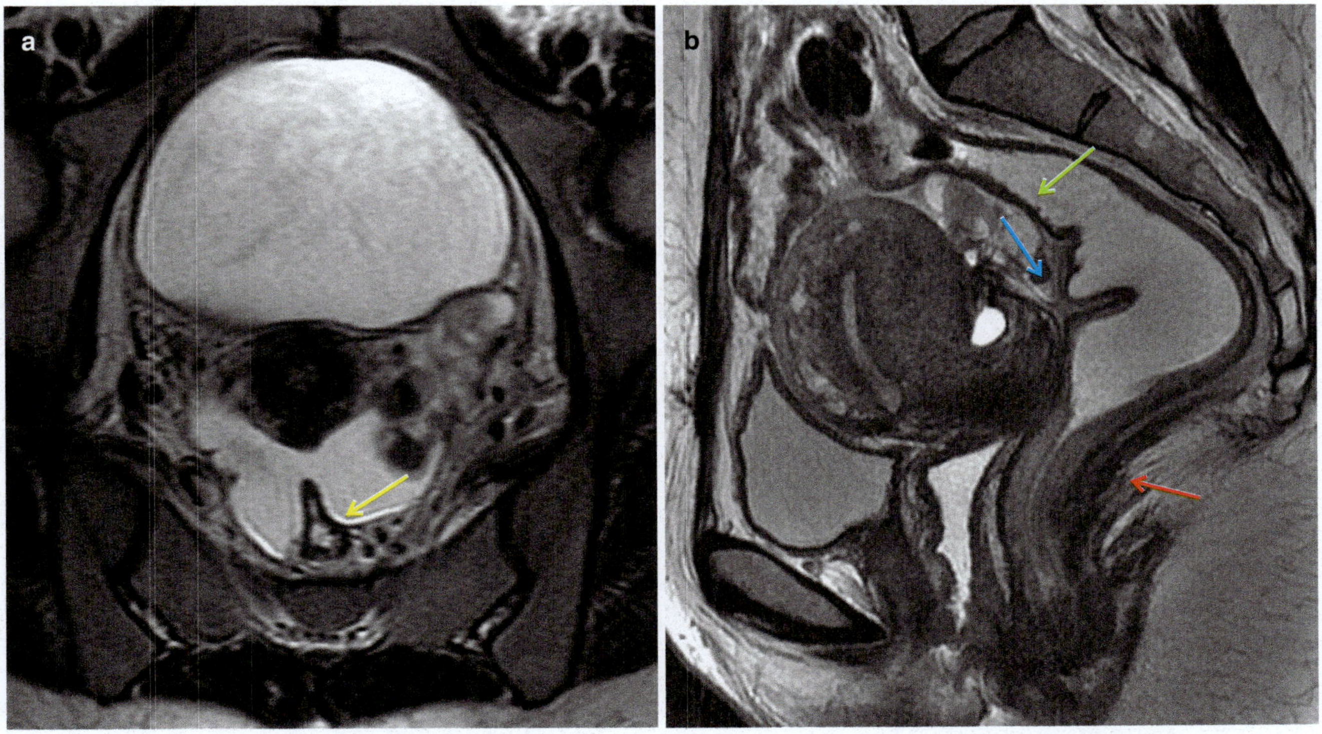

Fig. 4.123 The anterior (green arrow) and lateral sections of the upper rectum (yellow arrow) and part of the middle section are covered by a thin layer of visceral peritoneum to the peritoneal reflection (blue arrow). This analysis was possible because of the peritoneal fluid in the endometriosis (note hematic levels in the sagittal plane between the uterus and rectosigmoid). Note posterior impression by the levator ani muscle, forming the anorectal junction (red arrow). T2-weighted sequences. (**a**) Coronal short axis. (**b**) Sagittal

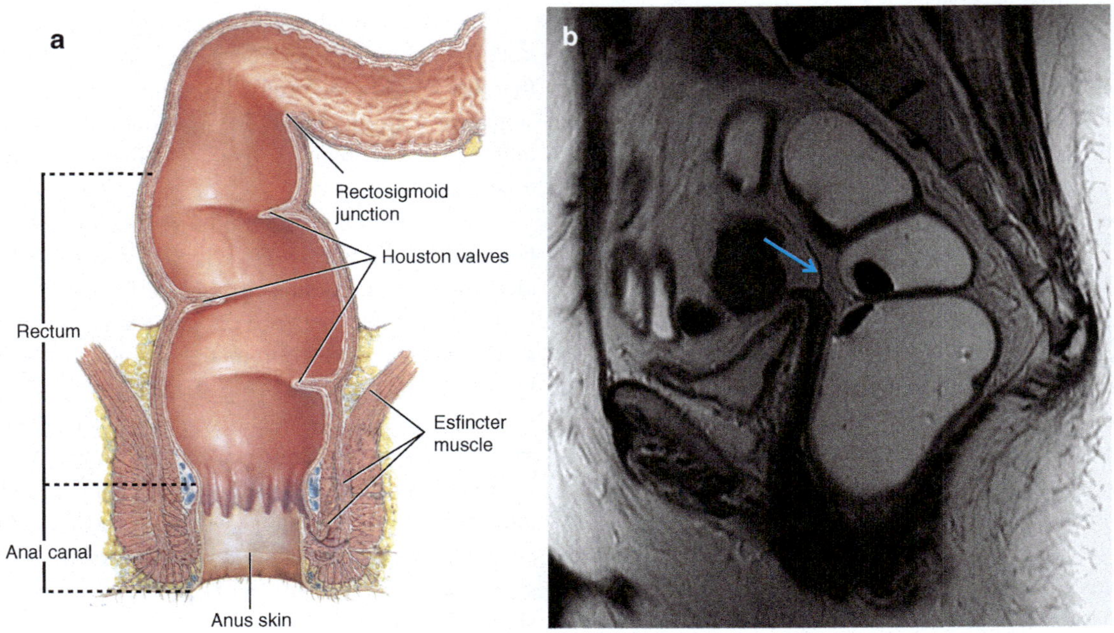

Fig. 4.124 Houston or rectal valves. There are generally two to three valves that segment the organ into upper, middle, and lower parts and facilitate the identification of its junction with the sigmoid. (**a**) Diagram (Netter). (**b**) T2-weighted sequence. Sagittal. Note peritoneal reflection (arrow)

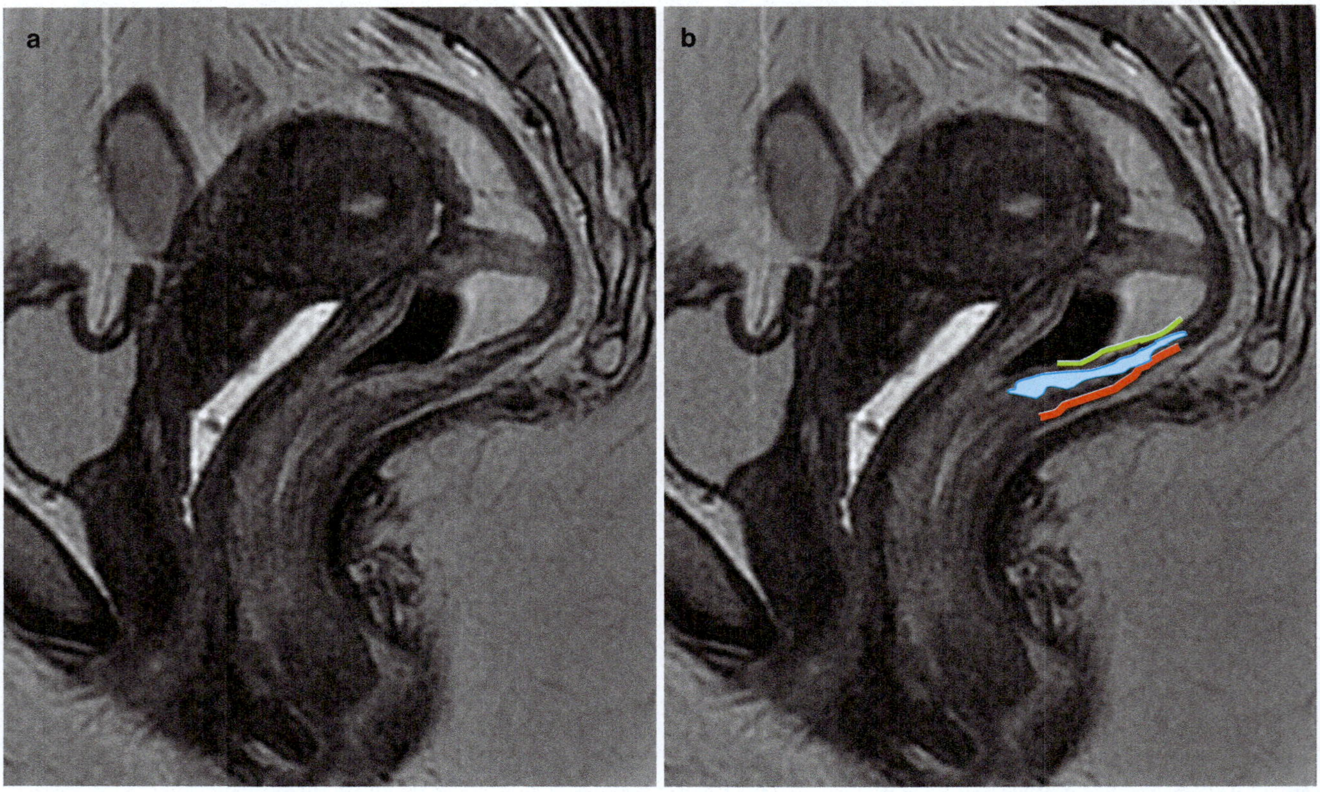

Fig. 4.125 Utility of rectal preparation. The irritative effect on the wall provokes thickening of the mucosa and submucosa, facilitating identification of the layers: (1) mucosa, an internal hypointense thin line following the lumen (green); (2) the submucosa, which appears as a thicker band with hyperintense signal (blue); (3) the muscularis propria with hypointense signal (red). (**a**, **d**) T2-weighted sequences. (**a**, **b**) Sagittal. (**c**, **d**) Coronal short axis. (**a**, **c**) Reference images for (**b**, **d**)

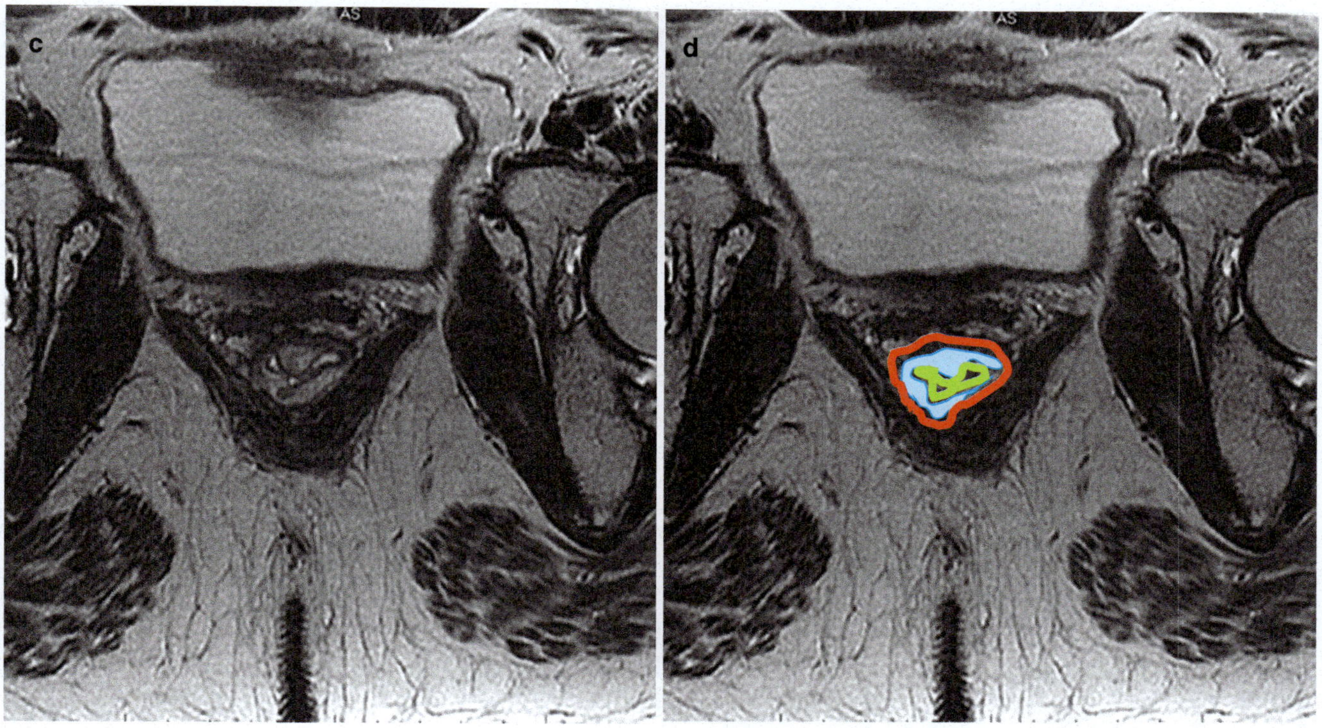

Fig. 4.125 (continued)

4.2.6.2 Most Common Aspects of Intestinal Endometriosis

Intestinal involvement is expected in every 5 of 12 women with endometriosis and in up to 31% of patients with deep endometriosis. It is commonly associated with deep lesion in other sites of the pelvis, and it is estimated that half of the patients with severe endometriosis have some degree of intestinal endometriosis (Fig. 4.126) [5, 8, 45, 49].

The most affected areas are the rectum and sigmoid, and the pattern of lesion distribution by decreasing order is the rectum (96%), the sigmoid (38, 7%), the ileus (22.7%), the cecum (10.7%), the appendix (10.7%), and the omentum (4%). In addition, multifocal intestinal involvement is common, identified in half the patients [1].

The high frequency of other intestinal lesions in patients with rectosigmoid lesions justifies a careful intestinal examination, since the number and location of these lesions determine the operative treatment (Fig. 4.127) [45].

Intestinal endometriosis implants are usually located in the serosa; however, with the progression of the disease, there is penetration into the wall, causing parietal thickening (Table 4.8 and Fig. 4.128).

The endometrial glands and stroma infiltrate the adjacent fibromuscular tissue and cause proliferation of smooth muscle and fibrosis, resulting in the formation of solid nodules. The mucosal layer is usually spared, since the pattern of growth of the implanted ectopic tissue is extramucosal parietal (Fig. 4.129) [50].

However, in larger lesions, there may be involvement of the mucosa, and there are rare reports in the literature of rupture of the loop in pregnant patients (Fig. 4.130) [51].

The involvement is asymmetrical, predominantly on the anterior face, producing adhesion and wrinkling on the wall of the affected loop (Fig. 4.131).

This alteration, together with the inflammatory response and cyclic hemorrhage, can lead to adherence, stenosis, and intestinal obstruction (Fig. 4.132) [5].

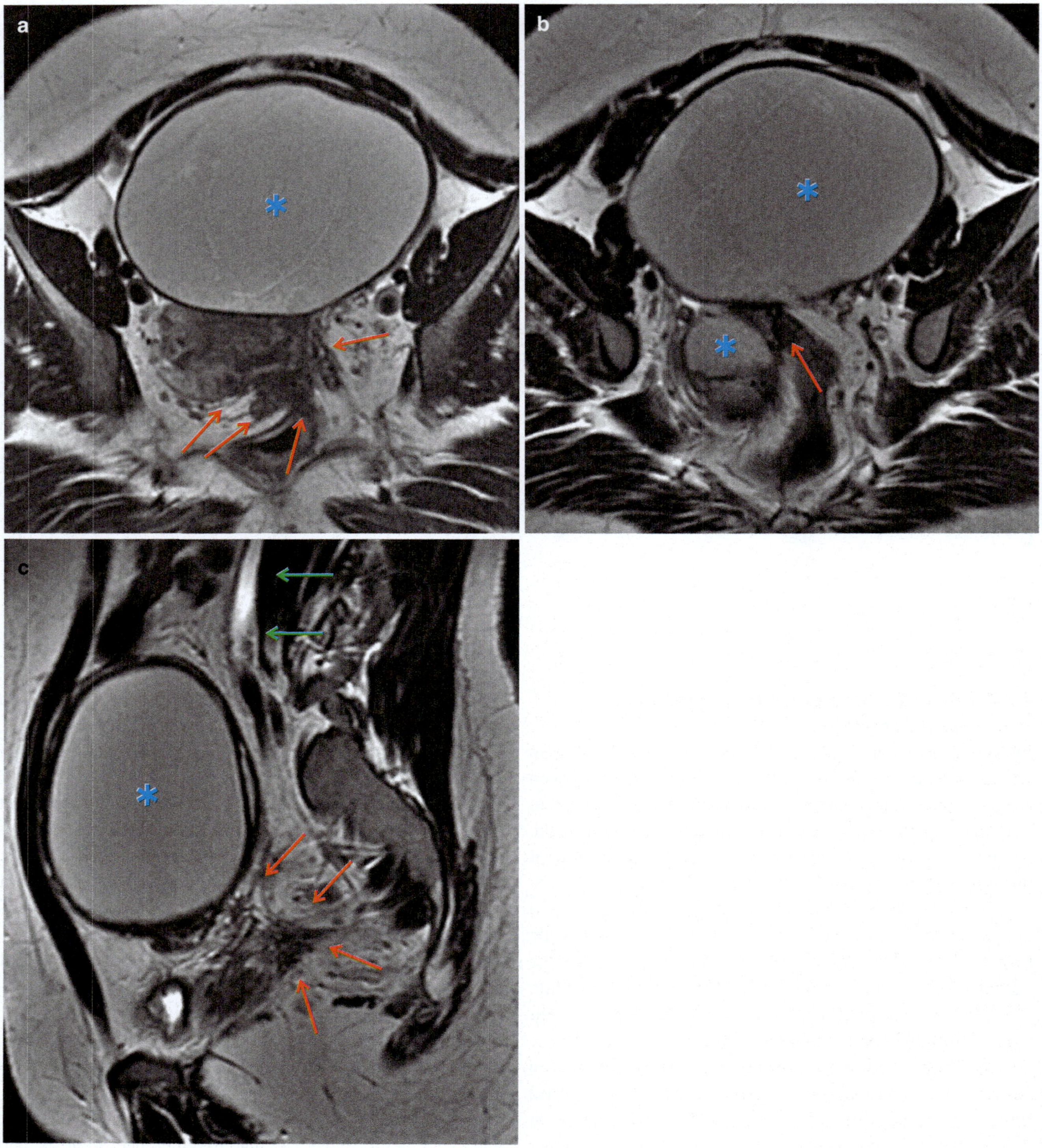

Fig. 4.126 Severe deep lesion (red arrows), multifocal, involving the rectum, sigmoid, right parametrium, and bilateral endometriomas (*) being large on the left, causing dilation of the ureter (green arrows). (**a**–**c**) T2-weighted sequences. (**a**, **b**) Coronal oblique. (**c**) Sagittal

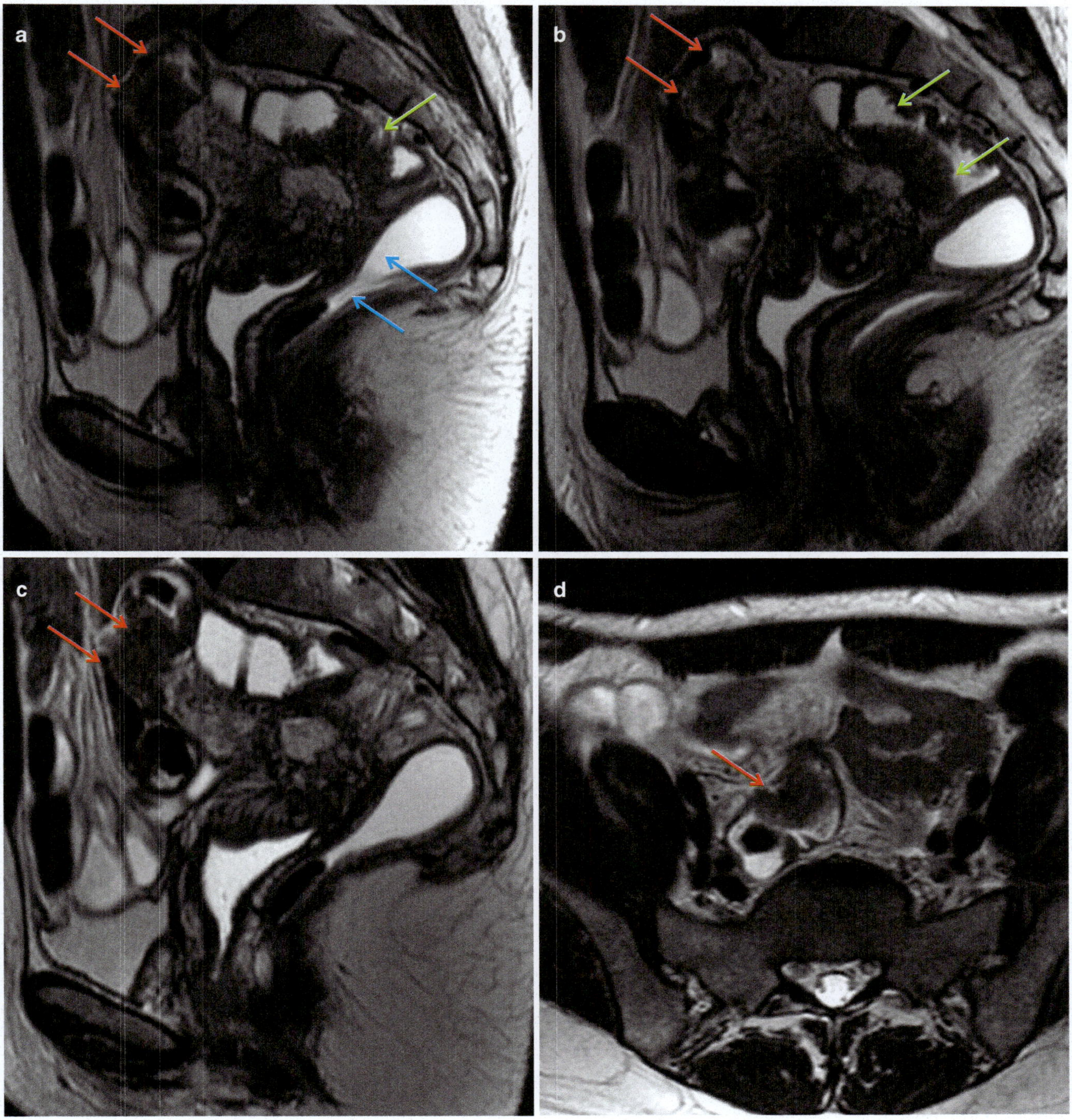

Fig. 4.127 High frequency of multifocal intestinal lesions. In this patient, three lesions were identified, one in the rectum (blue arrows) and two in the sigmoid (green and red arrows). T2-weighted sequences. (**a–c**) Sagittal. (**d–f**) Axial

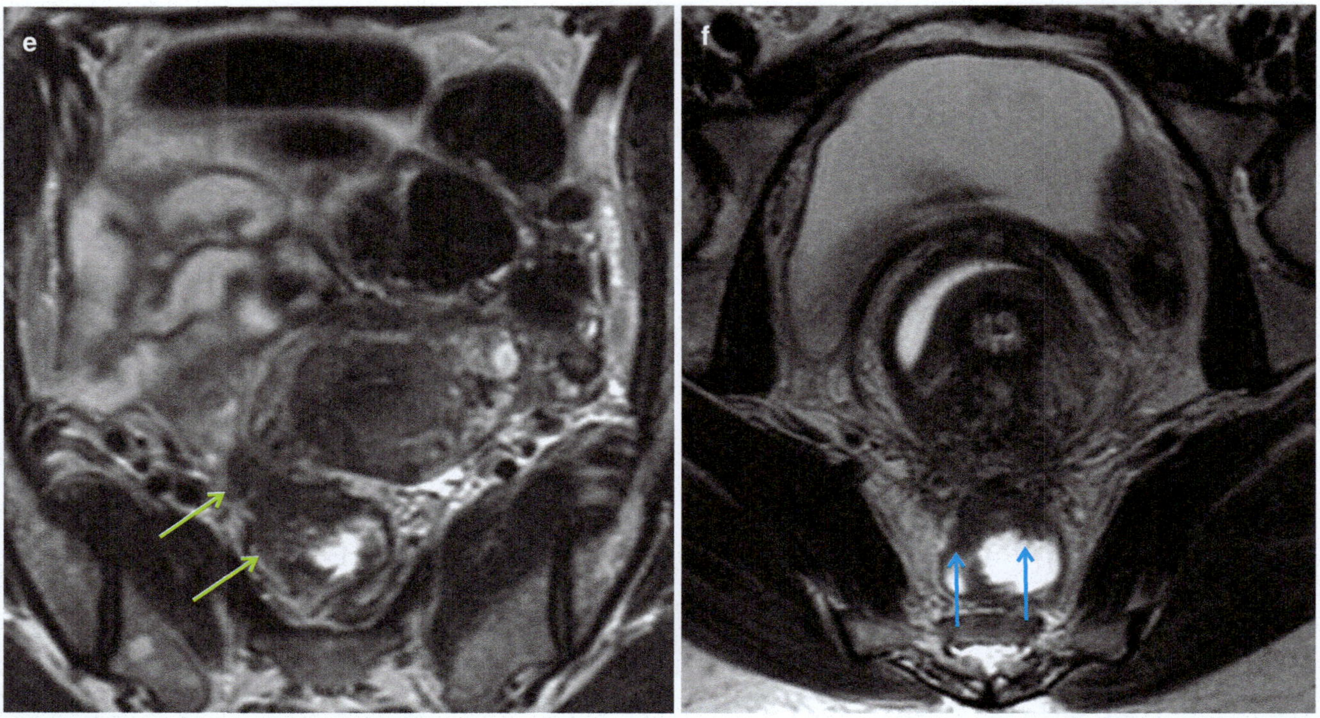

Fig. 4.127 (continued)

Table 4.8 Progression of the intestinal lesion

Superficial implant in the serosa
Proliferation with infiltration in the intestinal wall
Fibrous reaction
Transmural involvement with unaffected mucosa
Stenosis and adherence—Obstruction
Involvement of the mucosa
Rupture—Rare

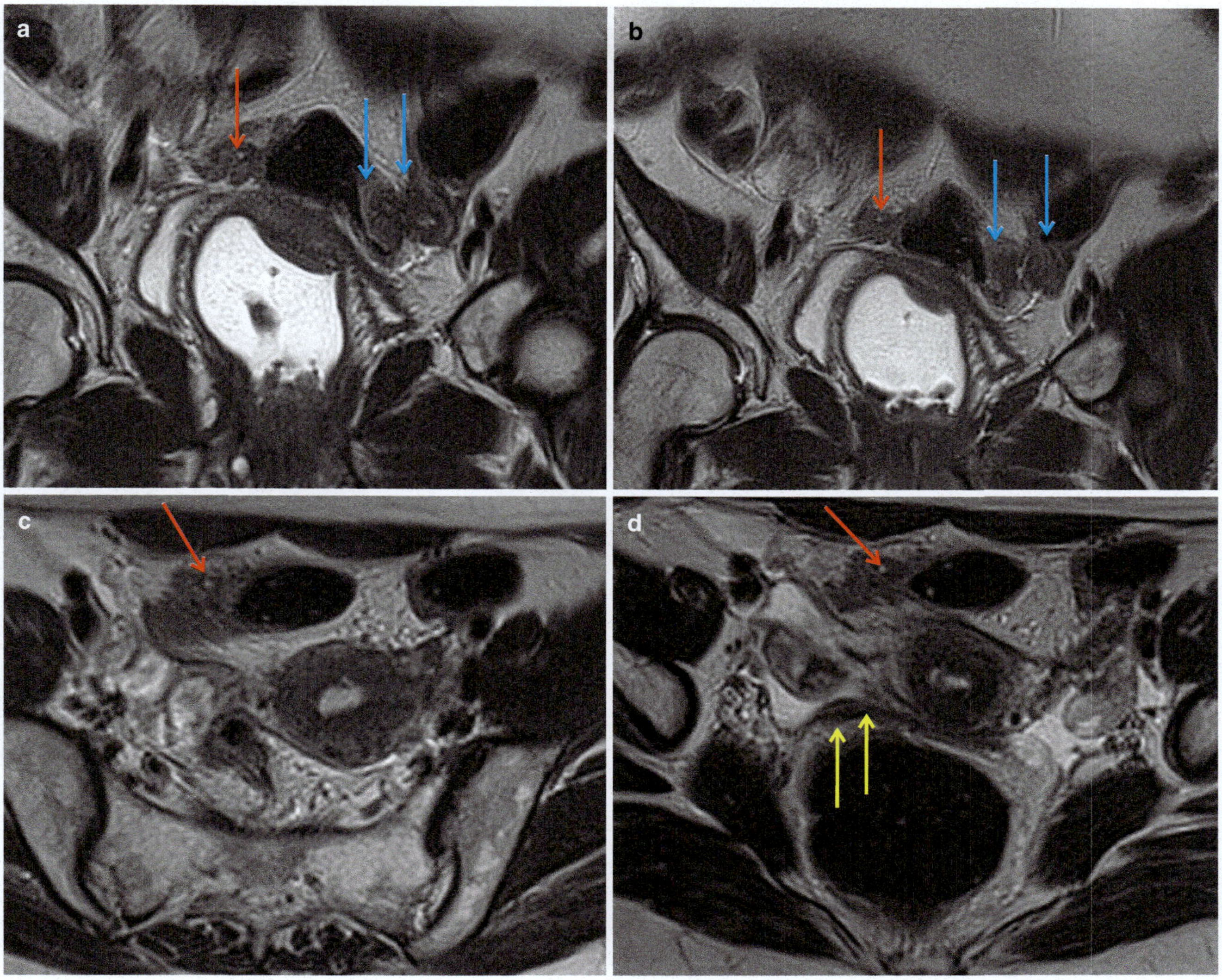

Fig. 4.128 Implant of intestinal endometriosis located in the serosa. Discrete hyperintense foci on the wall of the loop (red arrows). Note additional deep intestinal lesion, next to the descending colon (blue arrows), and the right uterosacral ligament, thickening (yellow arrows). (**a–g**) T2-weighted sequences. (**a**, **b**) Coronal, short axis. (**c–e**) Axial. (**f**, **g**) Sagittal

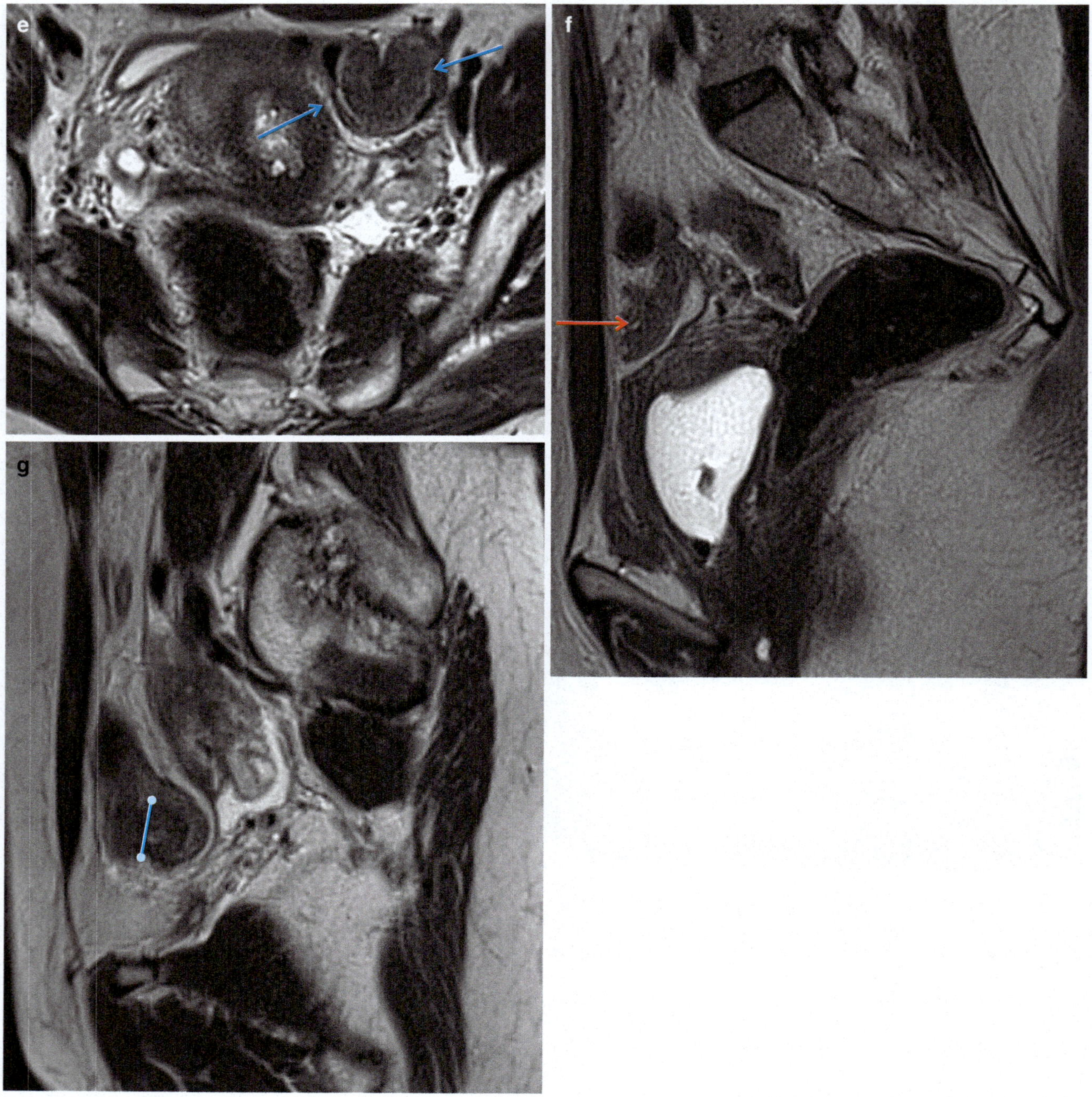

Fig. 4.128 (continued)

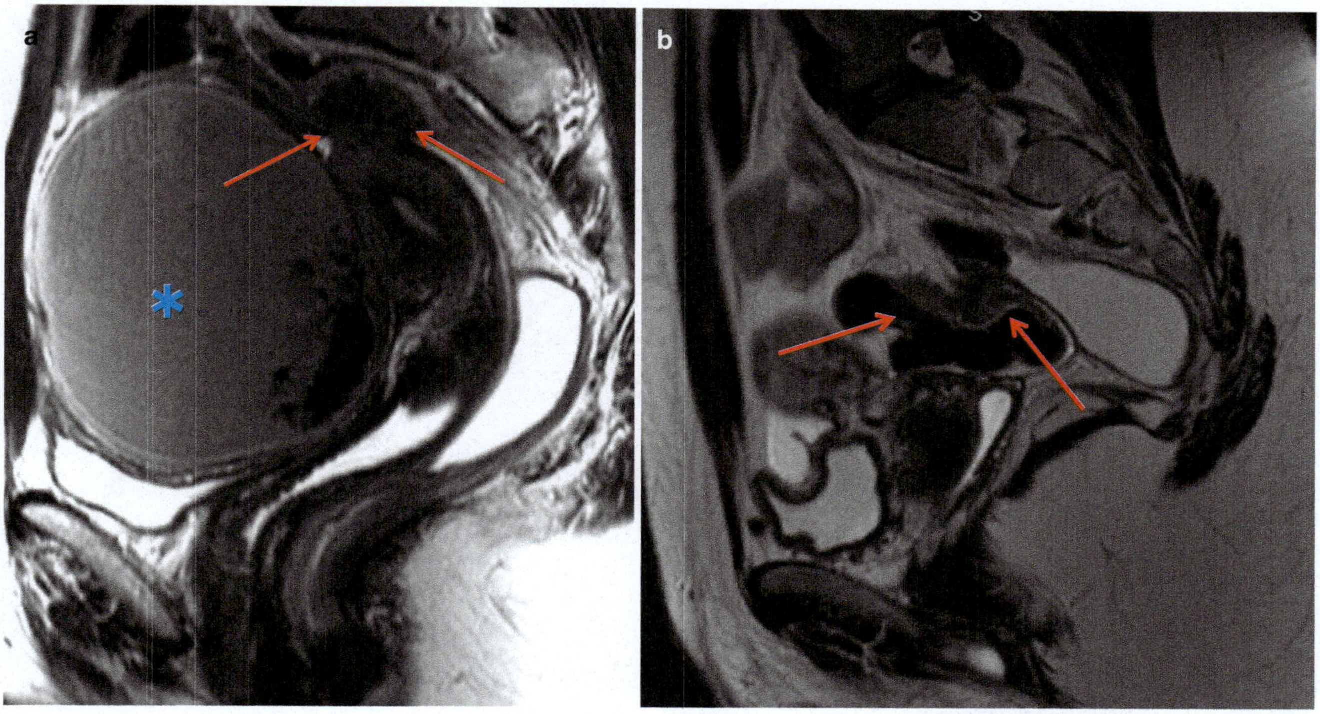

Fig. 4.129 Extramucosal parietal lesion in the sigmoid in two patients. Note the nodule that surrounds the outer layer of the loop (red arrows). The mucosal/submucosal layer is spared by the extramucosal growth pattern of endometriosis and maintains a hyperintense signal on T2. Large endometrioma with clot in **a** (*). (**a**, **b**) T2-weighted sequences. Sagittal

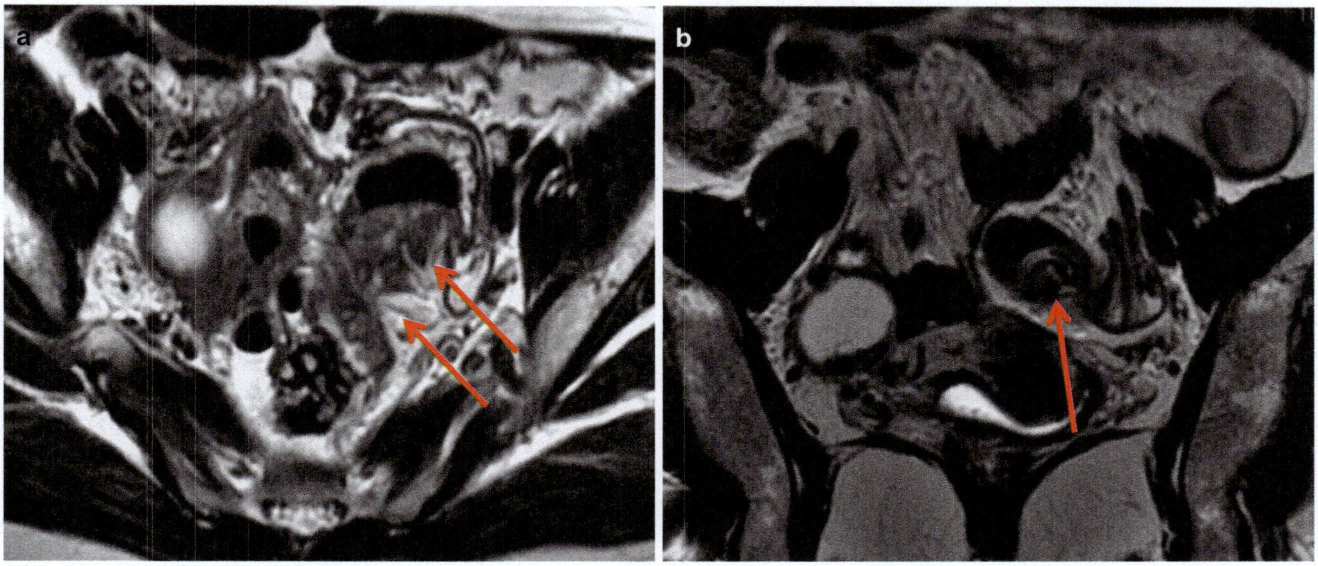

Fig. 4.130 Lesion with involvement of submucosa/mucosa, causing sigmoid stenosis. Note the change in the signal of the loop throughout the wall thickness of the affected segment, no hypersignal identified on T2 continuous of the submucosa/mucosa. There is significant parietal thickening with a reduction in the intestinal lumen (arrows). T2-weighted sequence. (**a**) Axial. (**b**) Coronal short axis. (**c**) Sagittal. (**d**) Pathology of the piece revealing hemorrhagic endometriosis foci near the intestinal mucosa

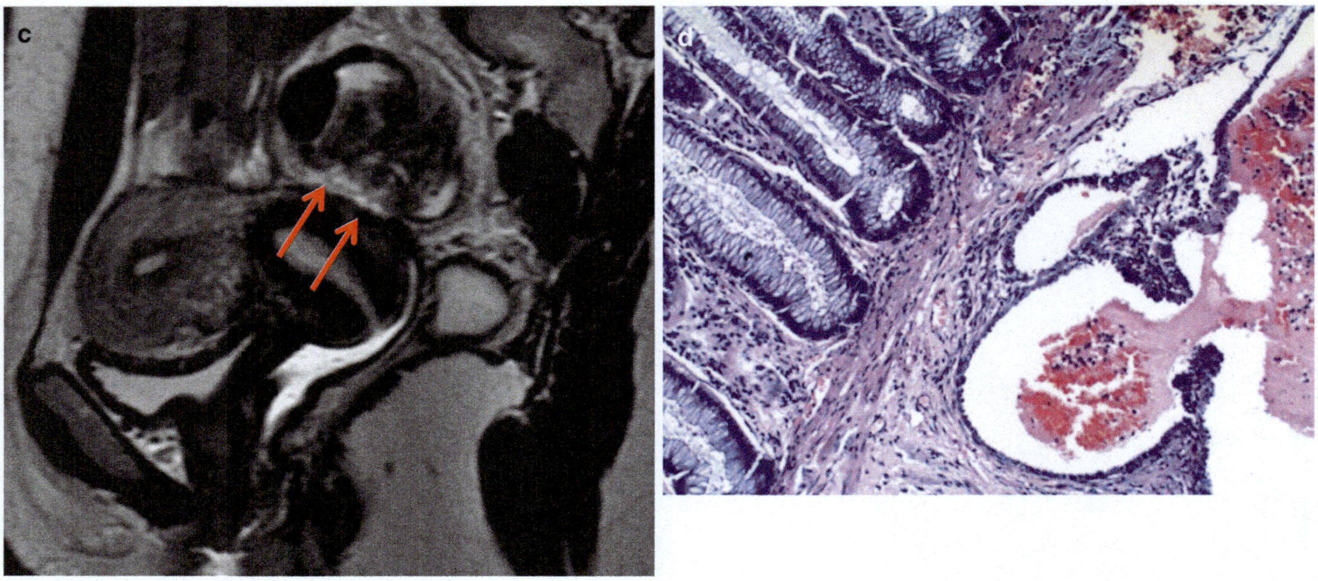

Fig. 4.130 (continued)

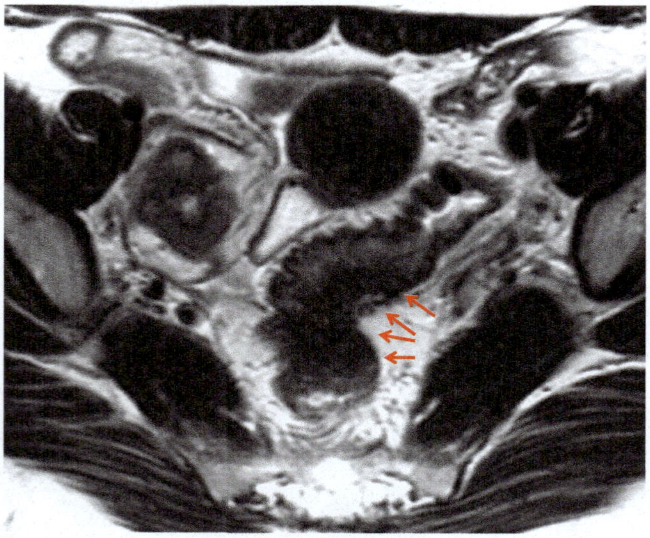

Fig. 4.131 Asymmetric involvement, causing adhesion and wrinkling on the wall of the affected loop. (sigmoid—arrows) T2-weighted sequence. Axial

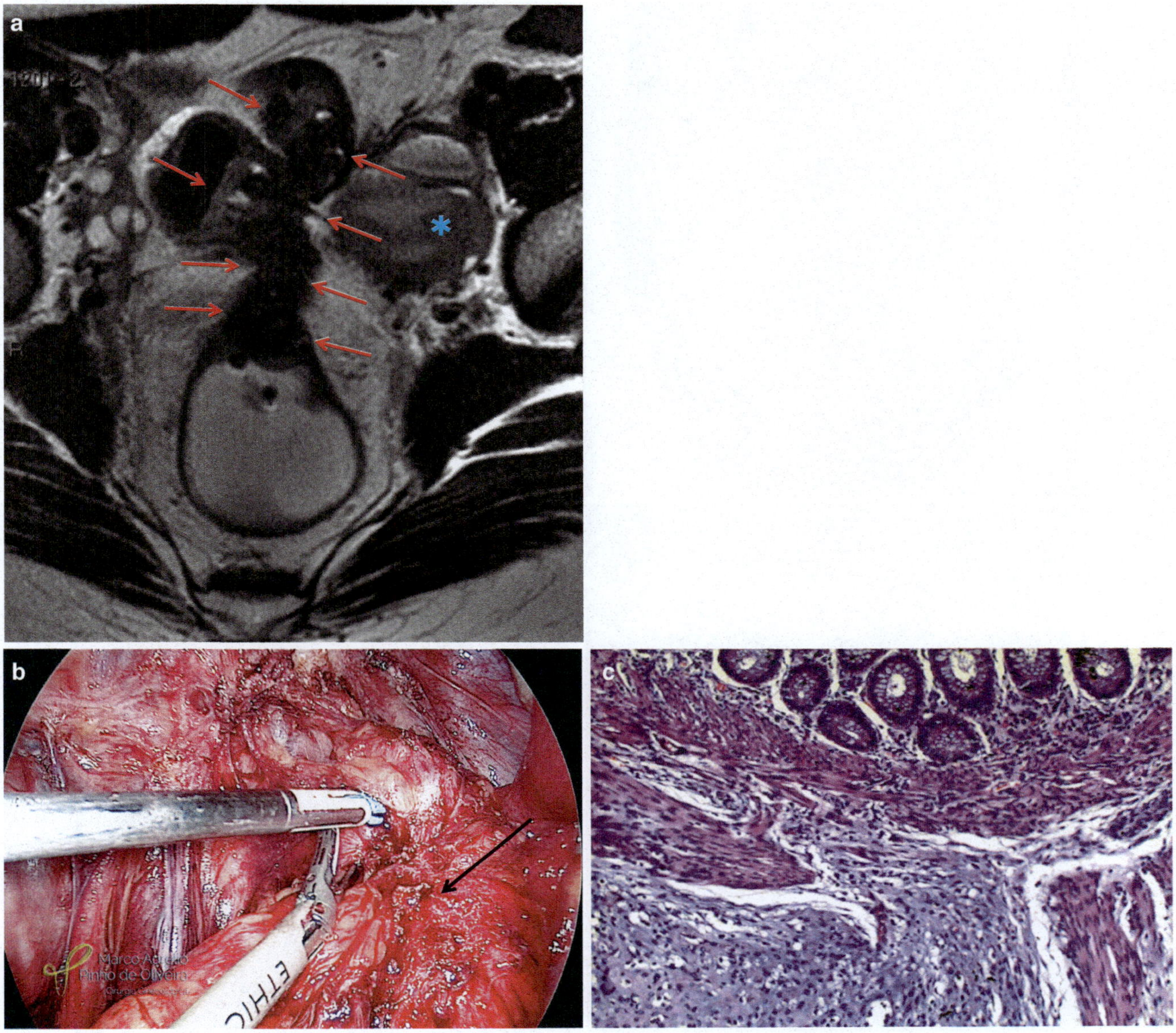

Fig. 4.132 Stenosis determined by endometriotic lesion of the left lateral wall of the sigmoid (arrows). Note endometrioma (*) adjacent to left intestinal lesion. (**a**) T2-weighted sequence. Axial. (**b**) Laparoscopy. Extensive sigmoid lesion. (**c**) Microscopy (100×) demonstrating fibrosis and lymphoplasmocytic infiltrate alongside the intestinal glands

4.2.6.3 Clinical Symptoms

The intestinal symptoms have their origin in two main mechanisms: (a) mechanical, by obstruction and luminal stenosis, and (b) physiological, by infiltration of the intestinal nerve plexus, with damage to the interstitial cells of Cajal [52, 53].

The clinical picture includes dyspareunia, dysmenorrhea, constipation, diarrhea, dyskinesia, abdominal distension, painful bowel movements, and mucus in the stool and may be correlated with the menstrual cycle. Cyclic rectal bleeding is less common [50, 54].

As the symptoms are nonspecific, the condition is often diagnosed as irritable bowel syndrome.

4.2.6.4 Resonance and Laparoscopic Findings

The MRI aspect of the deep lesion in the rectum and sigmoid is asymmetric parietal thickening, forming a nodule, which corresponds to the abundant fibrous tissue and fibromuscular hyperplasia identified in the histological examination (Fig. 4.129).

Due to these characteristics, the lesion has a hypointense signal on the T2-weighted sequence and intermediate on T1 and is highlighted by gadolinium (Fig. 4.133).

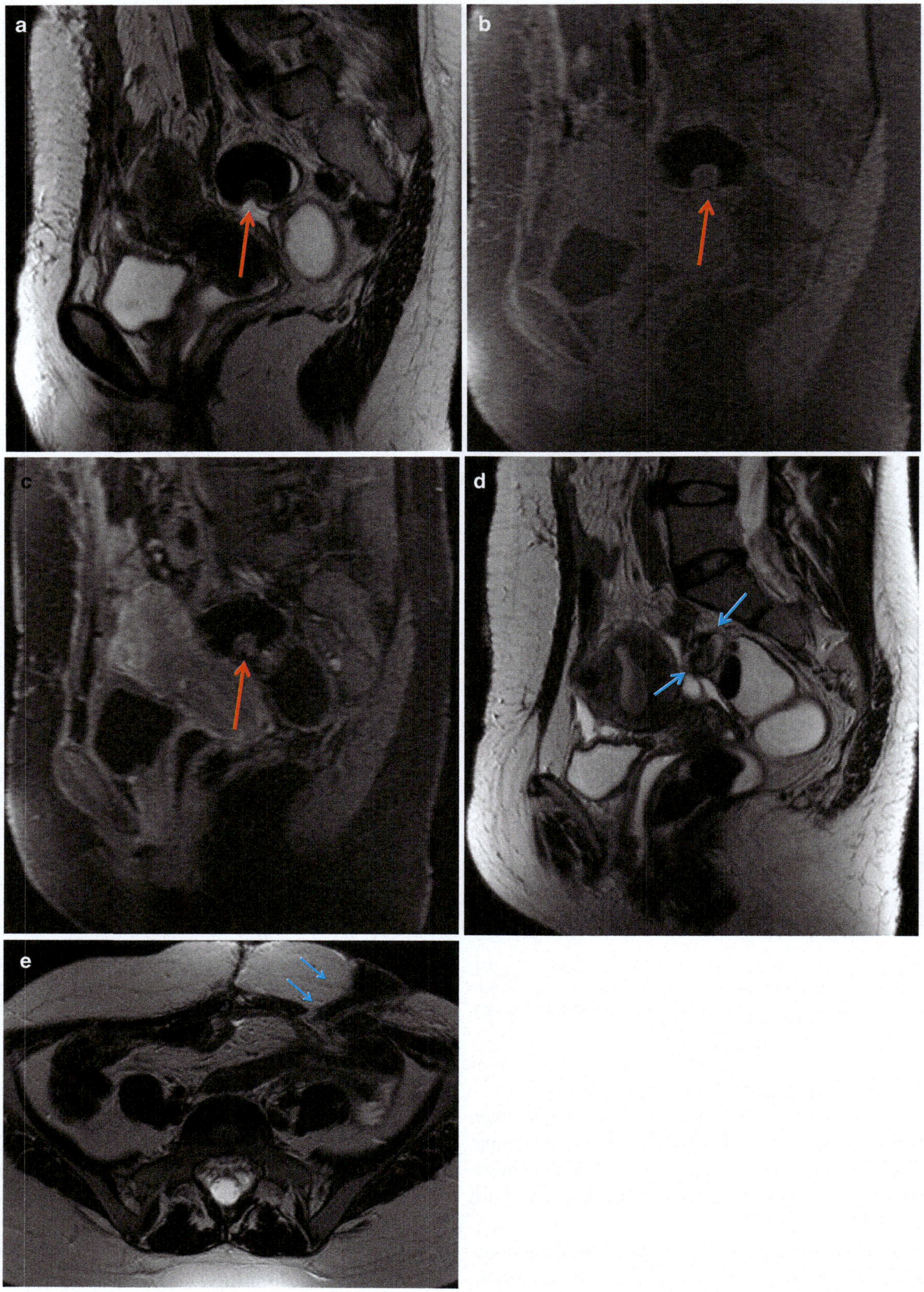

Fig. 4.133 Typical lesion in upper rectal segment (arrows **a**, **c**), residual (after emergency surgery on bowel obstruction caused by endometriosis) with hypointense signal on T2-weighted sequence (**a**, **d**, **e**), intermediate in T1 (**b**), and highlighted by gadolinium (**c**). Note post-surgical findings of the resected intestinal site (arrows in **d**) and left colostomy (arrows in **e**). (**a**–**d**) Sagittal. (**e**) Axial

When ectopic, endometrial tissue can be identified, with hyperintense foci on T2- and hypointense on T1-weighted images; when associated with bleeding, there is a hyperintense signal on T1- and T2-weighted images (Fig. 4.134).

This pattern of involvement has been described in the literature, with the "mushroom sign" in the upper section, considered a specific finding in rectum and sigmoid endometriosis. This signal is observed on T2-weighted images and characterized by extramucosal parietal nodules with hypointense signal in the lower segment (the hypertrophic muscle itself), covered by a thin layer with hypersignal (in unaffected mucosa and submucosa or with edema) (Fig. 4.135) [55].

With the progression of the lesion, there is adhesion formation, and the loop has a fringed appearance on the wall, which may make it difficult to properly evaluate the longitudinal extension of the lesion. The greater the penetration of the lesion, the greater the possibility of reduction of the size of the intestinal lumen; however, intestinal obstruction is uncommon (Figs. 4.131 and 4.132) [28].

Some characteristics of the lesion should be described by the radiologist, as they will directly impact the choice of conservative and surgical treatments.

The most important descriptive criteria are a lesion length of >3 cm, involvement of more than 40% of the circumference of the strap, penetration to the mucosa, stenosis of the lumen, a distance of <6 cm from the anal margin, and multiple lesions (Table 4.9).

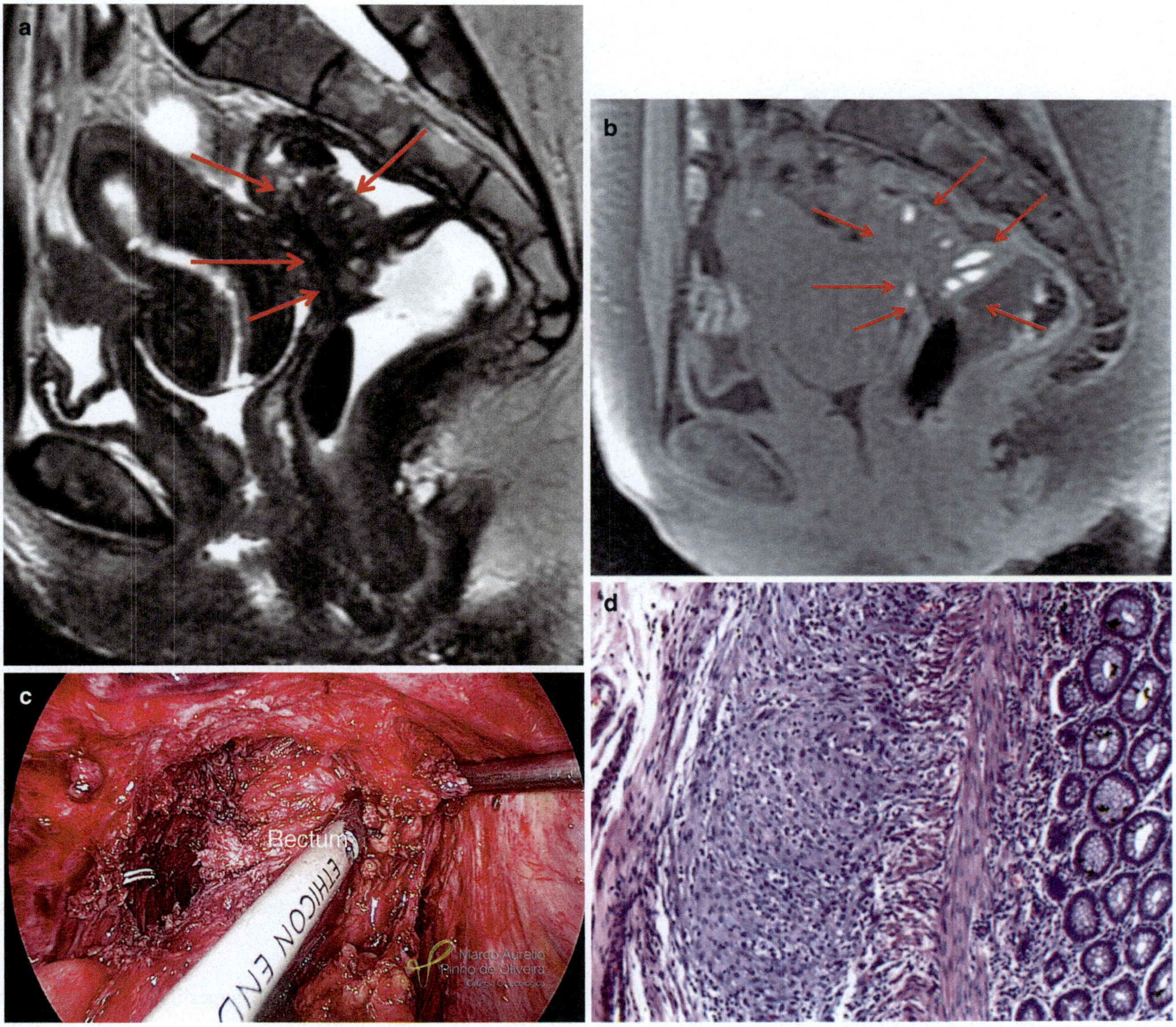

Fig. 4.134 Extensive ectopic endometrial tissue associated with bleeding, hyperintense foci in the T2-weighted sequence (arrows in **a**) and T1 (arrows in **b**). (**a**, **b**) Sagittal. (**c**) Laparoscopic evidence of resection of rectal nodule. (**d**) Marking and fixation of the sigmoid lesion with suture. (**e**) Microscopy. Rectum with endometrioid foci and decidual reaction. On the right, observe the glandular intestinal mucosa (100×)

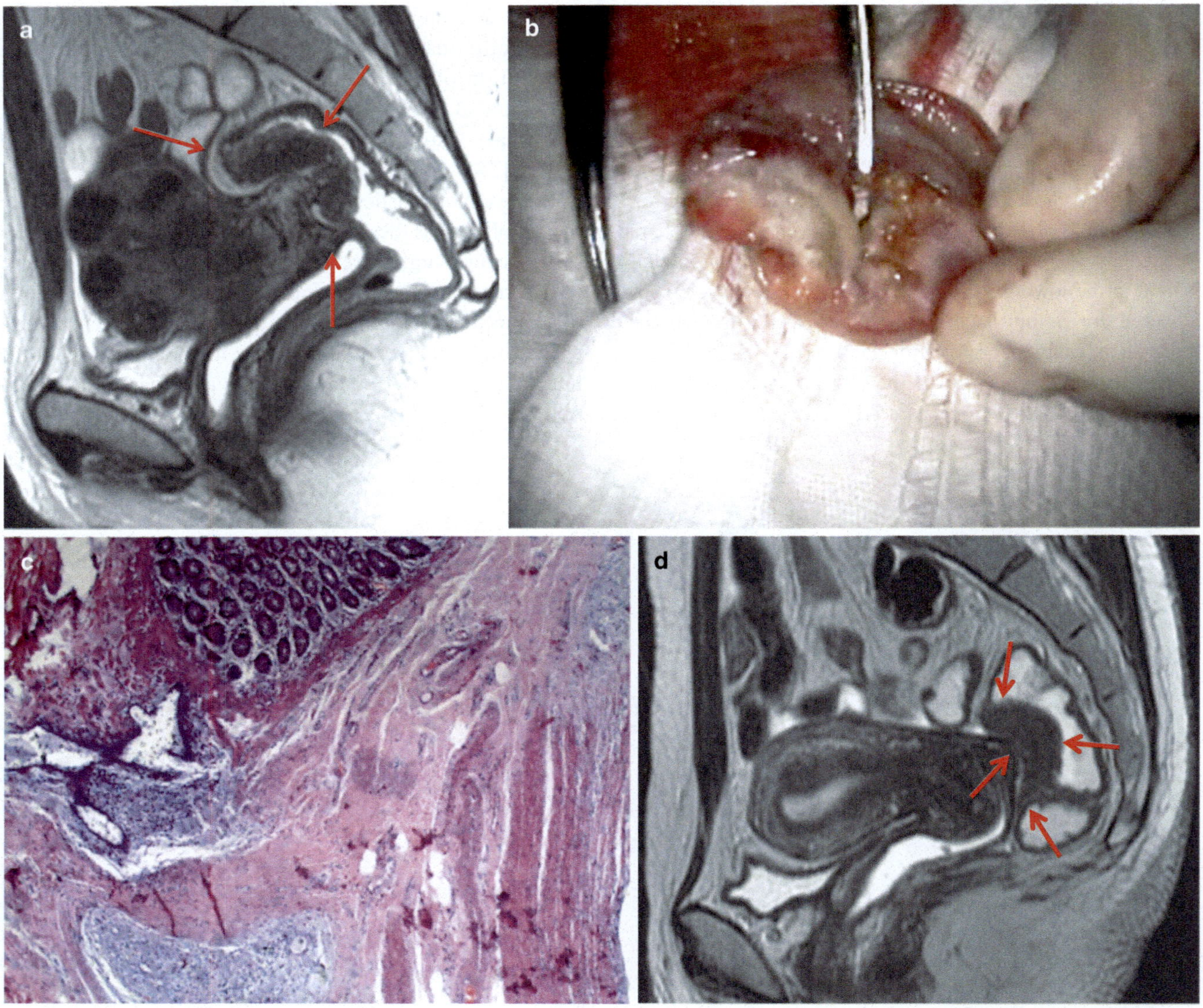

Fig. 4.135 (**a**) "Mushroom sign" observed on T2-weighted images (arrows—**a** and **d**) extramucosal parietal nodule with hyposignal in the rectum (hypertrophic muscularis propria), covered by thin hyperintense layer (preserved mucosa and submucosa or with edema). (**b**) Macroscopic aspect of lesion. (**c**) Microscopy (40×) with two foci of endometriosis next to the intestinal mucosa. (**d**) Compare with this lesion. Note the absence of thin hyperintense layer in T2 (arrows) due to mucous involvement. (**a**, **d**) Sagittal

Table 4.9 Criteria for describing intestinal lesion

Longitudinal involvement of the intestinal wall
Location on the organ's circumference—("located between the 12 o'clock and 4 o'clock position")
Depth of infiltration of intestinal wall
Mucosal/submucosal involvement
Degree of stenosis (reduced intestinal lumen and obstruction)
Distance to the anal margin
Number of lesions (multifocality)

4.2.6.5 Treatment Comments

The follow-up of intestinal endometriosis depends on the nodule size, the degree of stenosis of the lumen, and the symptoms experienced by patients.

In asymptomatic patients, wait-and-see treatment may be applied, excluding those with risk of intestinal occlusion. In other cases, the treatment of intestinal endometriosis depends on age, desire to maintain fertility, severity, and complications of the disease [56–58].

The choice of surgical technique is based on the characteristics of the lesions, such as size, depth of intestinal wall infiltration, mucosal preservation, percentage of infiltrated intestinal circumference, degree of stenosis, distance to the anocutaneous margin, and number of lesions.

Basically four types of techniques are used in this approach [1]:

1. **Surface resection (shaving):** superficial lesions of the serosa with little penetration of the wall removed with scissors or diathermy excision (Fig. 4.136).
2. **Simple discoid resection:** single lesions with up to 3 cm in intestinal extension, with involvement of up to 40% of

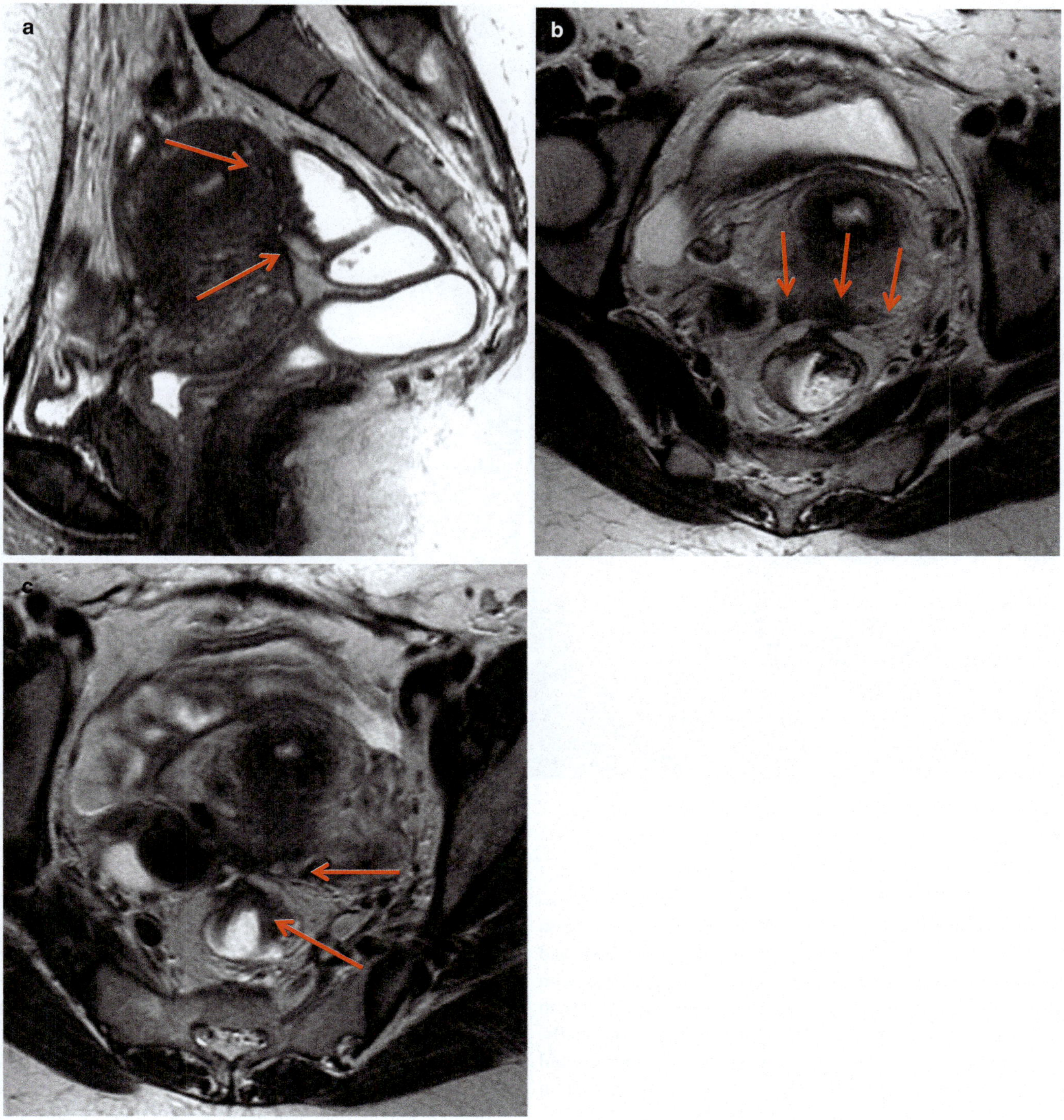

Fig. 4.136 (**a**–**c**) T2-weighted sequences. Retrocervical endometriosis (arrows in **b**) with superficial lesion of the upper rectal serosa segment with little penetration of the intestinal wall (arrows **a**, **c**). (**a**) Sagittal. (**b**, **c**) Axial. (**d**–**f**) Laparoscopy. (**d**) Obliteration of posterior cul-de-sac (arrow). (**e**, **f**) Resection of endometrial nodule by the shaving technique. (**g**) Microscopy. Endometrial foci with abundant cytogenetic stroma in the intestine (400×)

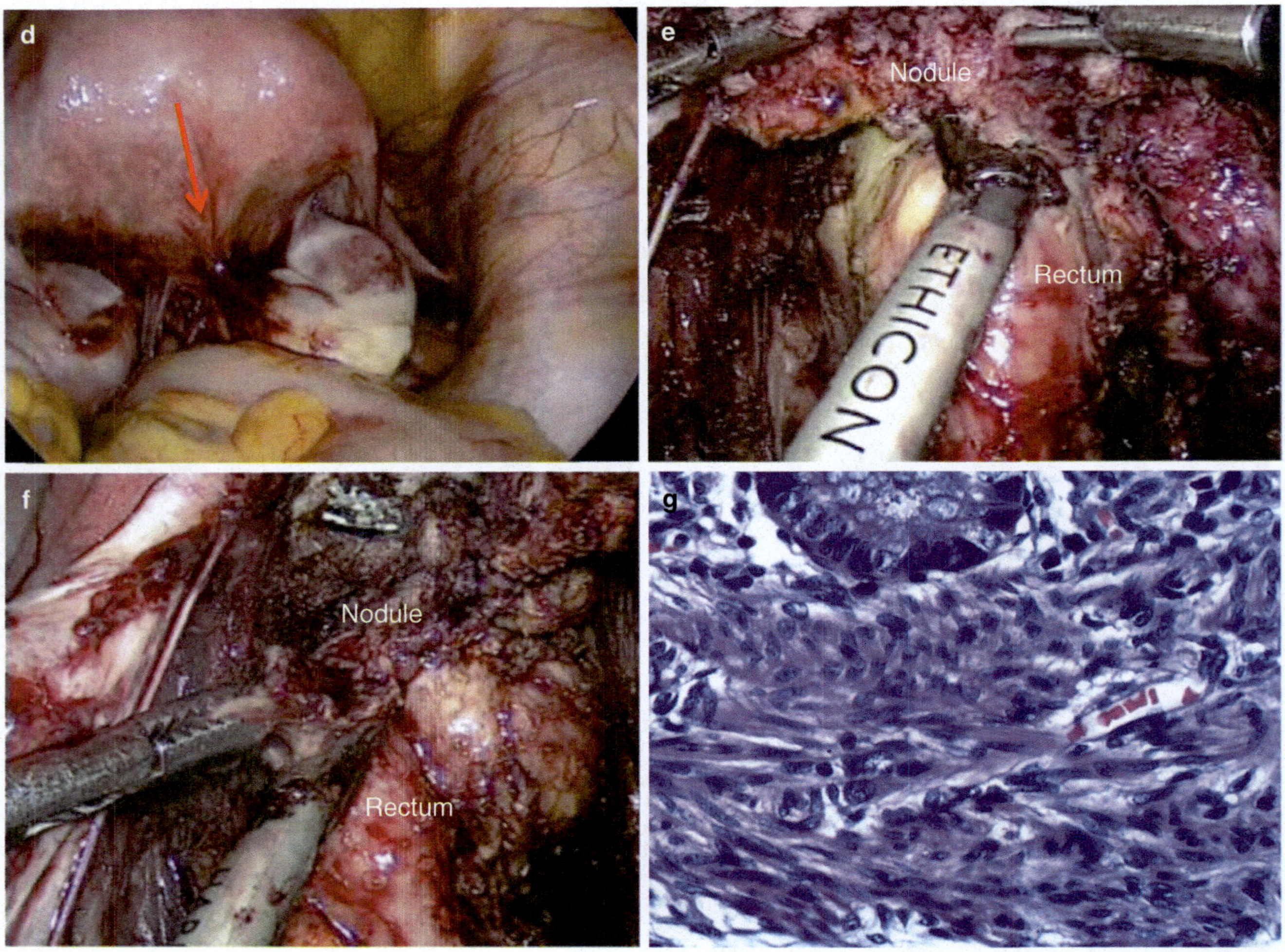

Fig. 4.136 (continued)

its circumference, and penetrating into the mucosa (Fig. 4.137). The technique may be manual (incision and transverse aperture to the lumen, lesion removal with scissors or diathermy, followed by suturing) or with mechanical suture (circular stapler inserted transanally, opened to 3 cm, closed, and triggered, causing discoid resection anterior of the wedge, in nodules up to 2 cm in diameter to prevent positive margins) (Fig. 4.137).

3. **Double discoid resection (double circular stapling):** single lesions with involvement of up to 40% of the intestinal lumen and extending up to 4 cm. Two circular stapler shots are made, the first removing part of the lesion and the second all the other remaining disease (including the previous stapling) (Fig. 4.138) [59].
4. **Segmental resection:** multiple intestinal lesions (multifocal) extending until the submucosa and mucosa, lesions with a longitudinal extension greater than 5 cm, and lesions with extension in circumference of more than half the lumen (Fig. 4.139).

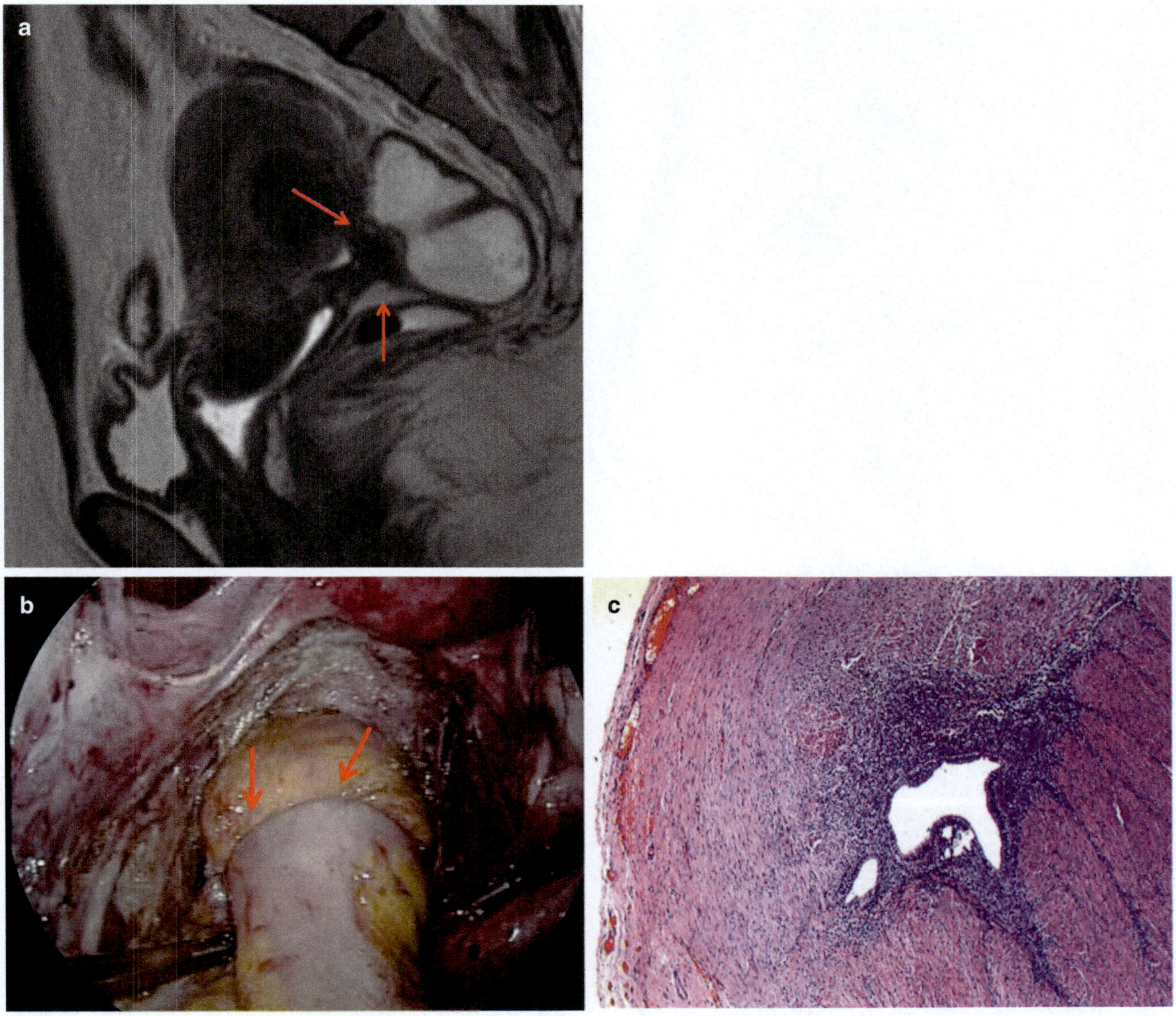

Fig. 4.137 (**a**) Single intestinal lesion less than 3 cm in length (arrows). T2-weighted sequence. Sagittal. (**b**) Laparoscopy. Simple discoid resection, sparing the mucosa. (**c**) Microscopy of the discoid resection with central endometriotic foci

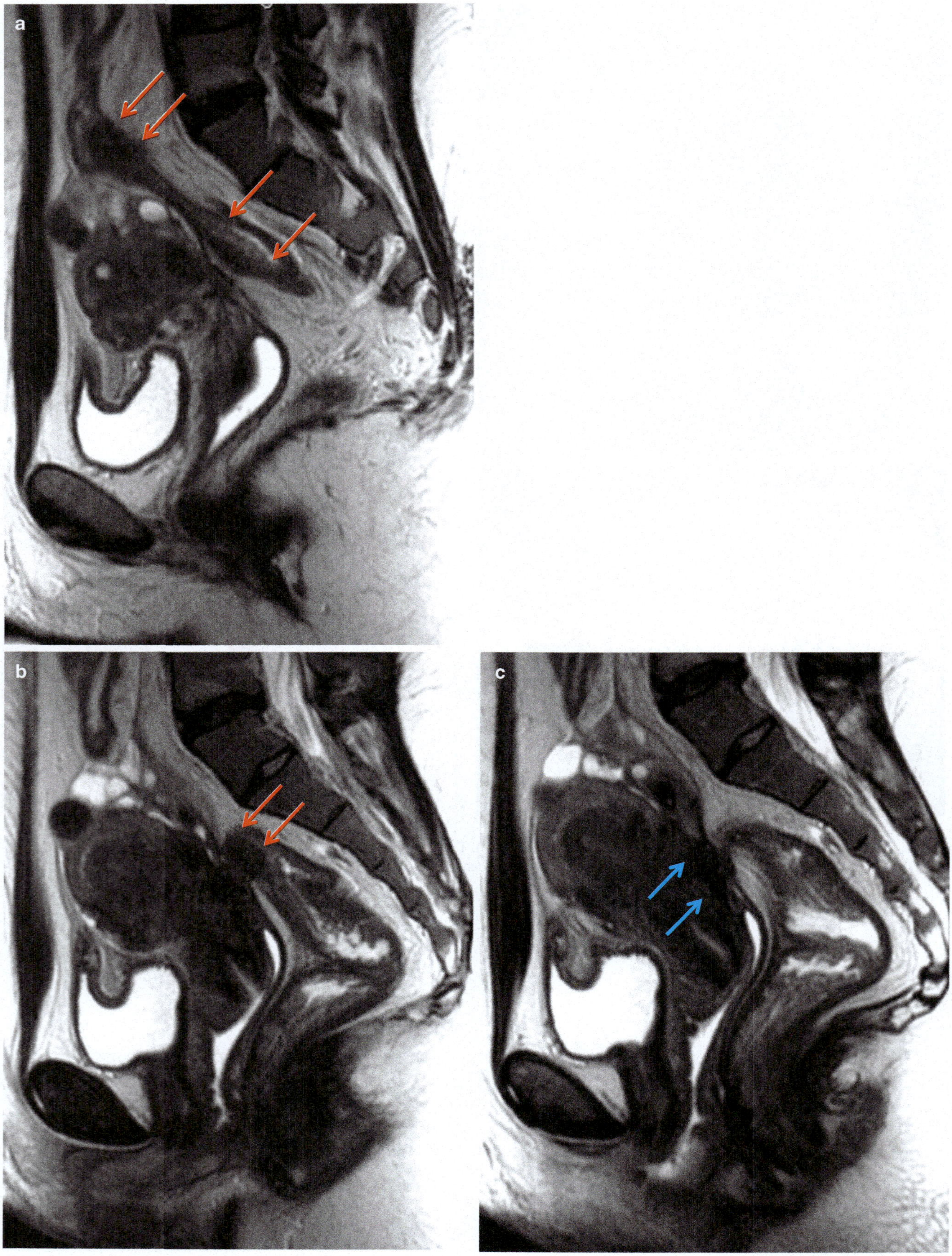

Fig. 4.138 (**a–c**) Posterior lesion with extensive involvement of the rectum and sigmoid (red arrow) and retrocervical lesion (blue arrows). (**d–f**) Double discoid resection (double circular stapling). (**d**, **e**) After the first circular stapling. (**d**) Note residual distal lesion. (**e**) Complete inclusion of the proximal section of the lesion. (**f**) Aspect of the second circular stapling. (**g**, **h**) Microscopy of the anastomotic ring with large endometriosis foci (40× and 100× magnification). (**i**) MRI post-anastomosis procedure (arrows). (**a–c**, **i**) T2-weighted sequences. Sagittal

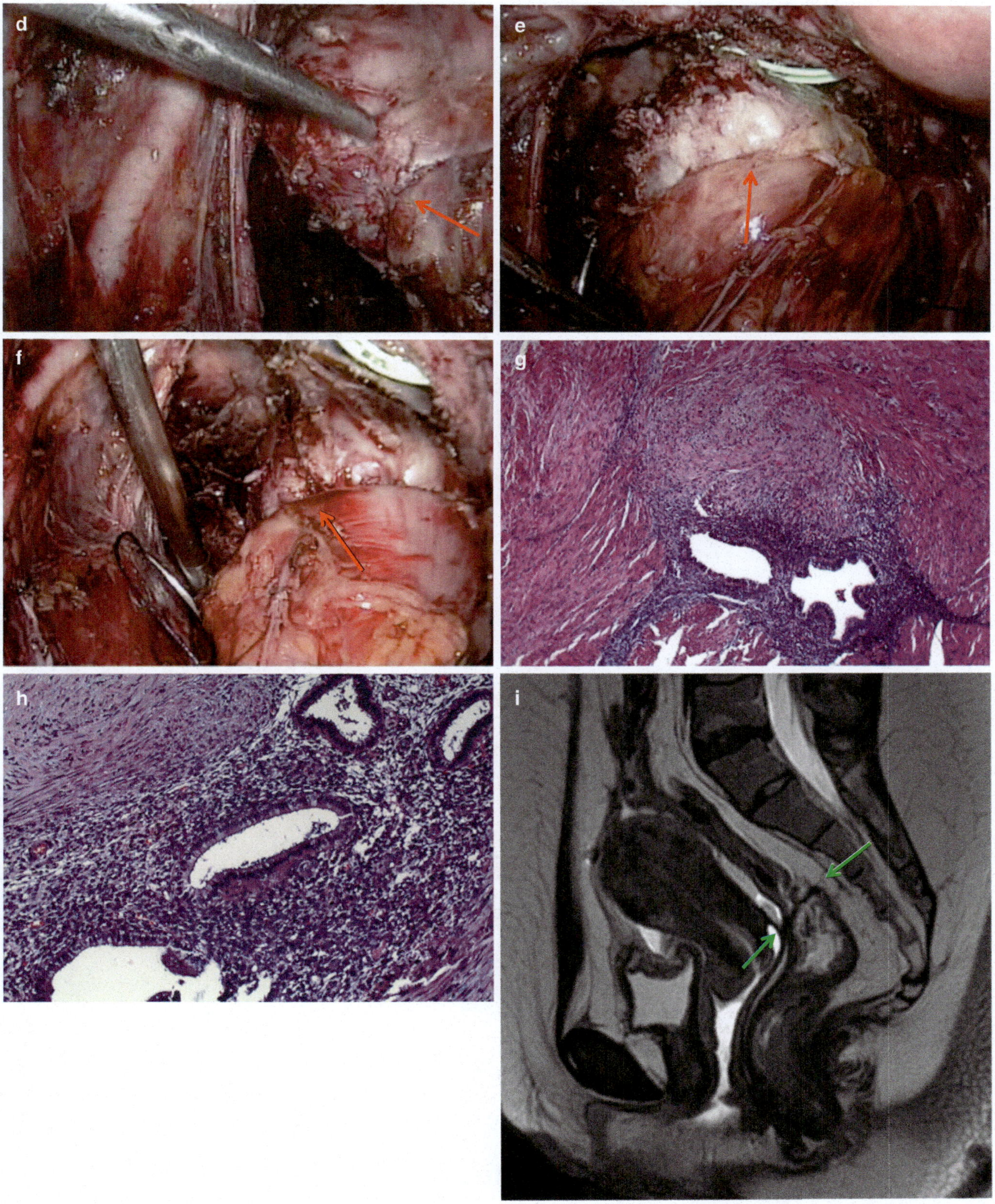

Fig. 4.138 (continued)

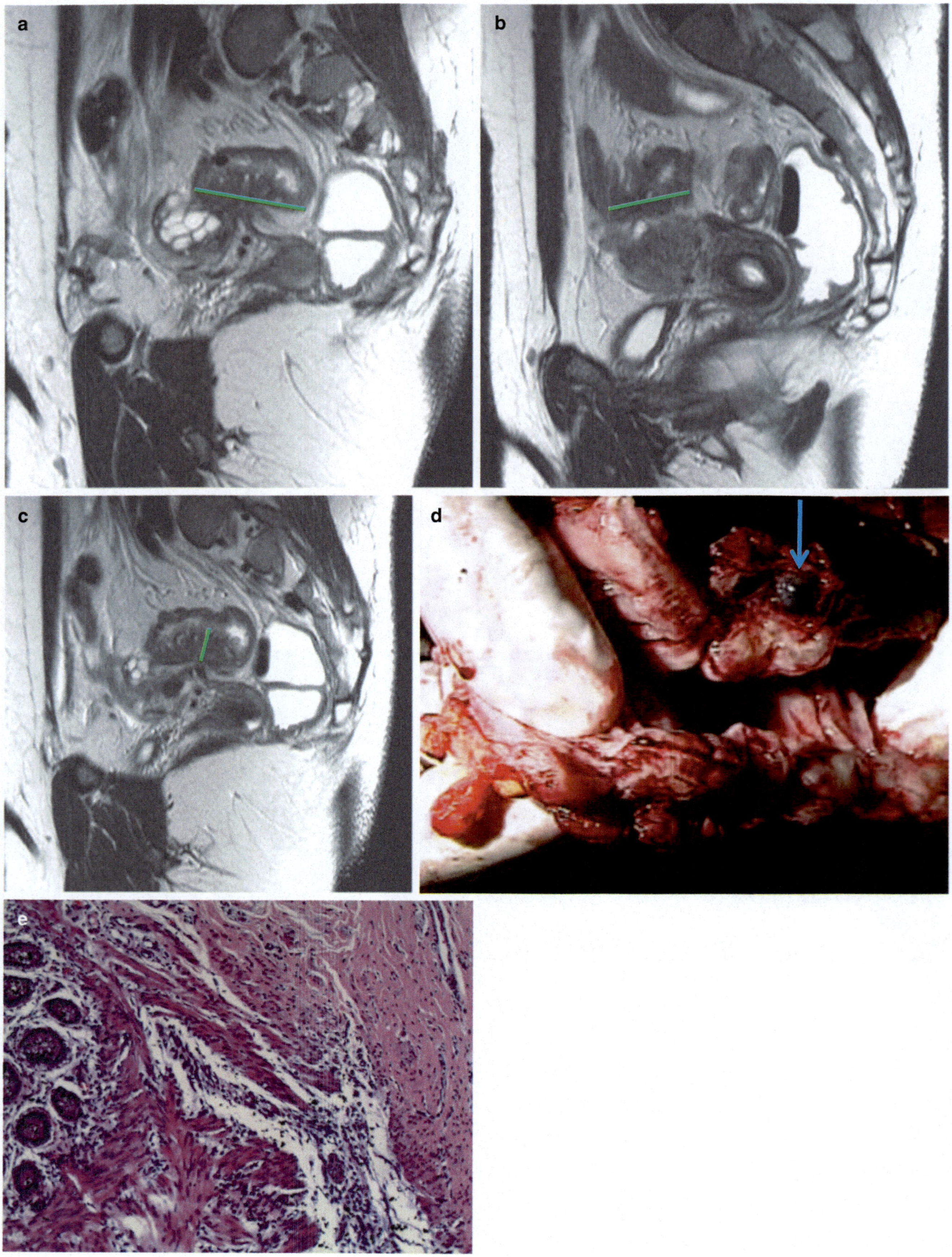

Fig. 4.139 Segmental resection. (**a–c**) Multiple intestinal lesions (multifocal) extending into the submucosa and mucosa. T2-weighted sequences. Sagittal. (**d**) Specimen after segmental resection of the sigmoid. (**e**) Microscopy showing the proximity of the endometriotic tissue to the intestinal glands

4.3 Lateral Compartment

This compartment is one of the most important of the pelvis, because the region is rich in nerve and vascular bundles, and being next to the ureter makes surgical treatment challenging. The same complexity is observed in MRI. Lesions may be discrete and go unnoticed; however they may compromise important structures, such as the ureter (Fig. 4.140).

Included in this compartment are the parametrium, the paracolpos, the ureter, the hypogastric nerve, and the ovarian fossa and floor.

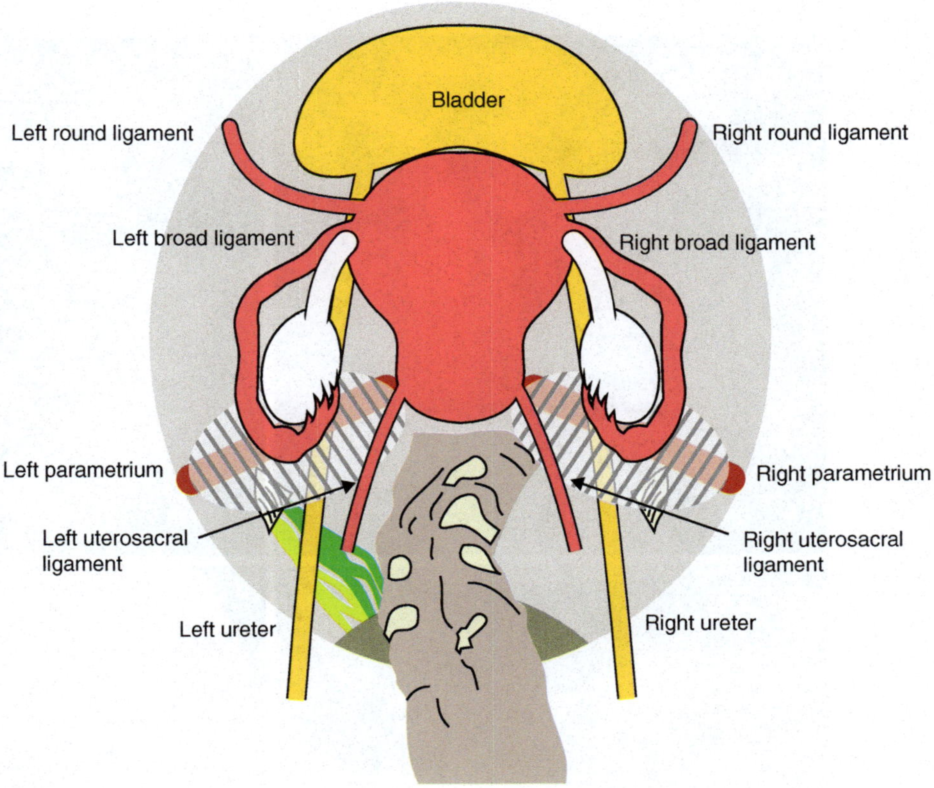

Fig. 4.140 Pattern of extension of deep endometriosis of the lateral compartment: (1) Anteriorly: uterine artery and ureter. (2) Posteriorly: rectum and sigmoid. (3) Inferiorly: hypogastric nerve, inferior hypogastric plexus, and levator ani muscle. (4) Laterally: ovarian fossa. Note that the scheme is based on the laparoscopic view, where the left side corresponds to the right of the MRI and vice versa

4.3.1 Parametrium and Paracolpos Anatomy

It is defined as a cellular connective tissue located between the layers of the broad ligament. It is medially contiguous with the lateral margins of the uterus, superiorly with the vagina, laterally with the parietal fascia, inferiorly with the cardinal ligaments, and anteriorly with the bladder.

Thus, the parametrium delineates the lateral edges of the uterus, and paracolpos, the superior third of the vagina, and extends laterally into the side walls of the pelvis (Fig. 1.4).

The parametrium and paracolpos are important anatomical landmarks, containing the uterine and vaginal vessels, the lower hypogastric nerve, being crossed by the ureter at the junction with the uterine artery and before entering the trigone (Figs. 1.4 and 4.141).

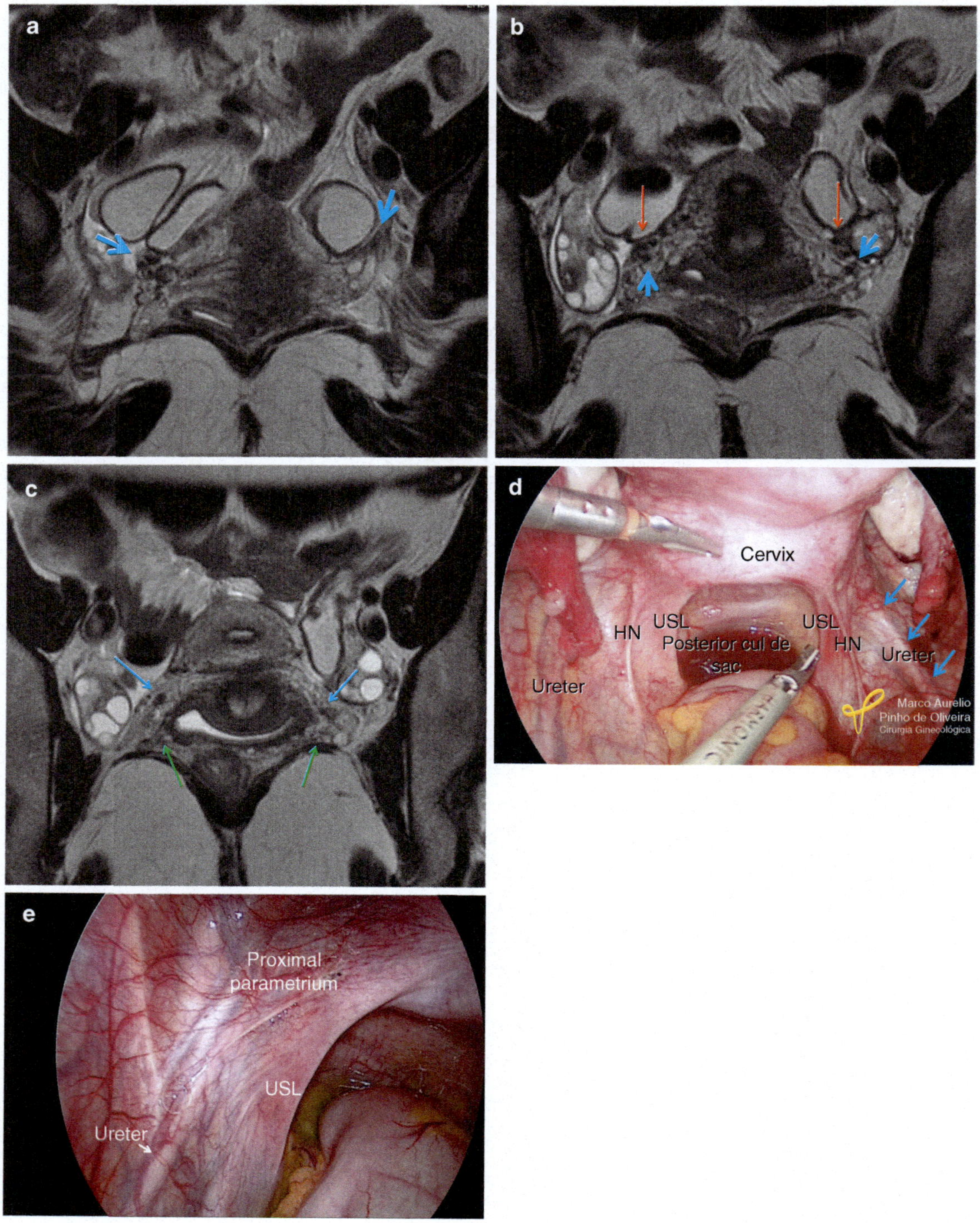

Fig. 4.141 The ureter superiorly crosses the parametrium (blue arrows), where it crosses the uterine artery (red arrows), before entering the trigone vesical. Located immediately superior and lateral to the hypogastric nerve (green arrows). (**a**-) T2-weighted sequences. Short coronal axis. (**d**, **e**) Laparoscopy

The thickening of the parametrium at the base of the broad ligament, in the plane of the cervix, is called the transverse cardinal or cervical ligament. This is a prominent connective tissue which is part of the pericervical ring, along with the uterosacral ligament (more detail in the section on the pelvic floor). Some authors denominate this ligament as the paracervix (Fig. 4.142) [60].

In MRI, the parametrium and the paracolpos present signal intensity predominantly similar to fat, hyperintense on T1 and T2. However, the signal is nonhomogeneous with small hypointense bands on T2-weighted images, especially in the plane of the cervix because of parametrial thickening in the cardinal ligament, important for uterine support (Fig. 4.143).

The vascular structures, lymphatics, nerves, and ureter contribute to the heterogeneous signal, with the first two, being enhanced by gadolinium.

All acquisition plans are excellent for analysis of the parametrium and paracolpos. The authors have a preference for the coronal axis and sagittal short axis of the uterus.

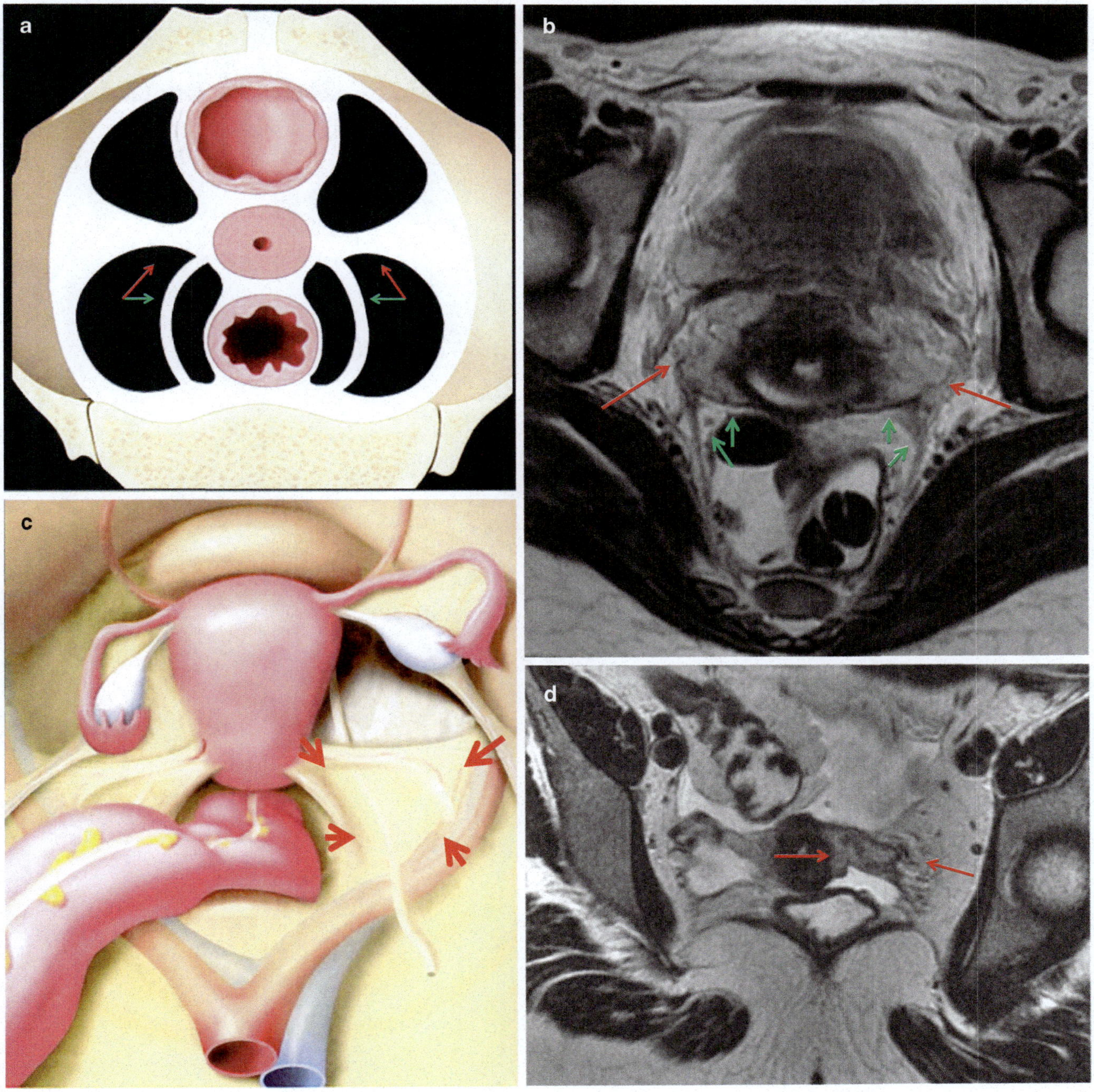

Fig. 4.142 The cardinal ligament represents the thickening of the parametrium, located in the cervical plane (red arrows), with prominent connective tissue. (**a**) Scheme. (**b**) Axial. (**c**) Scheme. (**d**) Coronal short axis. (**e**) Scheme. (**f**, **g**) long axis. (**a**, **b**, **f**, **g**) T2-weighted sequences. Blue arrow on the ureter (Diagrams taken from Ferdelle MP et al. Diagnostic and Surgical Imaging Anatomy. Chest, Abdomen, Pelvis, Lippincott Williams & Wilkins, 2006. pp. 85, 86)

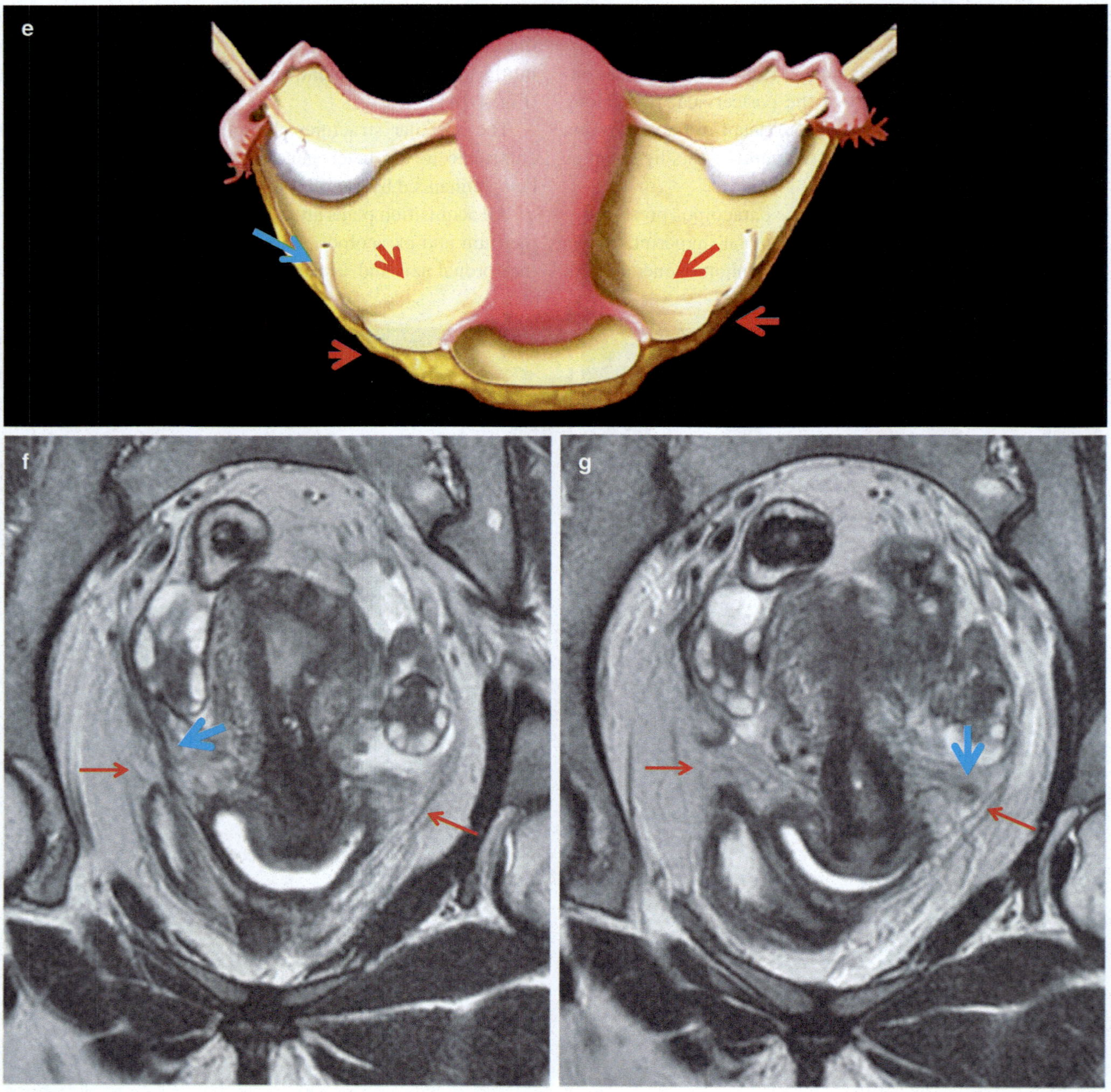

Fig. 4.142 (continued)

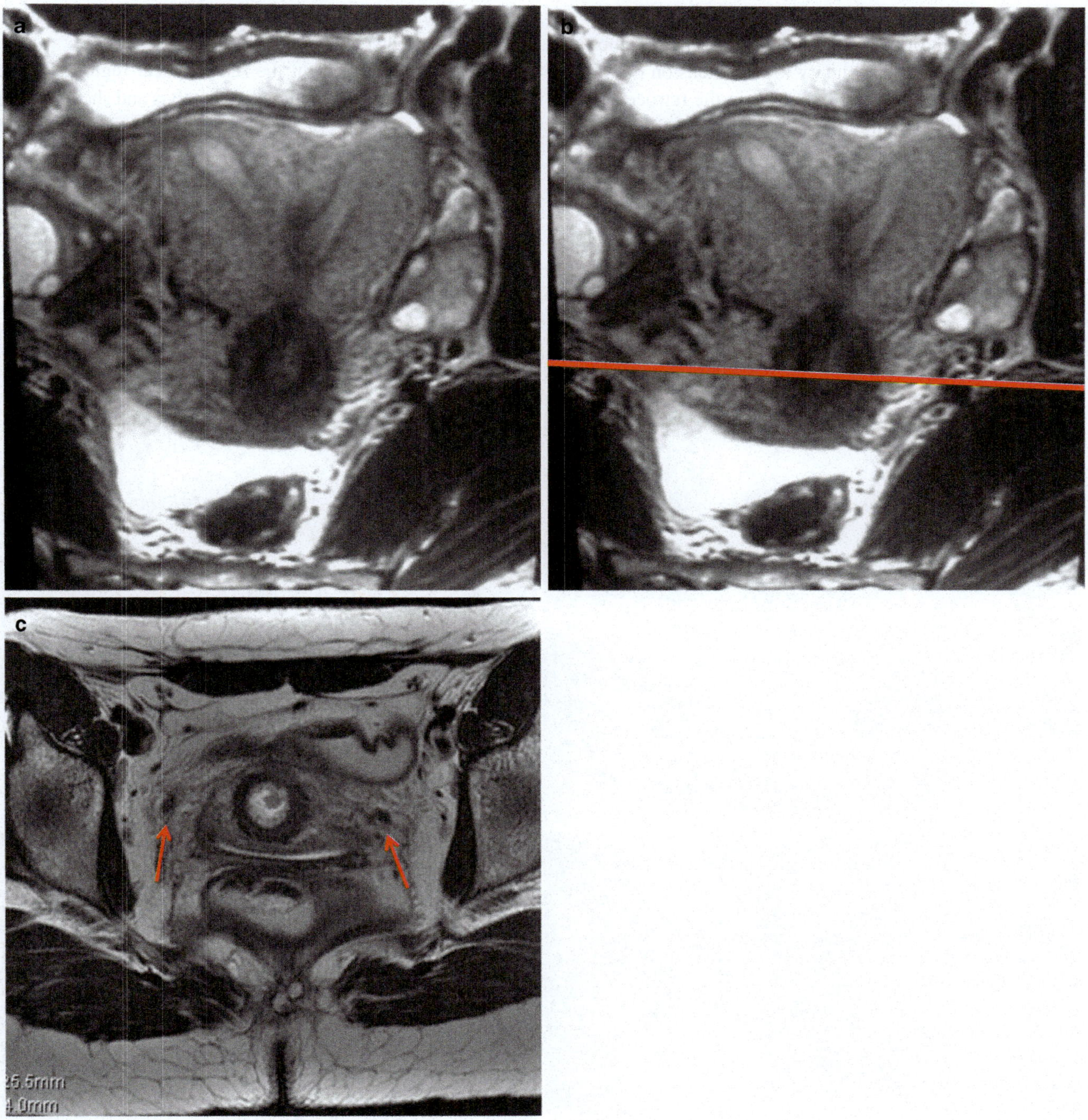

Fig. 4.143 The parametrium has hyperintense signal on T2-weighted images, nonhomogeneous, with small hypointense bands on T2 in the cervical plane. Note that the ureters have a superior path in the parametrium (red arrows). (**a**–**c**). T2-weighted sequences. (**a**, **b**) Axial, **b** at the ureter level. (**c**) Coronal short axis

4.3.1.1 Common Aspects of Deep Endometriosis

The involvement of deep endometriosis in the parametrium and the paracolpos is secondary to the extension of a lesion centered on the uterosacral ligament, in the retrocervical or the rectovaginal septum regions.

The pattern of these lesions may be different.

When centered on the uterosacral ligament, the lesion has a lateral, asymmetric location in the pelvis and penetrates anteriorly into the parametrium and the paracolpos. Sometimes the lesion is small but severe because it may rapidly involve the uterine artery, ureter, and lower hypogastric nerve (Fig. 4.144).

The lesion centered on the retrocervical region and the rectovaginal septum is median in the pelvis and shows lateral extension to the uterosacral ligament and, consequently, to the parametrium (Fig. 4.145).

Ectopic implantation of endometrial cells along the lateral and posterior aspects of the ovary and ovarian fossa may have posterior extension and adhere and also infiltrate the parametrium (Fig. 4.146).

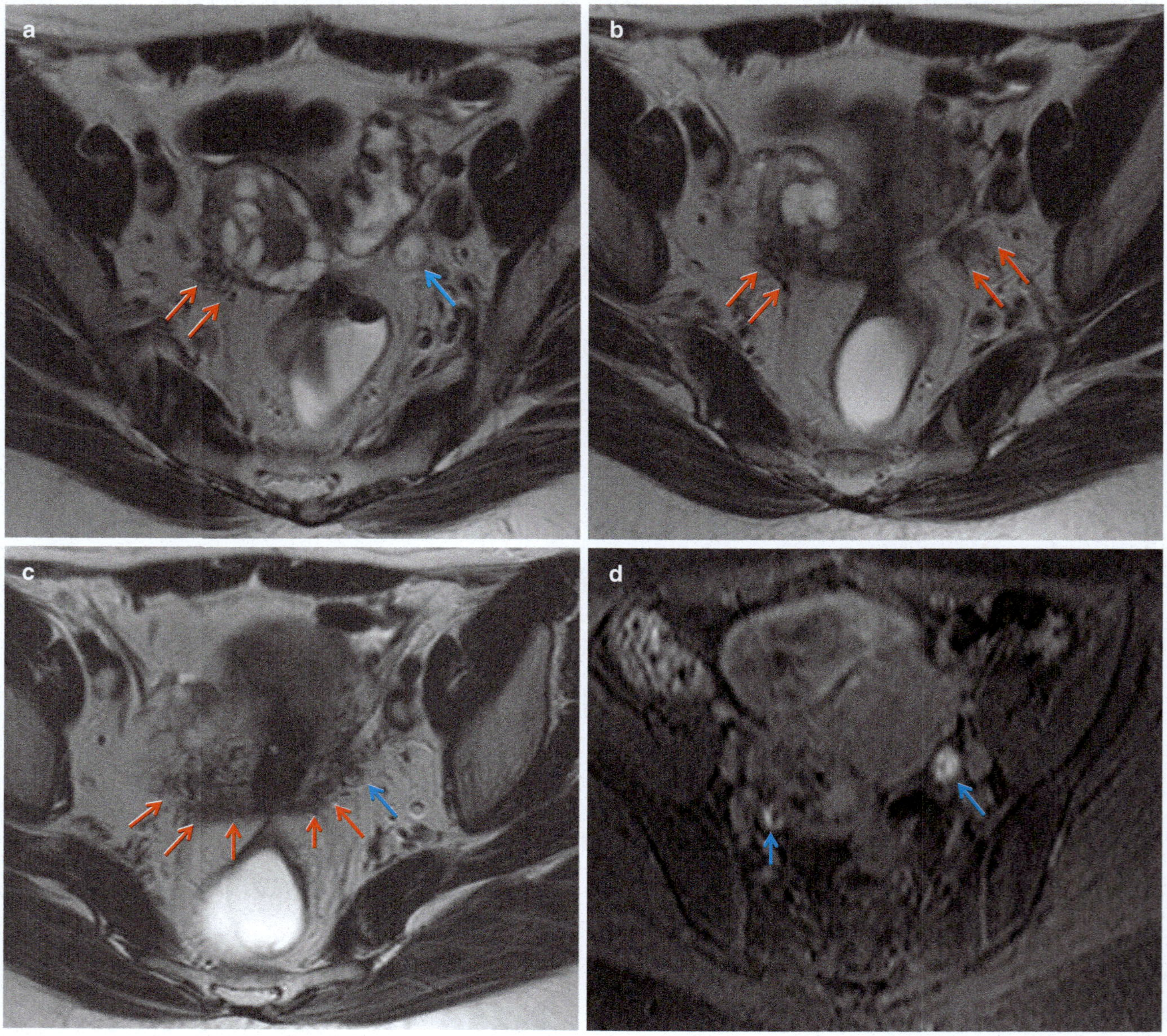

Fig. 4.144 Bilateral uterosacral ligament lesion (red arrows), with a little penetration in the upper parametrium, involving the ureter, causing severe dilation to the left (blue arrows). (**a–c**, **e–g**) T2-weighted sequences. (**a–c**) Axial. (**e–g**) Coronal. (**d**, **h**) MRI Urography. (**d**) T1-weighted sequence. Axial. (**h**) MIP, oblique posterior view

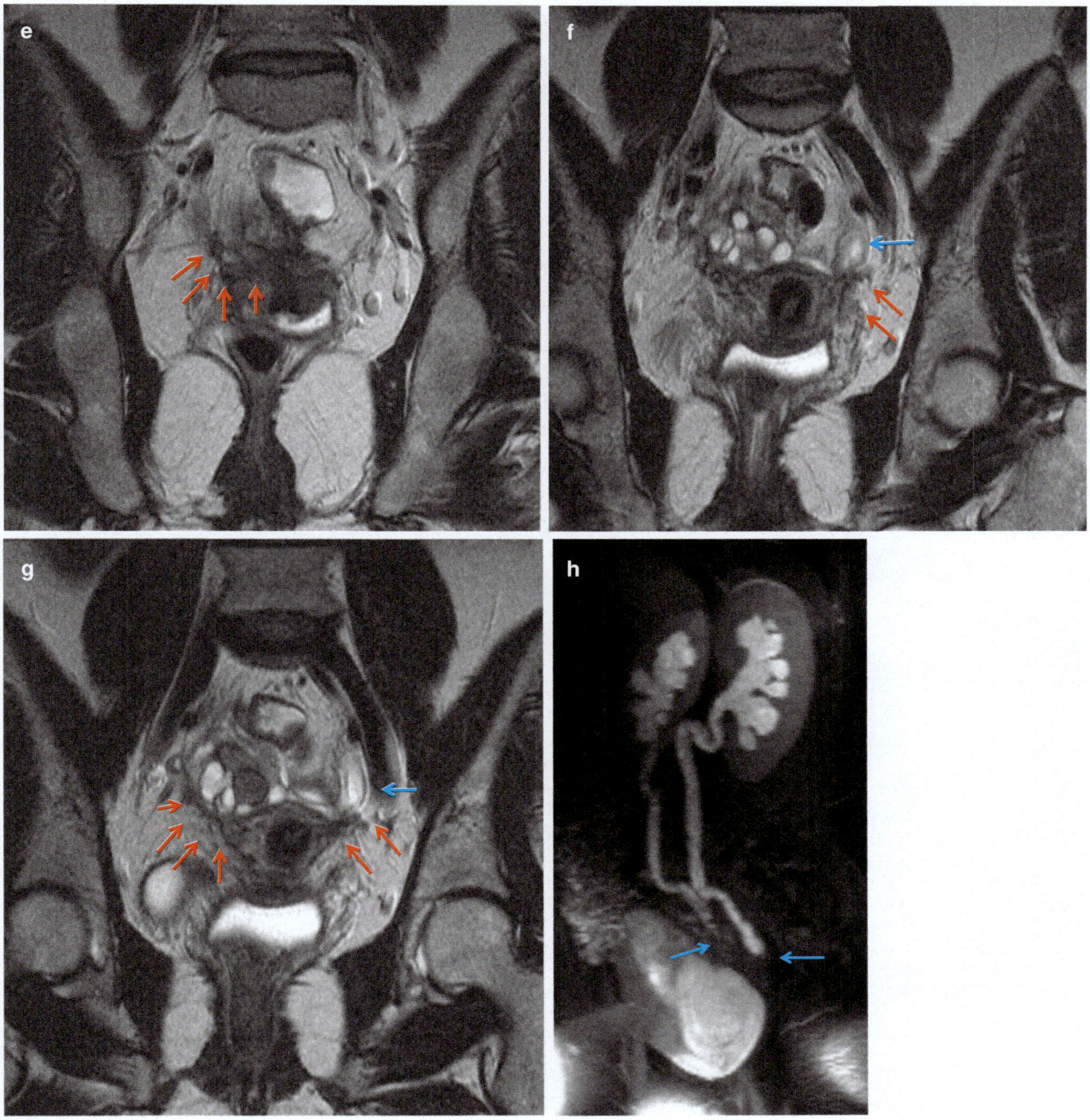

Fig. 4.144 (continued)

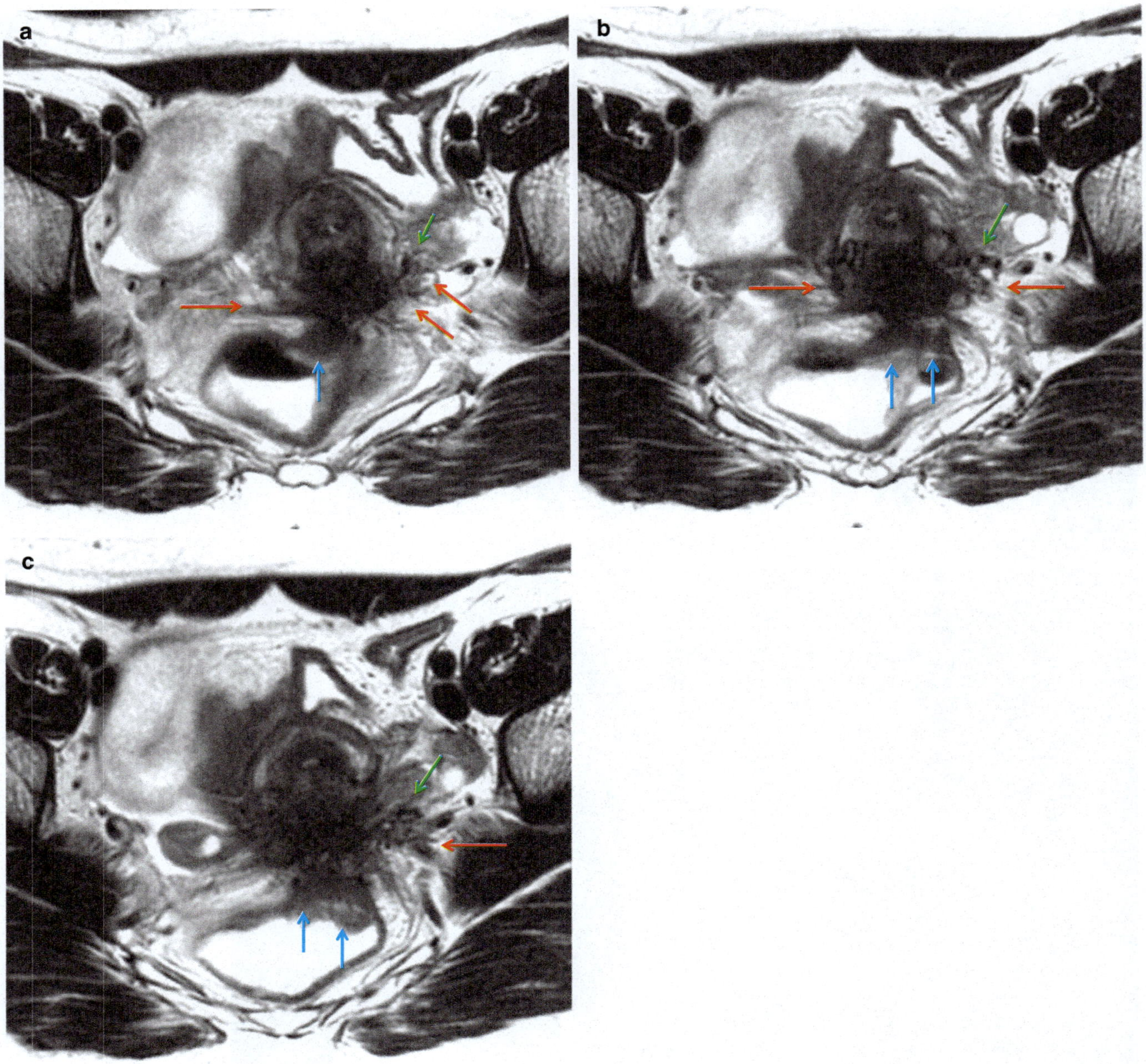

Fig. 4.145 Retrocervical and rectovaginal lesion, with lateral extension to the uterosacral ligaments and the left parametrium (red arrows) involving the left uterine artery (green arrows). Notice extension to the rectum (blue arrows). (**a**–**e**) T2-weighted sequences. (**a**–**c**) Axial. (**d**, **e**) Sagittal

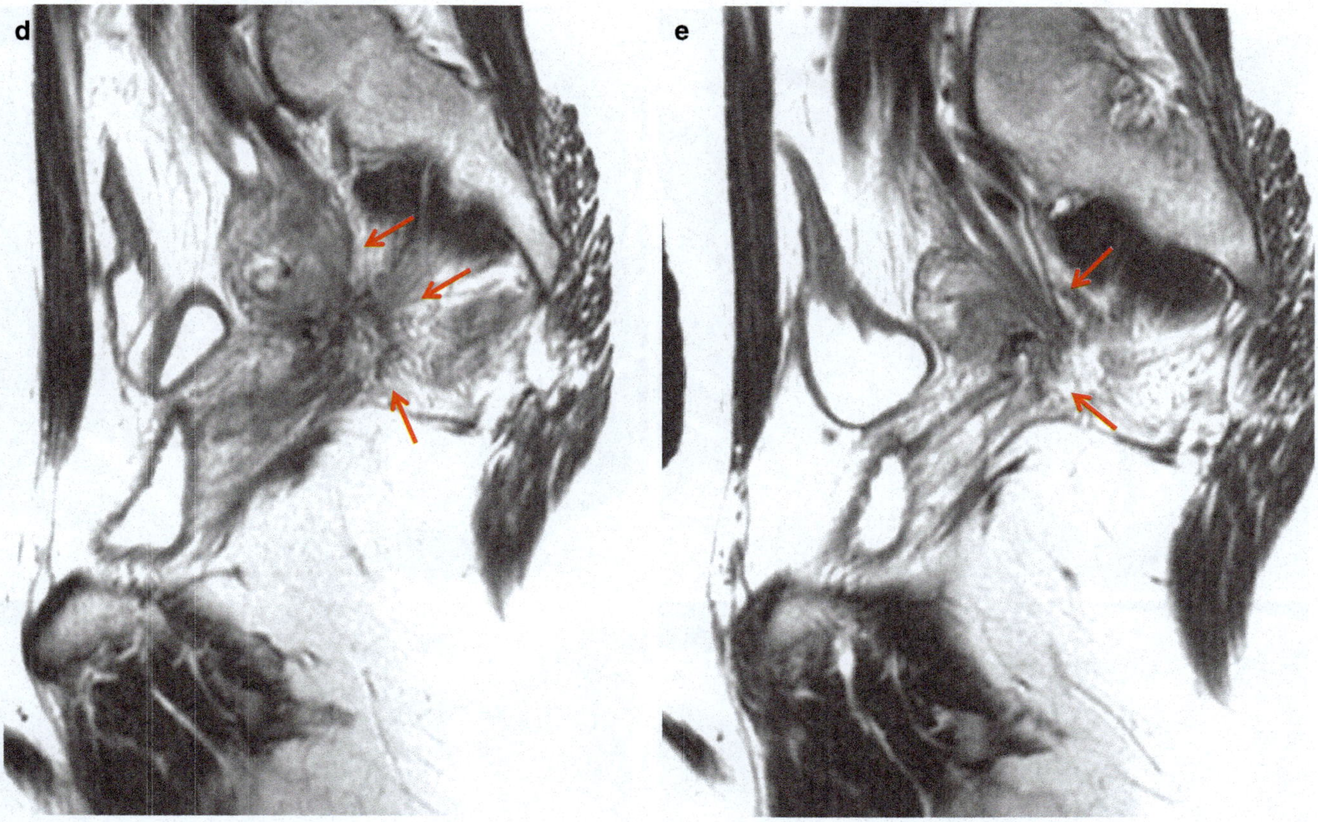

Fig. 4.145 (continued)

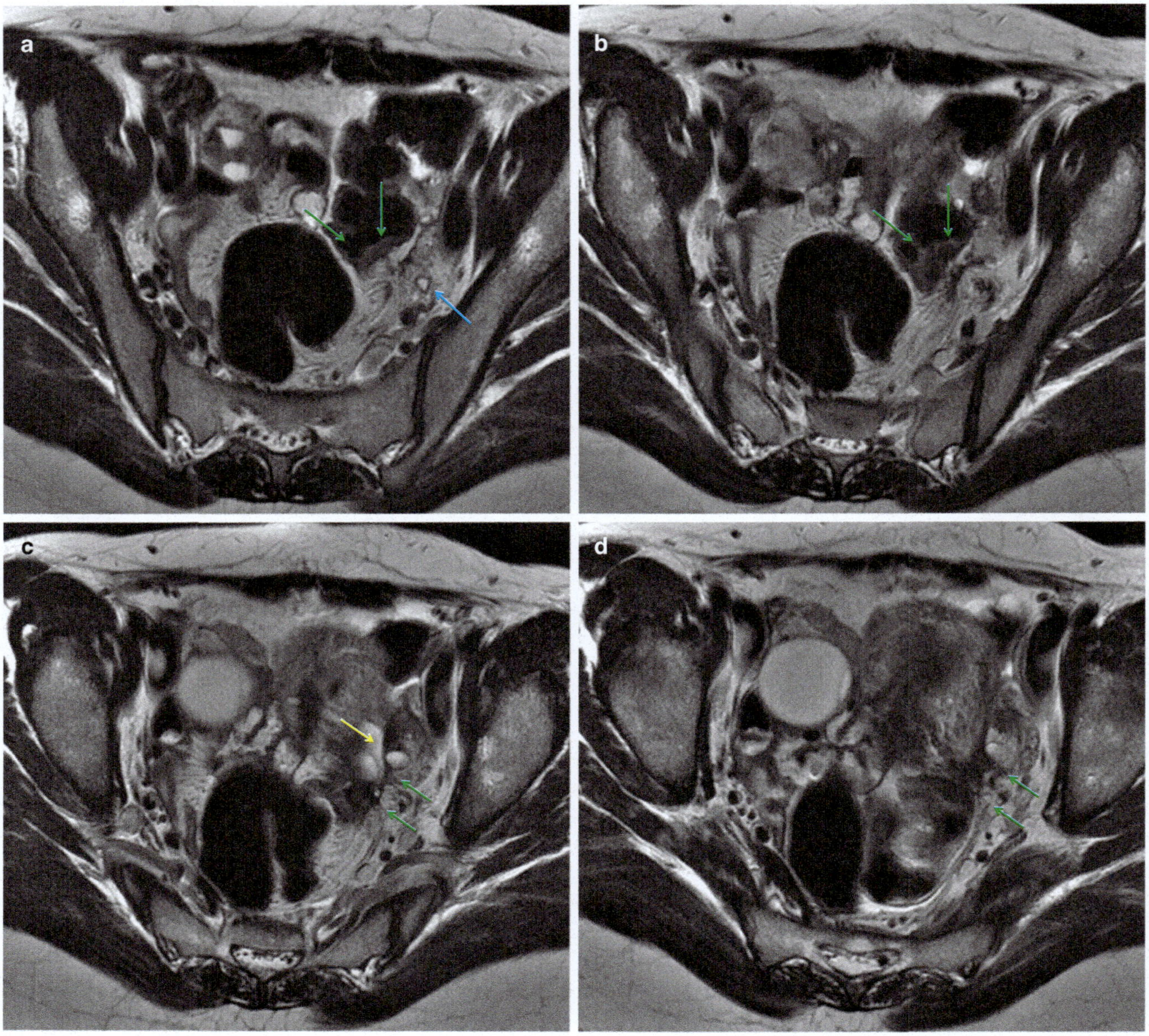

Fig. 4.146 Deep lesion along the lateral and posterior aspect of the ovary and in the left ovarian fossa (yellow arrow), with posterior extension, infiltrating the parametrium and the sigmoid (green arrows). Note proximity to the ureter (blue arrow). (**a**–**j**) T2-weighted sequences. (**a**–**e**) Axial. (**f**–**j**) Coronal short axis

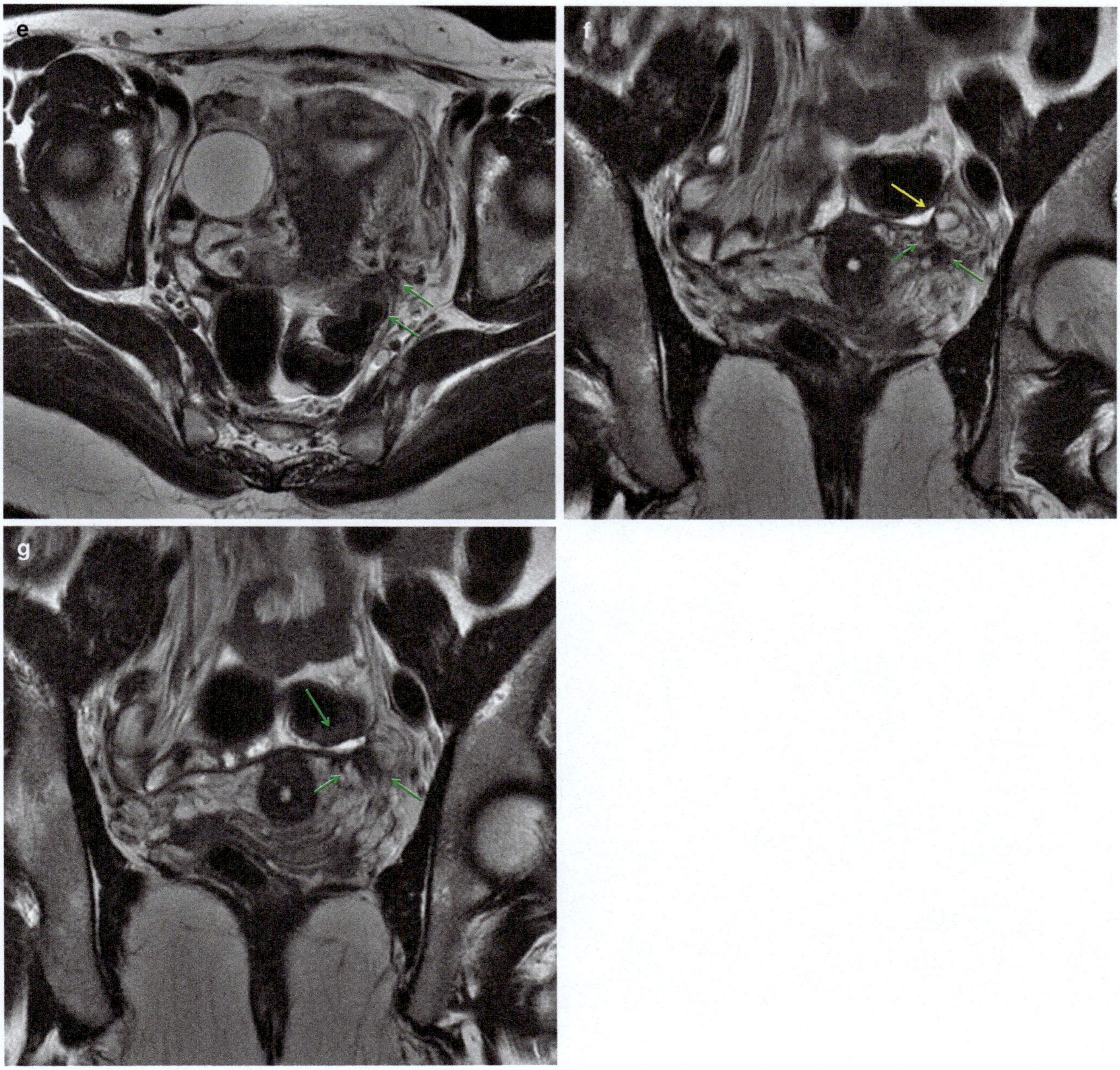

Fig. 4.146 (continued)

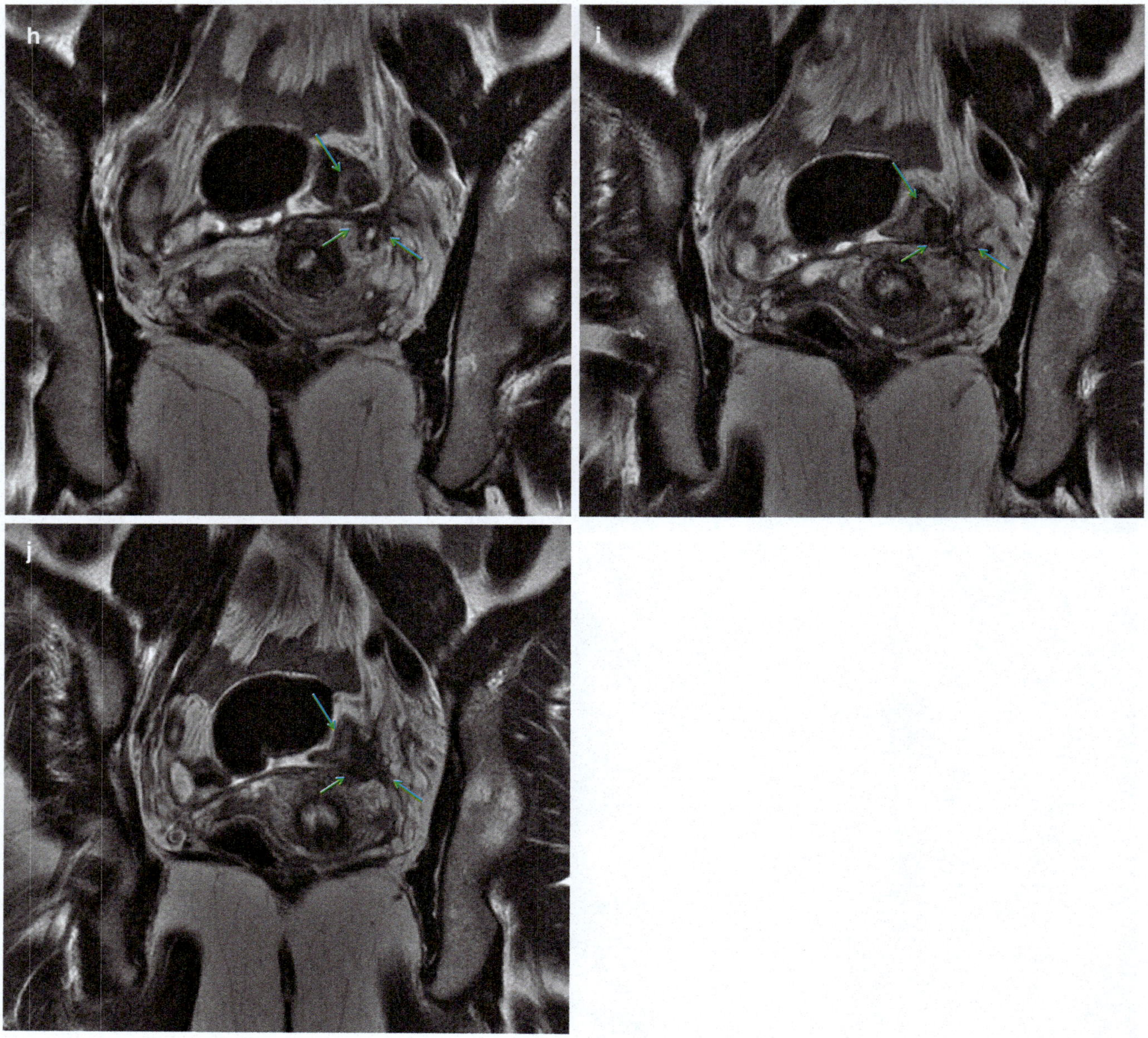

Fig. 4.146 (continued)

4.3.1.2 Clinical Symptoms

The clinical picture does not differ from other endometriosis of the posterior compartment, with chronic pelvic pain in women of reproductive age, in addition to dyspareunia and dysmenorrhea.

Ureteral involvement is often asymptomatic. However, when there is extension to the hypogastric nerve, the patient may present low back pain.

These lesions usually have clinical expression, with nodules and pain along the uterosacral ligaments, sensitivity and pain to touch in the uterus and adnexa, as well as fixed uterine retroflexion.

4.3.1.3 MRI and Laparoscopic Findings

The appearance of deep endometriotic lesions is similar to those in endometriosis of the uterosacral ligament, retrocervical region, and rectovaginal septum and ovarian fossa, ill-defined, infiltrative, lesion predominantly hypointense on T1- and T2-weighted sequences and enhanced by gadolinium, as in most cases there is a predominance of fibrosis. However, the signal intensity may vary according to the amount of ectopic endometrial tissue (Figs. 4.144, 4.145, and 4.146).

On the other hand, the morphology and the ease of identification of the parametrial lesion depend on the primary lesion. For example, a lesion centered on the uterosacral ligament may be discrete, but may penetrate the parametrium and present as ligament thickening (>0.5 cm), being better identified by MRI in the coronal and sagittal planes (Figs. 4.144 and 4.147).

On the other hand, lesions in the retrocervical region and the septum with larger nodules up to 6 cm, with easy identification in all planes, include the parametrial lesion (Figs. 4.145 and 4.146).

One of the complications of parametrial involvement is the involvement of the uterine artery and mainly extrinsic ureteral obstruction, dilation of the collecting system, and loss of renal function.

Therefore, whenever there is a parametrial extension, the radiologist must identify the uterine artery, an elongated and winding discrete structure, with absence of signal on T1- and T2-weighted sequences (due to rapid flow) and early enhancement by gadolinium (Fig. 4.148).

The ureter is presented as a well-defined structure, tubular or round (depending on the acquisition plane), hypointense on T2. When there is dilation, it is possible to identify the hyperintense fluid on T2. For further details of the anatomy and pathology of the ureter, see the section on lesions of the anterior compartment/ureter (Figs. 4.71 and 4.149).

In the paracolpos, just below the ureter and uterosacral ligament, the ratio of the lesion to the inferior hypogastric nerve, described below (Fig. 4.150), should be evaluated.

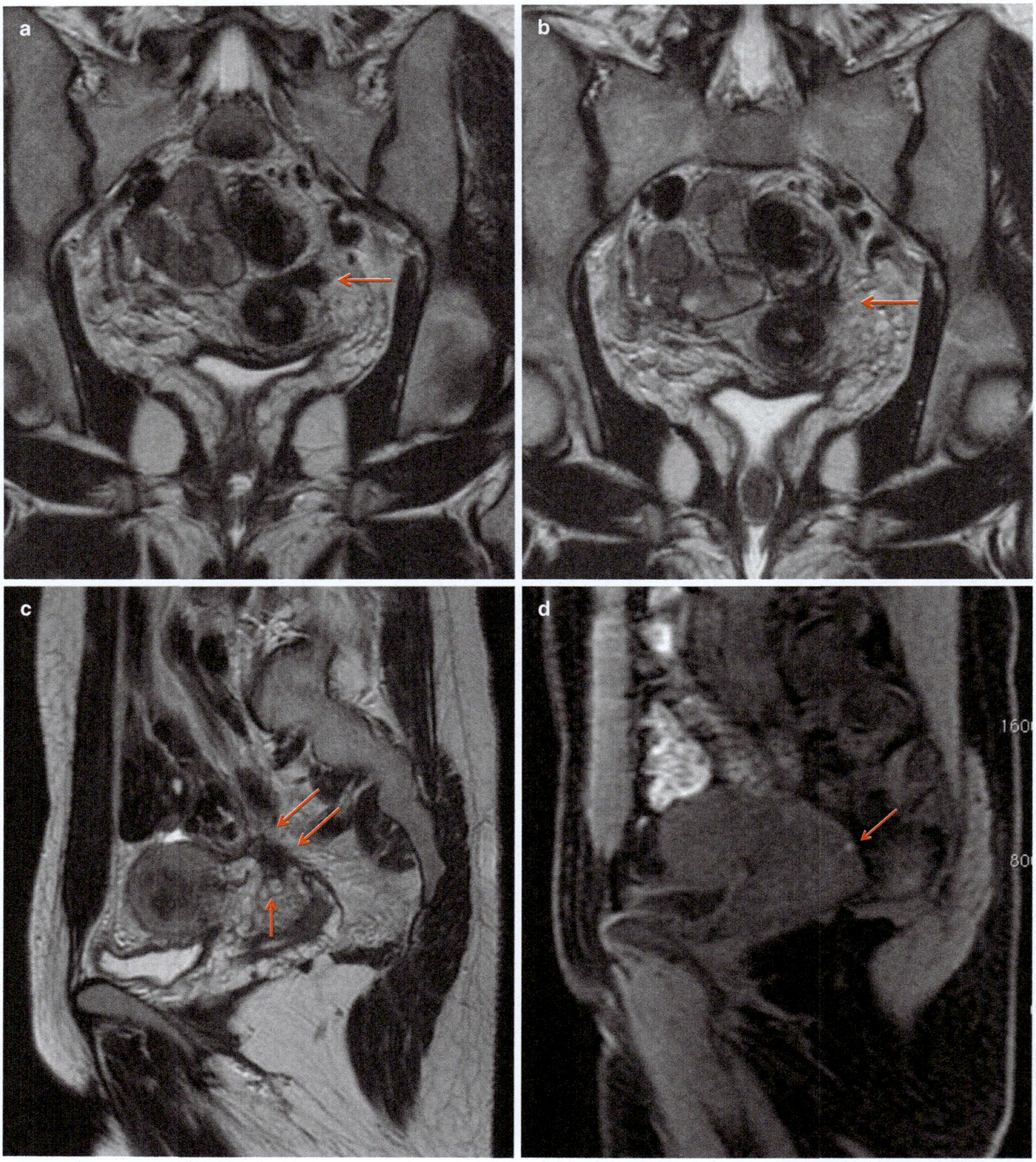

Fig. 4.147 (**a**–**d**) Lesion centered on the left uterosacral ligament penetrating the parametrium, touching the uterine artery (red arrows), with bleeding foci (arrow in **d**). (**e**, **f**) Comparison with normal parametrium (within the green outline). Notice the blue arrows in the superficial lesion in the ileum (hyperintense focus in T2). (**a**–**c**, E, **f**) T2-weighted sequences. (**d**) T1-weighted sequence with fat suppression. (**a**, **b**, **f**) Short axis. (**c**, **d**, **e**) Sagittal

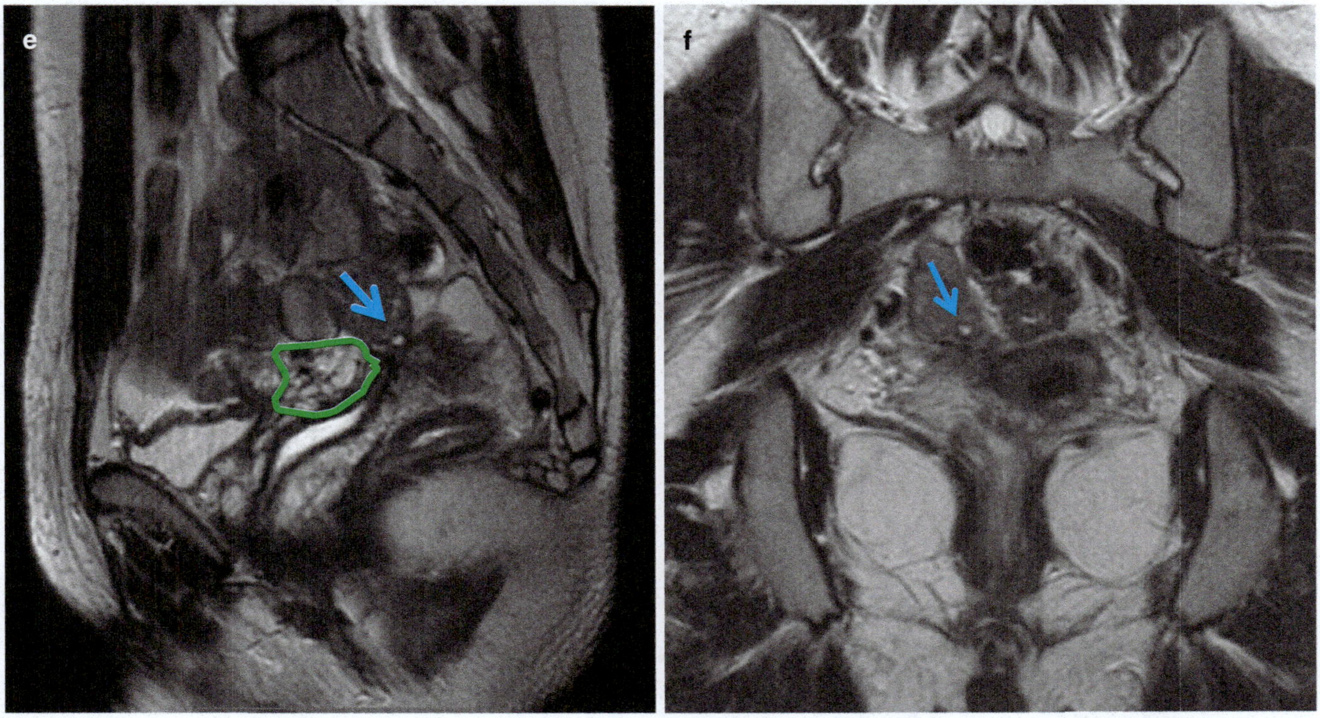

Fig. 4.147 (continued)

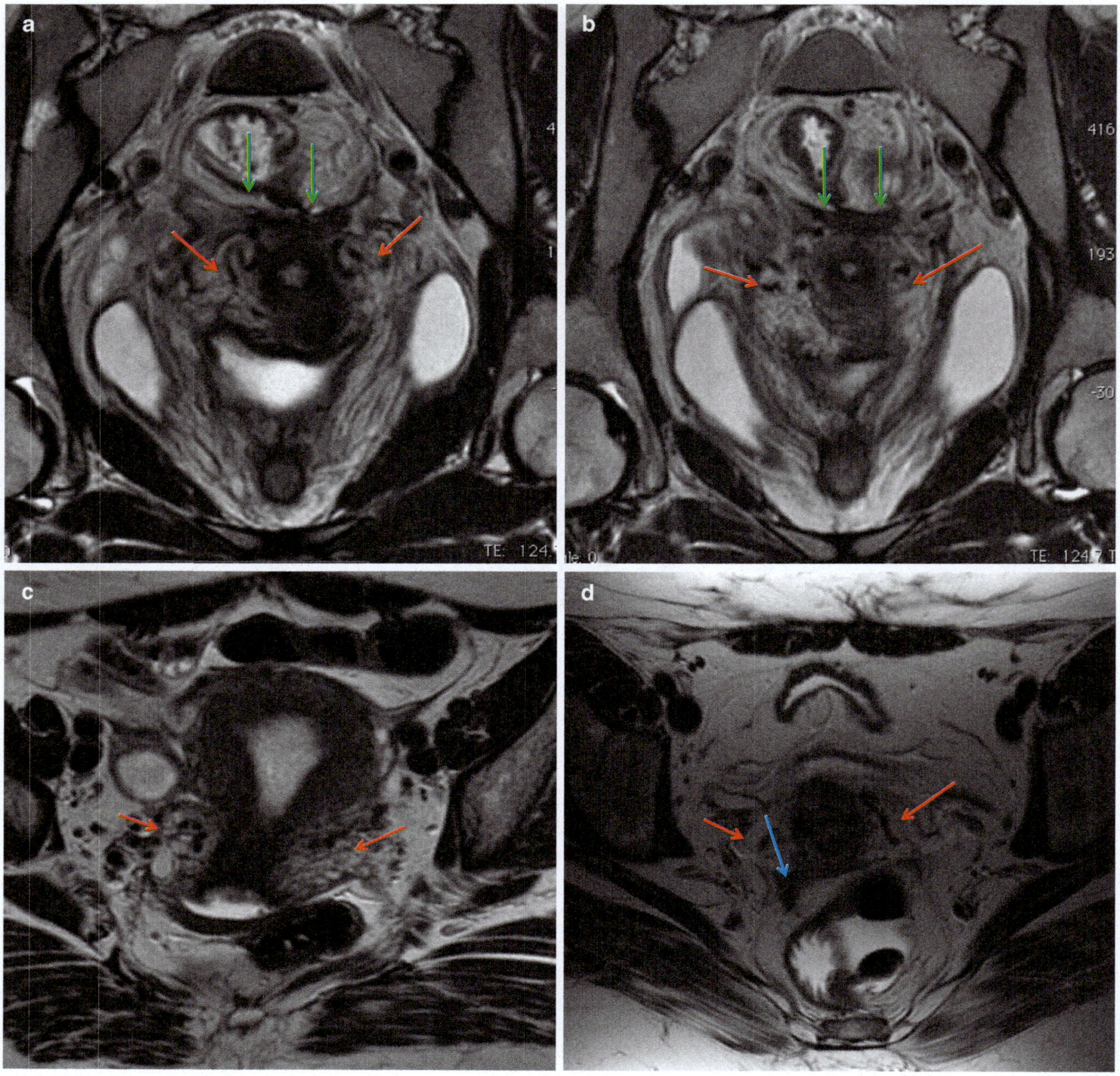

Fig. 4.148 Identification of the uterine artery in the parametrium. Discrete elongated structure and with absence of signal in T2-weighted sequences due to rapid flow (red arrows). Note a small retrocervical lesion (green arrows on **a**, **b**) and on the right uterosacral ligament (blue arrow in **d**). T2-weighted sequence. (**a**, **b**) Coronal short axis. (**c**) Coronal long axis. (**d**) Axial

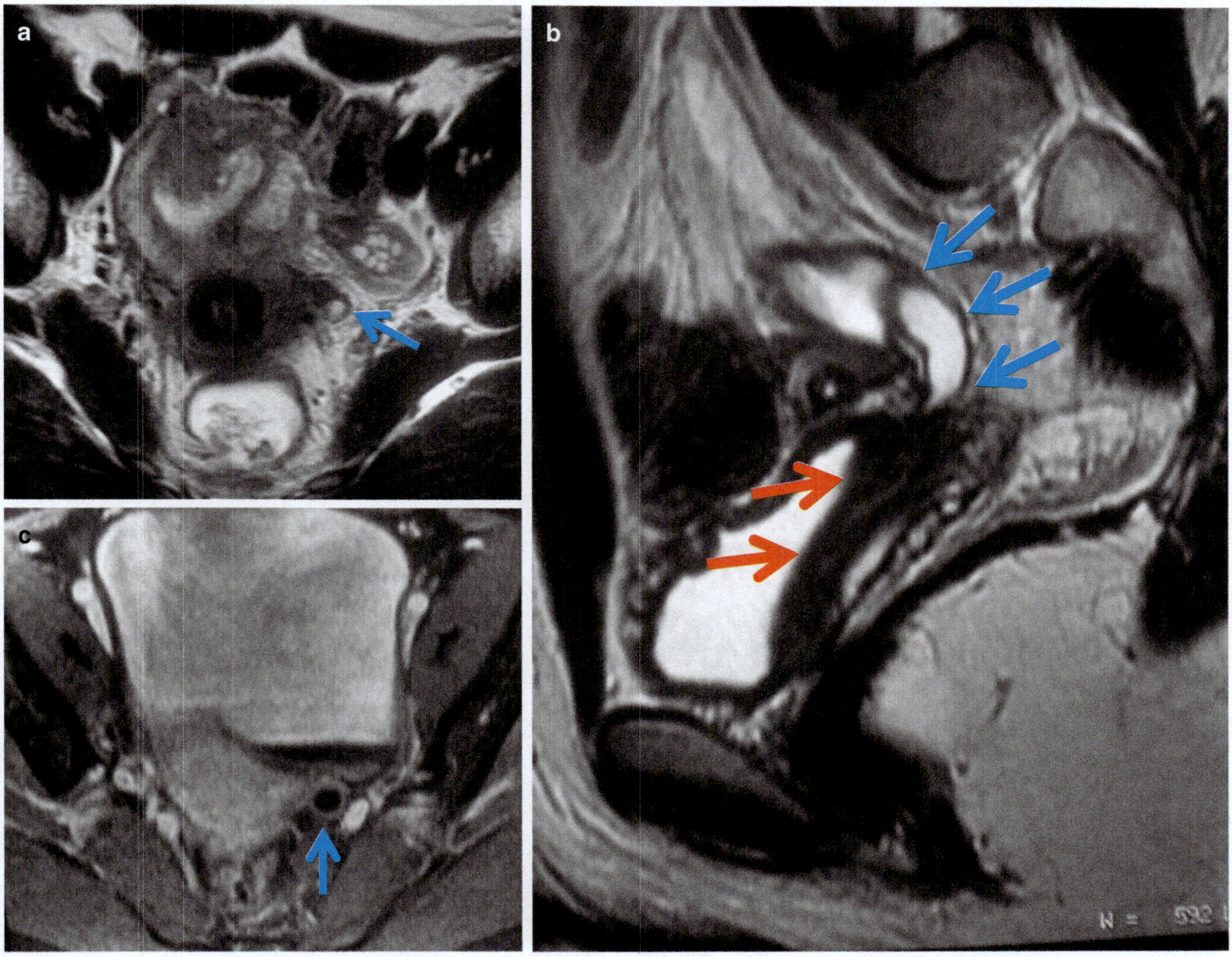

Fig. 4.149 The ureter is a well-defined structure, with a hypointense wall in the T2-weighted sequences (blue arrows in **a**, **b**), being tubular in the sagittal plane (**b**), and round in the axial plane (**a**). When dilated, the liquid inside is hyperintense on T2 (arrows **a**, **b**) and the ureter presents discrete parietal enhancement (arrow **c**). In this case, the obstruction is caused by a vesical lesion with extension to the ureteral ostium (red arrows). (**c**) T1-weighted sequence with gadolinium. Axial

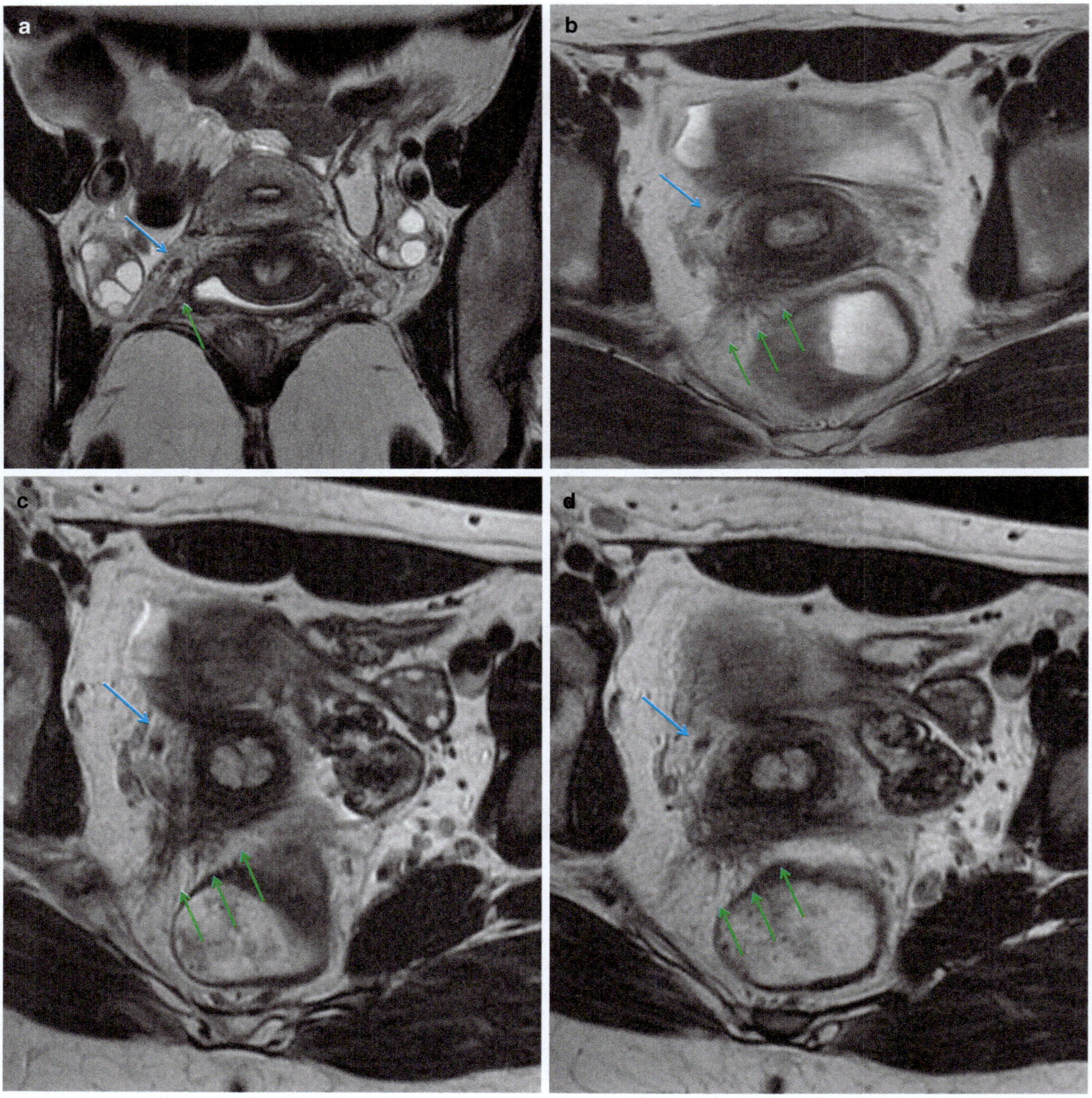

Fig. 4.150 In the paracolpos, just below the ureter (blue arrows) and uterosacral ligament, the relationship between the lesion and the hypogastric nerve and the inferior hypogastric plexus (green arrows) should be evaluated. (**a**) Anatomy. (**b**–**m**) Deep right uterosacral ligament lesion with significant inferior extension to the paracolpos, involving the nerve and plexus (green arrows) in the axial plane (**b**–**g**), sagittal (**h**–**j**) and coronal short axis (**k**–**m**). Also notice mesorectal and discrete involvement of the parametrium with the cleavage plane with the ureter (blue arrows)

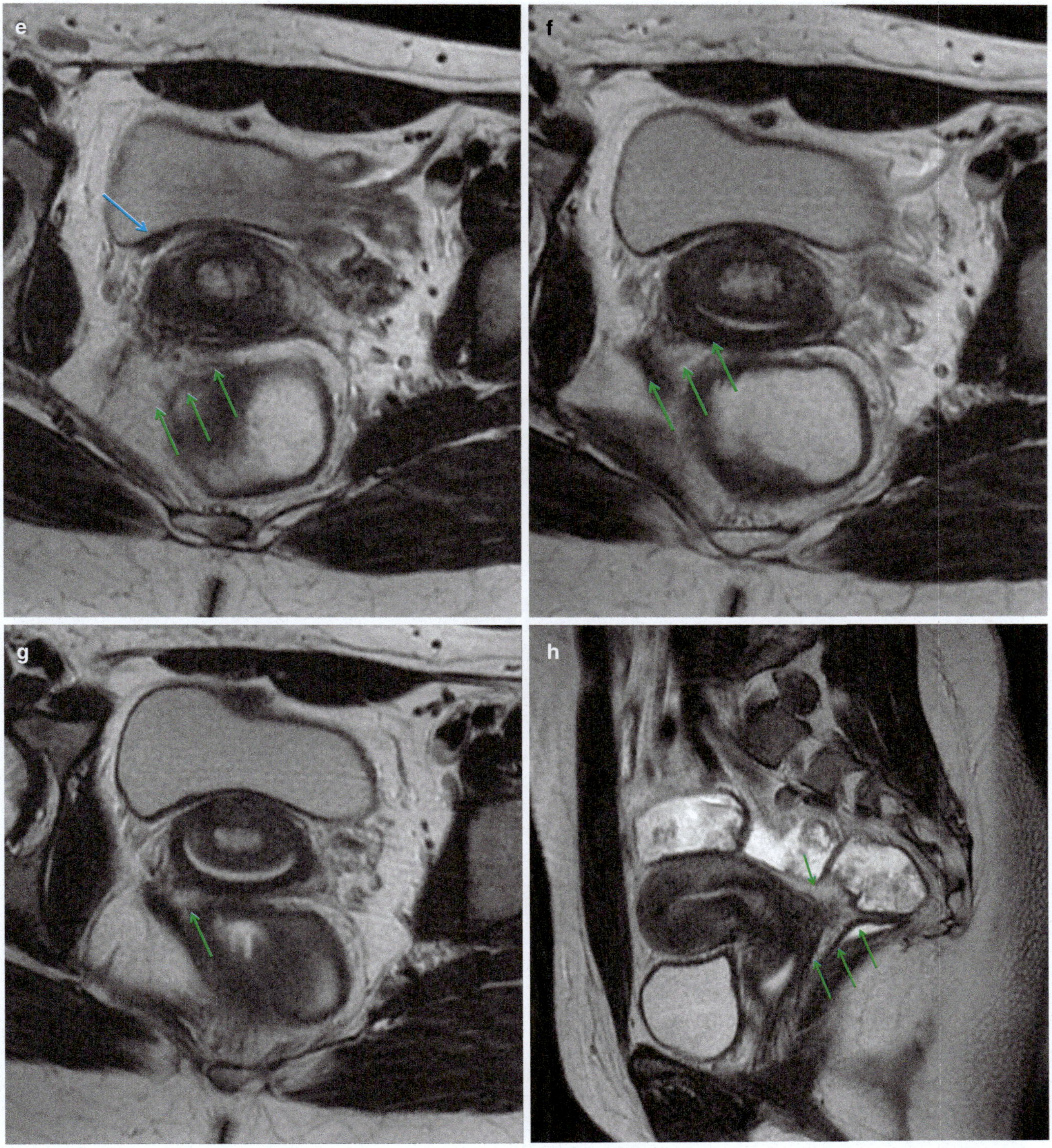

Fig. 4.150 (continued)

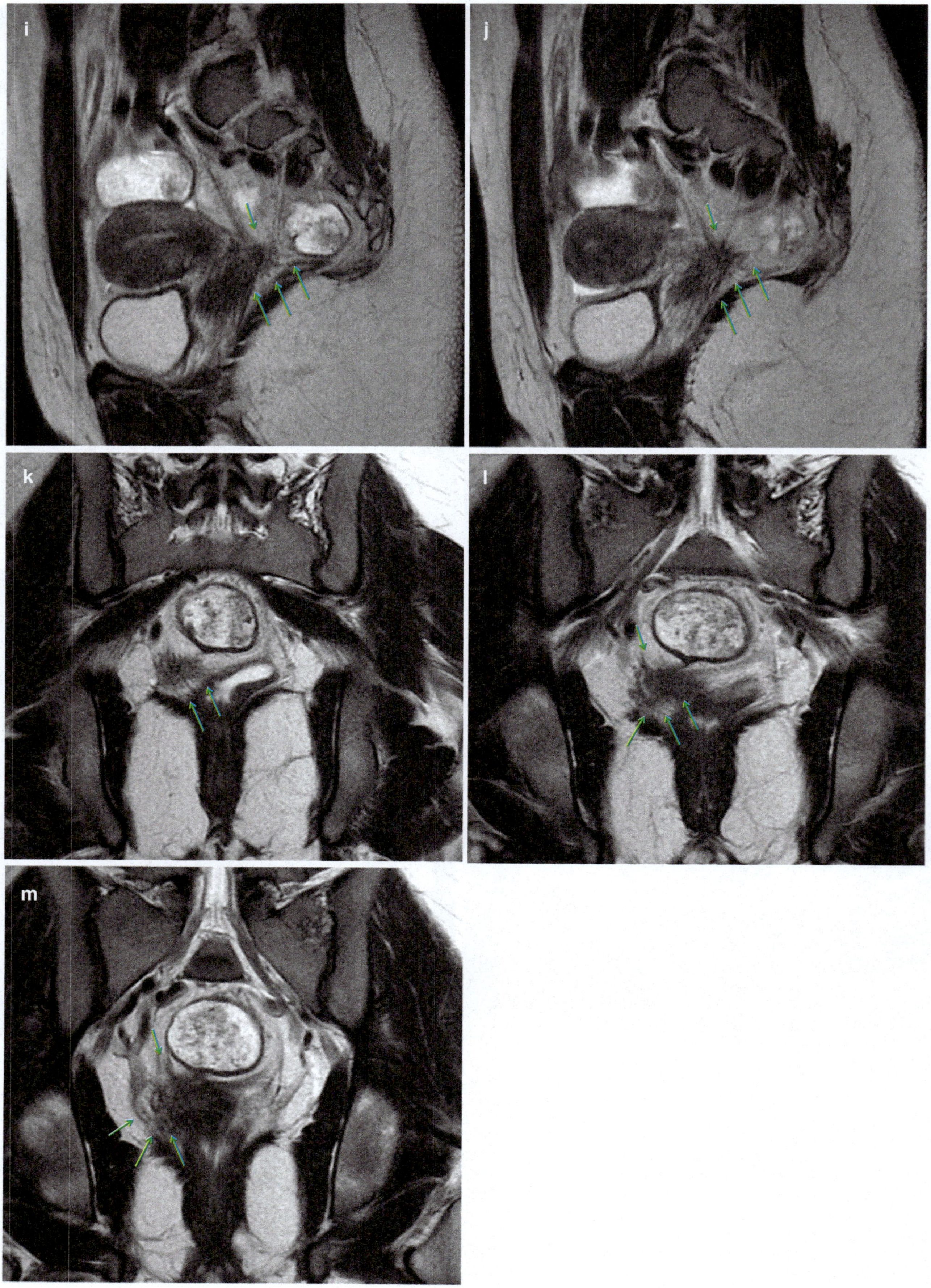

Fig. 4.150 (continued)

4.3.1.4 Treatment Comments

The surgical treatment of parametrial endometriosis is challenging because the region is rich in nerve and vascular bundles. In some situations the uterine artery must be isolated and sometimes sacrificed for a satisfactory parametrectomy. Although there is a need for bilateral ligation of the uterine arteries and damage to fertility is possible, this does not seem to be very significant according to published studies on bilateral ligation of the uterine arteries in women desiring to undergo laparoscopic myomectomy (Fig. 4.151).

However, bilateral parametrectomy should be avoided if at all possible, as nerve damage may be irreversible and cause definitive loss of bladder emptying capacity. Patients may require permanent intermittent bladder catheterization. Therefore, surgeons may choose to completely remove the most affected side and spare the nerves on the least affected side, even if this means the persistence of some of the disease.

4.3.2 Ureter

Not infrequently the ureter is also affected on the same side as the parametrium. The patient may present with hydroureter and/or hydronephrosis.

In some situations it is possible that only ureterolysis is required, but other cases may require segmental resection of the ureter with terminoterminal anastomosis or even ureteral reimplantation.

Further details are given in the specific section on lesions of the ureter in the anterior compartment.

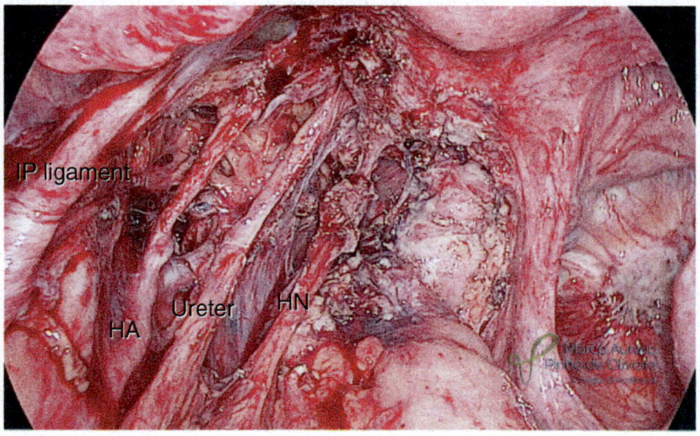

Fig. 4.151 Laparoscopy—appearance after resection of left parametrial nodule

4.3.3 The Pelvic Autonomic Nerves: Hypogastric Nerve and Plexus

4.3.3.1 Anatomy

The visceral nervous system is composed of sympathetic and parasympathetic fibers. The superior hypogastric plexus, originating from para-aortic sympathetic trunk, receives innervation from the thoracic and lumbar splanchnic nerves and gives rise to two hypogastric nerves. They carry the proprioception sensations of the bladder, rectum, and uterus and sympathetic signals whose main action is to contract internal urethral and anal sphincters [61].

Beneath the promontory, the upper hypogastric plexus gives rise to the hypogastric nerves. The left and right hypogastric nerves follow the common and internal iliac arteries into the pelvis. They have an anterior, medial, and inferior trajectory, insinuating itself in the retroperitoneum, bordering the sacrum, and later maintaining close contact with the sigmoid and rectum in the pararectal space. They are located medially to the ureters and lateral to the uterosacral ligaments. By carefully dissecting the retroperitoneum, starting near the promontory, the hypogastric nerve can be identified and avoid unnecessary injuries (Fig. 4.152).

The sympathetic fibers of the hypogastric nerves merge parasympathetic fibers of the pelvic splanchnic nerves coming away from S2, S3, and S4 to form the inferior hypogastric plexus.

Between the rectum, the broad ligament, and the paracolpos, there is the formation of the inferior hypogastric plexus, a triangular structure, which gives rise to several visceral efferent branches, to the bladder, vagina, uterus, and rectum, with two trunks crossing inferiorly the uterine artery and the ureter. The reference point of the two trunks is the ureter. The lateral trunk, vesical, inferiorly accompanies the ureter until the bladder. The medial trunk follows the uterine artery, bordering the vagina, and subdivided into anterior and posterior. The anterior portion innervates the vagina and crosses the ureter in the plane of the uterine artery, and the posterior portion inferiorly follows the ureter and penetrates the posterior vagina and rectum (Fig. 4.153).

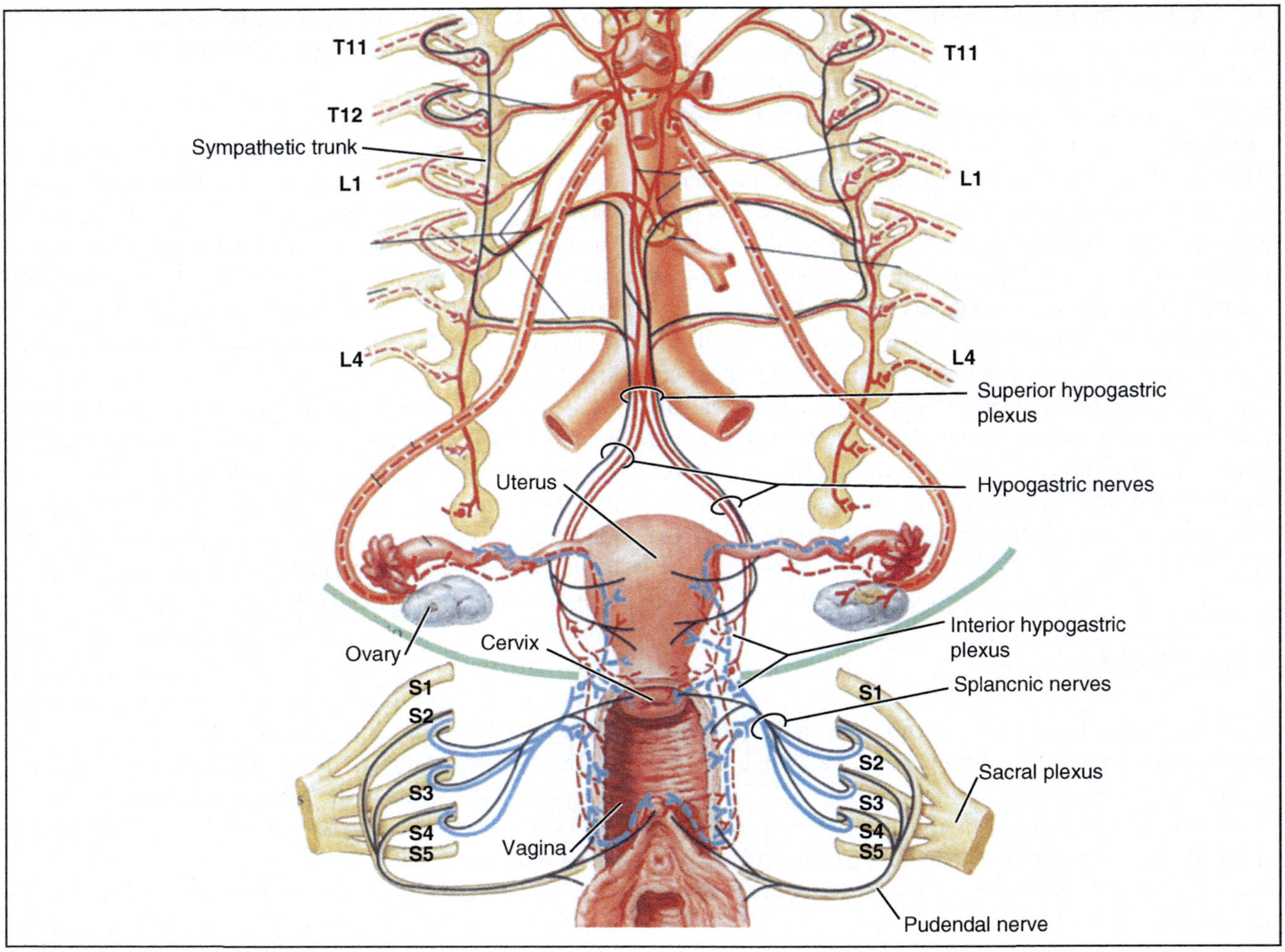

Fig. 4.152 Hypogastric nerves. Anterior, medial, and inferior trajectory, insinuating itself in the retroperitoneum. They are situated medially to the ureters and laterally to the uterosacral ligaments (arrows). (**a**) Diagram from Ferdelle MP et al. Diagnostic and Surgical Imaging Anatomy: Chest, Abdomen, Pelvis. Lippincott Williams & Wilkins, 2006, pp. 85, 86. (**b**) Laparoscopy identifying the hypogastric nerve (blue arrow) and the relationship with uterosacral ligament (blue arrow) and ureter. (**c**) Diagram from Mauroy B. et al. Systematization of the vesical and utero vaginal efferences of the female inferior hypogastric plexus (pelvic): applications to pelvic surgery on women patients. Surg Radiol Anat 2007; 29: 209-217. Lateral view. Note that the rectum was removed and the uterus, vagina (gray), and bladder were pulled anteriorly to allow identification of the nerve (yellow). (**d–g**) Sagittal T2. Note ureter (blue), uterosacral (red), parametrium (green), and topography of the nerve (yellow)

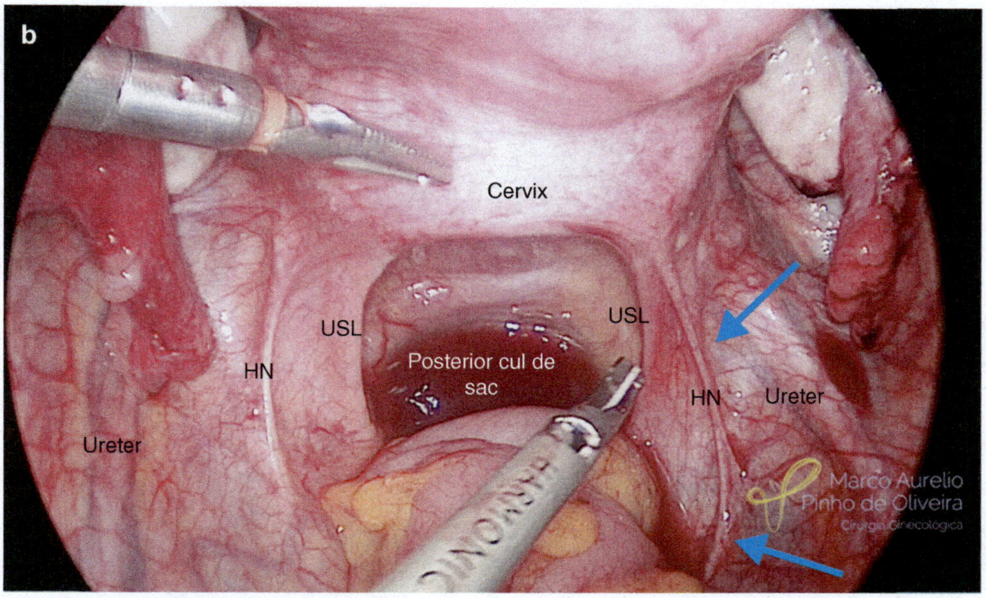

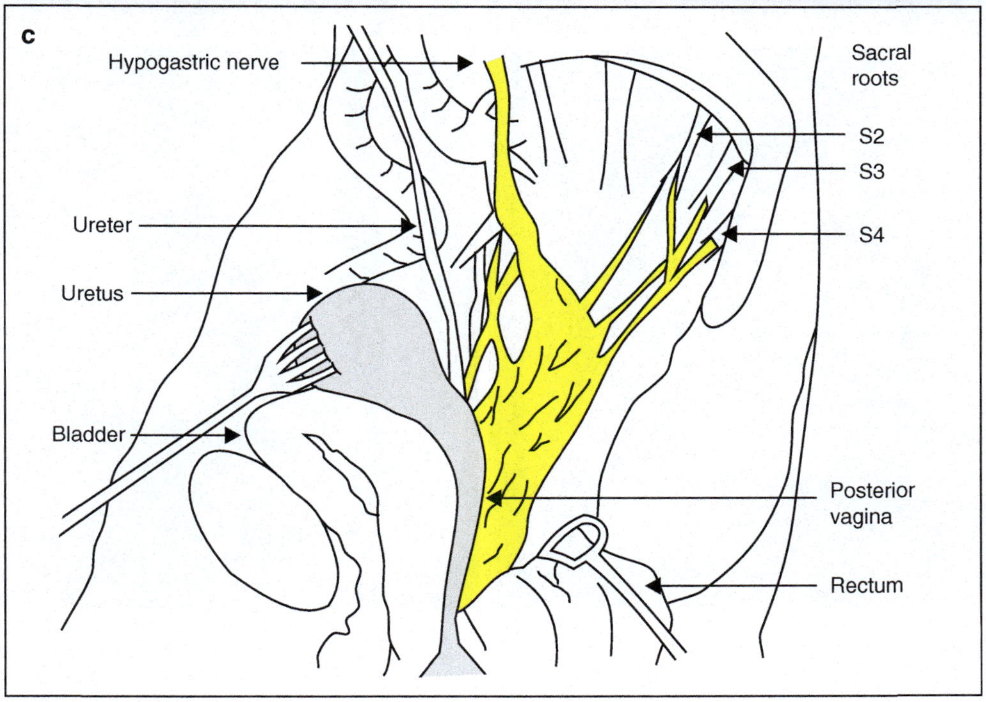

Fig. 4.152 (continued)

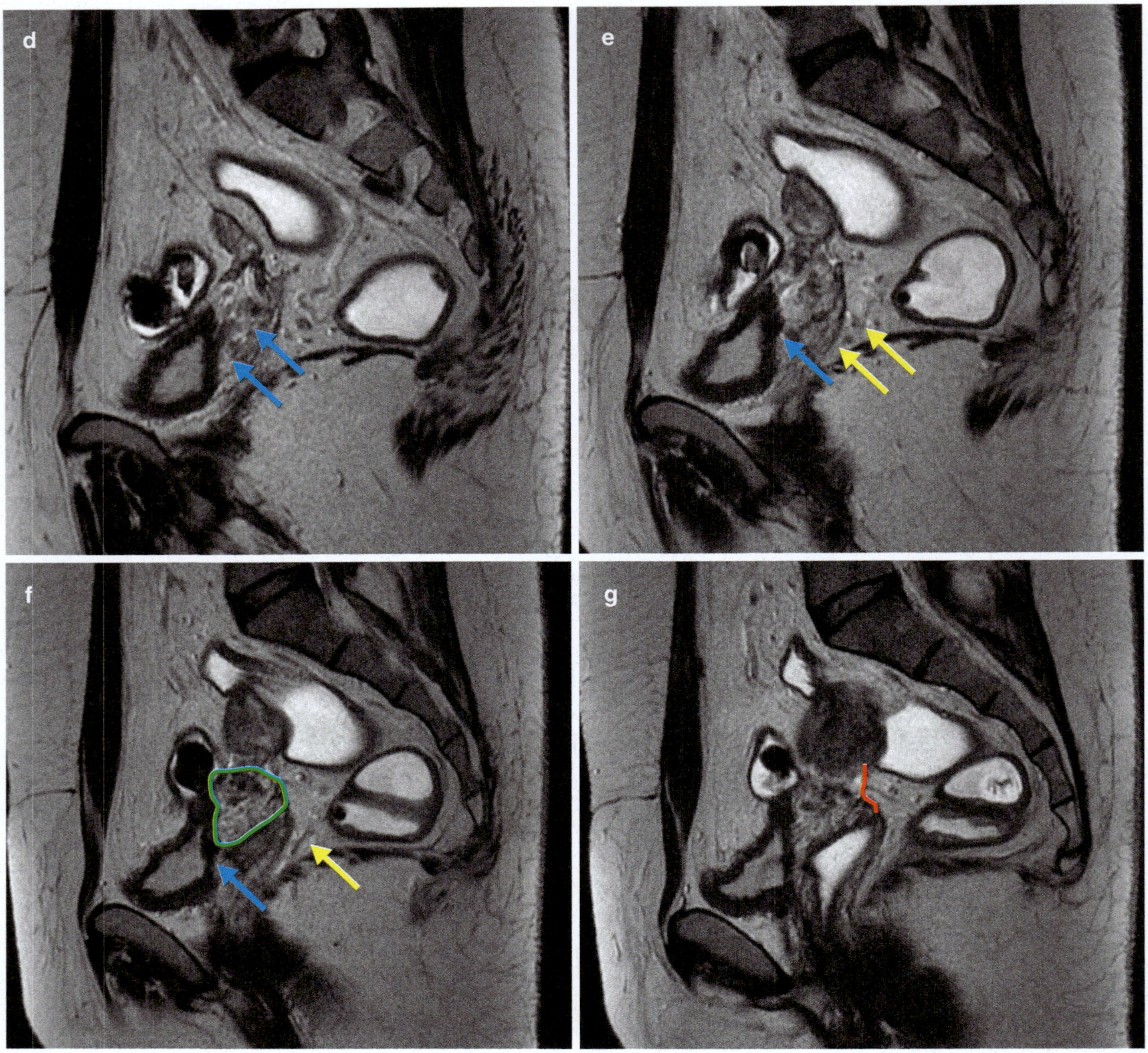

Fig. 4.152 (continued)

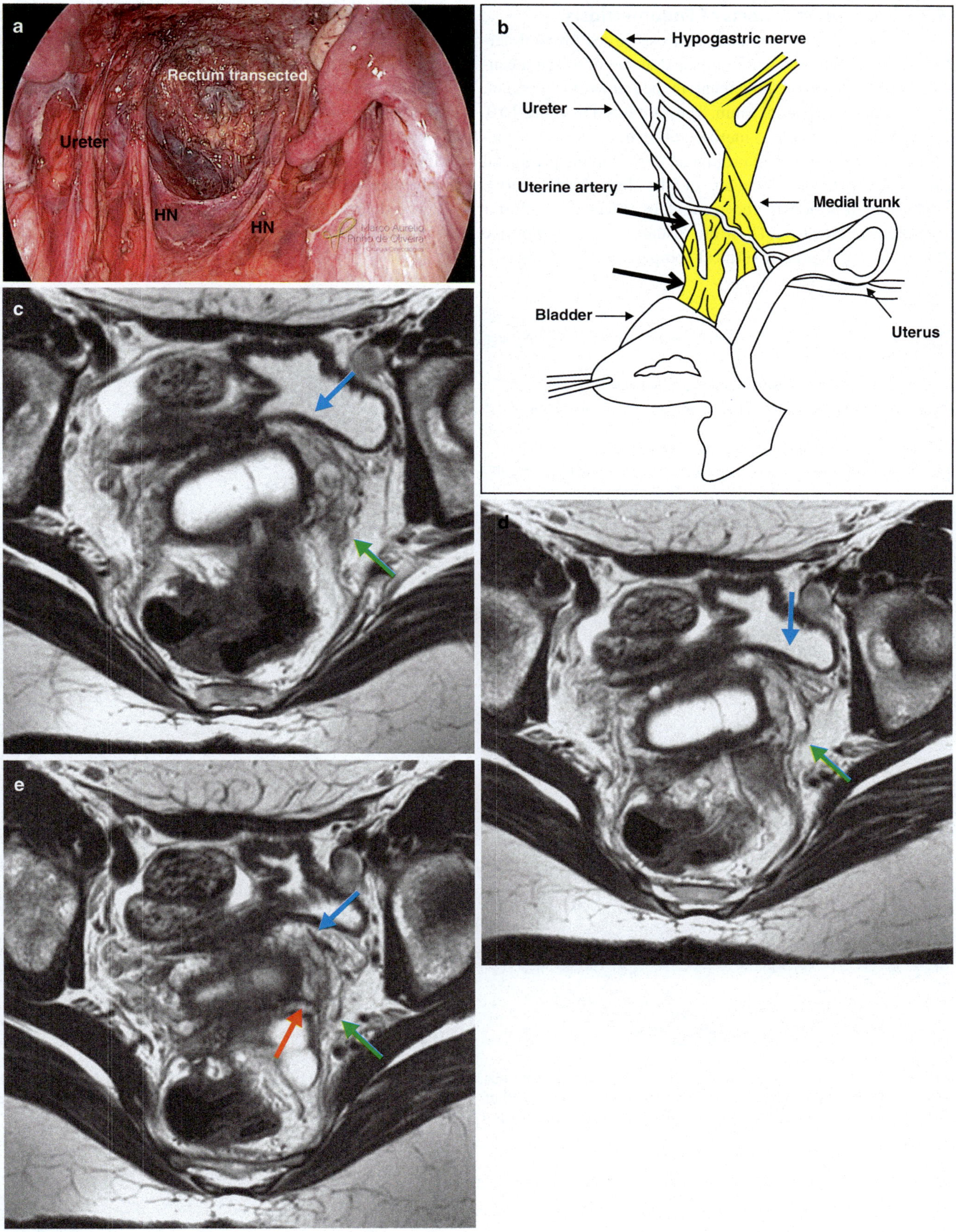

Fig. 4.153 Path of the hypogastric nerve. Two trunks crossing inferiorly the uterine artery and the ureter, with the ureter as the reference point (blue arrows). Note uterosacral (red arrow on **e**), medial to the hypogastric nerve (green arrows in **c–e**). Right side uterosacral lesion with normal left side. (**a**) Laparoscopy identifying the hypogastric nerve bilaterally and its relationship with the ureter. (**b**) from Mauroy Scheme B. et al. Systematization of the vesical and uterovaginal efferences of the female inferior hypogastric plexus (pelvic): applications to pelvic surgery on women patients. Surg Radiol Anat 2007; 29: 209-217 (**c–e**) T2-weighted sequences. Axial

4.3.3.2 Common Aspects of Endometriosis

The involvement of deep endometriosis in the visceral nervous system can be related to the extension of a lesion centered on the uterosacral ligament, in the retrocervical region, or in the anterior parametrium. They are listed in Table 4.10.

A lateral extension of uterosacral ligament lesion or rectovaginal or retrocervical prominent nodule to the pararectal space leads to involvement of the hypogastric nerve. Extension of lesion to the paracolpos affects the inferior hypogastric plexus. They are usually large, infiltrative lesions and with greater surgical complexity (Fig. 4.154).

An anterior parametrium lesion with involvement of the ureter near the bladder trigone can affect the lateral trunk of the inferior hypogastric plexus.

There is a rare form of hypogastric nerve and lumbosacral plexus lesion presentation, with an infiltrative nodule, lateral and posterior in the pelvis, between the acetabulum and the piriformis muscle (Fig. 4.155). In addition, pelvic nerve involvement may occur adjacent to the sciatic nerve, related to a well-defined cystic or diverticulum formation that allows the implantation of endometrial cells (Fig. 4.156) [61].

Table 4.10 Common aspects of visceral nervous system deep endometriosis

Lateral extension of the uterosacral ligament lesion
Lateral extension of the rectovaginal or retrocervical prominent nodule
Anterior parametrium lesion, near the bladder trigone
Infiltrative lesion or nodule centered on the lateral and posterior wall

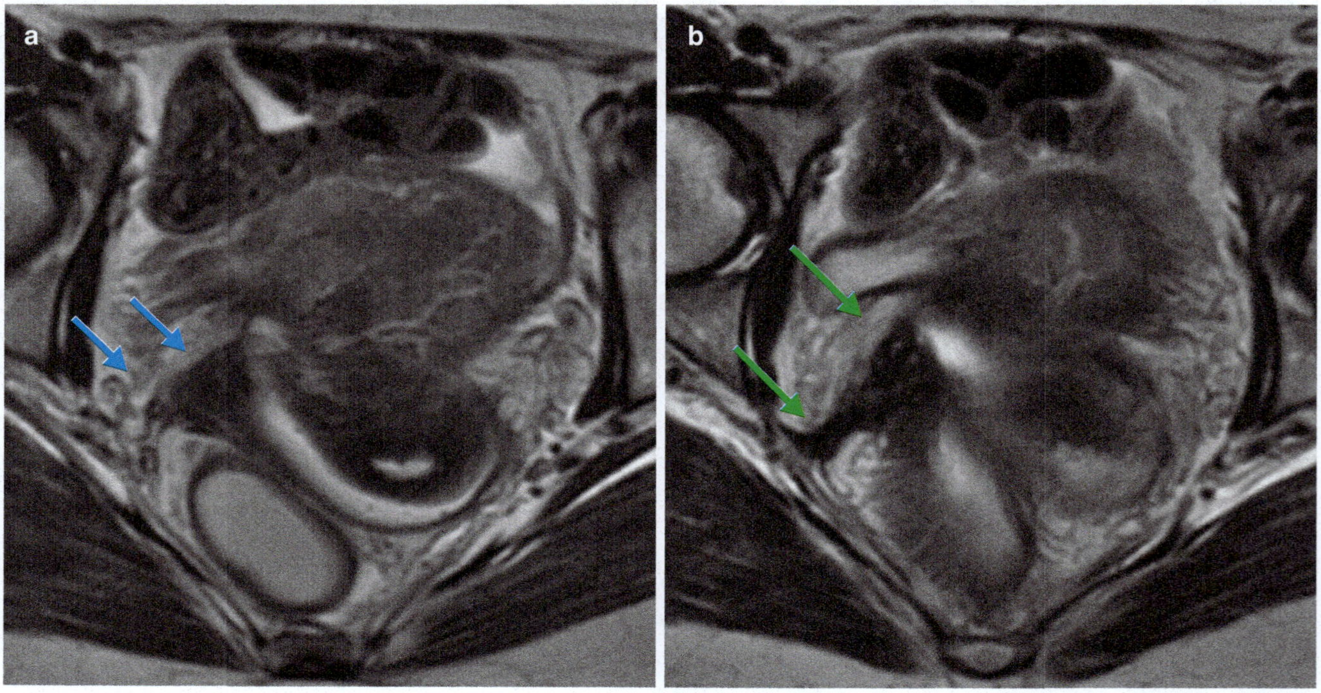

Fig. 4.154 Extension of lesion of the right uterosacral ligament (blue arrows), involving the paracolpos and extending to the lateral wall of the pelvis (green arrow). The lesion is predominantly fibrous, with discrete hyperintense foci on T2-weighted sequences (**a–b**, **d–f**) and T1 with fat saturation (arrow on **c**). Note inferior relation to the uterine artery (red arrows). (**a–c**) Axial. (**d**) Sagittal. (**e**, **f**) Short axis

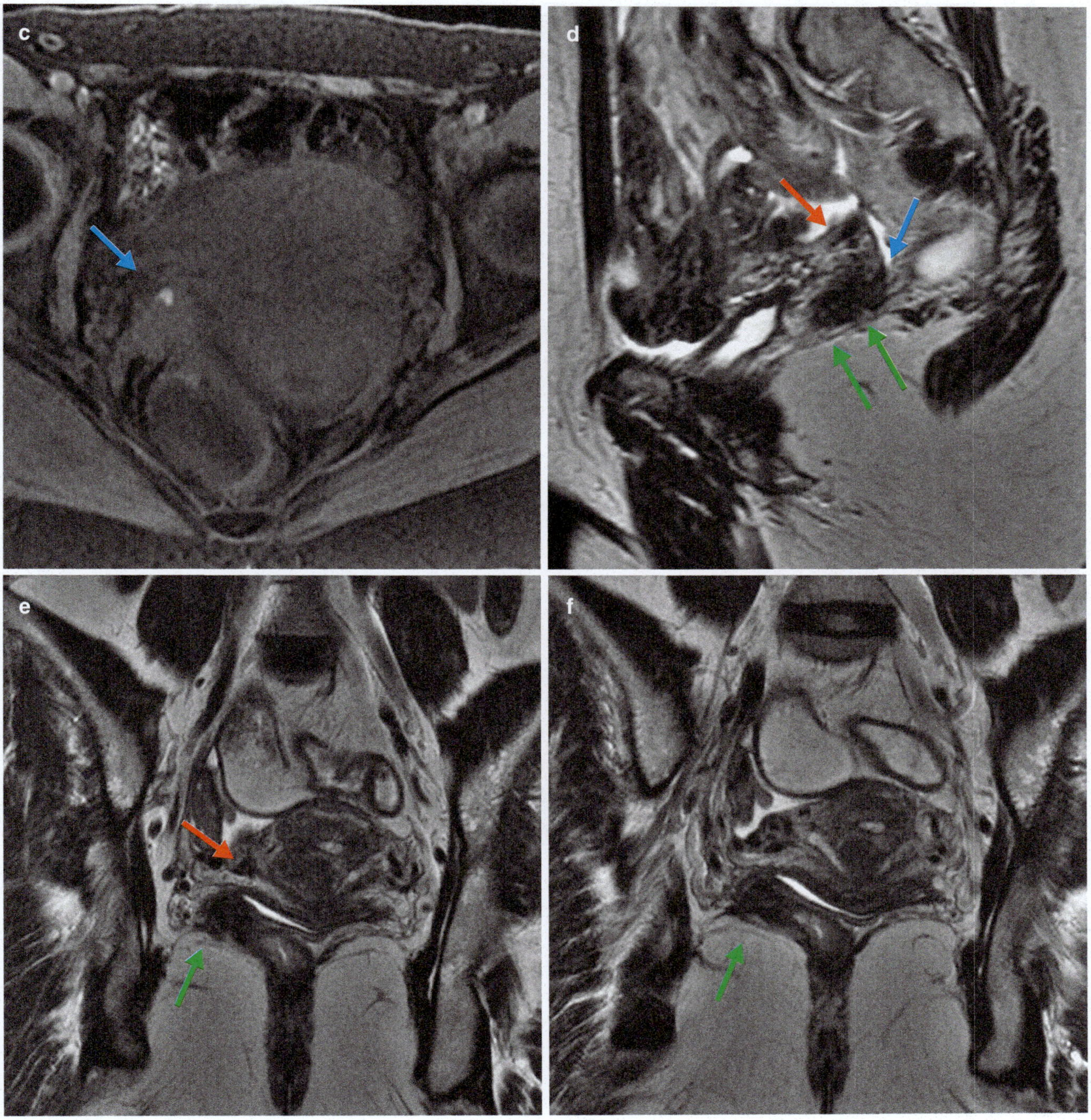

Fig. 4.154 (continued)

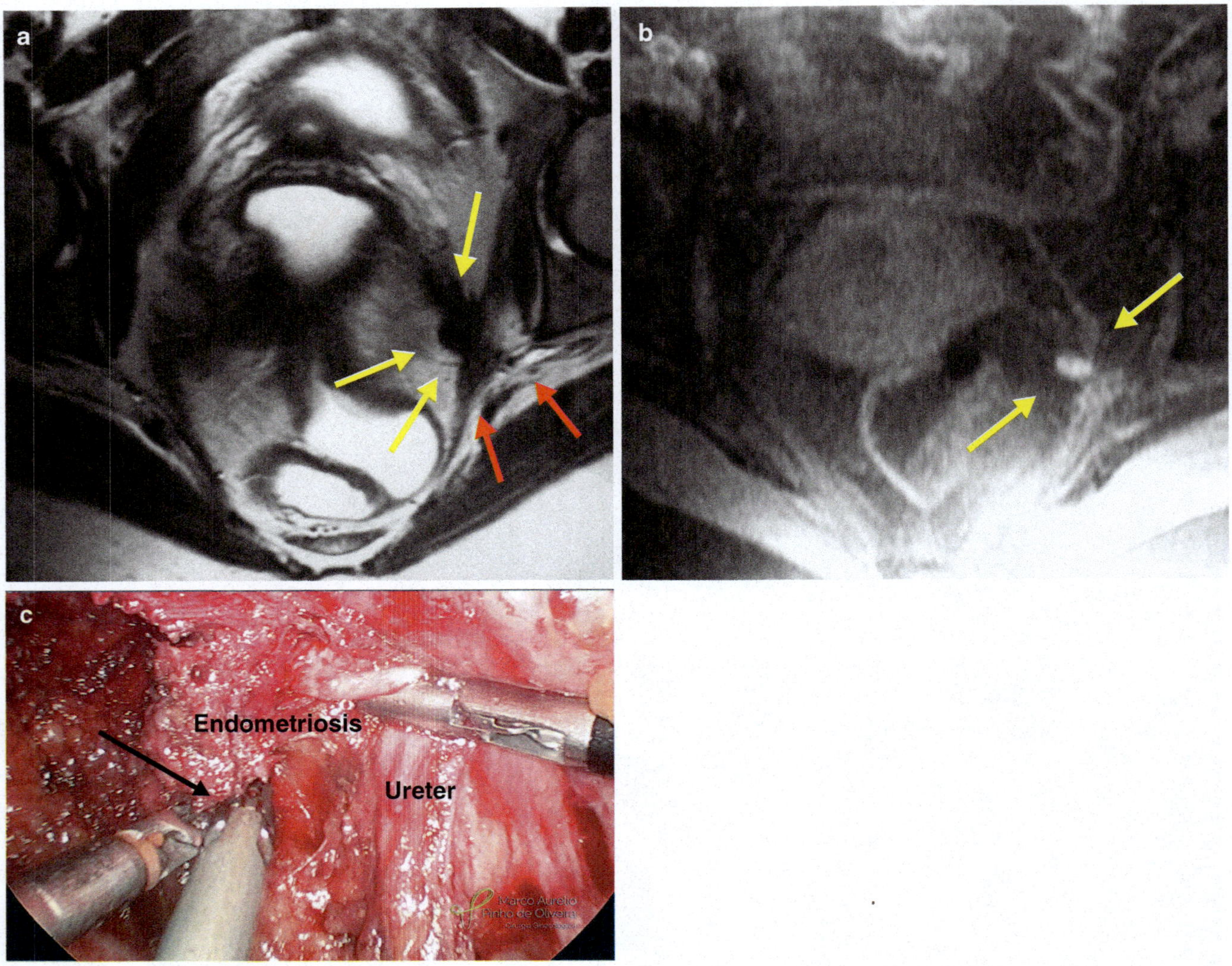

Fig. 4.155 (**a**–**c**) Case 1: Infiltrative small lesion, centered on the left and posterior lateral wall of the pelvis, affecting the hypogastric nerve (yellow arrows), as well as with proximity to the sciatic nerve (red arrow). Note the prevalence of fibrosis (hypointense on T2-weighted sequence [**a**]) and bleeding foci (hyperintense on T1-weighted fat suppression [**b**]). (**c**) Laparoscopy identifying involvement of hypogastric nerve (arrow). (**d**–**h**) Case 2: Infiltrative lesion on the left posterior lateral wall of the pelvis (arrows), following the hypogastric nerve pathway, as well as the lumbosacral plexus, correlating with the pain site (cutaneous marker in the sagittal plane—red arrow in **g**), with superficial involvement of the vagina and rectum (**d**). There is a predominance of fibrosis (hypointense in T2-weighted sequences [**d**, **g**]), without bleeding (intermediate signal in T1-weighted sequence with fat saturation [**e**]) and with discrete enhancement by gadolinium (**f**). (**a**, **b**, **d**–**f**) Axial. (**g**) Sagittal. (**c**) Laparoscopy for reference

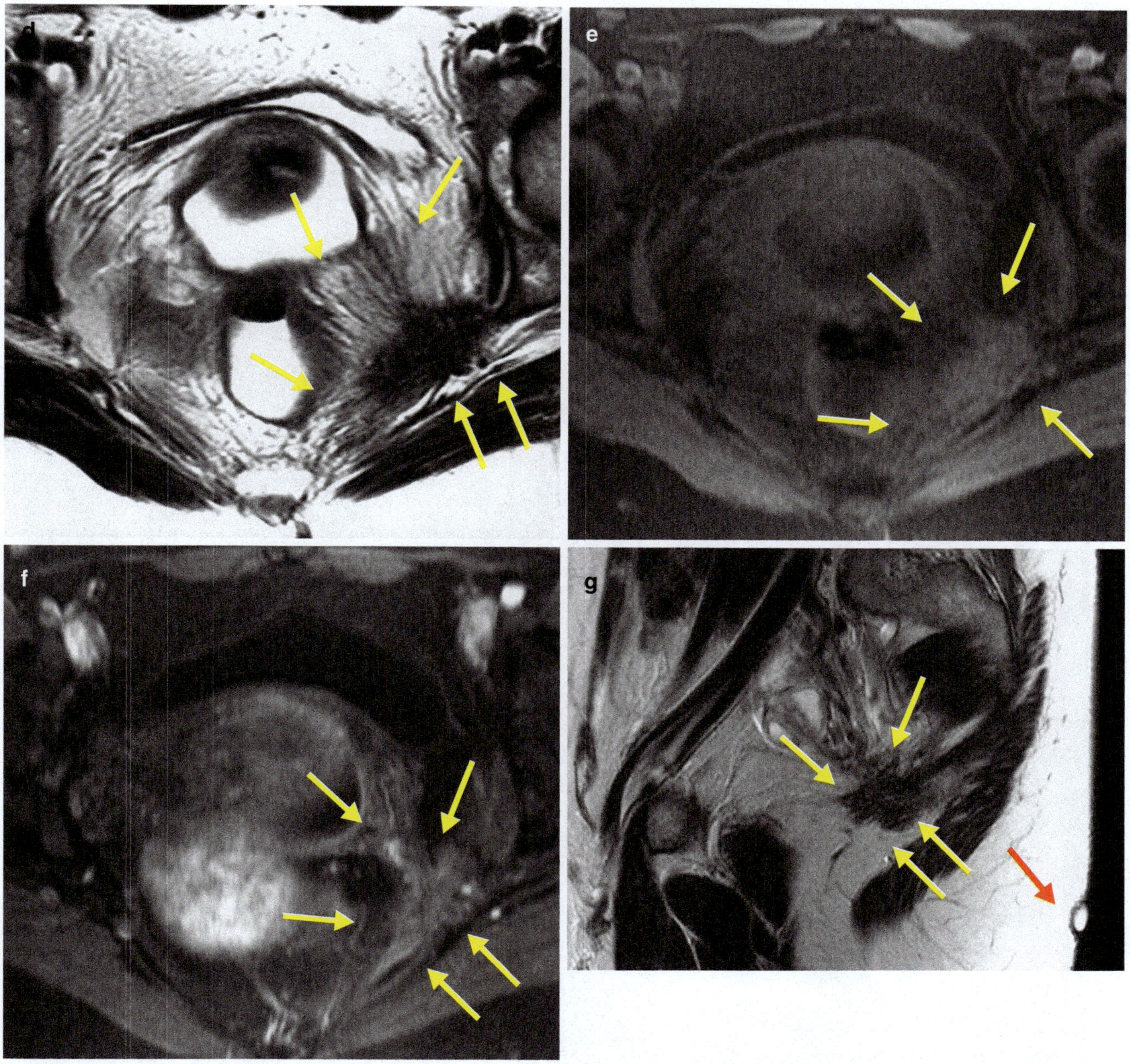

Fig. 4.155 (continued)

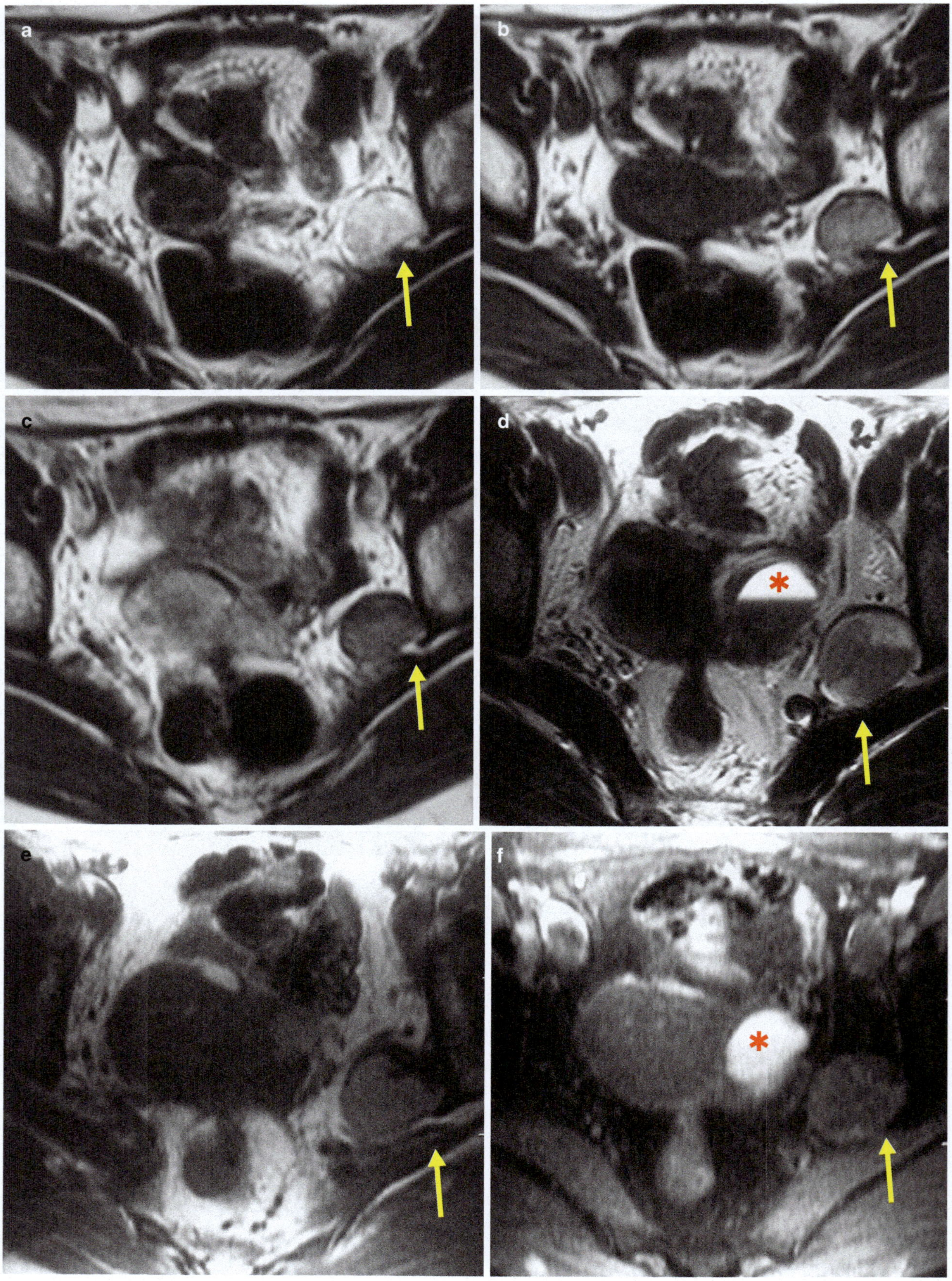

Fig. 4.156 Diverticulum adjacent to the hypogastric and lumbosacral plexus. Well-defined lesion, lateral and posterior to the left of the pelvis, between the acetabulum and the piriformis muscle (arrows). There was an increase in the lesion between the first examination (**a–c**) and the second one (**d–f**) and hyposignal appearance on the T2-weighted sequence (compare with **d**), hypersignal persisting in T1 (**b**, **c**, **e**, **f**). (**a–f**) Axial. Note the endometrioma in the left ovary (*), in the second examination

4.3.3.3 Clinical Condition

The main symptom is pain. This may have different patterns due to the relationship with the nerve, with greater intensity, and spread to the sacral, lumbar, and lower limb regions. Sciatica is typically cyclical and occurs during the menstrual period, 1–2 days before or after the first day of the period. The pain is intense and progressive and can become constant. In more advanced cases, it may be accompanied by motor deficit. Early diagnosis and treatment are important in order to avoid permanent neurological damage [62].

4.3.3.4 MRI and Laparoscopic Findings

For neural involvement to be suspected, an understanding of the anatomy and pathway of the nerves in the pelvis by MRI, described above, is extremely important.

Two types of MRI lesions can be observed, namely:

(a) **Irregular or spiculated nodules** in the path of the nerves of the pelvis or extending to it.
   - Extensive lateral involvement of the uterosacral ligament, in the cervical portion with inferior extension to the paracolpos with proximity to the hypogastric nerve and inferior hypogastric plexus, respectively (Fig. 4.157)
   - Extensive lateral involvement of the uterosacral ligament, including the sacral portion, in proximity to the sacral nerves (Fig. 4.158)
   - Posterior compartment lesion with extension to the paracolpos and inferior hypogastric plexus involvement (Fig. 4.159)
   - Lateral anterior compartment lesion with proximity to the distal portion of the ureter, adjacent to the trigone, the reference point of the lateral trunk (Fig. 4.160).
   - The intensity of this type of lesion is similar to others described in the posterior compartment, with a predominance of fibrosis and lack of glandular tissue.

(b) **An endometrioma-like cystic lesion**, with old hematic content, hypointense in the T2-weighted sequence, hyperintense in the T1-weighted sequence, with a hypointense halo (a fibrous capsule composed of granulation tissue with hemosiderin-filled macrophages), and without enhancement by gadolinium (Fig. 4.156)

The differential includes neurogenic benign tumors (neurinoma and neurofibroma) which tend to have an intermediate signal in the T1- and T2-weighted sequences and are enhanced by gadolinium (Fig. 4.161) [62].

However, despite the excellent ability of laparoscopy and MRI to identify deep lesions, there may be discrepancies between the severity of the disease detected by these methods and the degree of pain. Tractography, pathology, and nerve integrity assessed by MRI have identified microstructural abnormalities in the sacral nerve that may be the basis for understanding this phenomenon [63].

4.3.3.5 Comments on Treatment

Pelvic innervation is complex, being a very important factor in the success of infiltrative endometriosis surgery. Thus, neurolysis has become a fundamental procedure in these patients in order to preserve bladder, sexual, and fecal functions. Injury to a nerve in the pelvis can cause urinary and fecal incontinence, evacuatory difficulties, and bladder atony.

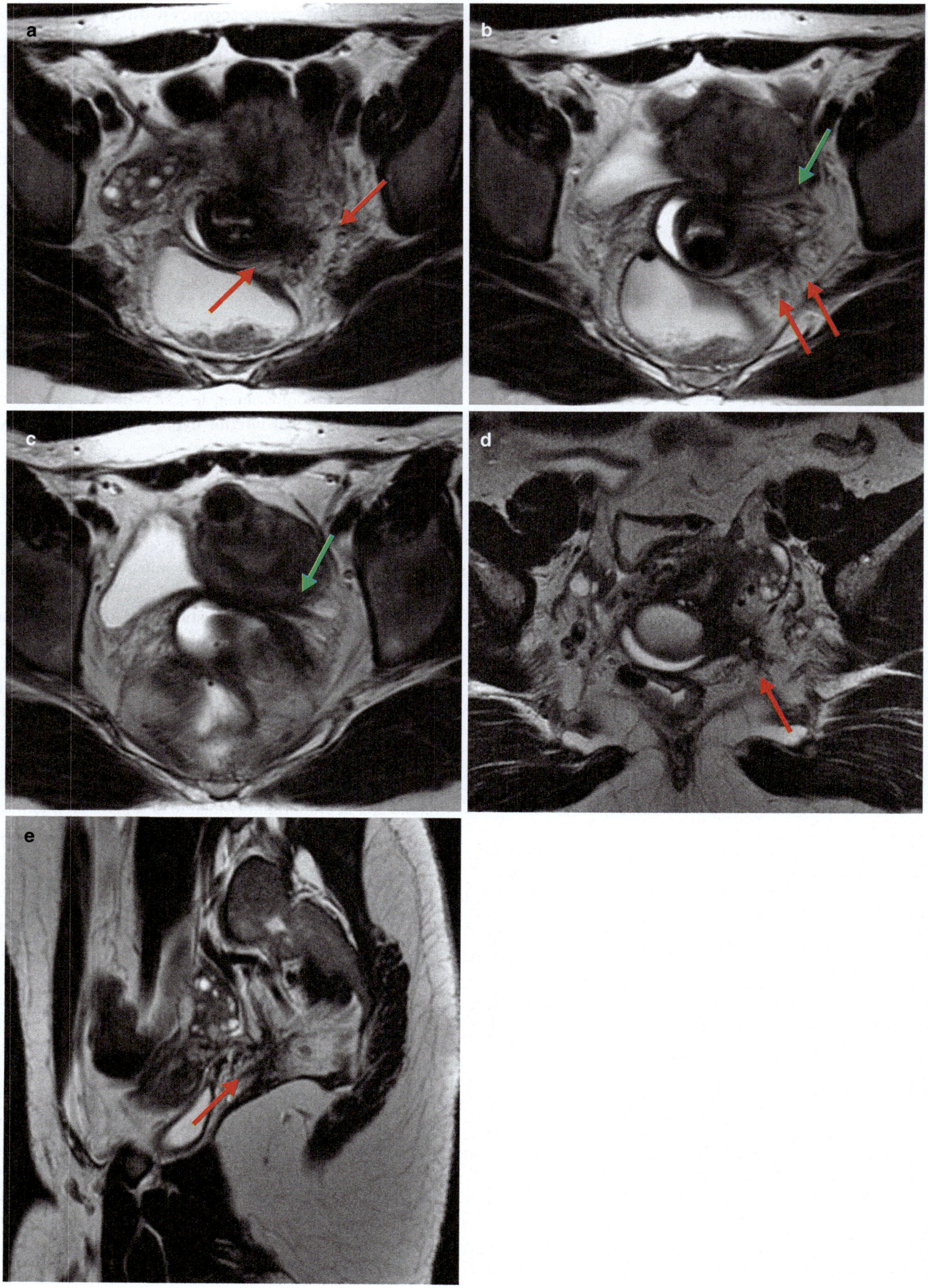

Fig. 4.157 Extensive lateral involvement of the left uterosacral ligament, in the cervical section extending to the paracolpos close to the hypogastric nerve and lower hypogastric plexus (red arrows). Note preserved ureter (green arrows) (**a**–**e**) T2-weighted sequences. (**a**–**c**) Axial. (**d**) Coronal oblique. (**e**) Sagittal

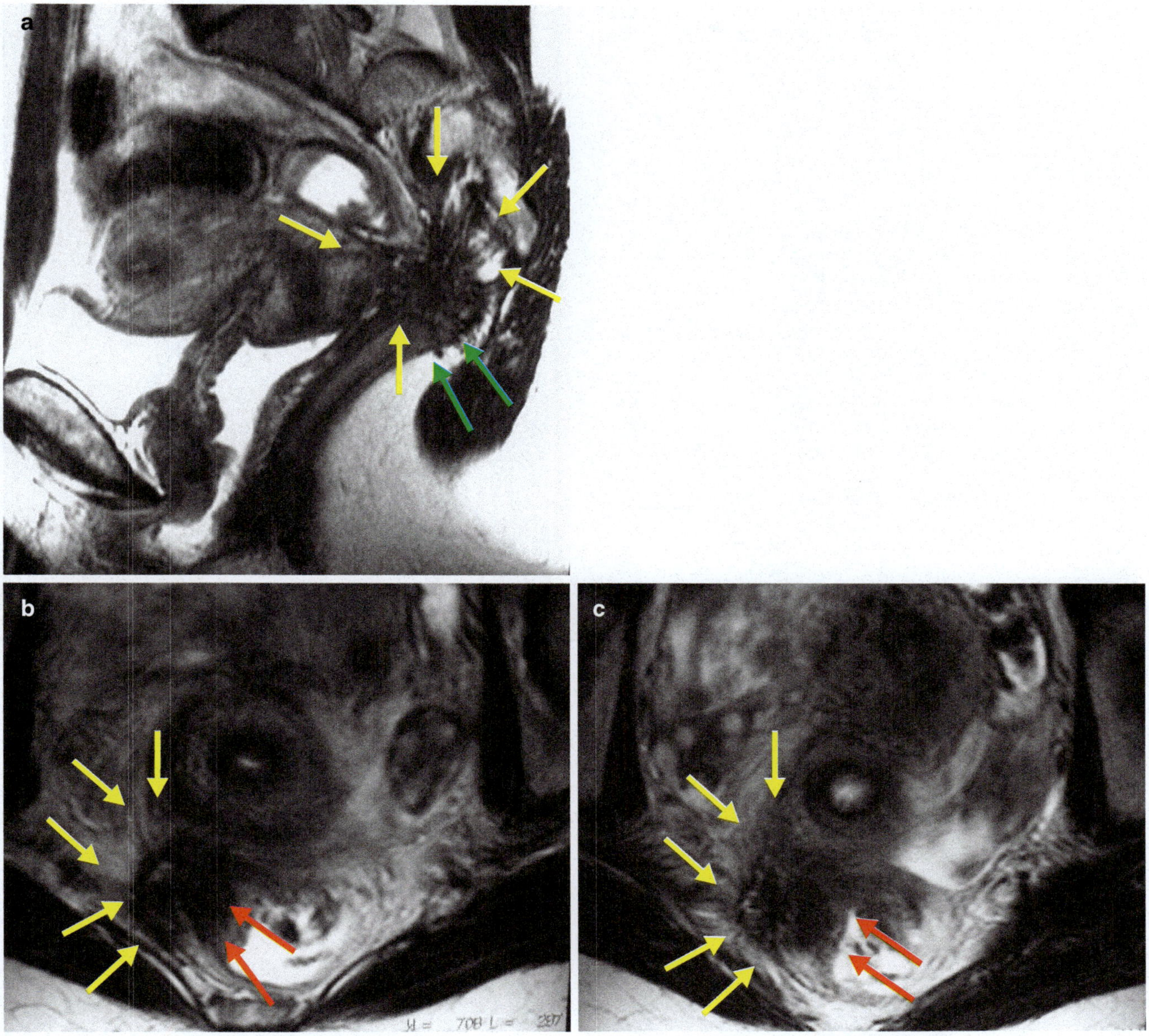

Fig. 4.158 Extensive lateral involvement (yellow arrows) of the right uterosacral ligament to the sacral section close to the sacral roots. Ligamentous lesion forming an irregular nodule, with rectal involvement (red arrows in **b**, **c**) and near the levator ani muscle (green arrow in **a**). (**a**–**c**) T2-weighted sequences. (**a**) Sagittal. (**b**, **c**) Axial

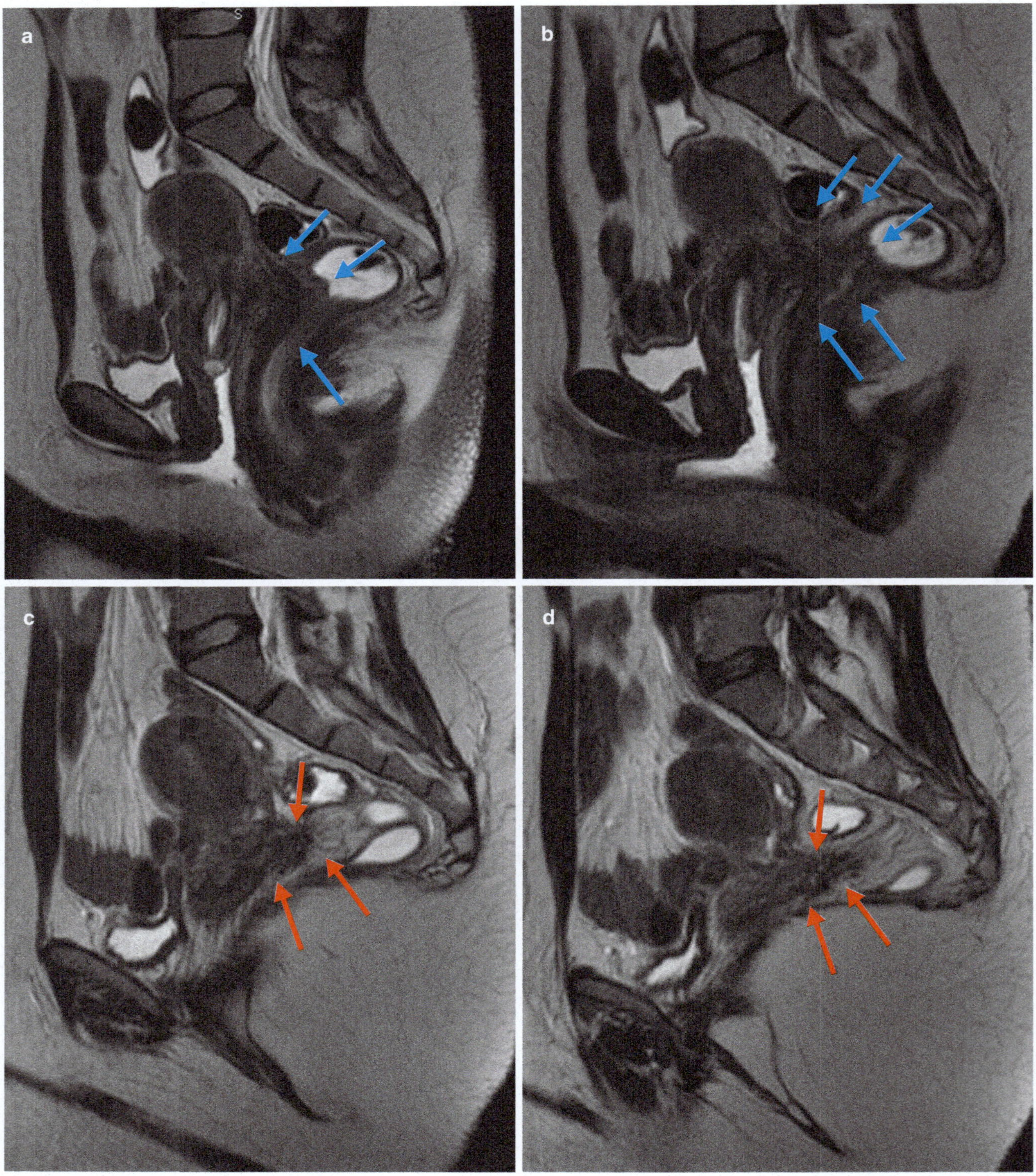

Fig. 4.159 Extensive deep lesion of the rectovaginal septum (blue arrows **a**, **b**) extending to the paracolpos (red arrows in **c**, **d**). (**a**–**d**) T2-weighted sequence. Sagittal. Note rectal and vaginal involvement in (**a**, **b**)

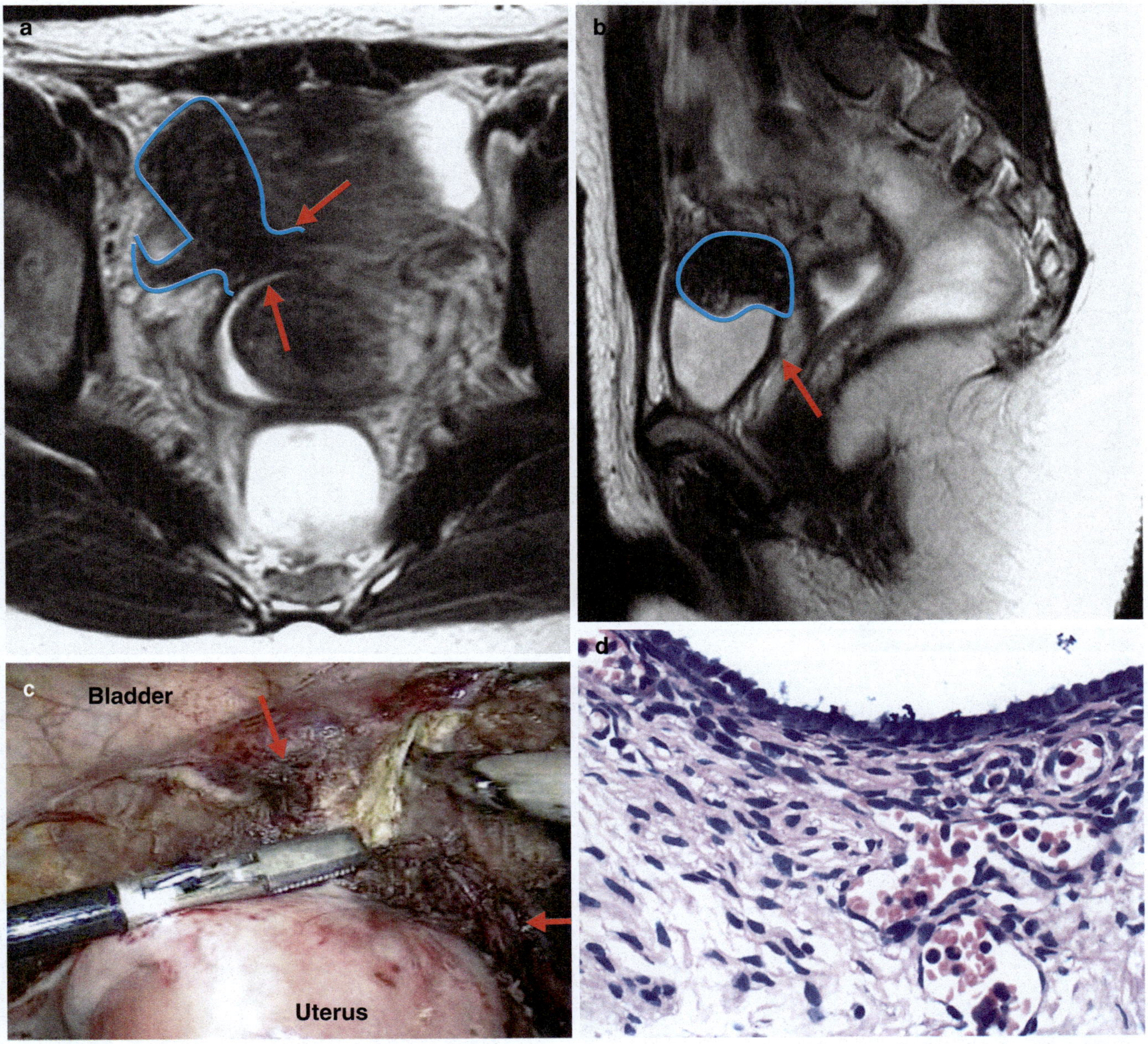

Fig. 4.160 Lesion in right anterior compartment (blue trace) near the distal section of the ureter, adjacent to the trigone vesical (red arrows). T2-weighted sequence. Axial. (**b**) Sagittal. (**c**) Laparoscopy during resection of the endometriotic nodule in the bladder dome and in the paravesical space. (**d**) Microscopy. Endometriotic foci and dilated capillaries (400×)

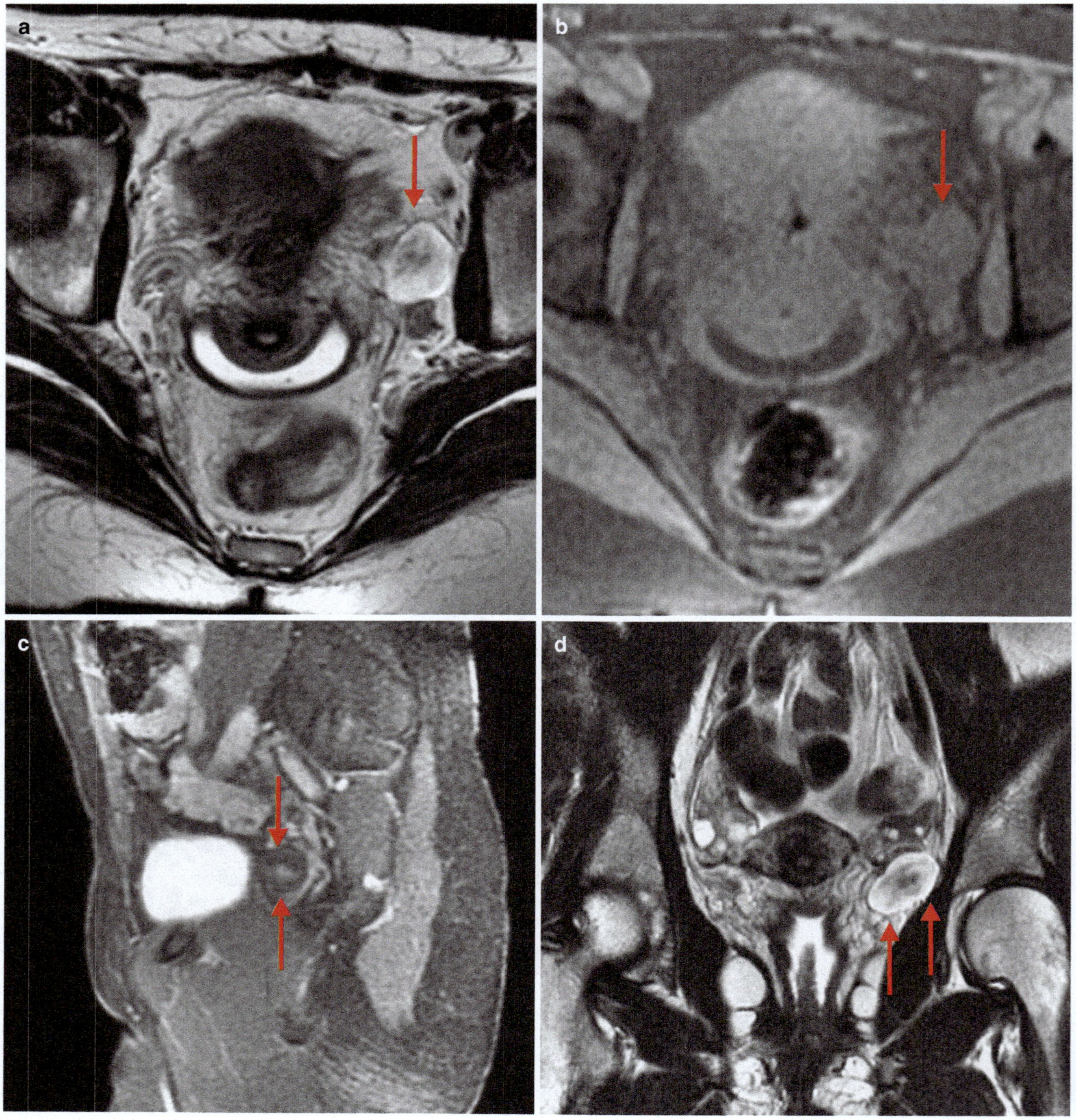

Fig. 4.161 Left extraperitoneal benign neurogenic tumor (arrows). Well-defined ovoid nodule, isointense on T1-weighted sequences (**b**) and hyperintense on T2 (**a**, **d**), enhanced by gadolinium (**c**) located inferior to the left of the adnexa and between the parametrium and the lateral wall of the pelvis. (**a**, **b**) Axial. (**c**) Sagittal. (**d**) Coronal

4.3.4 Pelvic Floor

4.3.4.1 Anatomy

The pelvic floor is a complex integrated system of multiple layers (muscular and fascial) that provides active and passive support. The support of the structures arises from the fixation of the muscles, fascias, and ligaments to the pelvis bone. Fascias and ligaments give passive support, while the muscles, especially the levator ani, provide active support.

The pelvic floor has three layers: the pelvic fascia and the pelvic and urogenital diaphragms, from upper to lower levels, respectively.

The pelvic fascia is a delicate and special structure that surrounds and maintains the support of the pelvic viscera. It is formed by a continuous endopelvic connective tissue that covers the viscera under the peritoneum to the pelvic diaphragm and inserts laterally into the bony pelvis (Fig. 4.162) [35].

It is subdivided into (1) the pubocervical fascia, between the bladder and the vagina;(2) the rectovaginal fascia, between the vagina and rectum;(3) the cardinal ligament, which extends from the cervix to the lateral wall of the pelvic cavity;(4) the paracolpos at the vaginal level, which extends from the vagina to the lateral wall of the pelvic cavity; and (5) the tendinous arch, which is a lateral fascial condensation [37]. Both the cardinal ligament and the paracolpos were described in the lateral compartment in the treatment of deep endometriosis.

The pubocervical fascia is a transverse layer extending from the pubis to the cervix, involving the bladder, urethra, and vagina, from the pericervical ring to the perineal membrane of the urogenital triangle (Fig. 4.162).

The rectovaginal fascia is a layer attached to the lower surface of the posterior and anterior vaginal walls of the rectum, suspended by the cardinal and uterosacral ligaments, distally by the perineal body and laterally by the tendinous arch. It supports the posterior compartment. Between this fascia and the rectum are the rectovaginal space and the pararectal space, important planes for dissection [35].

The cardinal ligament forms, together with the uterosacral pericervical ring, an important system of complex support for the uterus and the upper 1/3 of the vagina (Fig. 4.163). Ligaments are a thickening of the fascia [35].

The pelvic diaphragm comprises the levator ani and the coccygeal muscles. These muscles are easily visible in MRI, and our main emphasis will be on the levator.

The levator ani is the main muscle of the pelvic diaphragm, keeping the basal tone constant and closing the urogenital gap. It is inserted into the pubis and laterally into the tendinous arch of the levator ani. It is complex and subdivided according to the visceral insertions, such as the pubococcygeus and iliococcygeus (Fig. 4.164) [64].

The pubovisceral or pubococcygeus muscle and the puborectalis muscles have a U-shaped appearance, with fibers originating from the inner face of the pubis, encompassing the urethra, vagina, rectum, and anal canal. The puborectalis suspends the rectum by surrounding the anorectal junction. The pubococcygeal part is larger, Y-shaped, with insertion in the coccyx (levator plate). It is important for floor support and evacuation, and it is little affected by endometriosis (Fig. 4.164) [35].

The least dynamic component is the iliococcygeus. Located above the pubococcygeal muscle, it originates from the tendinous arch of the levator ani along the lateral wall of the pelvis and subsequently extends to the rectum (Figs. 4.164 and 4.165).

However, for endometriosis it is very important, just like the levator plate. Both are the most affected sites of the pelvis floor.

The urogenital diaphragm is caudal to the pelvic and anterior diaphragm, the perineal body, and the external anal sphincter. It has a triangular configuration between the lateral pubic bones and the posterior perineal body. It is comprised of the deep transverse perineal muscle and the urethral and urethrovaginal sphincters (Table 4.11 and Fig. 4.166).

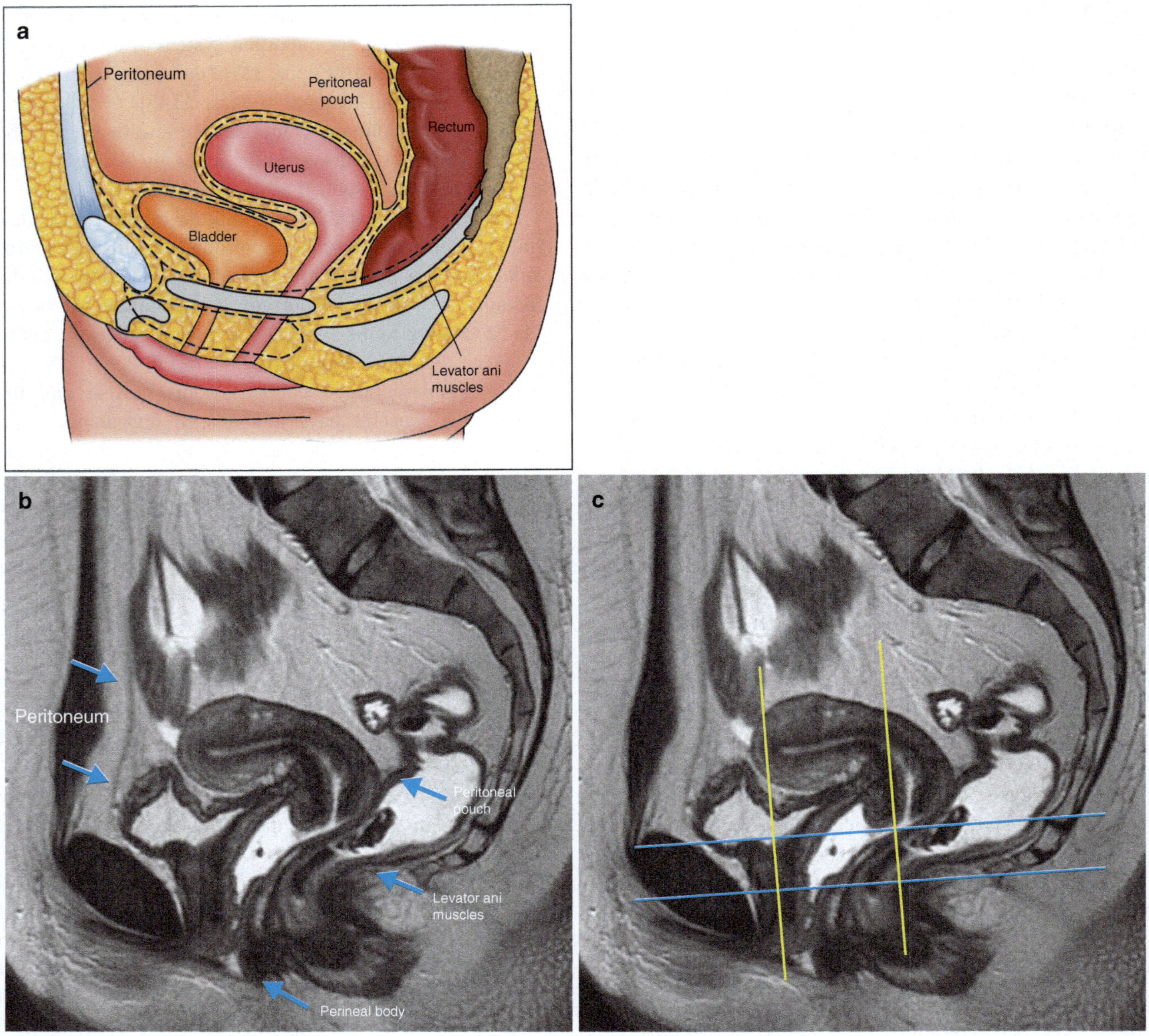

Fig. 4.162 Pelvic fascia. Formed by continuous pelvic connective tissue (dashed line), it covers the viscera under the peritoneum, extending inferiorly to the pelvic diaphragm (levator ani muscle and perineal body) and inserts laterally into the bony pelvis (arrows). Displays hyperintense signal on T2 (**b**, **d**–**g**). (**a**) Diagram for reference (**b**). (**b**, **c**) Sagittal. (**c**) Reference of axial and coronal images. (**d**, **e**) Axial in the plane of the pubocervical fascia. (**f**, **g**) Coronal of the fascia in the plane of the cervix and vagina (**f**) and urethra and bladder (yellow arrows **g**). T2-weighted sequences. Note deep bladder injury (red arrow **g**)

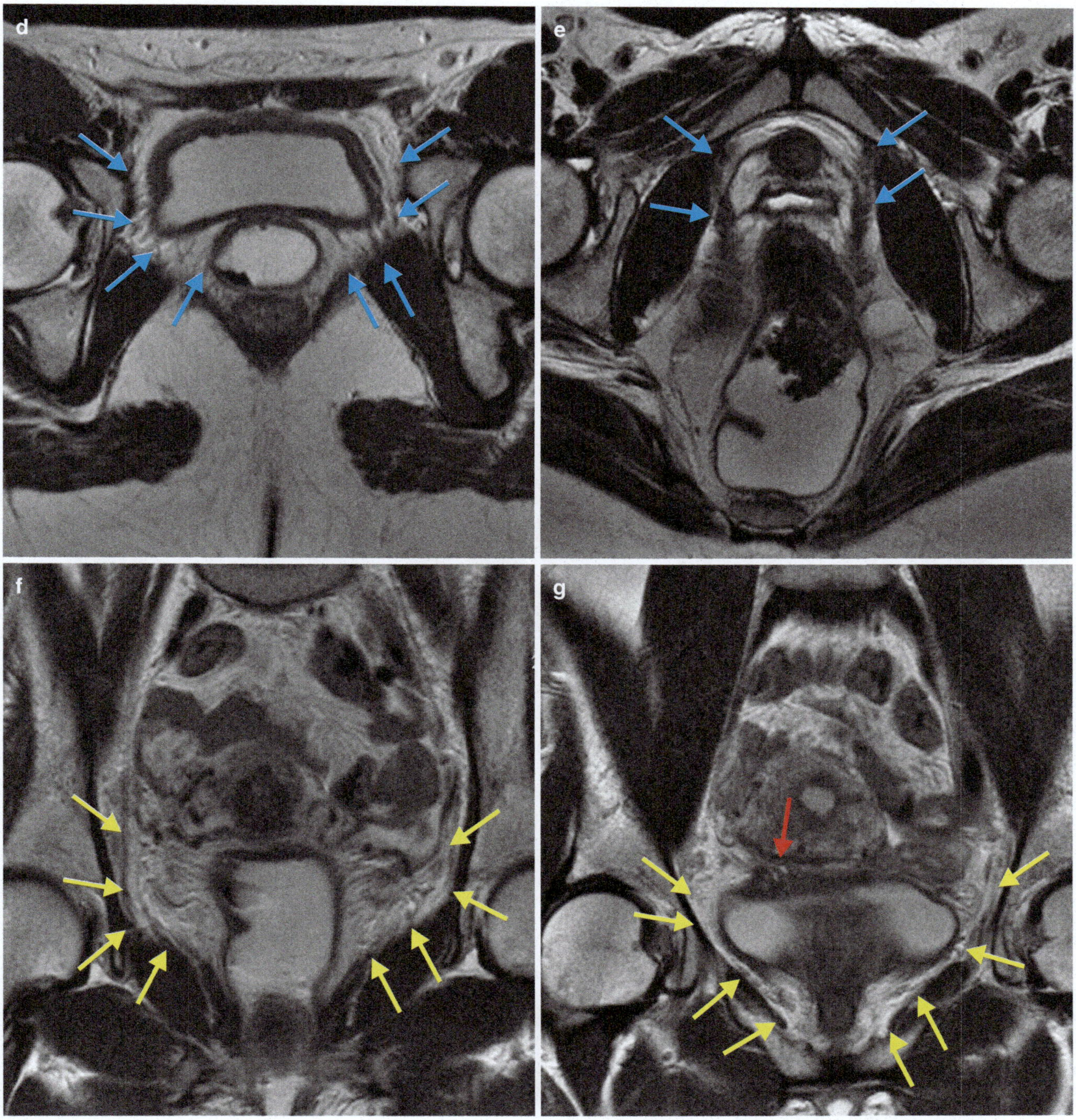

Fig. 4.162 (continued)

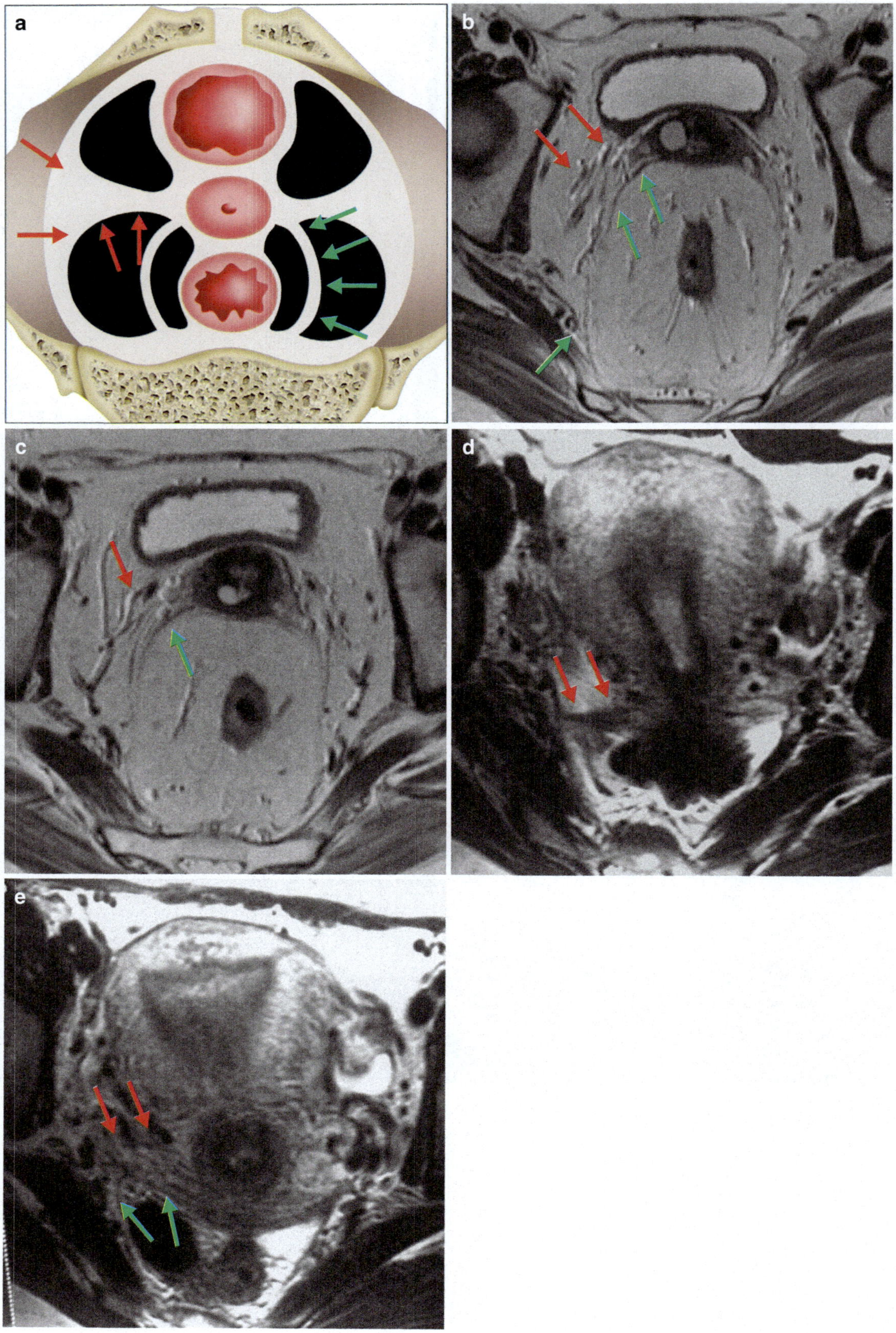

Fig. 4.163 Ligaments are a thickening of the fascia. The uterosacral (green arrows in **a–d**) and cardinal ligaments (red arrows **a–d**) form the pericervical ring, the support system for the uterus, and the upper third of the vagina. The cardinal ligaments merge laterally with the parietal fascia of the lateral pelvic muscles and the uterosacral ligaments with the presacral fascia (**a**). (**a**) Diagram from Ferdelle MP et al. Diagnostic and Surgical Imaging Anatomy: Chest, Abdomen, Pelvis. Lippincott, Williams & Wilkins, 2006. pp. 85, 86. (**b–d**) T2-weighted sequence. Axial

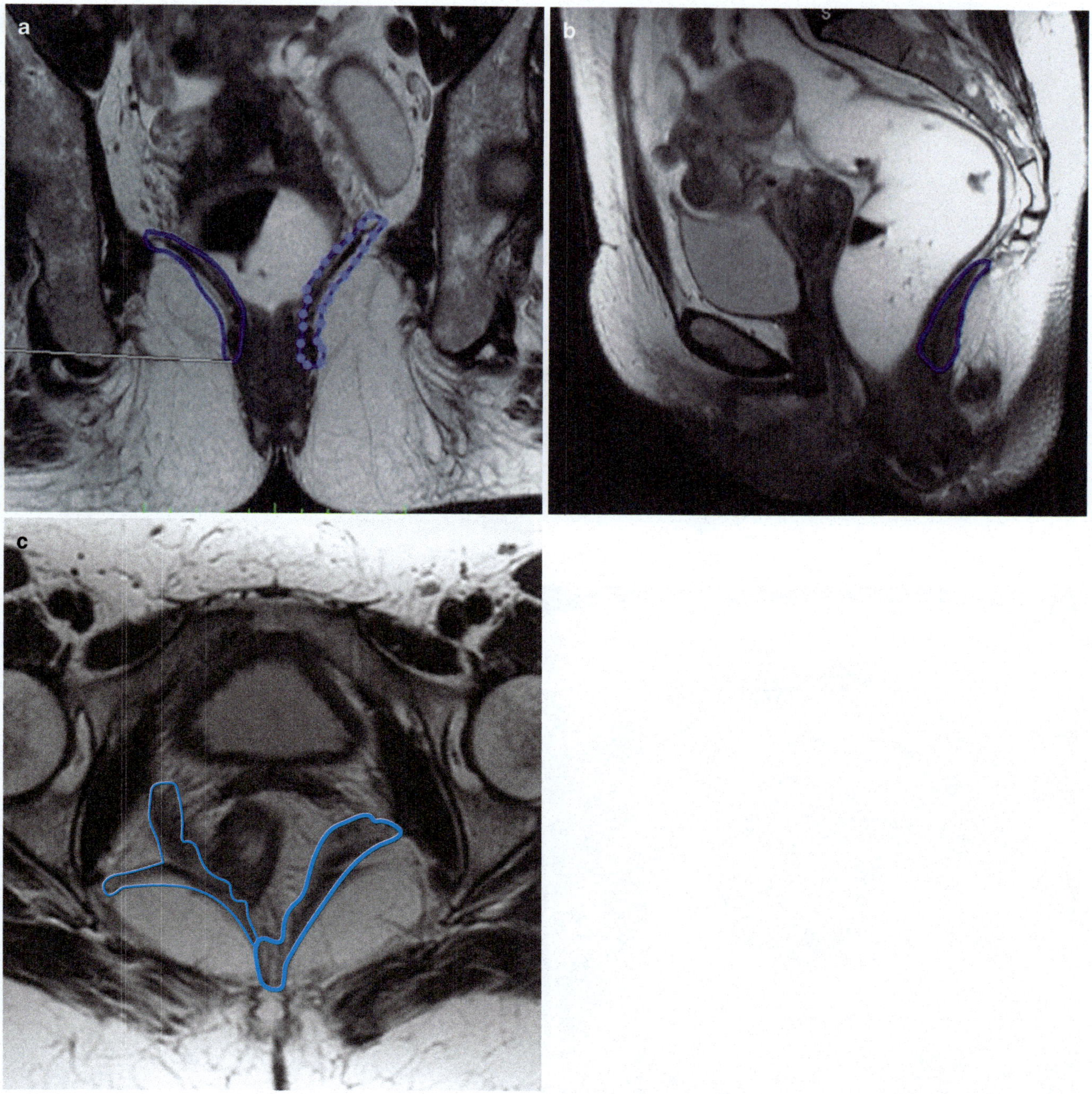

Fig. 4.164 The levator ani, the main muscle of the diaphragm, is subdivided according to its visceral insertions, as the puborectal, pubococcygeal, and iliococcygeal (**a**, **b** in blue). (**c**, **d**) Iliococcygeal outlined in blue. (**e**, **f**) Puborectal outlined in blue. (**a**–**c**) T2-weighted sequences. (**a**) Coronal. (**b**) Sagittal. (**c**–**f**) Axial

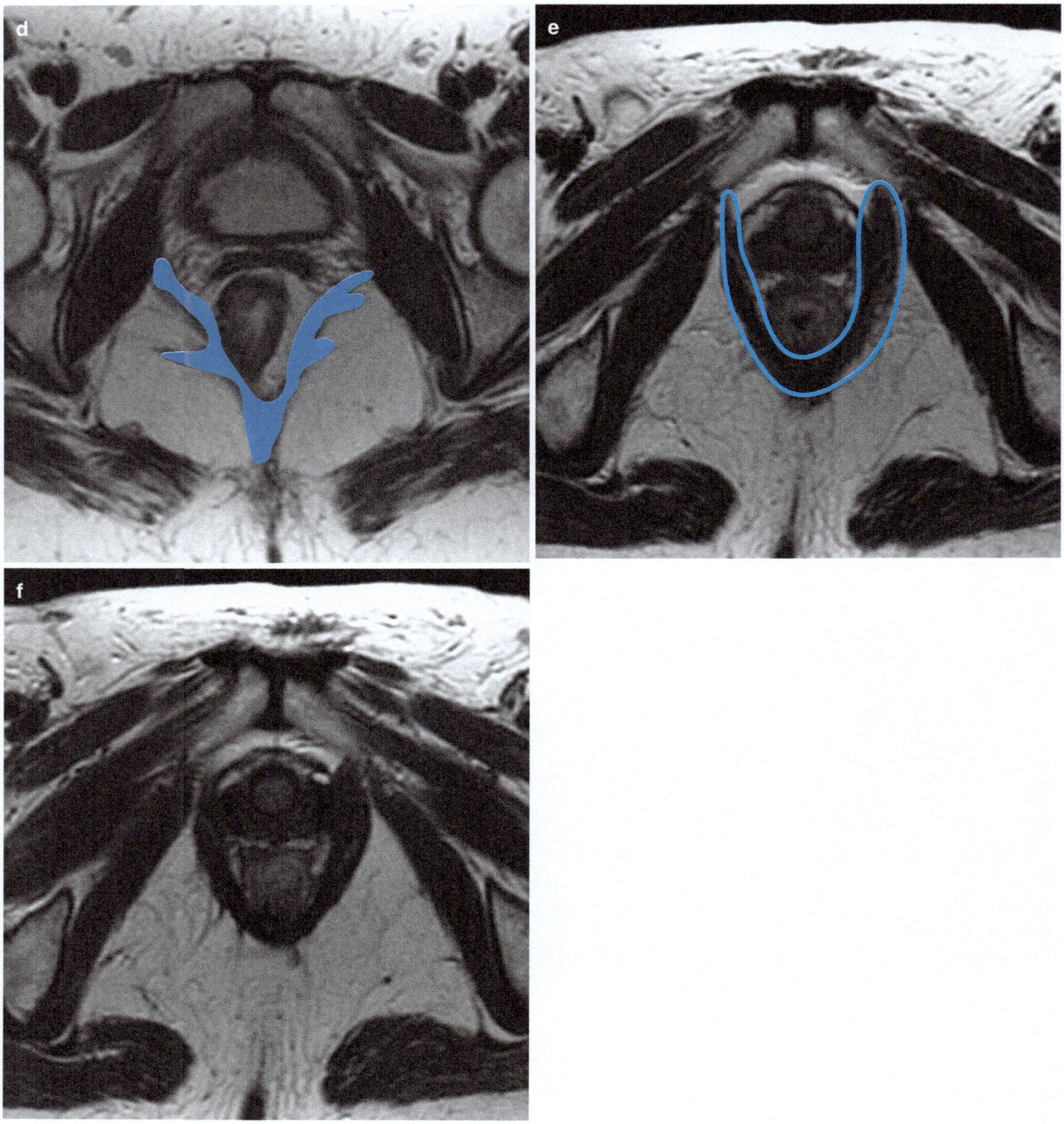

Fig. 4.164 (continued)

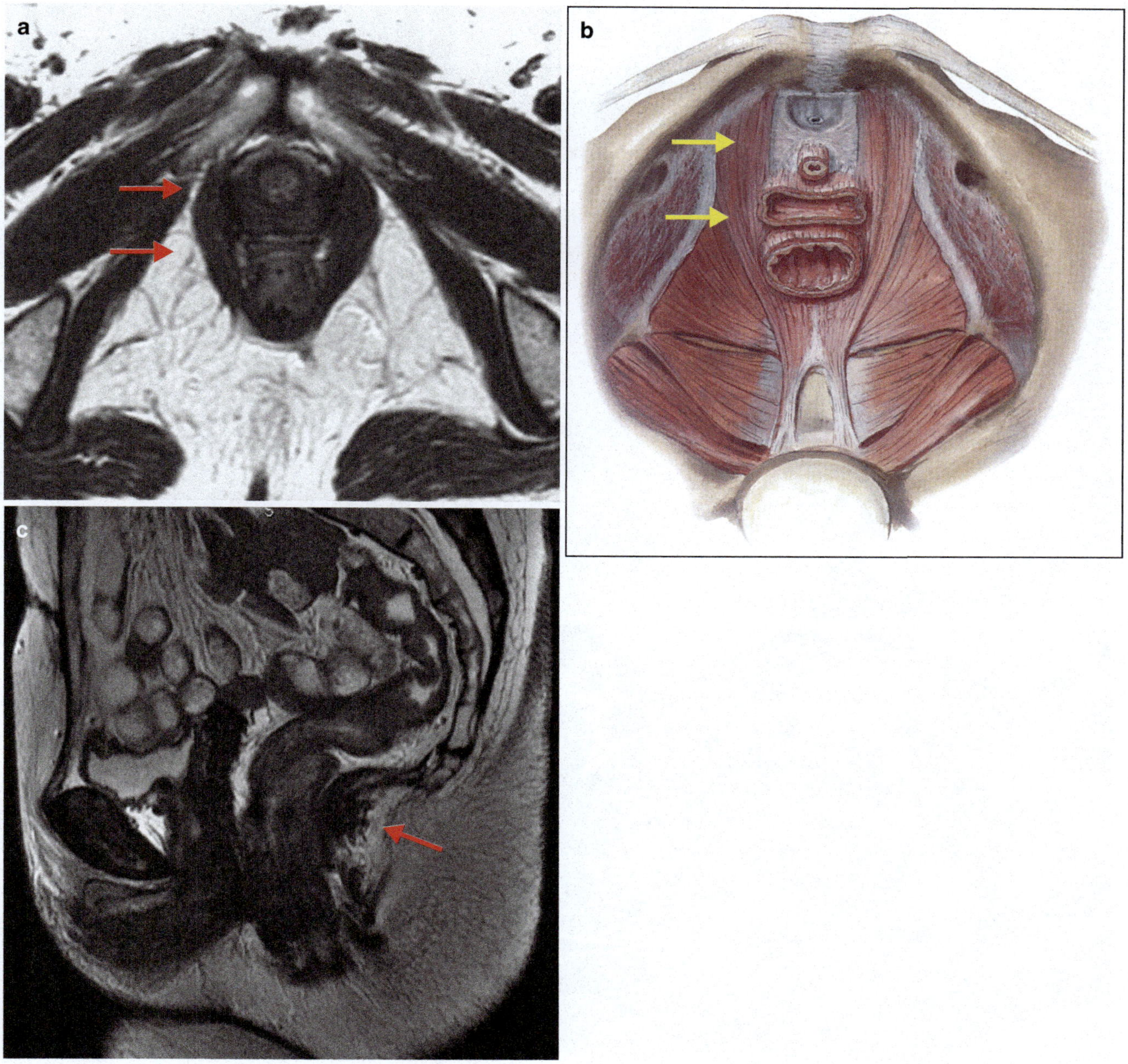

Fig. 4.165 Puborectal and pubococcygeal components of the levator ani (arrows in **a**, **b** and shaded in **h**). It has a U-shaped appearance and involves the urethra, vagina, rectum, and anal canal (**a**, **b**). Iliococcygeal component. Easily seen in the coronal (**d**), sagittal (**e**), and axial (**f**) planes on T2-weighted sequences. Extension with fan-like appearance of this muscle (arrows in **f**, **g**) and posterior insertion of the levator ani plaque in **e** (arrow). (**a**, **c**–**f**) T2-weighted sequences. (**a**, **d**) Axial. (**c**, **e**) Sagittal. (**b**, **g**) Anatomy. (**h**) Laparoscopy after dissection of the floor, with identification of the levator ani beyond the piriformis

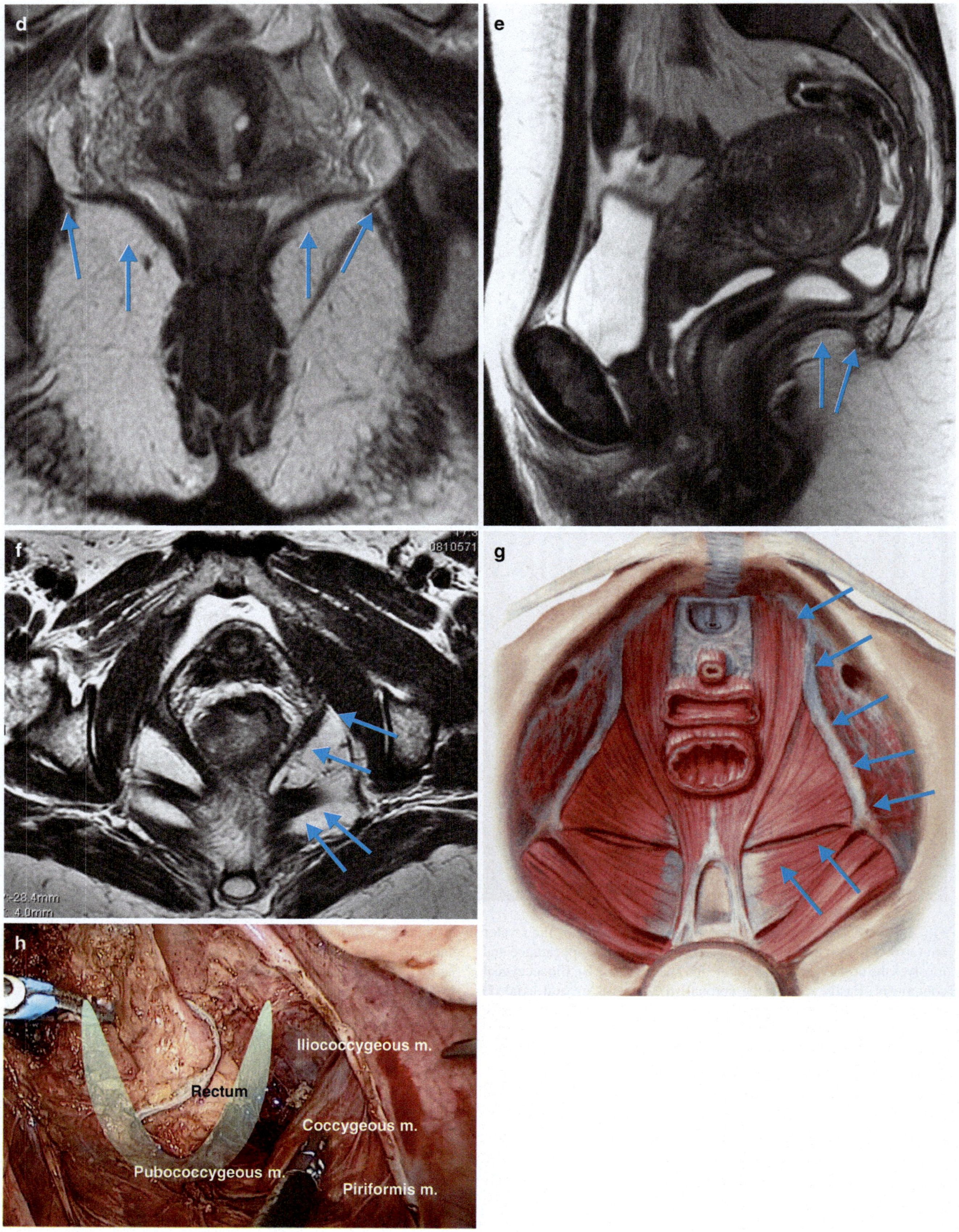

Fig. 4.165 (continued)

Table 4.11 Pelvic floor components

Pelvic fascia	The pubocervical fascia The rectovaginal fascia The parametrium (included in the lateral compartment) The paracolpos (included in the lateral compartment) The tendinous arch
Pelvic diaphragm	The levator ani (puborectal, pubococcygeal and iliococcygeus) and coccygeal
Urogenital diaphragm	Deep transverse perineal muscle Urethral and urethrovaginal sphincters

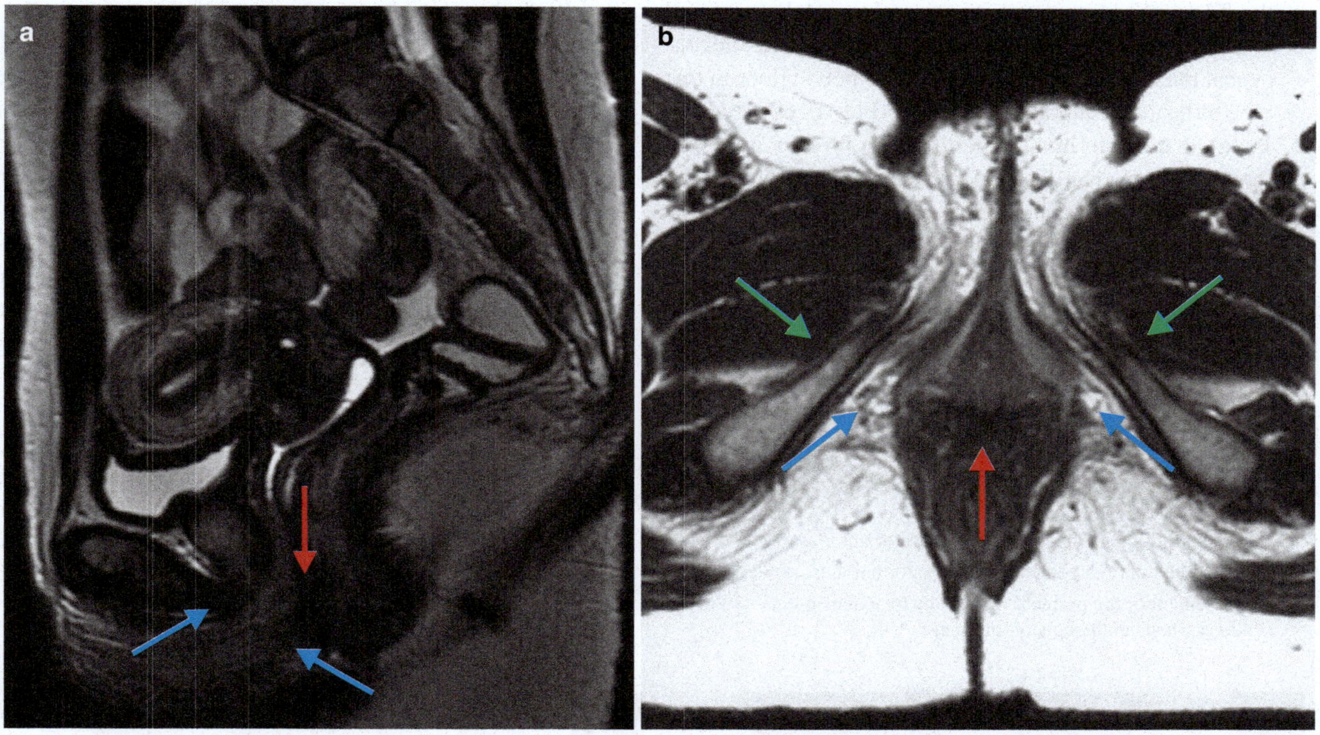

Fig. 4.166 (**a**) The urogenital diaphragm (blue arrows) is caudal to the pelvic diaphragm and anterior to the perineal body (red arrows) and the external anal sphincter. (**b**) It has a triangular configuration between the lateral pubic bones (green arrow) and the posterior perineal body (red arrows). It may be affected by deep endometriosis when there is an episiotomy scar. (**a**, **b**) T2-weighted sequences. (**a**) Sagittal. (**b**) Axial

4.3.4.2 Most Common Aspects of Endometriosis in MRI and Laparoscopic Findings

Little is found in the literature on the description of endometriosis of the pelvic floor. In our experience, the involvement follows four patterns (Table 4.12).

1. **Involvement by inferior extension of lesion of the rectovaginal septum**: usually the lesion is large and infiltrative, with a predominance of fibrosis (hypointense in the T2-weighted sequence and with an intermediate signal in the T1, with discreet enhancement by gadolinium) and inferior spicules that touch and may penetrate the iliococcygeal muscle. The involvement of the pelvic floor in this type of lesion is lateral, paramedian (Fig. 4.167).
2. **Isolated midline involvement of the levator ani**: very rare, with a median location between the insertion of the levator plate and the anococcygeal ligament. The lesion is well delimited and unilocular and shows a signal intensity similar to that of an endometrioma, with a well-delimited cyst containing mostly old blood, hyperintense in the T1-weighted sequence, and hypointense in the T2-weighted sequence, without enhancement by gadolinium (Fig. 4.168).

   The differential diagnosis is a congenital retrorectal cyst originating in the primitive intestine, located at the retrorectal space, in relation with the coccyx. Among the possibilities for a unilocular congentital cyst are included dermoid and epidermoid cysts. However, endometriosis is located outside the retrorectal space, below the anococcygeal ligament insertion (Fig. 4.169).
3. **Isolated lateral involvement of the levator ani muscle**: very rare and characterized by a lateral lesion, involving the iliococcygeal muscle, with proximity to the lateral wall of the pelvis, sacral roots, and the sciatic nerve. Usually the lesion is poorly delimited, with an infiltrative pattern and a predominance of fibrosis. Glandular tissue can be identified and helps the radiologist identify minor lesions (Fig. 4.170).
4. **Involvement of the perineal membrane by extension of endometriosis in the episiotomy scar**: this type of lesion occurs by implantation of ectopic endometrial tissue after normal delivery, in the episiotomy scar, with an incidence of 0.06–0.07%. It may be explained by the mechanical dissemination of viable deciduous endometrial cells transplanted during normal delivery with episiotomy or perineal injury, with subsequent growth [30].

Table 4.12 Most common aspects of pelvic floor endometriosis

– Involvement by inferior extension of lesion of the rectovaginal septum
– Isolated midline involvement of the levator ani muscle
– Isolated lateral involvement of the levator ani muscle
– Involvement of the perineal membrane by extension of endometriosis in the episiotomy scar

It occurs more in young multiparous women, and the lesion has an infiltrative aspect with a paramedian location near the midline, close to the perineal body, perineal membrane (perineal transverse muscle), and external anal sphincter (Fig. 4.171).

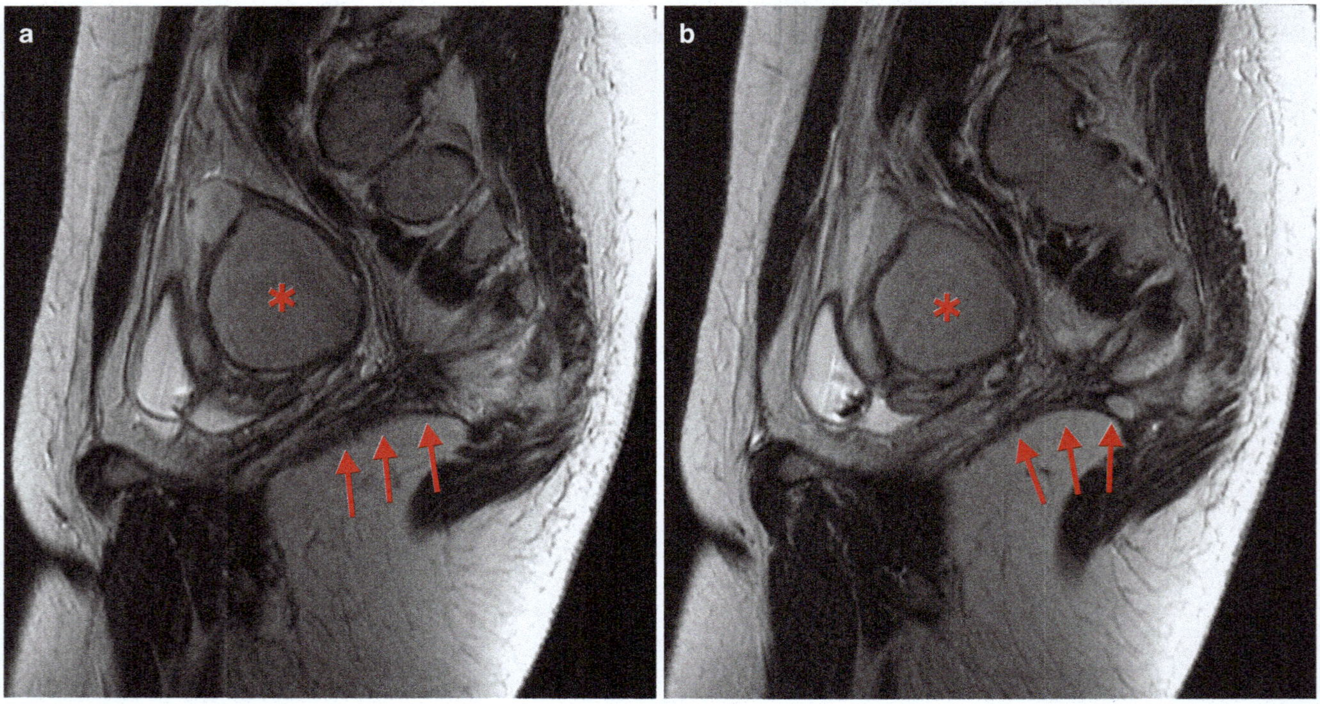

Fig. 4.167 Involvement by inferior extension of rectovaginal lesion. Infiltrative lesion with predominant fibrosis (hypointense on T2-weighted sequence and intermediary signal on T1, with slight gadolinium enhancement) with inferior spicules which touch the iliococcygeus muscle (red arrows). (**a–e**) T2-weighted sequences. (**a, b**) Sagittal. (**c**) Coronal short axis. (**d, e**) Axial. Note involvement of the uterosacral ligament (blue arrow in **e**), rectal (green arrow in **d, e**), and endometrioma (*)

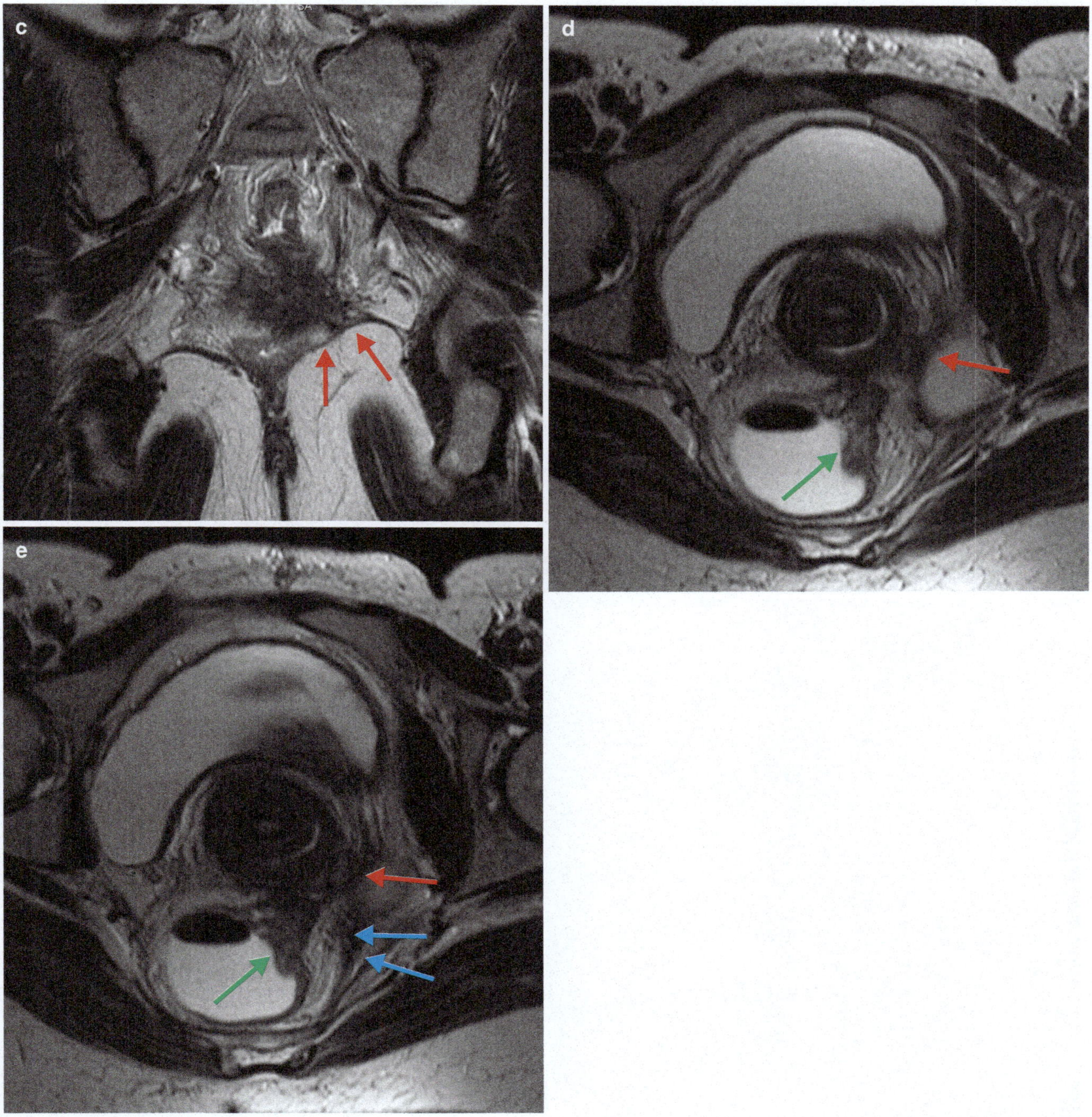

Fig. 4.167 (continued)

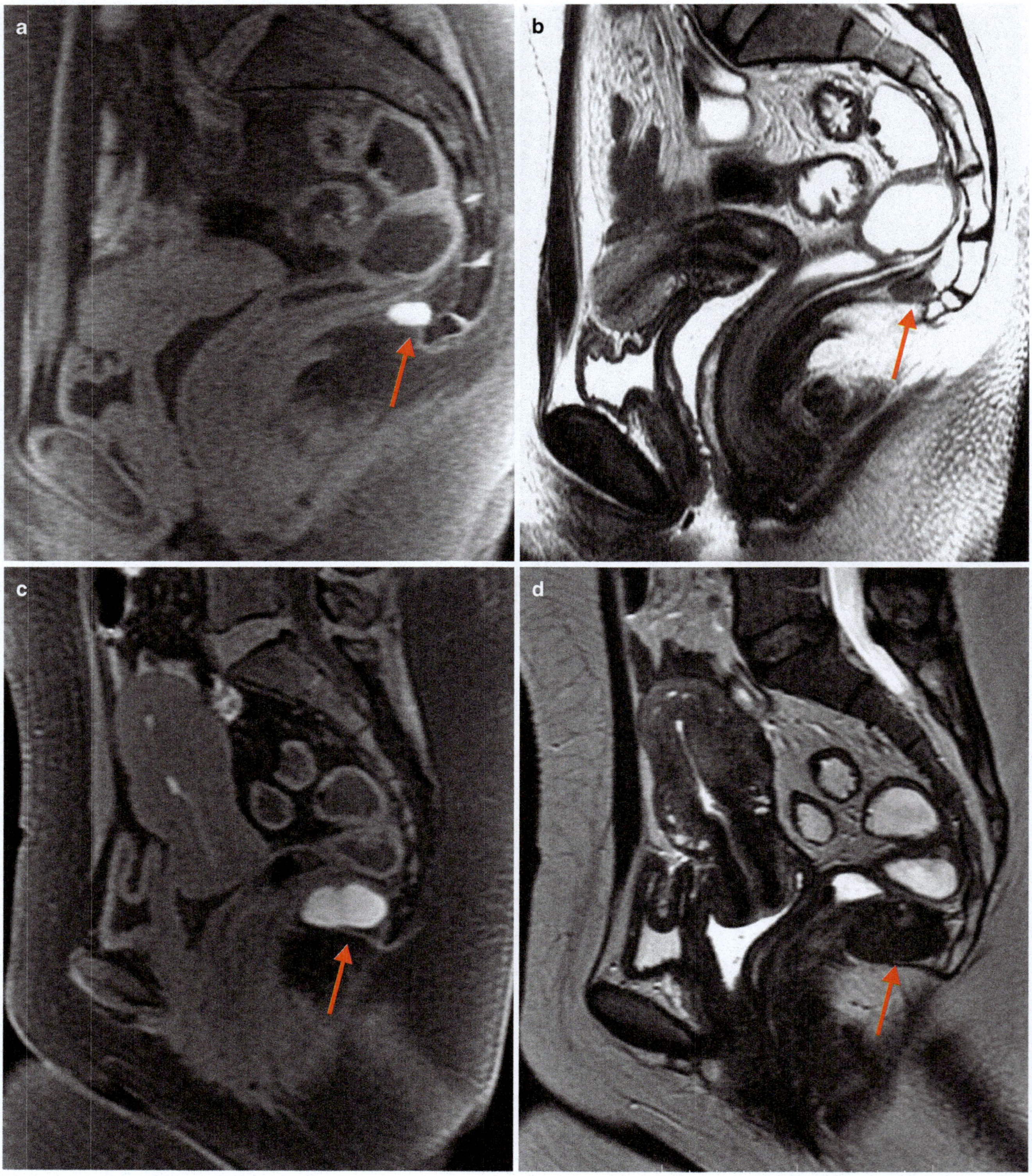

Fig. 4.168 Isolated involvement of the levator ani with central location, between the insertion of the levator ani plate and the anococcygeal ligament. Case 1 (**a**, **b**) and Case 2 (**c**, **d**). The lesion (arrows) is well defined, cystic, and unilocular, with a signal similar to that of endometrioma, hyperintense in T1-weighted sequences (**a**, **c**) and hypointense on T2 (**b**, **d**). (**a**–**d**) Sagittal

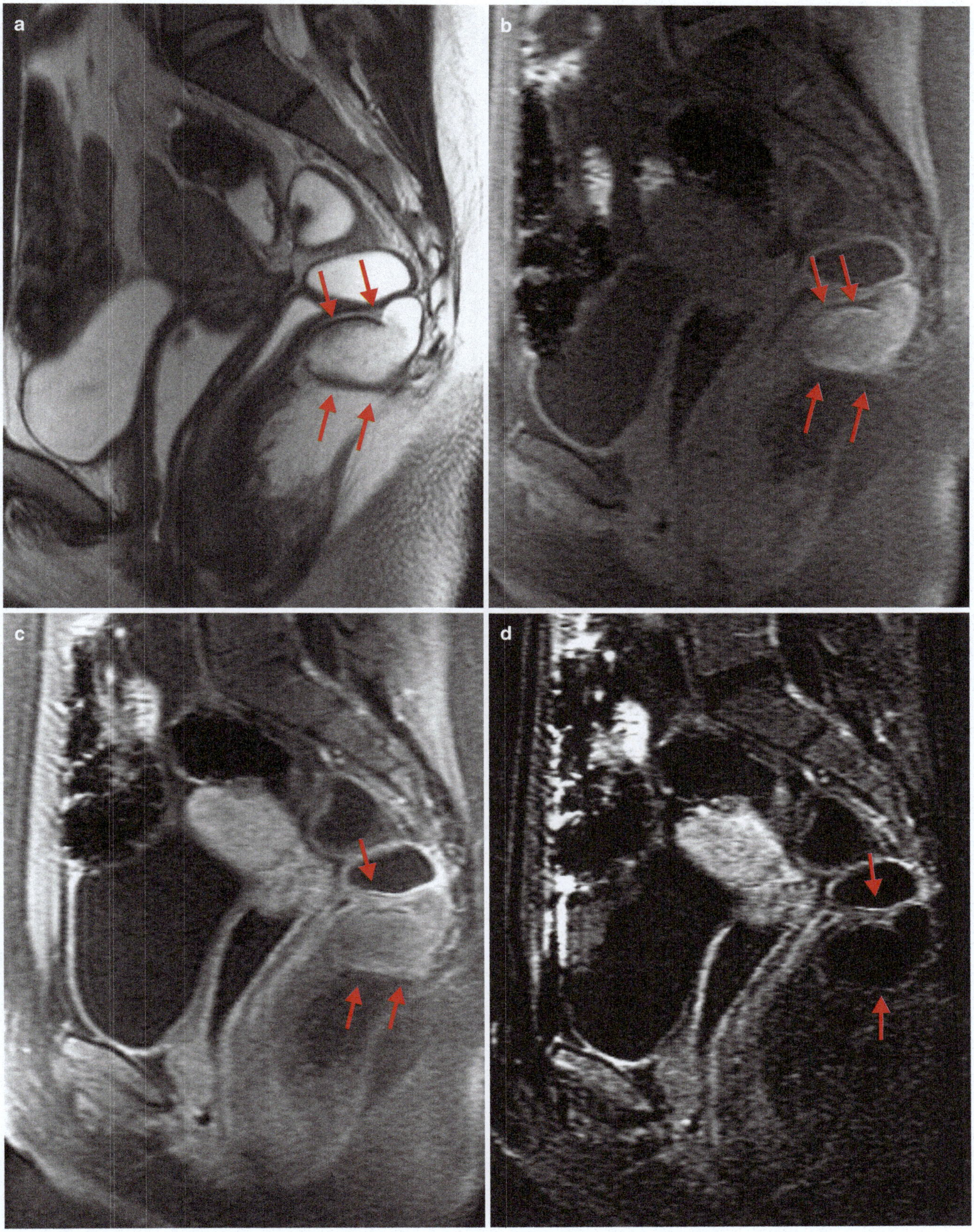

Fig. 4.169 Unilocular epidermoid cyst of the retrorectal space, hyperintense on T2-weighted sequences (**a**) and T1 (**b**, **c**), without enhancement by gadolinium (note the subtraction image [**d**]). (**a–d**) Sagittal. (**b–d**) T1-weighted sequences

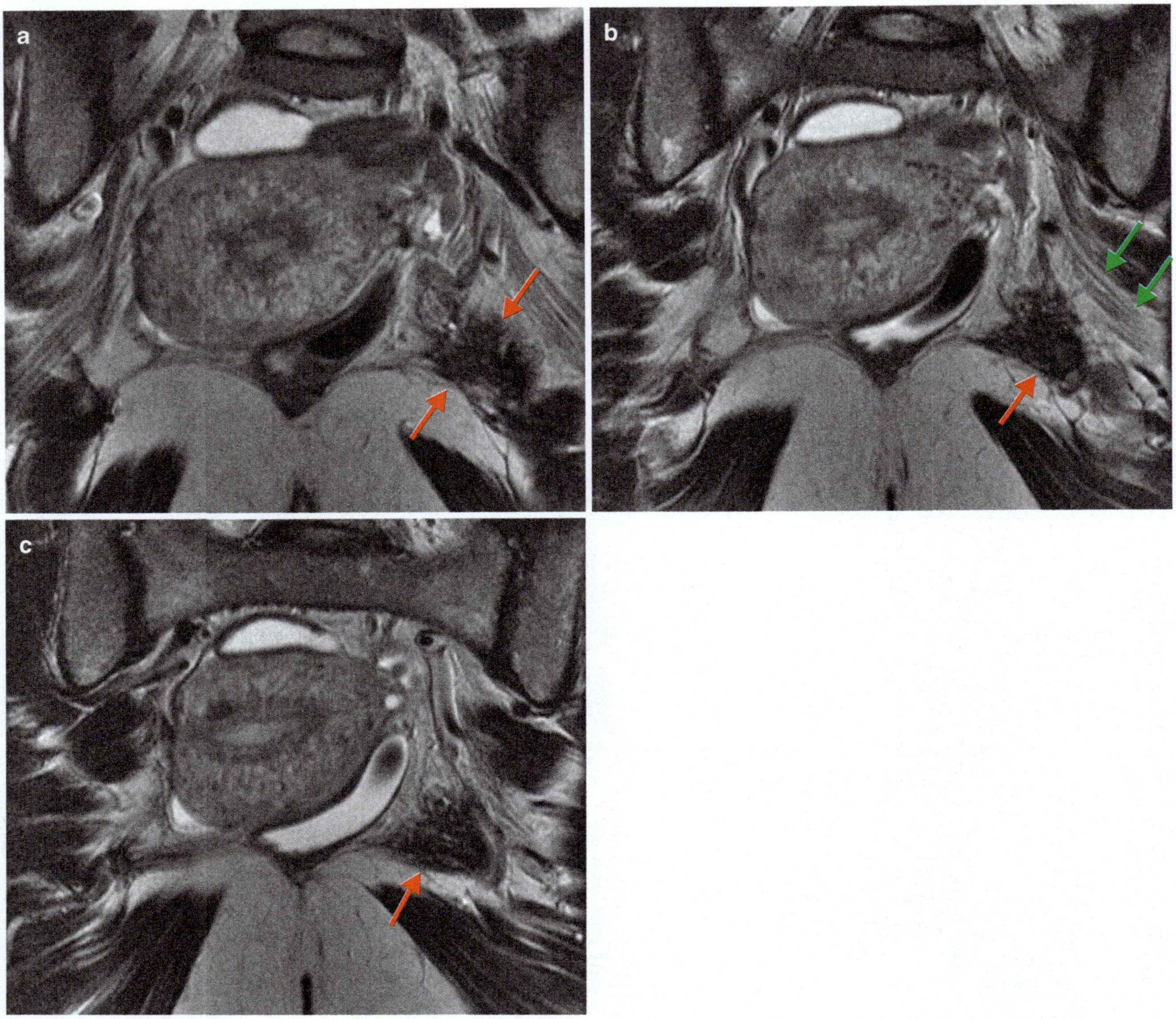

Fig. 4.170 Lateral isolated involvement on the left levator ani muscle. Lesion with infiltrative pattern and prevalence of fibrosis involving the iliococcygeus muscle (arrows) in close proximity to the side wall of the pelvis, sacral plexus, and sciatic nerve (green arrows in **b**). (**a**–**c**) T2-weighted sequences. Coronal

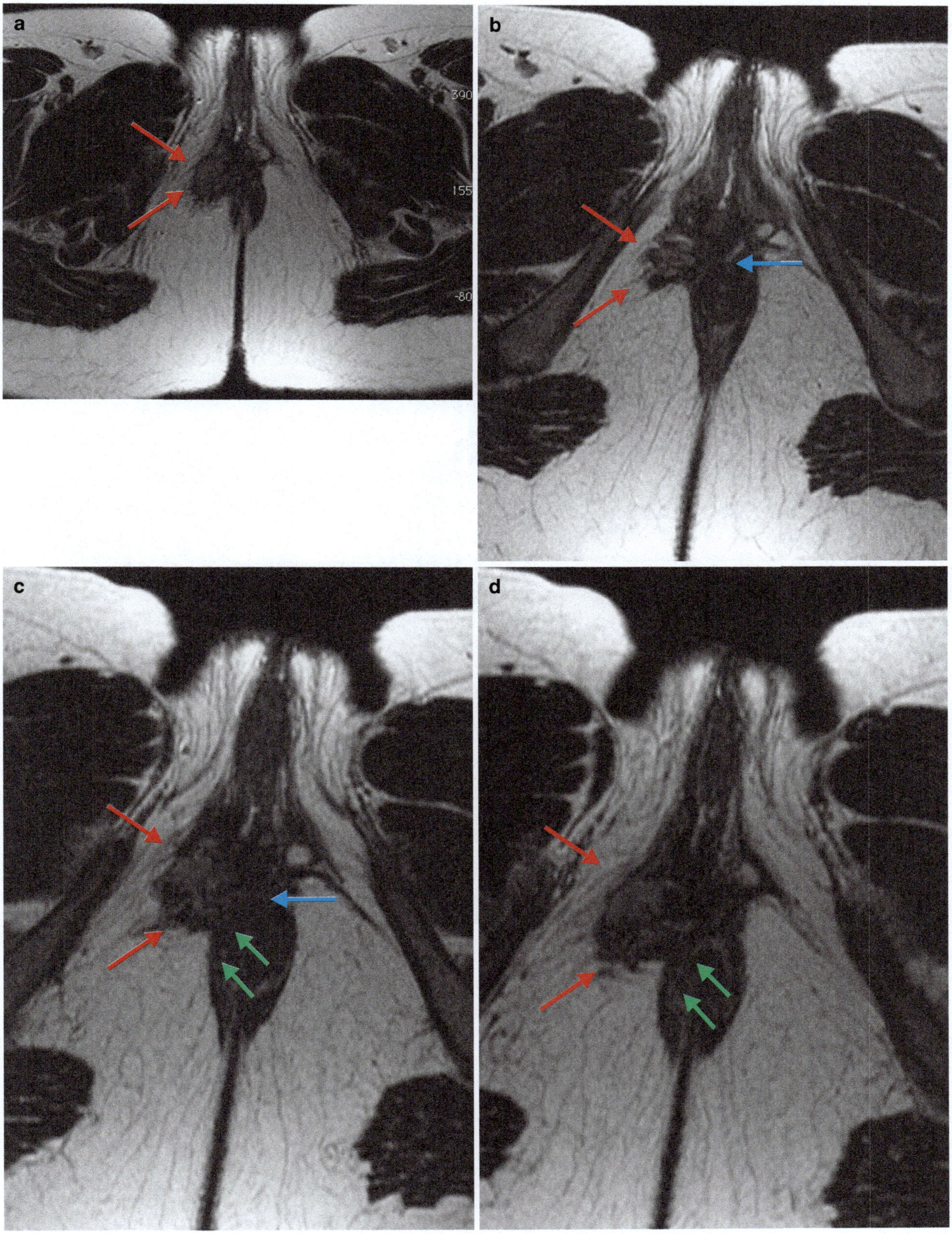

Fig. 4.171 Lesion of the urogenital diaphragm after episiotomy (red arrows). Slightly hyperintense infiltrative lesions on T2-weighted sequence with hemorrhagic foci (hyperintense on T1-weighted sequence [**f**]) and gadolinium enhancement (**g**), located at the right urogenital diaphragm, with slight involvement of the perineal body (blue arrow) and anal external sphincter (green arrow). (**a–e**, **h**) T2-weighted sequences. (**f**) T1-weighted sequence with fat saturation and **g** with gadolinium. (**a–f**) Axial. (**h**) Coronal

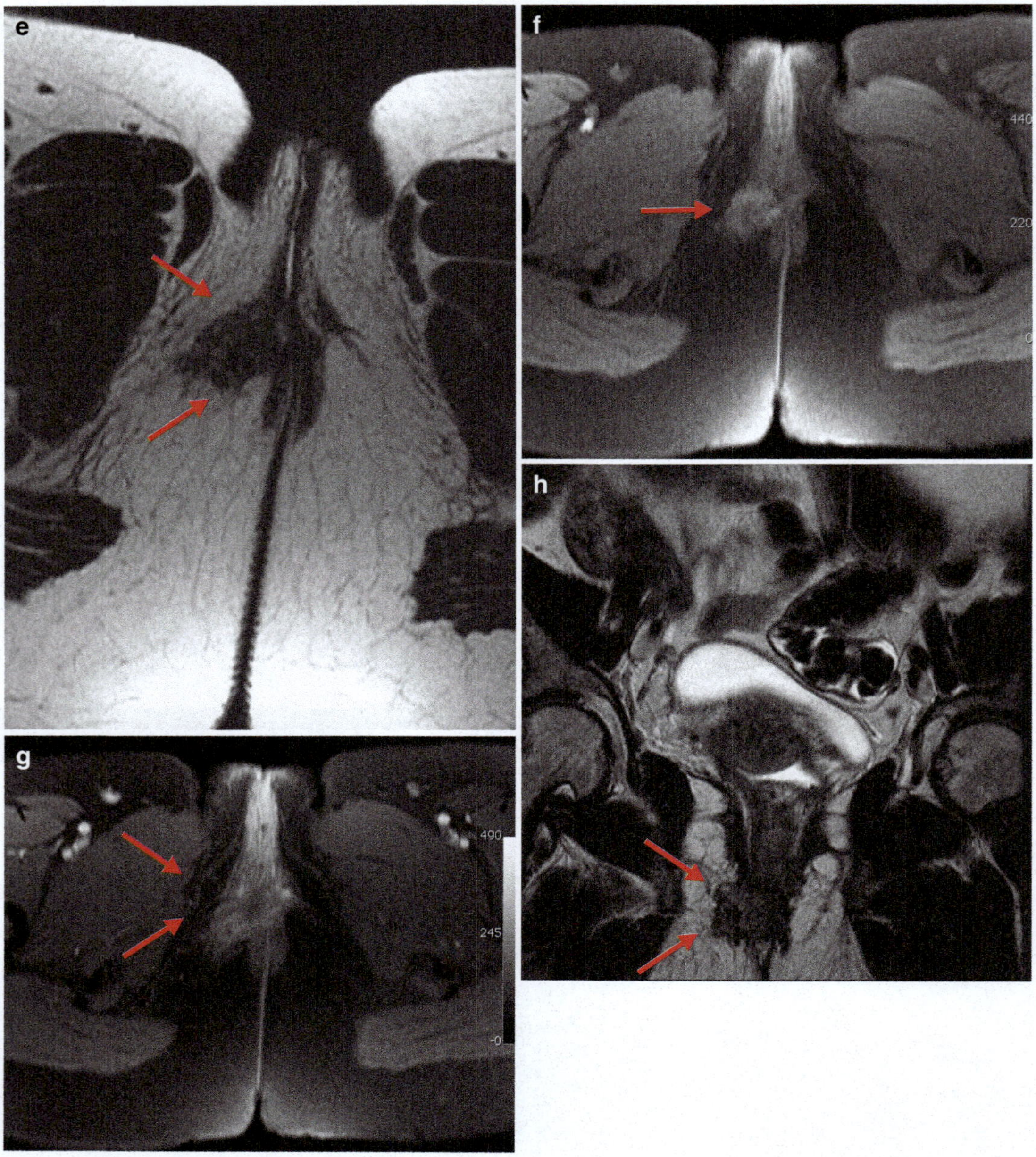

Fig. 4.171 (continued)

4.3.4.3 Clinical Presentation

The literature describes levator syndrome only as a consequence of pain in this region. This syndrome is little known, with diagnosis of exclusion related to chronic perianal pain, marked with defecation.

However, the clinical picture is not specific, except for vaginal delivery scar related to endometriosis, with intensified perineal pain during the menstrual cycle.

4.3.4.4 Comments on Treatments

The lesion must be resected and involves an increase in surgical complexity due to the need to operate in pelvic spaces where there are important structures, particularly nerves.

In the case of perineal lesion after episiotomy, a broad excision of the endometrial tissue is necessary, which may involve resection of part of the external anal sphincter [31].

4.3.5 Ovarian Fossa

It is important to emphasize that the authors chose to describe only deep lesions of the ovarian fossa. These lesions may arise from the contact with an ovarian endometrioma in this region.

However, ovarian endometrioma itself will not be addressed in this atlas, because of its complexity; it is usually studied separately, outside the topic of deep endometriosis.

4.3.5.1 Anatomy

The ovarian fossa is a shallow depression of the parietal, lateral, and posterior peritoneum in the pelvis, delimited superiorly by the external iliac vessels, anteriorly by the broad ligament and mesovarium, and posteriorly by the ureter and internal iliac vessels (Fig. 4.172) [65].

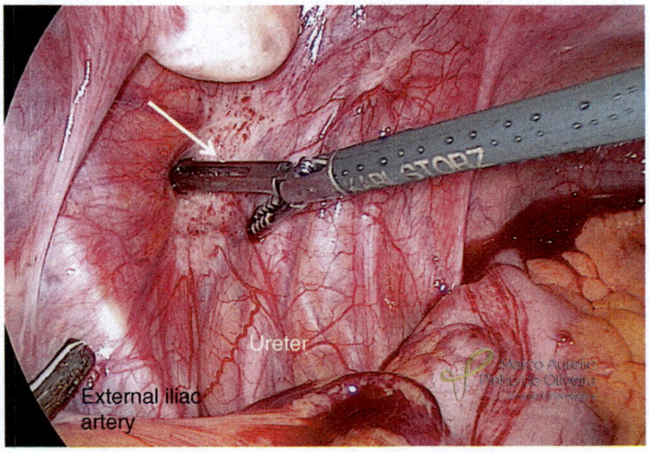

Fig. 4.172 Laparoscopy identifying lesion in the ovarian fossa. Lateral and posterior location, defined superiorly by the external iliac vessels, anteriorly by the broad ligament and mesovarium, and posteriorly by the ureter and internal iliac vessels

4.3.5.2 Common Aspects of Endometriosis

The ovarian fossa can be involved by the superficial ovarian bleeding and endometrioma, causing adherence of the fallopian tube and the ovary to the lateral wall of the pelvis, as well as the parametrium, the uterosacral ligament, and on the left side the sigmoid, promoting modification in the attachment position and ligament and intestinal retractions (Fig. 4.173).

This process may superficially involve the peritoneum of the ovarian fossa and develop into a deep lesion with penetration greater than 5 mm [66].

The deep involvement may extend laterally to the parieto-colic gutters, superior to the sigmoid, and inferior to the parametrium (Fig. 4.174).

4.3.5.3 Clinical Condition

Isolated ovarian endometriosis is usually asymptomatic. Thus, the presence of severe pain in a patient with endometrioma suggests coexistence of infiltrative endometriosis and adhesion. In these patients, the analysis of the images should be systematic because underestimation of the severity and extent of the infiltrative process is one of the main reasons for inadequate surgery [33].

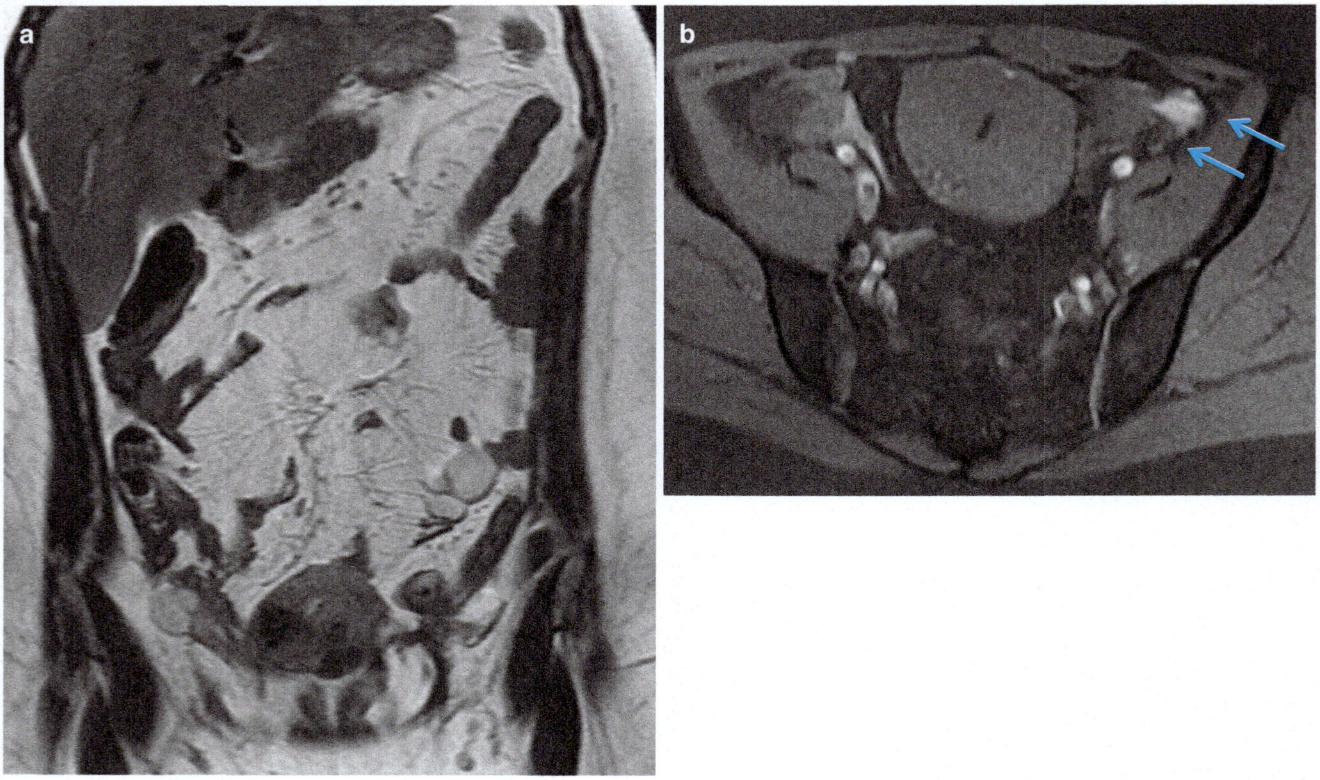

Fig. 4.173 Adherence on the left ovarian fossa, involving the fallopian tube and ovary, distorted by the deep endometrial process (arrows **b**–**d**), which also involves the descending colon, sigmoid, parieto-colic gutter, and the round ligament (arrows to **b**, **e**–**g**). (**a**, **c**–**f**) T2-weighted sequences. (**b**) T1-weighted with axial fat suppression (note bleeding). (**a**) Coronal of the abdomen and pelvis. (**c**–**e**) short axis. (**f**) Coronal long axis. (**g**) Laparoscopy showing extensive adhesions in the pelvis and toward the left ovarian fossa (arrows)

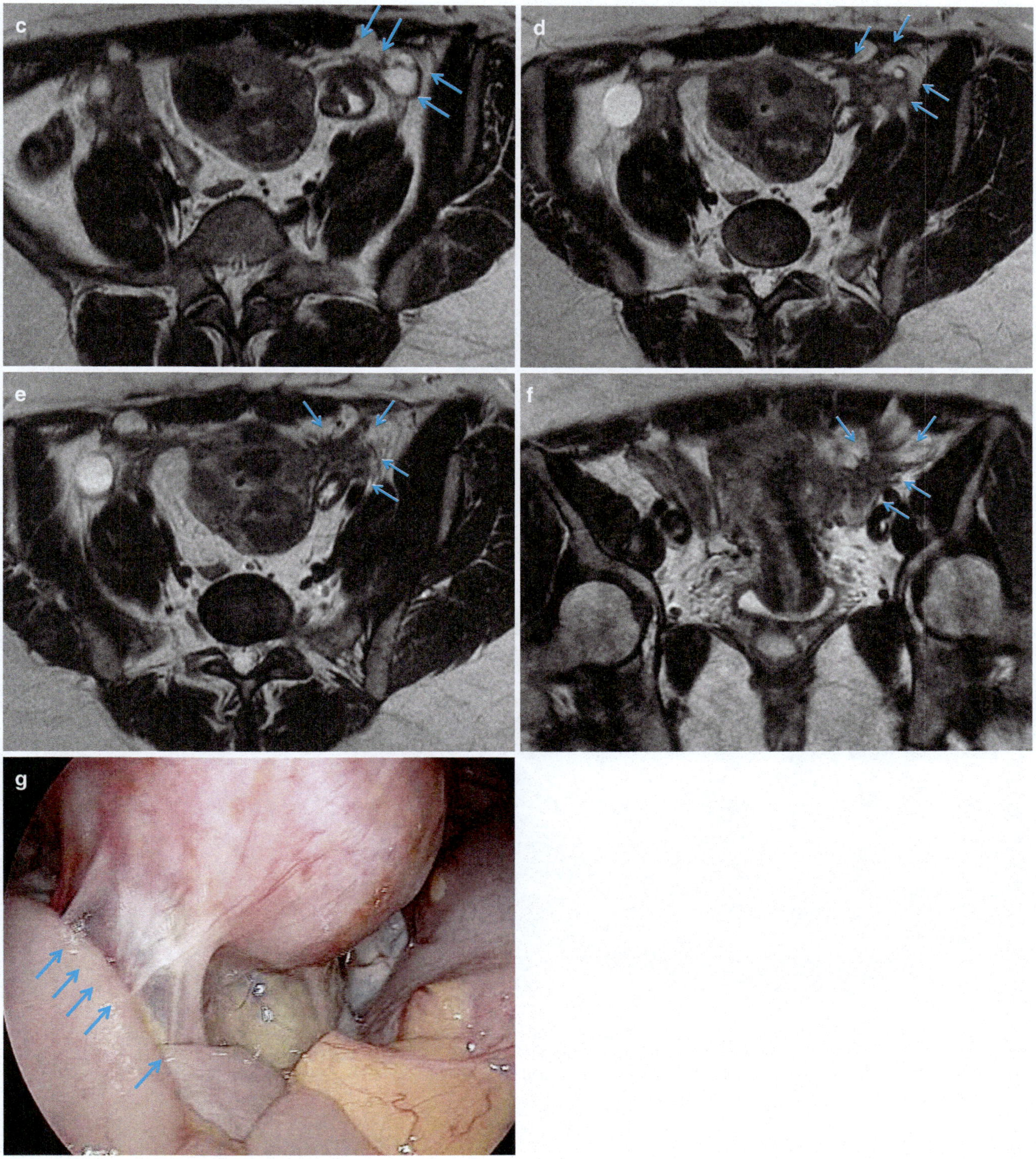

Fig. 4.173 (continued)

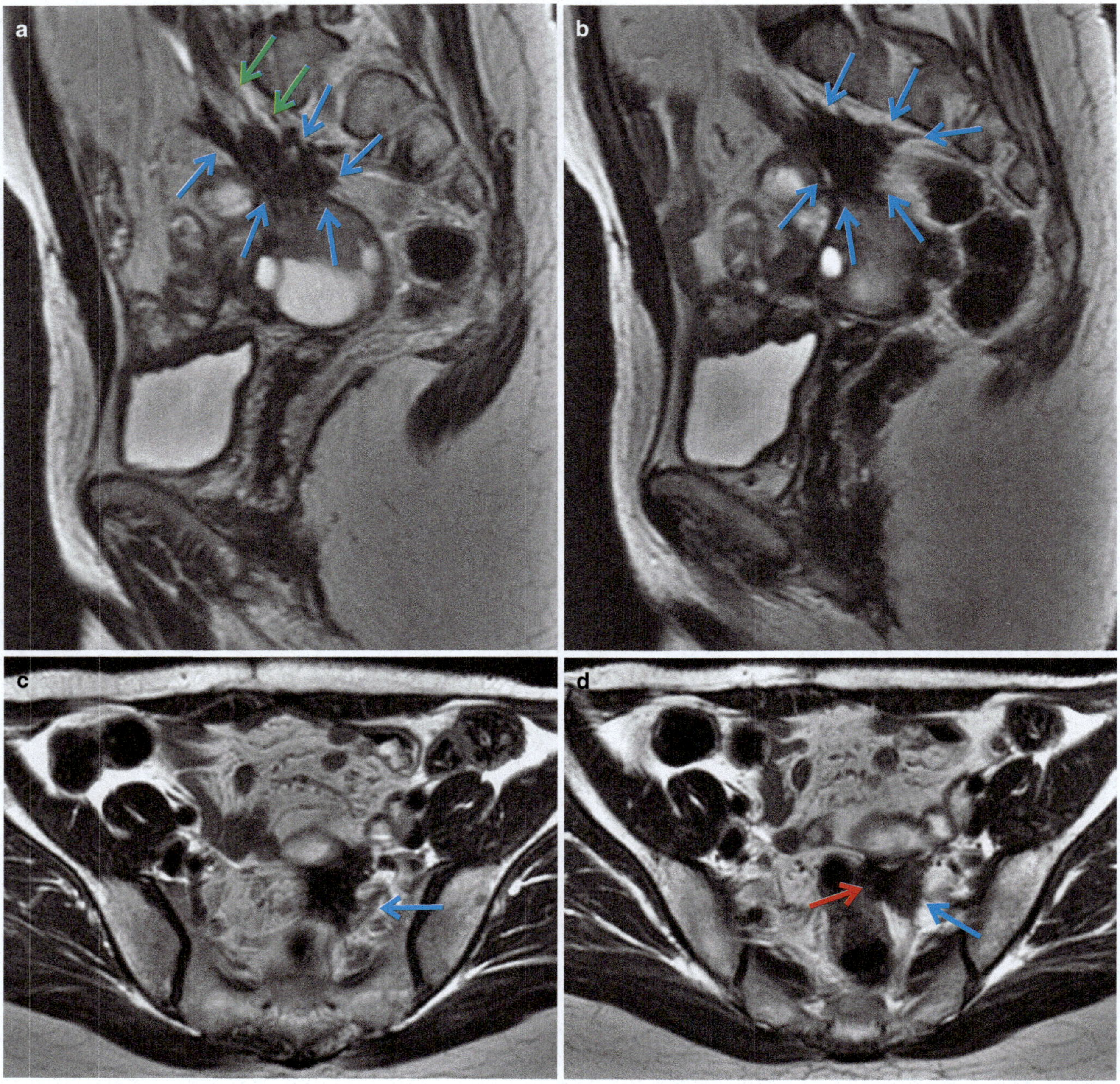

Fig. 4.174 Lesion in the left adnexa, involving the ovarian fossa, infiltrative, hypointense on T2 (blue arrows) with involvement of the sigmoid (red arrow in **d**) and near the ureter (green arrows in **a**) and vascular and presacral nerve structures. Endometrioma (*). (**a–d**) T2-weighted sequences. (**a**, **b**) Sagittal. (**c**, **d**) Axial. (**e–h**) Laparoscopy showing lesion (**e**), resection of the lesion, and ureterolysis (**f–h**)

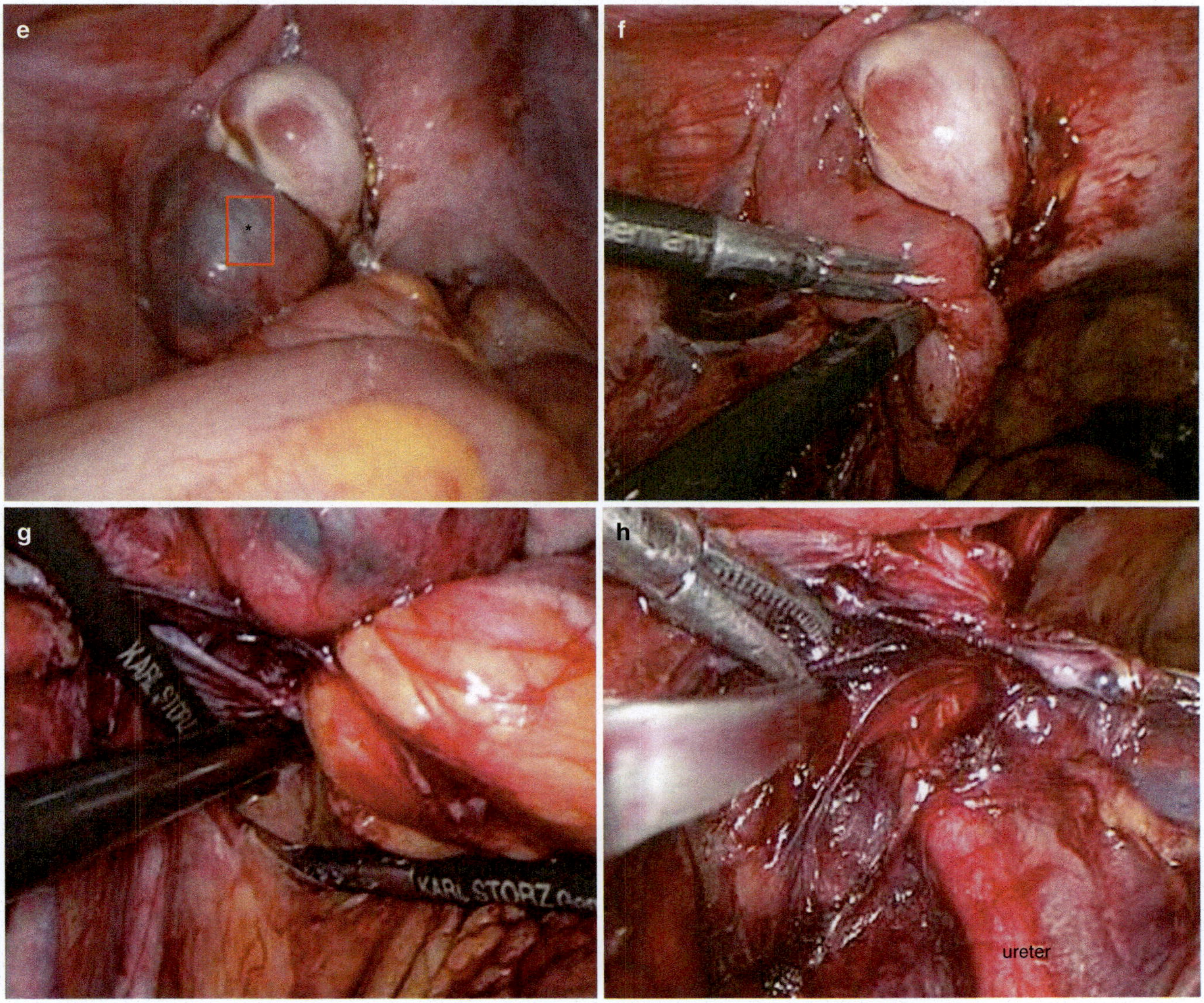

Fig. 4.174 (continued)

4.3.5.4 MRI and Laparoscopic Findings

Deep involvement in the ovarian fossa may go undetected by MRI and laparoscopy, especially when the lesions are small.

It is important to analyze the parietal peritoneum in the parieto-colic gutter, evaluate the parametrium, and especially look for any impairment of the ureteral tract to the vesical trigone, and the inferior hypogastric plexus and sigmoid branch just above the left ovary.

In the parieto-colic gutter, there is peritoneal thickening with subperitoneal penetration of the lesion, with proximity to the iliac vessels, and it is important to rule out thrombosis by vascular involvement (Fig. 4.175).

In the parametrium, the lesion may be small but aggressive, due to the greater probability of ureteral involvement, and of the vesical branch of the inferior hypogastric plexus (Fig. 4.176).

In the sigmoid the lesion promotes deep intestinal penetration, with the same characteristics as the other intestinal lesions, being able to evolve to luminal occlusion (Fig. 4.177).

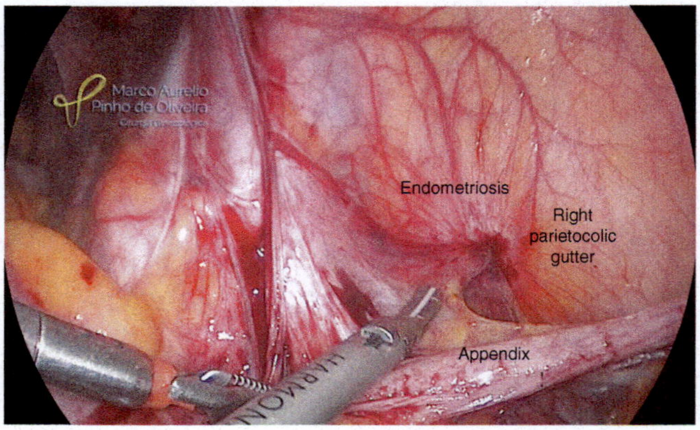

Fig. 4.175 Laparoscopy. Peritoneal thickening in the parieto-colic gutter with subperitoneal penetration of the lesion, close to the iliac vessels

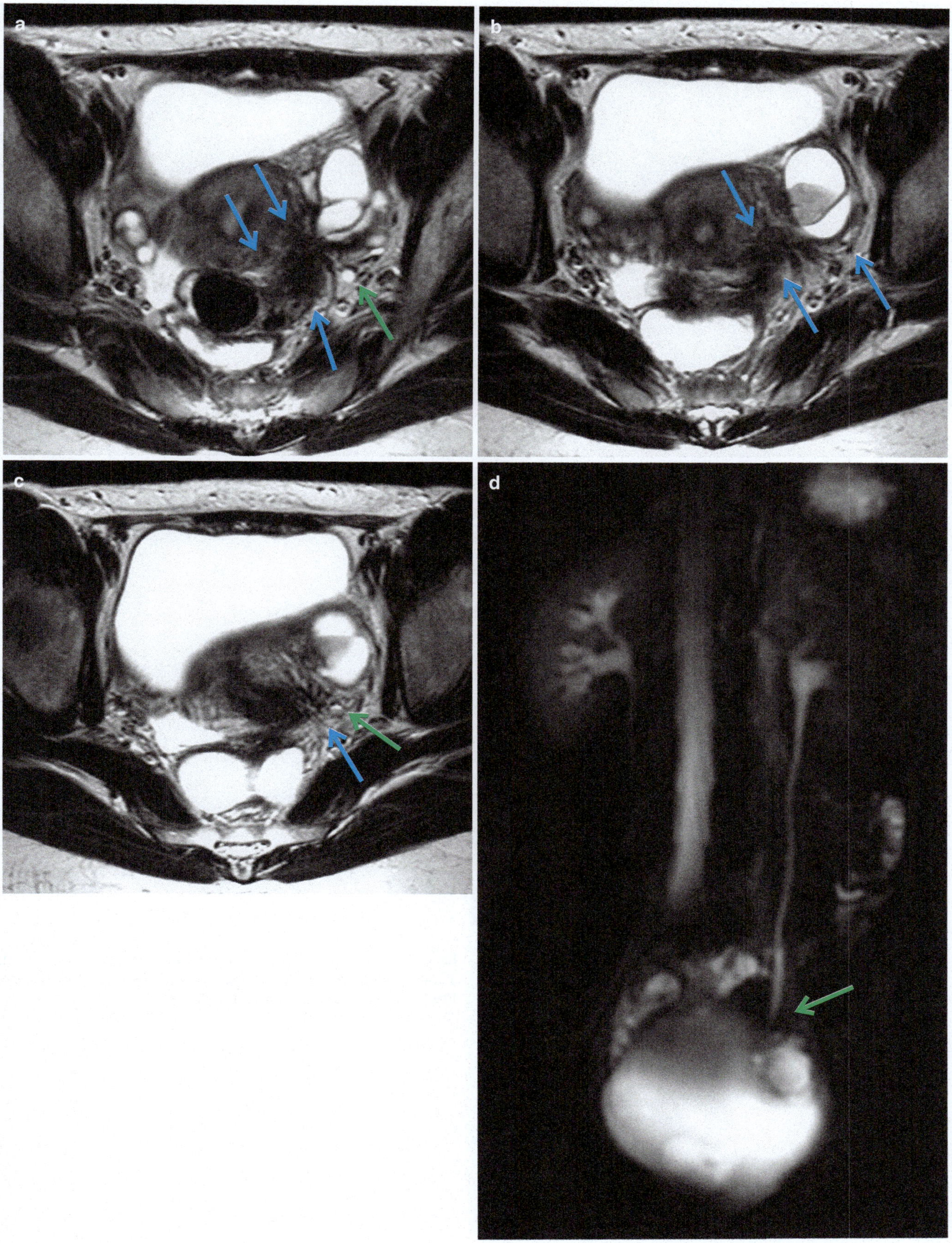

Fig. 4.176 Inferior extension in left parametrium (blue arrows **a**–**c**) with ureteral involvement (green arrows **a**–**c**) including dilation (green arrow **d**). (**a**–**c**) T2-weighted sequence. Axial. (green arrow in **d**) MRI urography

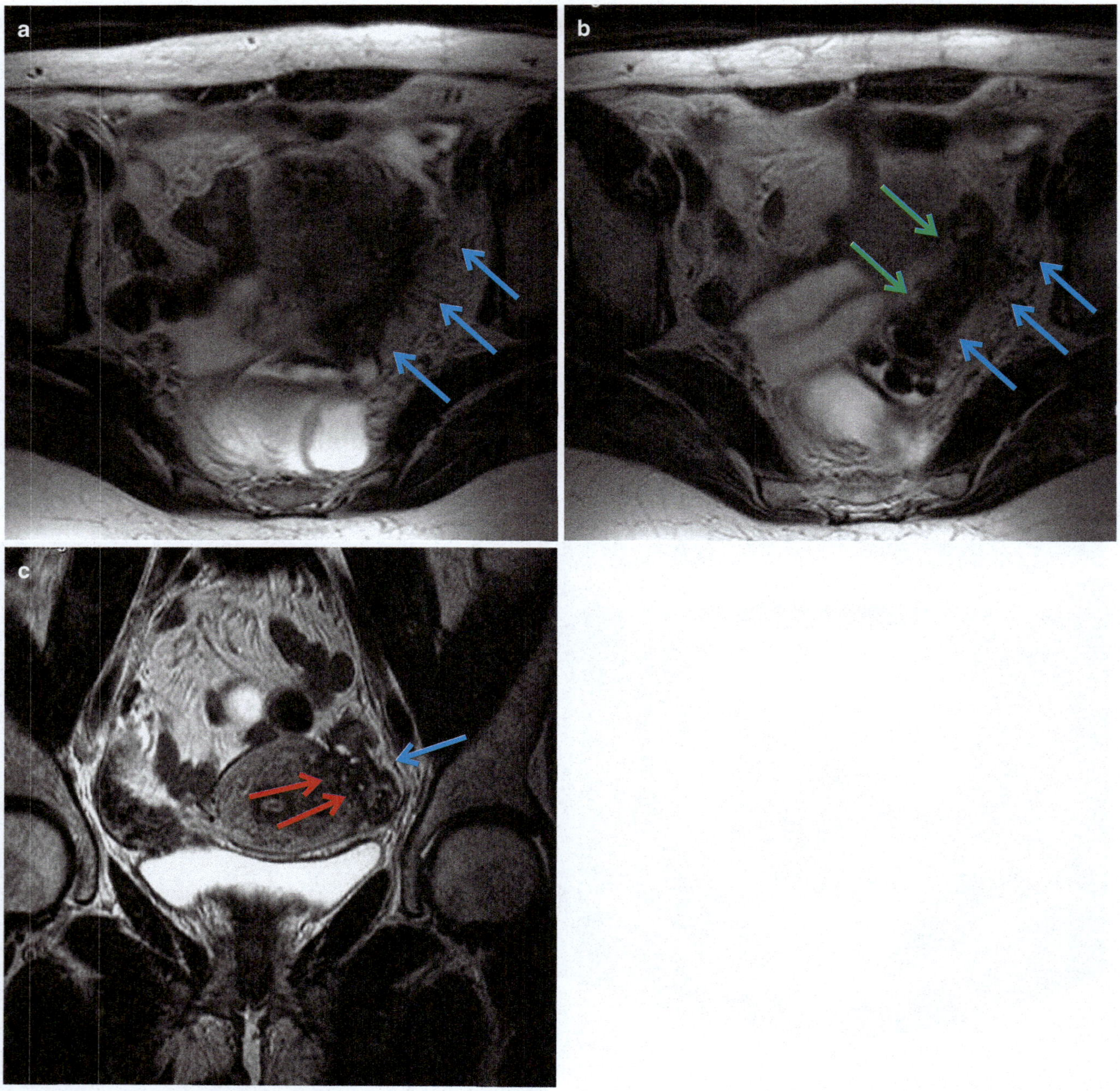

Fig. 4.177 Extensive lesion of the left ovarian fossa (blue arrows of **a–f**), with deep penetration into the sigmoid (green arrows in **b**, **f**), located between the 3 o'clock and 8 o'clock positions, reducing the lumen loop and involving the myometrium (red arrows in **c**). (**a–f**) T2-weighted sequences. (**a**, **b**) Axial. (**c–f**) Coronal. (**g**) Laparoscopy. Involvement of the sigmoid near the left ovary

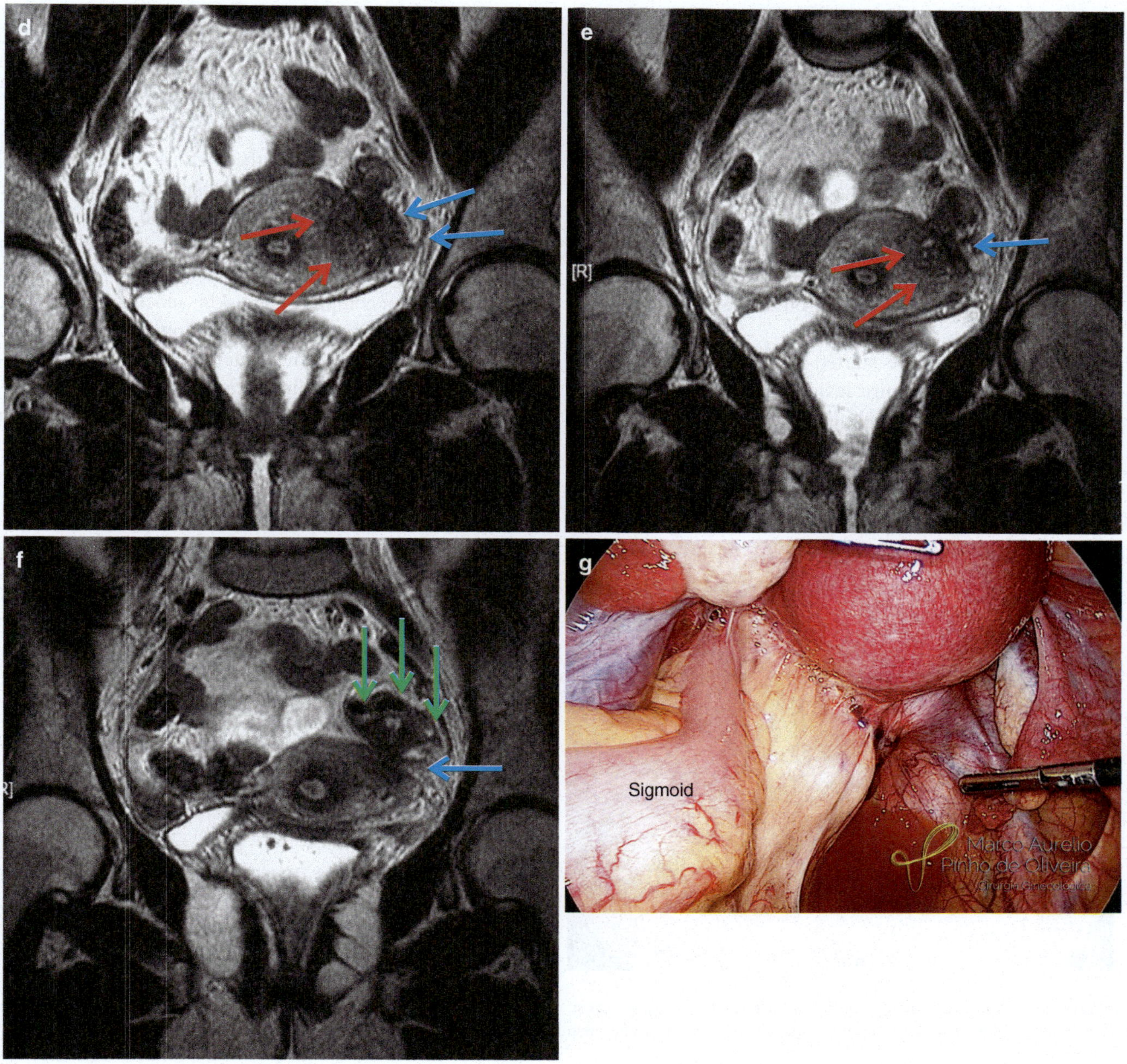

Fig. 4.177 (continued)

4.3.5.5 Comments on Treatment

It is important to expose the ovarian fossa during laparoscopy in advanced endometriosis surgery.

The deep lesion on the ovarian fossa topography should be resected with great care. It is very common for the ovarian endometrioma to be adhered to this location, and it should be initially released with great care so as not to cause unnecessary damage to the parenchyma.

Suspension of the ovaries is recommended for adequate exposure of the ovarian fossa using a single mononylon thread with a straight needle through the abdominal wall (Fig. 4.178).

Dissection should be started in an area unaffected by the disease, and the entire lesion should be removed. In some more extensive nodules, there may be ureteral involvement (already commented on in the anterior compartment section) and may extend to the hypogastric vessels and nerves.

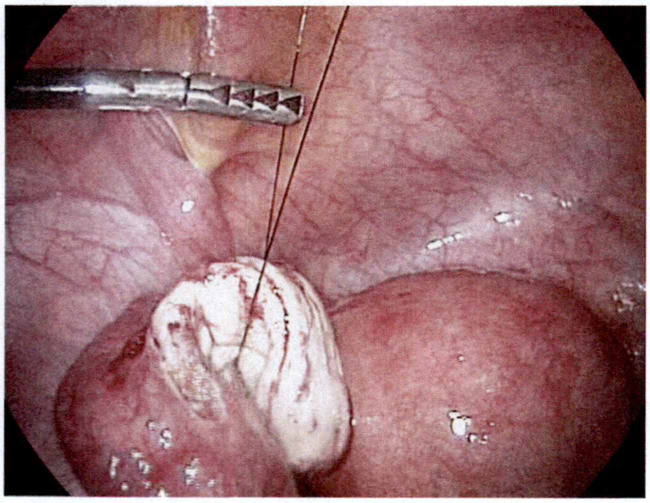

Fig. 4.178 Surgical manipulation of the left ovarian fossa. Laparoscopy demonstrating ovarian suspension for ovarian fossa exposure

4.4 Abdominal Wall

4.4.1 Cesarean Scar Line: Umbilicus

4.4.1.1 Anatomy

The anterior abdominal wall is the entrance to the abdominal cavity for the surgeon. The upper border comprises the xiphoid process and the costal arches and the lower, the pubic symphysis, the inguinal ligament, and the anterior superior iliac spine [9].

The layers that comprise it are skin; subcutaneous fat; the anterior fascia covering the rectus abdominis (medial) and oblique muscles, the external, internal, and transverse (lateral); the linea alba (a tendinous raphe between the abdominal muscles); the transversalis fascia that covers the posterior sheath of the rectus abdominis and the transverse oblique; and the preperitoneal space, which contains fat and connective tissue (Fig. 4.179) [9].

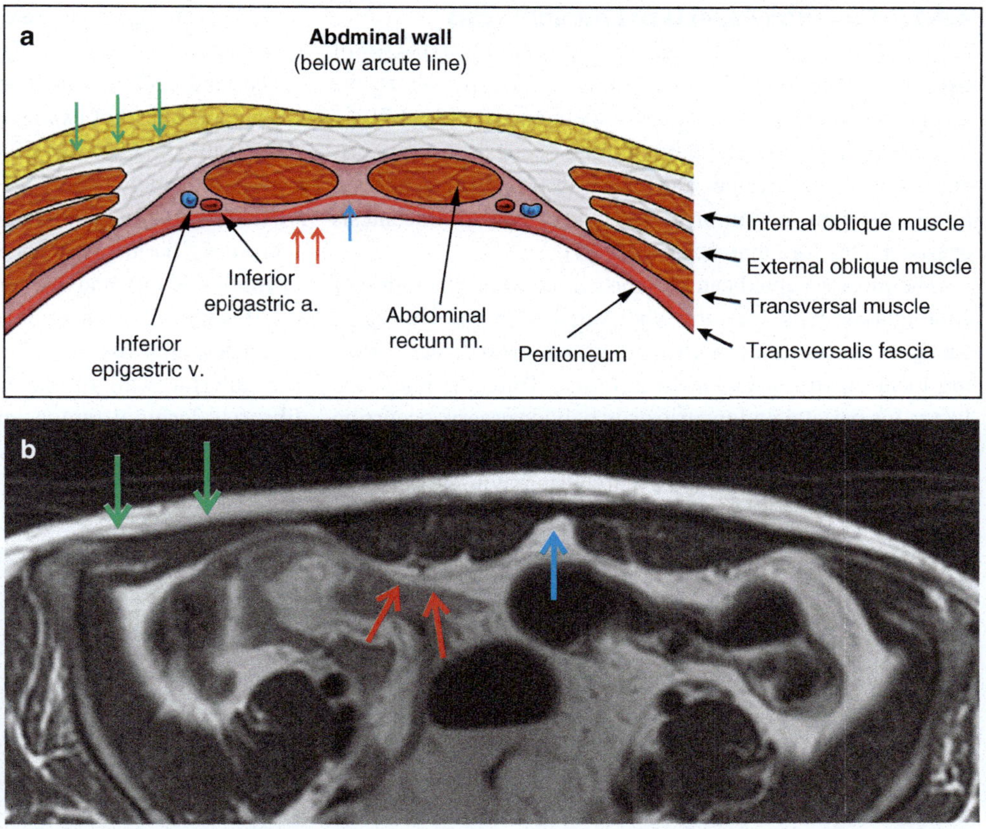

Fig. 4.179 (**a**) Schematic of the layers of the anterior abdominal wall. Skin and subcutaneous tissue; anterior layer of the fascia covering the rectus abdominis (white area, medial), transverse (lateral, green arrow) and oblique external and internal muscles (green arrow); linea alba (blue arrow); transverse fascia covering the posterior leaflet of the rectus abdominis and transverse oblique muscles; preperitoneal space, which contains fat and connective tissue (red arrow). (**b**) T2-weighted sequence. Axial

4.4.1.2 Common Aspects of Endometriosis

Although it is a rare presentation, representing 0.03–2% of extragenital endometrioses, parietal endometriosis is the most common location outside the pelvic cavity [26, 67].

Abdominal wall endometriosis can occur in several parietal sites, including the subcutaneous tissue, musculature, navel, cesarean section or hysterectomy, and amniocentesis or trocar sites for laparoscopy [68, 69].

The most accepted cause is the ectopic transplantation of endometrial cells into the abdominal wall by iatrogenic transport to scar tissue, with an immunological defect, allowing local growth of endometrial tissue. Thus, the main risk factor for parietal endometriosis is pelvic surgery, occurring in about 0.05% of patients submitted to cesarean section, in 1.6% to micro-cesarean, and 1% to hysterectomy [67, 70].

However, there are rare cases of spontaneous parietal endometriosis, such as in the umbilical scar.

Parietal endometriosis typically respects the muscular fascia and does not extend to the pelvic cavity. In addition, these patients generally have a lower incidence of endometriosis in the pelvic cavity (13%) (Fig. 4.180) [26, 71].

Differential diagnoses of umbilical nodules include metastasis, hernia, primary carcinoma, granuloma (pyogenic or foreign body), and urachal cyst. When caused by metastasis, it is known as the nodule of "Sister Mary Joseph" [72].

Differential diagnoses of nodules at other locations in the anterior wall of the abdomen include postoperative fibrosis, desmoid tumor, and rarely metastasis or primary lesion (Fig. 3.16).

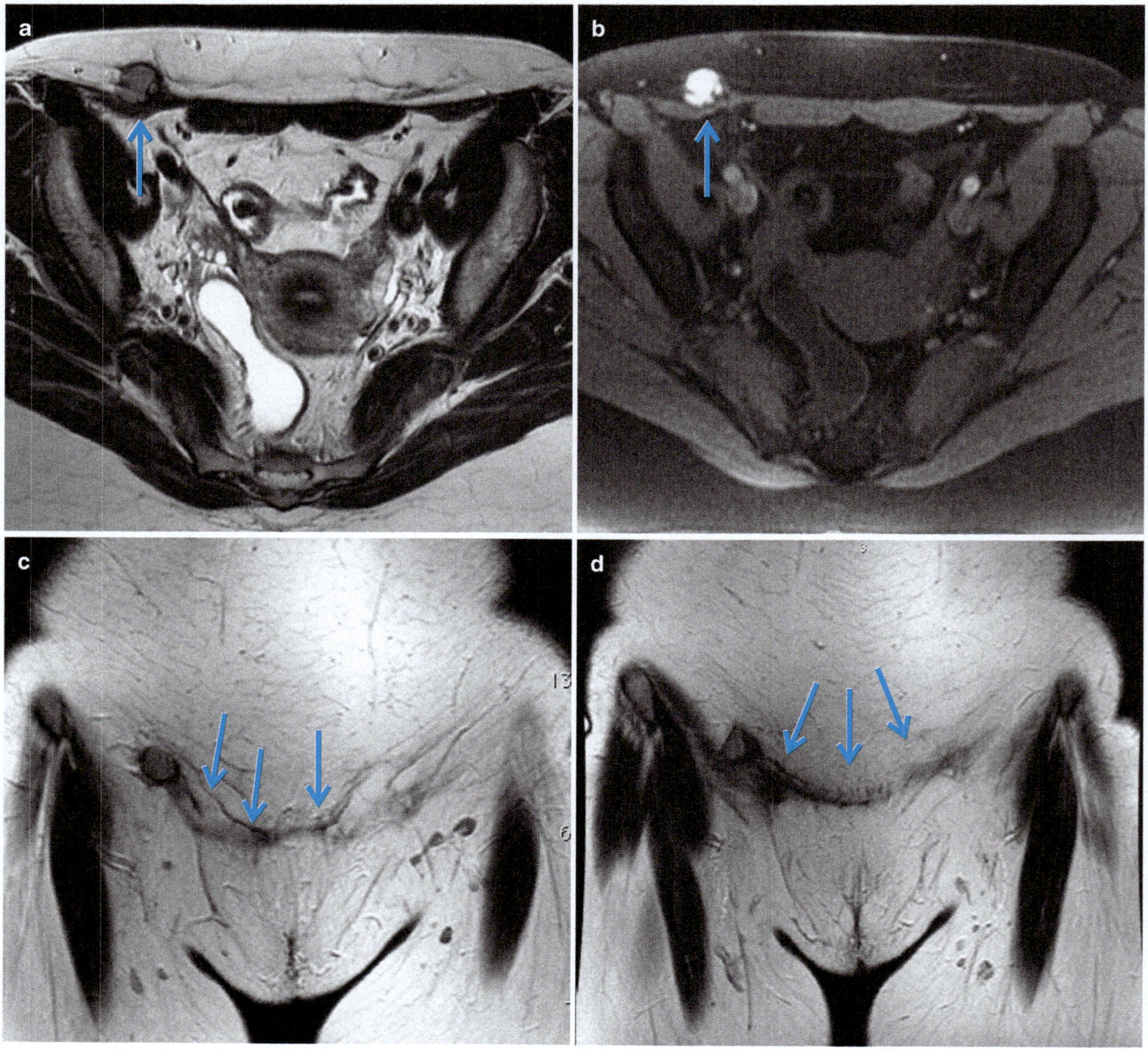

Fig. 4.180 Endometriosis in the subcutaneous and fascia of the right oblique muscle. The muscle lesion extends posteriorly and has minimal penetration into the muscle belly (arrows **a**, **b**). No extension to the pelvic cavity (**a**, **b**). Note the location adjacent to the cesarean scar (arrows on **c**, **d**) in correlation with marker (**d**). (**a**, **c**, **d**) T2-weighted sequences. (**b**) T1-weighted. (**a**, **b**) Axial. (**c**, **d**) Coronal

4.4.1.3 Clinical Condition

Symptoms can occur several weeks to years after surgery, with an average of about 30 months. Cyclical pain related to the menstrual cycle is an important diagnostic criterion but is present in only 25% of cases [26].

The lesion is palpable in about 96% of cases and may be visible when it occurs on the umbilical scar [71].

4.4.1.4 MRI and Surgical Findings

MR imaging protocol should be directed to the anterior abdominal wall and preferably using a cutaneous marker in order to guide the study on the clinically suspected area (Fig. 2.8).

The protocol uses sequences performed with the patient in apnea, since respiratory artifacts can impair the identification and analysis of the extent of the lesion in this topography.

As multiple lesions may occur, the field of view is larger. For more details see the section on examination protocols (Figs. 2.9 and 2.10).

The lesions may have a varied size and morphology, namely:

1. **Small nodules identified by bleeding or clinical examination**: poorly delimited, infiltrative nodules with a heterogeneous signal, predominantly hypointense in the T1-weighted sequence, with small, hyperintense foci due to bleeding (Fig. 4.181).
   For detection of lesions smaller than 1 cm, the T1-weighted sequence with fat suppression is essential.
   When the lesion is purely hypointense in the T1-weighted sequence, the detection can be difficult, and the intravenous use of gadolinium may help. In these cases, the differential diagnoses with postsurgical fibrosis and desmoid tumor are also difficult. The clinical picture may suggest a diagnosis of endometriosis (Figs. 2.10 and 3.16). An alternative is to include in the protocol the susceptibility-weighted imaging (SWI), a relatively new technique. This technique is able to detect the signal voids due to hemorrhagic materials in the endometriotic nodules.
2. **Bleeding cyst (endometrioma)**: this type of lesion has a heterogeneous signal, due to its cystic component and bleeding, being predominantly hyperintense in the T1- and T2-weighted sequences, when bleeding is recent, and with a hyperintense signal in T1 and a hypointense signal in T2 with old bleeding, similar to the ovarian endometrioma (Fig. 4.182).
3. **Purely solid mass**: infiltrative lesions with a predominance of fibrosis, with a hypointense signal in the T2-weighted sequence and intermediate in T1 and with enhancement by gadolinium. Bleeding foci are rare in this type of lesion (Fig. 4.183).
   The lesions can be bulky and the differential diagnosis of desmoid tumor more difficult if there is no bleeding.
4. **Mixed lesion**: usually larger lesions which combine the characteristics of a fibrotic mass with bleeding cysts.

The radiologist should detail some characteristics of the abdominal wall endometriosis lesion as they have a direct impact on the surgical technique (Table 4.13).

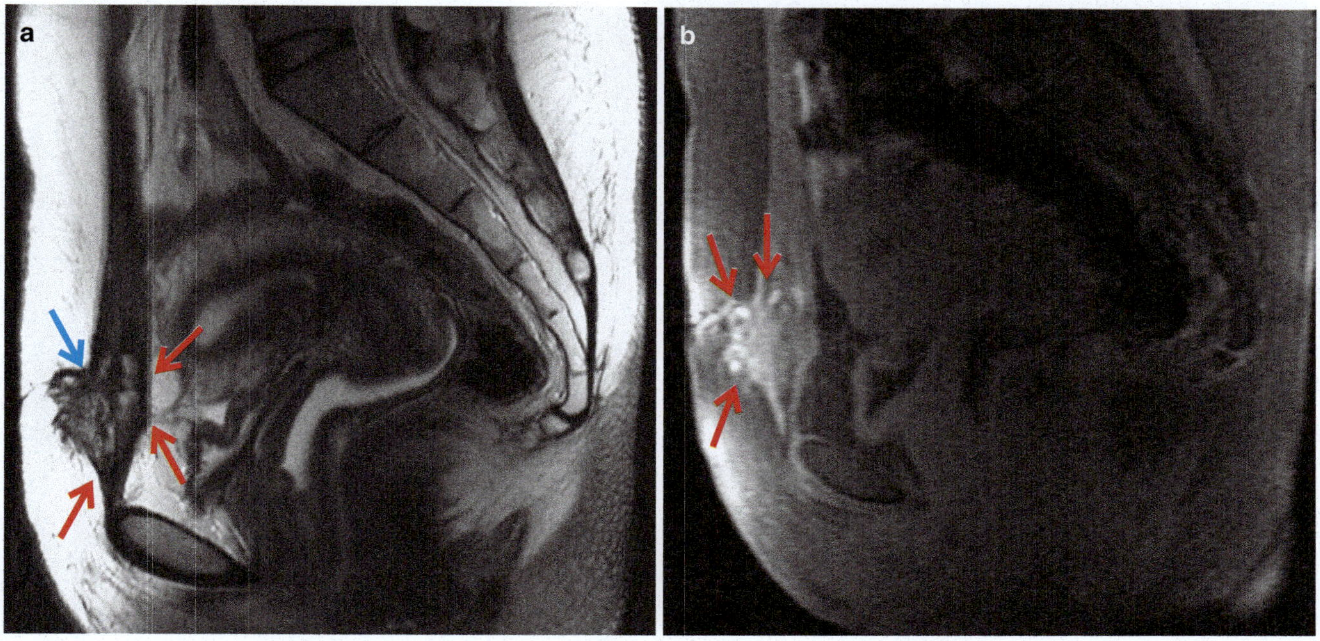

Fig. 4.181 Cesarean section scar nodule with subcutaneous, rectus abdominis muscle belly and the preperitoneal space extension, poorly defined, infiltrative, heterogeneous, predominantly hypointense on T2-weighted sequences, with multiple hyperintense foci of ectopic endometrial tissue (**a, c**) with hyperintense bleeding foci on T1-weighted (**b, d**) and intense enhancement (**e**). (**a, b**) Sagittal. (**c–e**) Axial. (**f**) Clinical examination of another patient

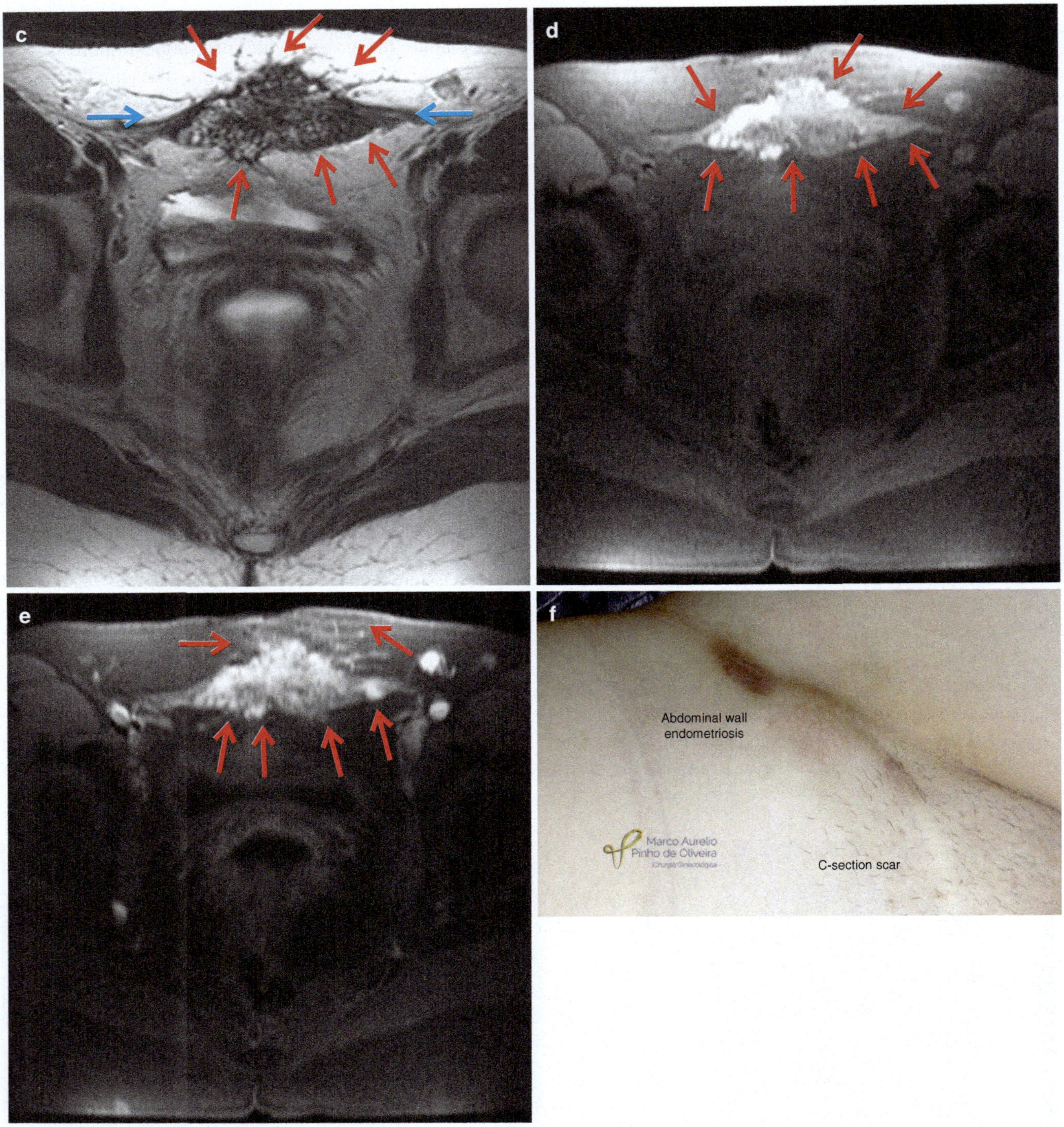

Fig. 4.181 (continued)

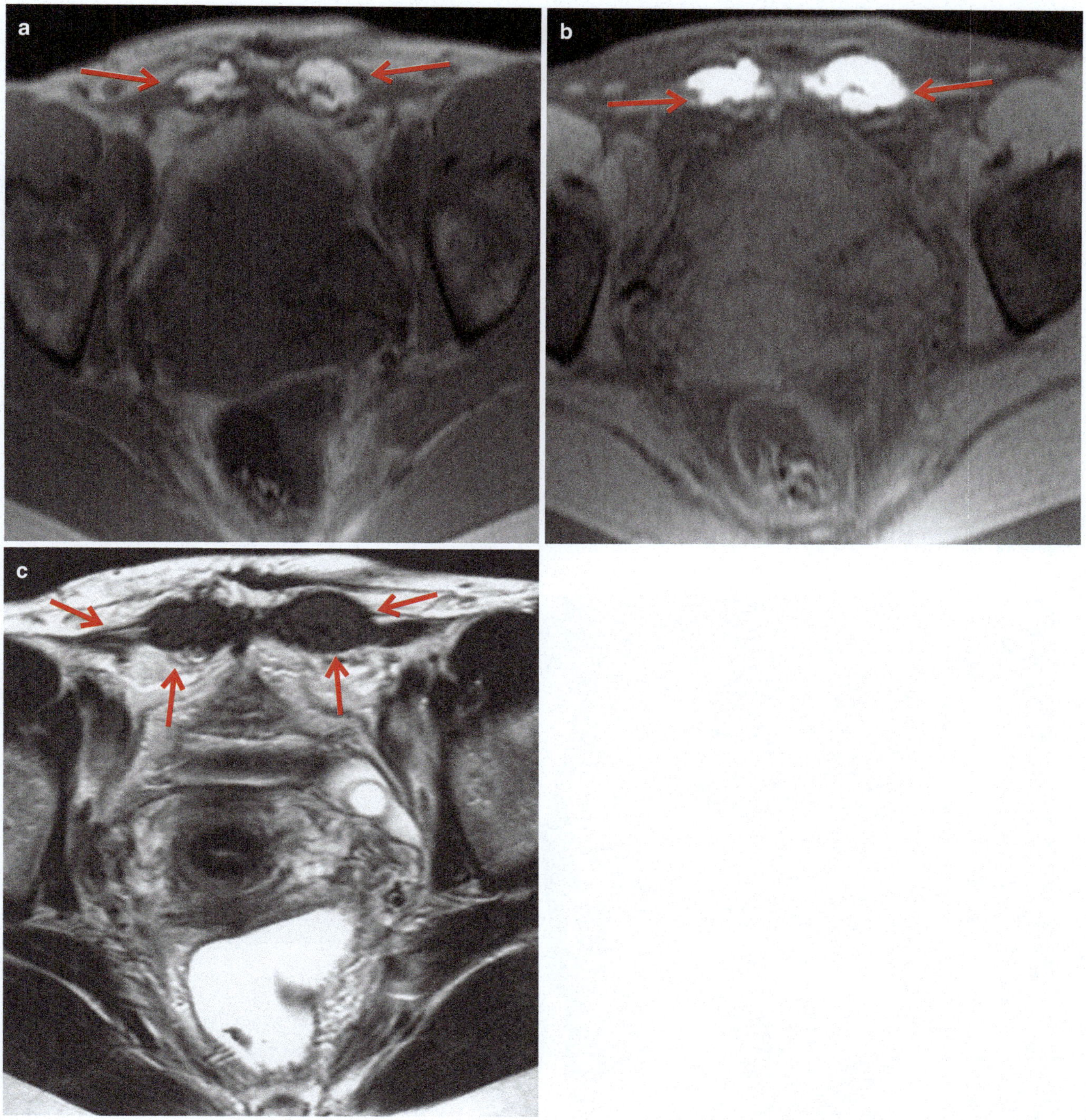

Fig. 4.182 Cysts with bleeding (wall endometriomas). Lesions with heterogeneous signal from cystic component and bleeding, predominantly hyperintense in T1-weighted sequences (**a**, **b**, **d**) and hypointense on T2 (**c**, **e**) by old blood, compromising the bilateral rectus abdominis, extending to the pubic symphysis (blue arrow **d**, **e**).(**a–c**) Axial. (**d–e**) Sagittal

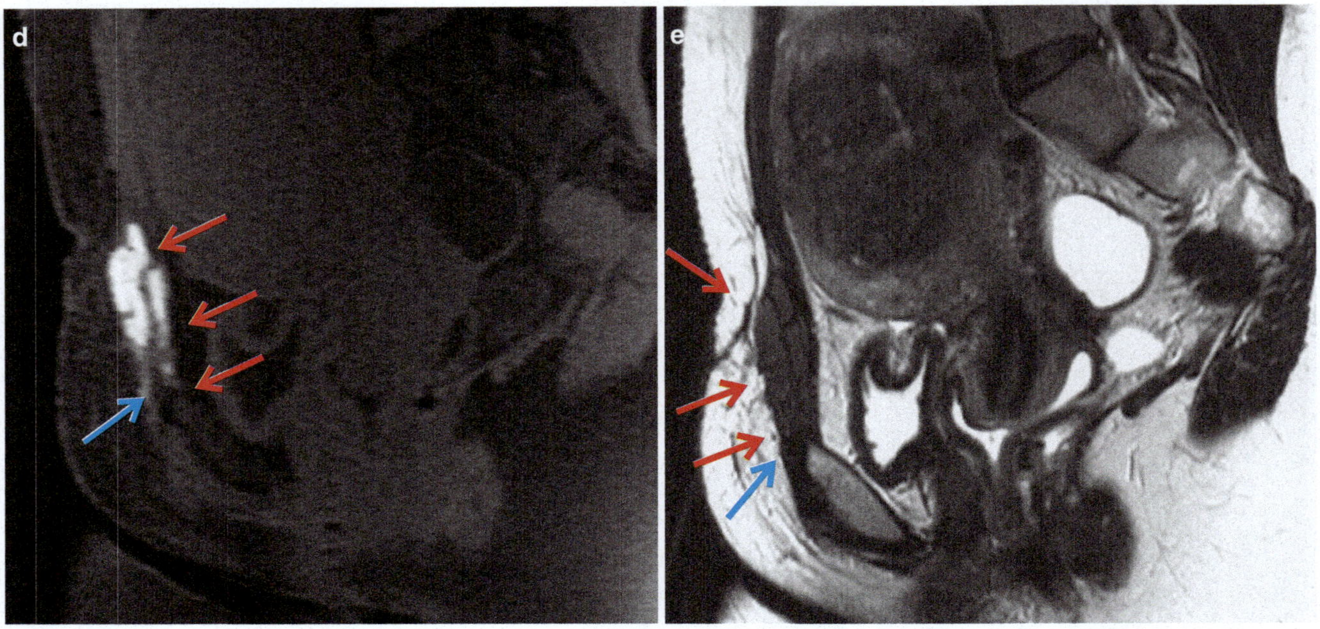

Fig. 4.182 (continued)

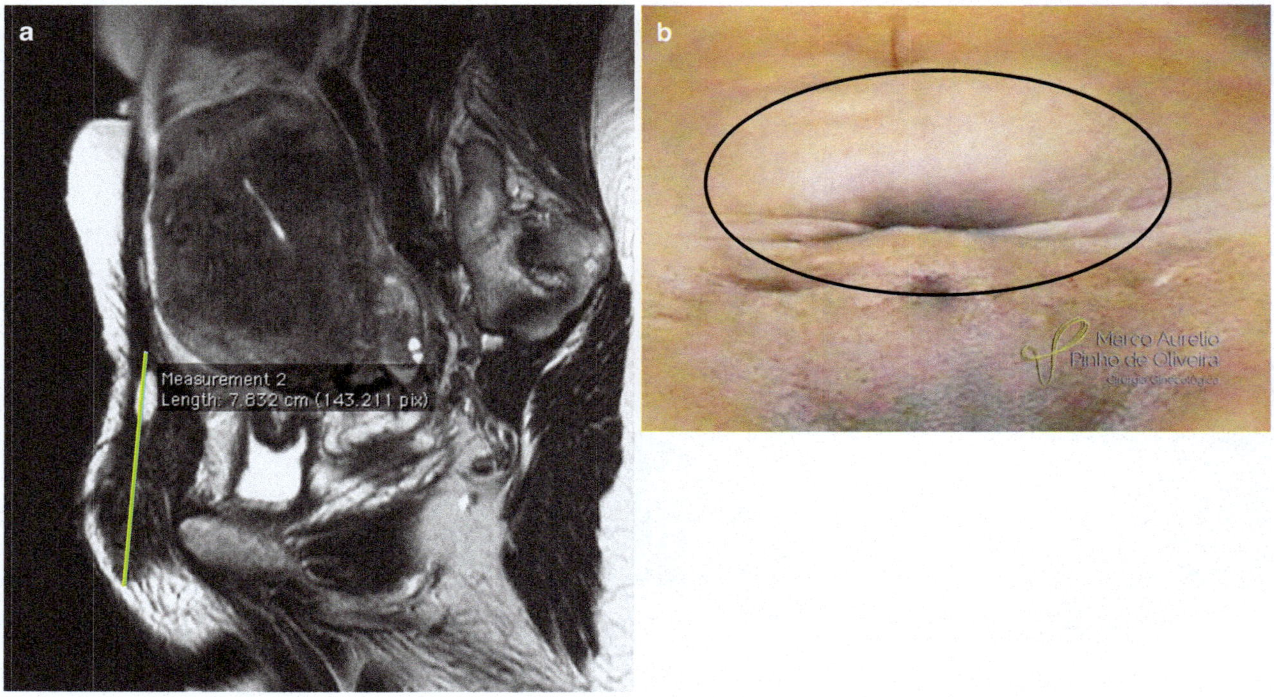

Fig. 4.183 Extensive infiltrative lesion (7 cm) extending from the skin to the muscle belly of the rectus abdominis (**a**) with greater involvement in the subcutaneous below the symphysis, with a predominance of fibrosis, hypointense signal on T2-weighted sequences (**a**) intermediate in T1 (**d**) and discrete gadolinium enhancement (**e**). Blood foci are rare (**a**) Sagittal. (**c–e**) Axial. (**b**) Clinical exam image

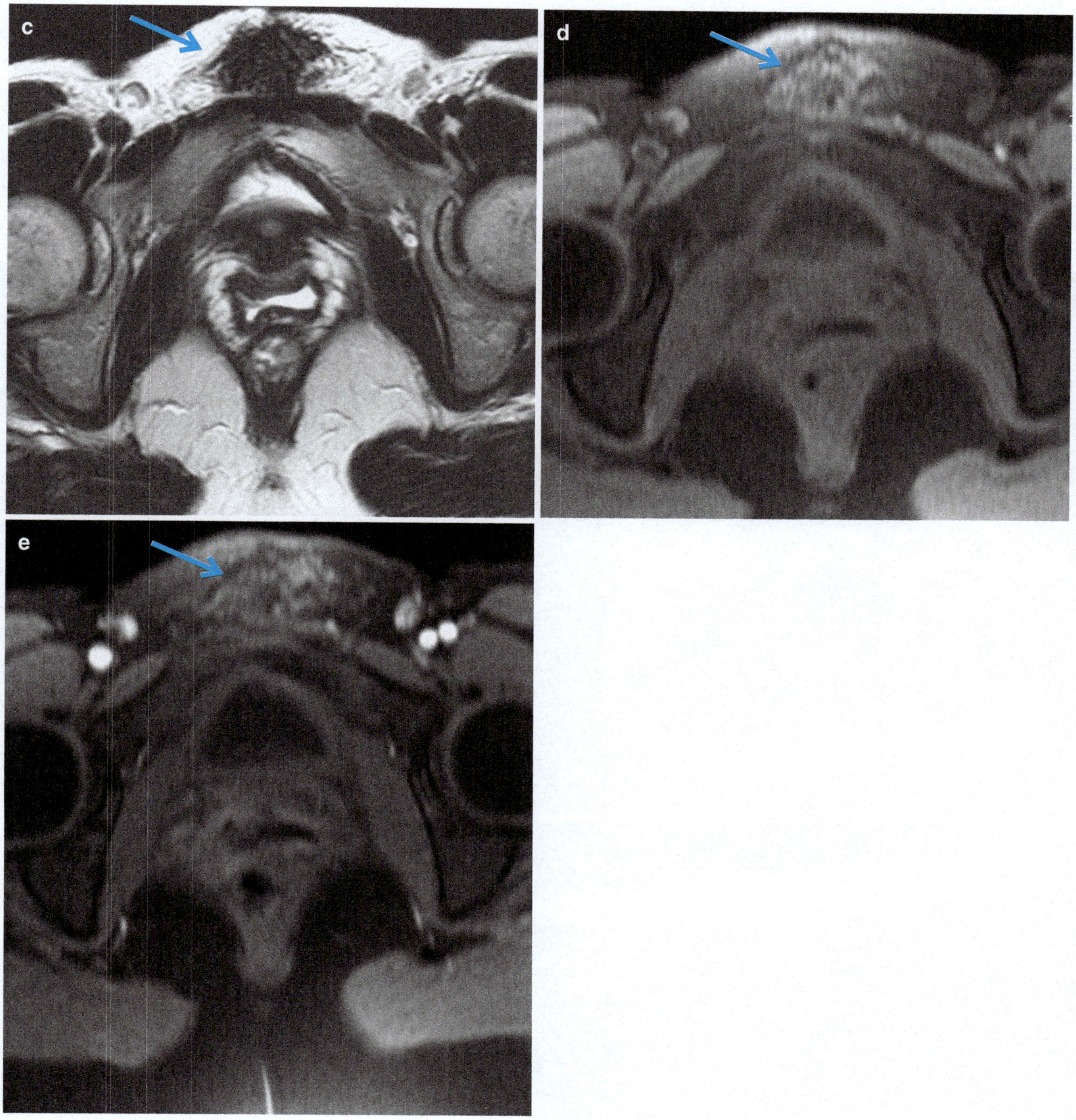

Fig. 4.183 (continued)

Table 4.13 Characteristics of the lesion that should be described in the report

Length of lesion on all axes	Defines the need to use abdominal mesh
Depth of infiltration of the abdominal wall	Significant in the complexity of the surgery, the use of a mesh, and access to the pelvic cavity, if there is penetration of the lesion beyond the preperitoneal space
Relation with anatomical structure	Reference point of the lesion for surgery, such as the pubic symphysis and iliac crest, especially for lesions without clinical expression

4.4.1.5 Comments on Treatment

Percutaneous aspiration and biopsy of these lesions should be avoided as there is a risk of dissemination along the needle path.

Treatment involves surgical excision of the entire lump, with lesion-free margins, in order to avoid recurrence. It may be necessary to use a mesh depending on the penetration and size of the lesion.

4.4.2 Inguinal Region or Canal of Nuck

4.4.2.1 Anatomy

The canal of Nuck is an embryological remnant of the vaginal process, an evagination of the parietal peritoneum, that accompanies the round ligament through the inguinal ring in the inguinal canal, obliterated shortly after birth (Fig. 4.184) [26].

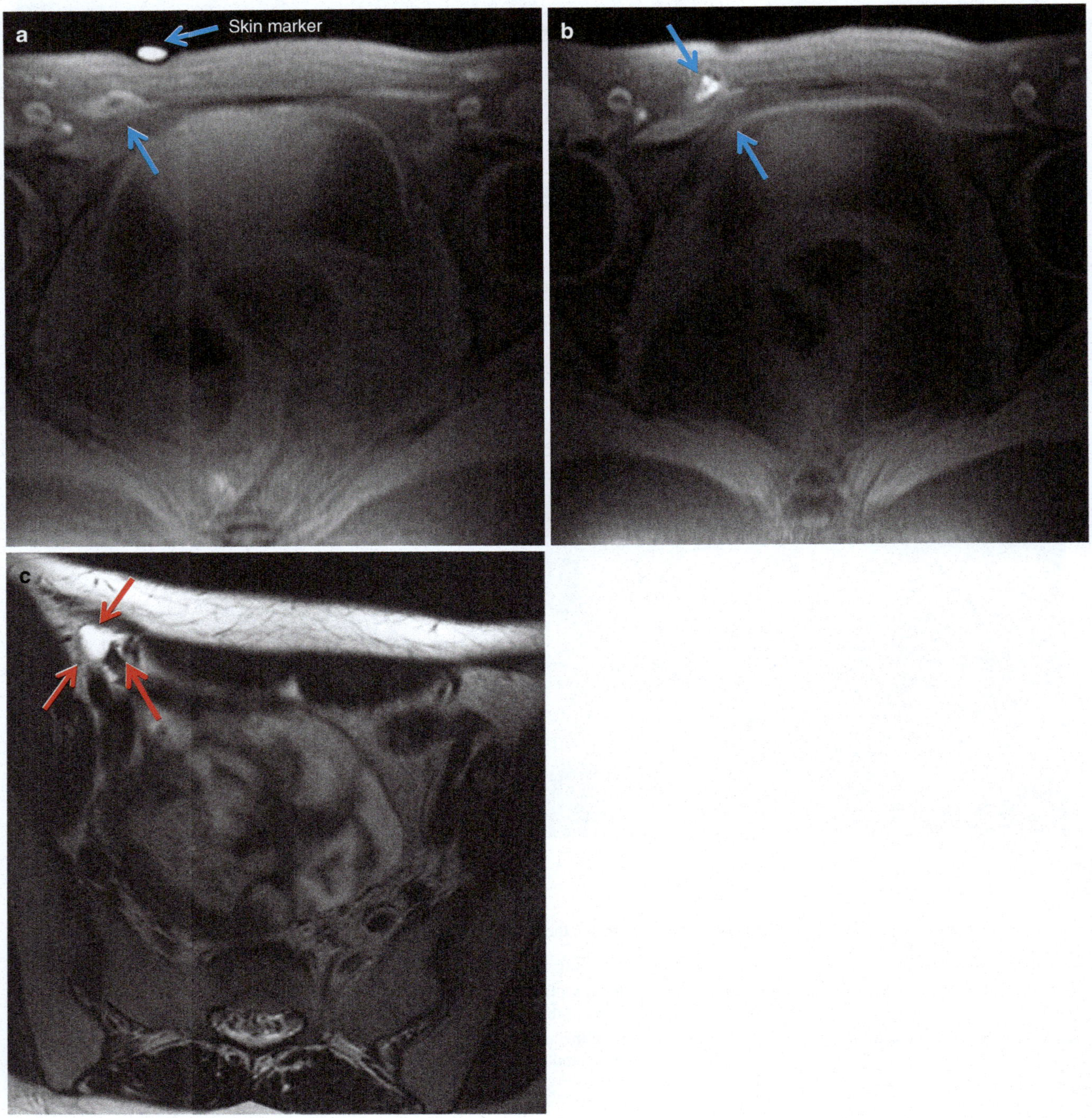

Fig. 4.184 The canal of Nuck is an evagination of the parietal peritoneum that follows the round ligament through the inguinal ring in the inguinal canal. Note liquid in the channel on the right (hyperintense on T2 **c**–**e**) associated with inguinal endometriosis (skin marker and blue arrows). (**a**, **b**) T1-weighted sequence, axial. (**c**–**f**) T2-weighted long axis

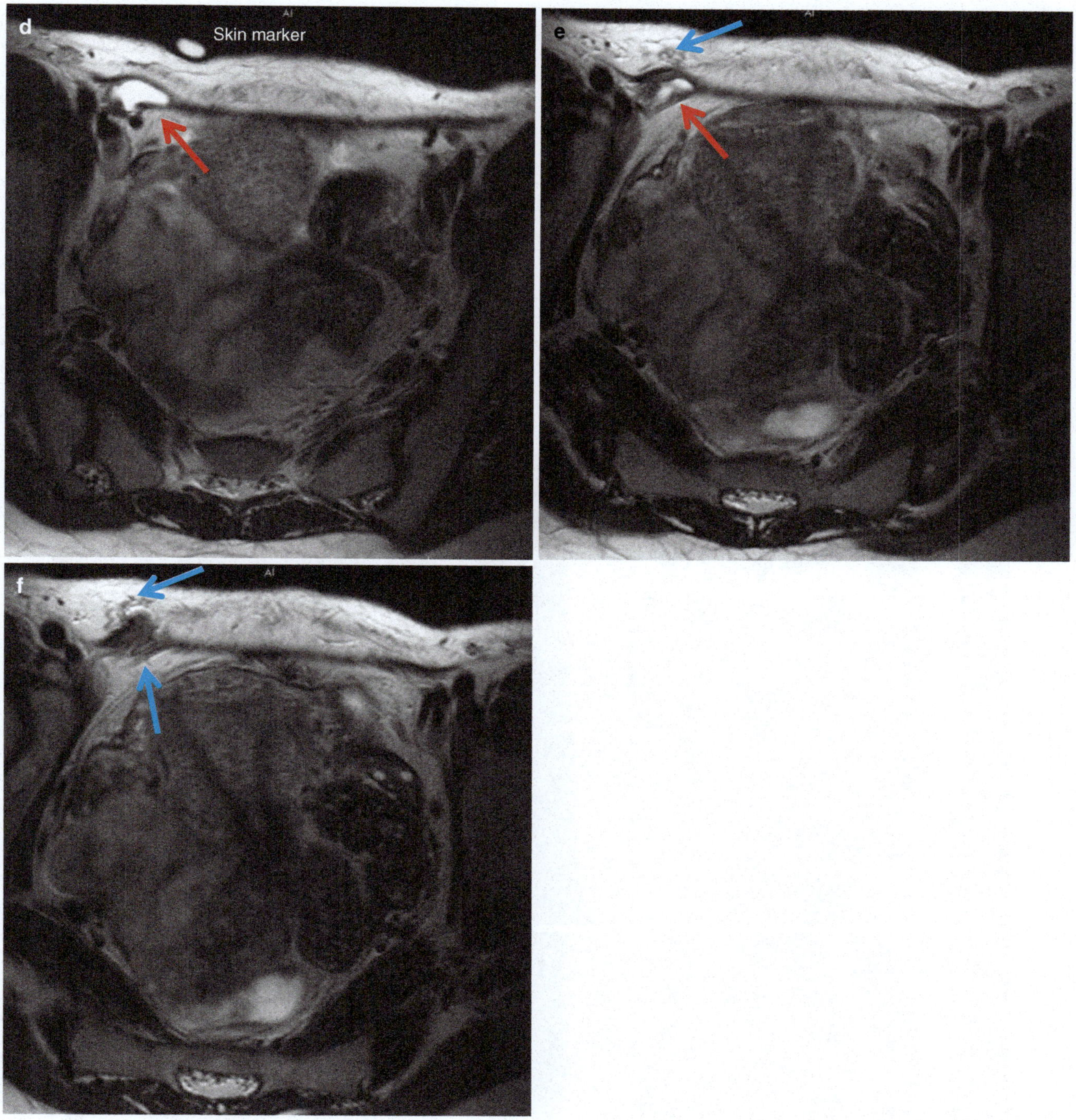

Fig. 4.184 (continued)

4.4.2.2 Common Aspects of Endometriosis

Involvement in this location is extremely rare. It can occur by the spread of pelvic endometriosis, through the round ligament, whose extraperitoneal portion extends through the inguinal canal.

On the other hand, the lesion may be isolated, without pelvic involvement, with dissemination of the endometrial tissue by the peritoneal flow through the canal of Nuck, which when present creates a communication channel between the peritoneal cavity and the inguinal canal, providing the most likely pathway for implantation of ectopic endometrial tissue in the inguinal region [24, 73].

According to the literature, there is a predilection for the right inguinal region [74].

4.4.2.3 MRI and Surgical Findings

The appearance of the lesion may vary. The most common is a solid infiltrative lesion with a predominance of fibrosis, hypointense in the T2-weighted sequence, with ectopic endometrial tissue hyperintense in T2, and with bleeding foci hyperintense on T1- and T2-weighted sequences. Usually, moderate enhancement occurs with gadolinium. This aspect of the lesion is very characteristic (Fig. 4.185).

However, multiloculated cystic lesions with heterogeneous content due to bleeding can be observed. The differential diagnoses in these cases are canal of Nuck hydrocele, inguinal hernia, abscess, and less commonly lesions such as hematoma. The hydrocele usually presents as a cyst without bleeding, and communication with the peritoneal cavity can be identified (Fig. 4.186) [73].

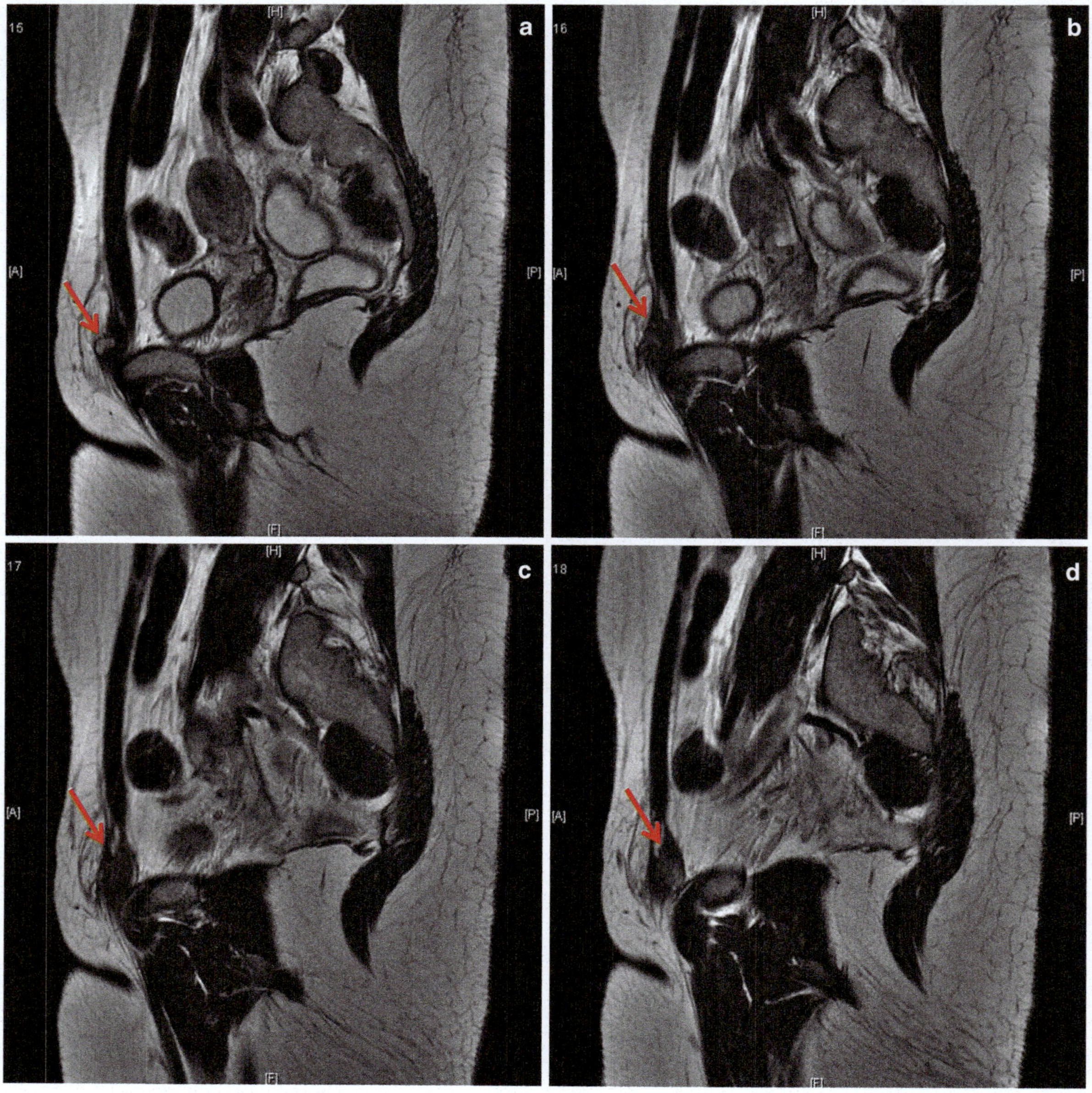

Fig. 4.185 Solid infiltrating lesion in the canal of Nuck (red arrows), with a predominance of fibrosis, hypointense on T2-weighted sequence (**a–j**), with ectopic endometrial tissue (hyperintense foci) and moderate enhancement with gadolinium (T1-weighted sequence with fat suppression and contrast [**k**]). Sagittal plane (**a–d**) and axial (**k–e**)

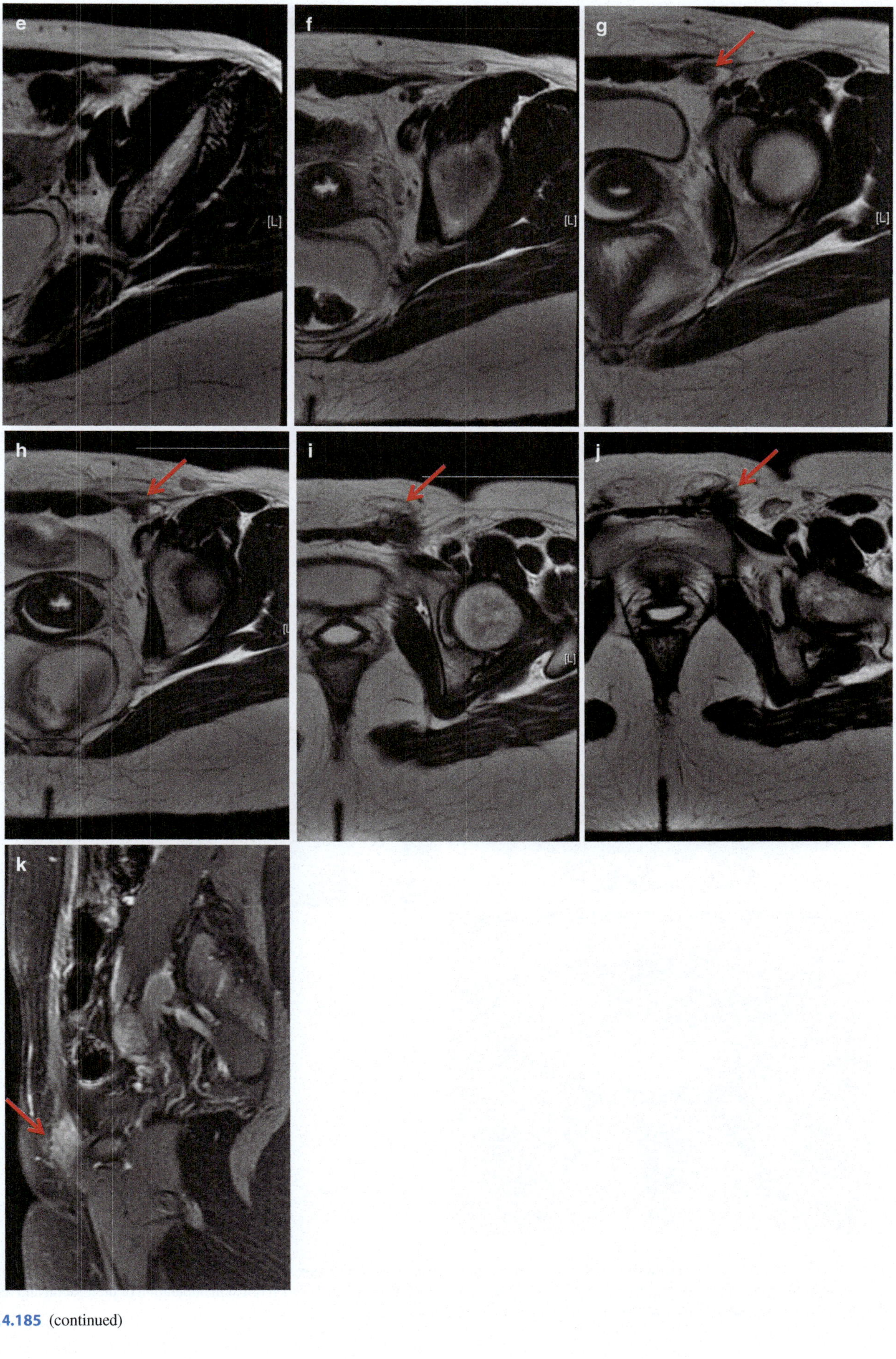

Fig. 4.185 (continued)

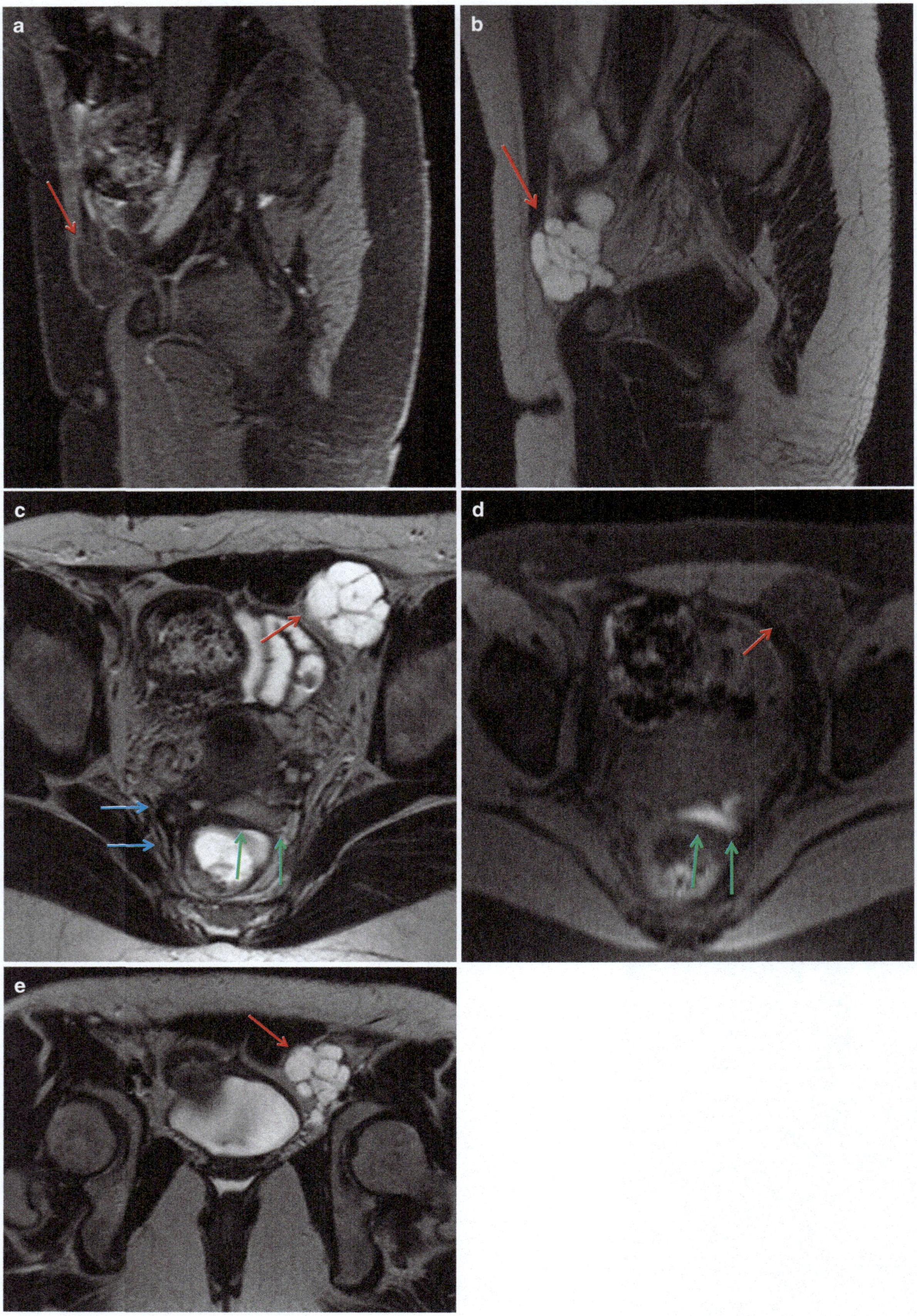

Fig. 4.186 Canal of Nuck cyst (red arrows). Multilocular cyst, hypointense on T1-weighted sequences (**d**) and hyperintense on T2 (**b**, **c**, **e**) with discrete parietal and septal enhancement (**a**). (**a**, **b**) Sagittal. (**c**, **d**) Axial. (**e**) Short axis. Note liquid with blood in posterior compartment (green arrows **c**, **d**) and surgical manipulation of uterosacral and rectum on the right (blue arrows in **c**)

4.4.2.4 Comments on Treatment

The treatment is similar to that of endometriosis of the anterior wall of the abdomen, with surgical excision of the entire nodule, with lesion-free margins, in order to avoid recurrence. It may be necessary to use a mesh.

4.5 Appendix, Cecum, and Terminal Ileum

4.5.1 Anatomy

The cecum and appendix are the first parts of the large intestine and are located at the right iliac fossa. The appendix is a narrow wormlike structure originating in the posterior wall of the cecum about 2 cm below the ileocecal junction and is not constant in its position. The length of the appendage varies from 2 to 20 cm (average of 2–9 cm) [75].

4.5.2 Common Aspects of Endometriosis

Deep intestinal endometriosis is defined when a lesion involves the muscularis propria of the intestine.

It affects up to 45.4% of women with extraintestinal infiltrative lesions and can be found from the small intestine to the anal border [76].

Endometriosis of the gastrointestinal tract is a more frequent than expected disease, with the rectum and sigmoid (72%) being the most affected areas, followed by the small intestine (7%), the cecum (4%), and the appendix (3%) [76].

Like Crohn's disease, enteric endometriosis may have multiple, discontinuous lesions in the colon and small intestine, interspersed with normal bowel.

Intestinal implants are usually located in the serosa but, when deep, penetrate into the muscle itself and cause fibrosis and parietal thickening, largely because of the smooth muscle hypertrophy surrounding the endometriosis foci (Fig. 4.187) [77].

The mucosal layer is usually spared, since the pattern of growth of the implanted ectopic tissue is extramucosal parietal and is rarely invasive [28].

The involvement is asymmetrical, predominantly on the antimesenteric face, determining adhesion and wrinkling on the wall of the affected loop. This change, together with the inflammatory response due to cyclic hemorrhage, can lead to adhesion and stenosis, resulting in intestinal obstruction (Fig. 4.188) [28].

Differential diagnoses are Crohn's disease, tuberculous enteritis, carcinoid tumors, small bowel lymphoma, and Behçet's disease [78].

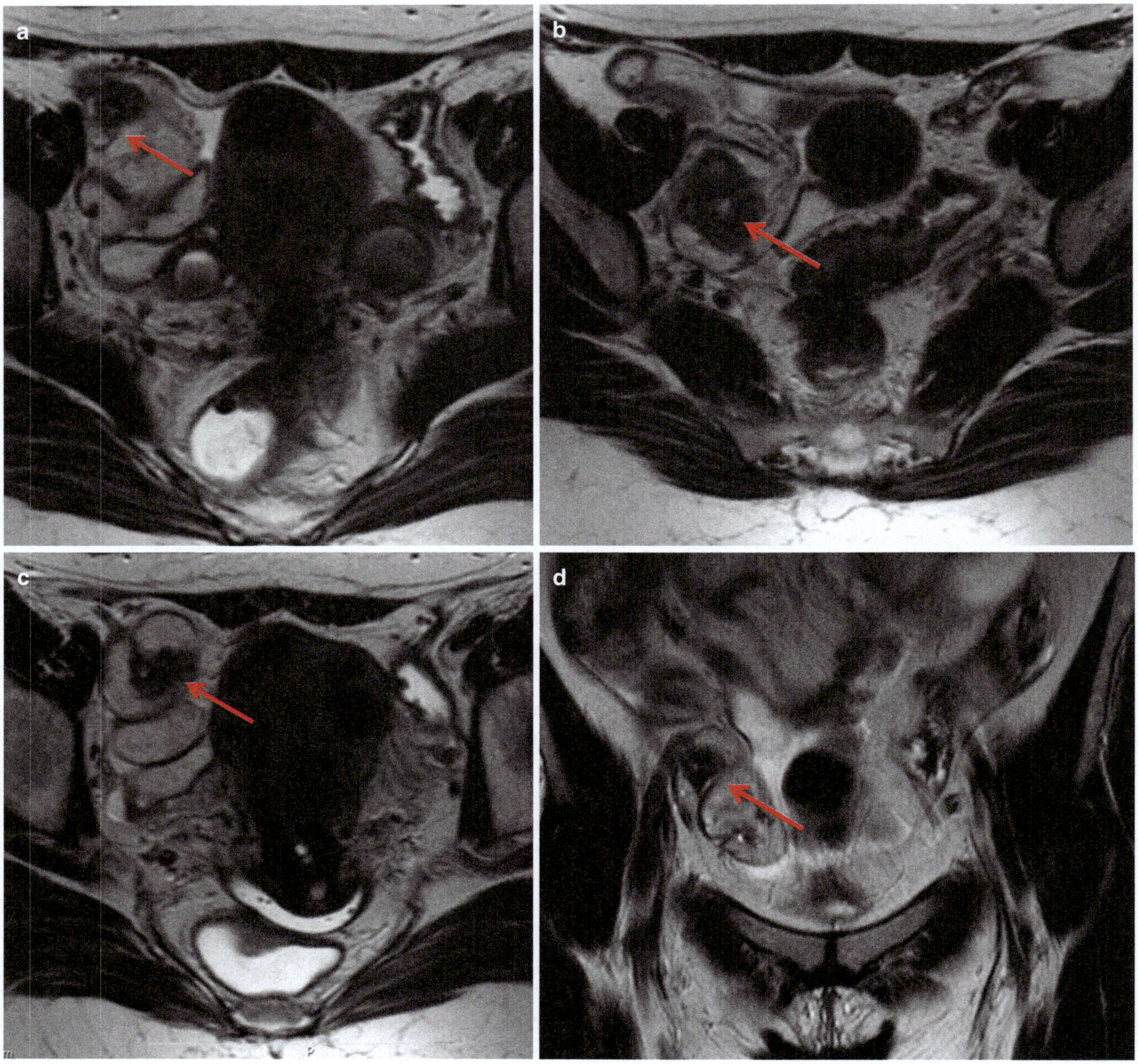

Fig. 4.187 Small bowel endometriosis with three discontinuous lesions in the ileum, interspersed with normal intestine. Deep implants, penetrating the muscularis propria, causing parietal thickening (arrows). T2-weighted sequences (**a**–**g**). (**a**–**c**) Axial. (**d**–**f**) Coronal. (**g**) Sagittal. (**h**) Laparoscopy identifying one of the ileal lesions. Note association with sigmoid endometriosis in (**b**), bilateral endometriomas in (**a**), and uterine leiomyomas

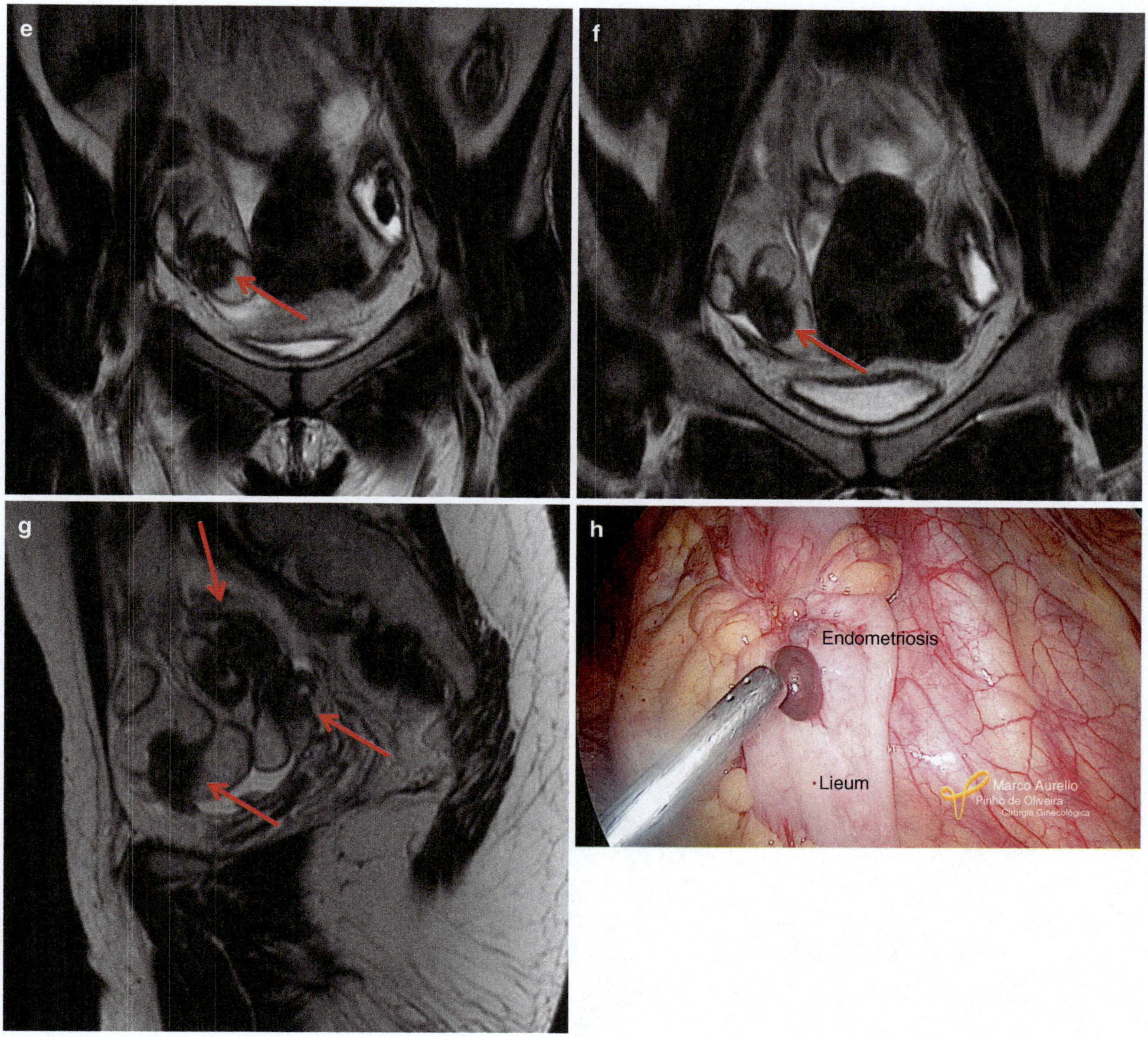

Fig. 4.187 (continued)

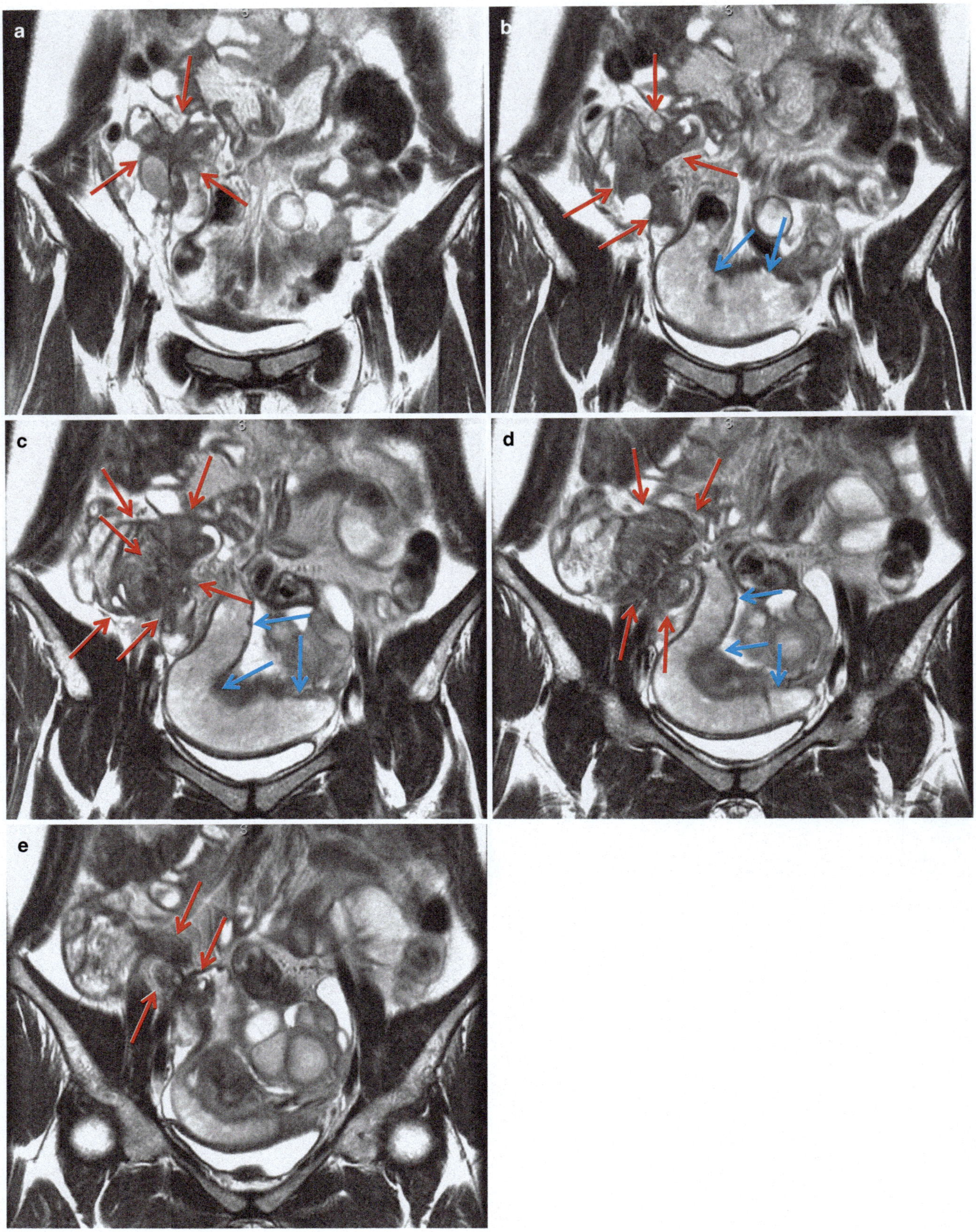

Fig. 4.188 Asymmetric involvement of the ileocecal valve and especially of the cecum (red arrows), causing parietal thickening, adhesion, distortion, and puckered aspect on the wall of the loop and stenosis, with dilation of the upright ilium (blue arrows **a**–**e**) and intestinal obstruction (**g**). T2-weighted sequence (**a**–**g**). (**a**–**f**) Coronal. (**g**) Axial. (**h**) Laparoscopy of the lesion

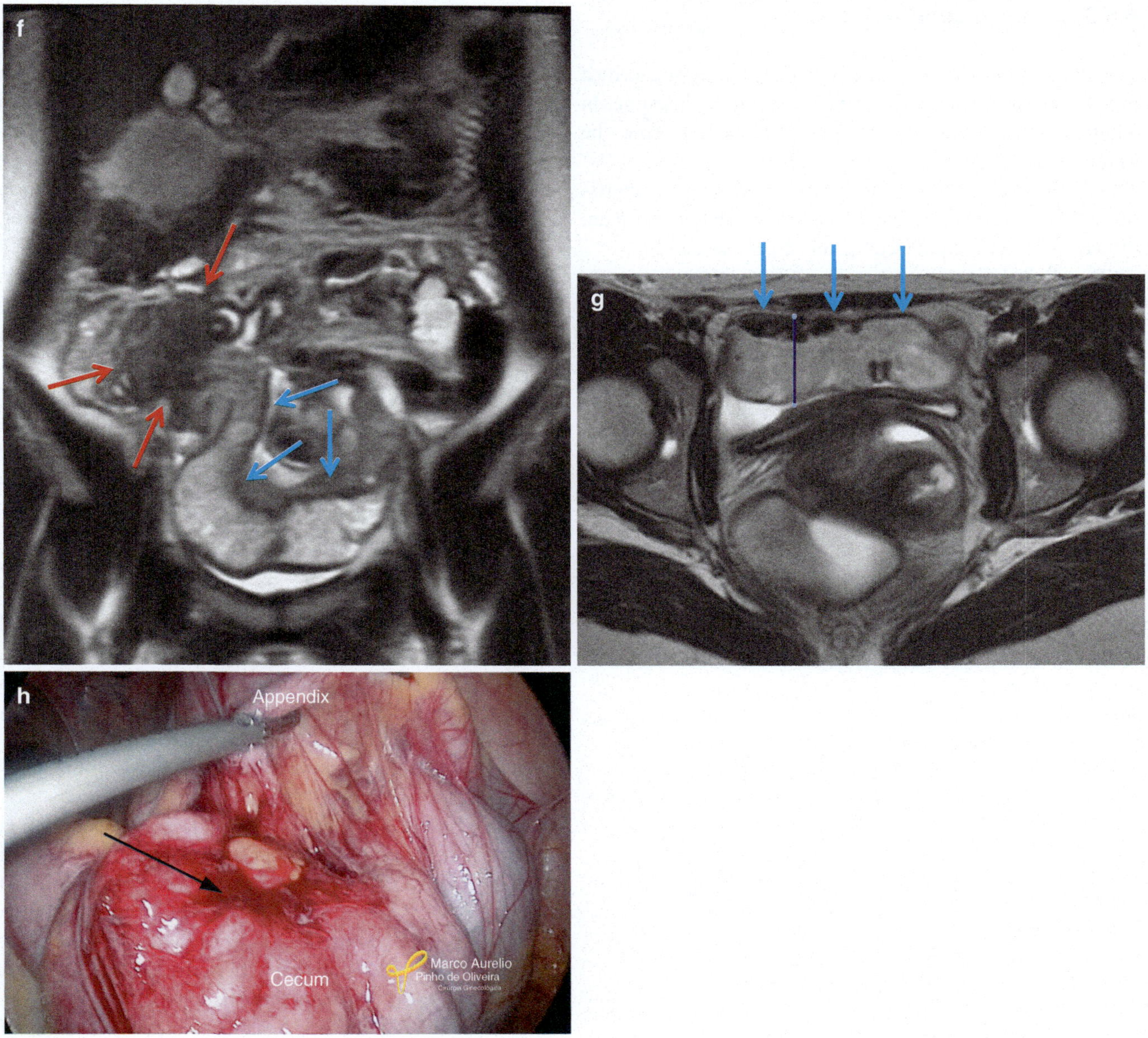

Fig. 4.188 (continued)

4.5.3 Clinical Condition

The classic picture of chronic pelvic pain and dysmenorrhea may be absent if the involvement is only in the intestine. In addition, superficial intestinal endometriosis may be asymptomatic.

Symptoms of intestinal endometriosis are not characteristic and include intermittent or persistent abdominal pain, bloody diarrhea, rectal bleeding, and constipation [79].

The clinical picture can be progressive with serious complications, such as intestinal obstruction and perforation [80].

However, despite its rarity, when affecting a woman of childbearing age, endometriosis should be included in the differential diagnosis.

4.5.4 MRI and Laparoscopic Findings

Because enteric endometriosis can have multiple lesions in the colon and the small intestine, the radiological evaluation should be systematic of all sites that can be affected, especially the rectum, sigmoid, cecum, appendix, and ileum.

To do so in MRI, it is necessary to study the abdomen in order to include the right iliac fossa. In some cases, however, it is possible to evaluate the cecal and pericecal regions in a study of the pelvis, when this segment is insinuated in this region. In the pelvis, the cecum can occupy the anterior compartment and, less frequently, the posterior compartment (Fig. 4.189).

Cecal, appendicular, and ileal intestinal lesions may be isolated, but these segments may be involved by direct extension of deep pelvic lesion. Thus, in endometriosis of the anterior compartment and the right ovarian fossa, it is very important to identify the integrity of these intestinal segments in order to exclude deep involvement (Fig. 4.189).

The superficial, serous involvement may go unnoticed by MRI, especially in the appendix (Fig. 4.190).

Deep implants are expressed by asymmetric parietal thickening on the antimesenteric face, sparing the mucosa, which progressively determines adhesion and wrinkling on the wall of the loop. When in the cecum, they promote retraction and deformity, especially at the base (Fig. 4.191).

Rarely, adhesions and fibrosis cause stenosis of the intestinal loop (Fig. 4.188) [80].

Signal intensity is low in the T2-weighted sequence and intermediate in the T1-weighted sequence, but may present bleeding foci (T1) or cysts (T2) due to ectopic endometrial tissue.

Appendiceal endometriosis may present with mucocele. However, there are only ten reported cases of appendix mucocele related to endometriosis. Hypertrophy of the smooth muscle of the appendix promotes obstruction of some of the glandular crypts, with increased mucin production. There is lumen dilation (15 mm) with circumscribed cystic lesion formation, with a hypointense or intermediate signal in the T1-weighted sequence and a hyperintense signal in the T2-weighted sequence, due to the high protein content (Figs. 4.191 and 4.192) [78, 81].

The presence of a nodule on the mucocele wall suggests an association with cystadenocarcinoma [78].

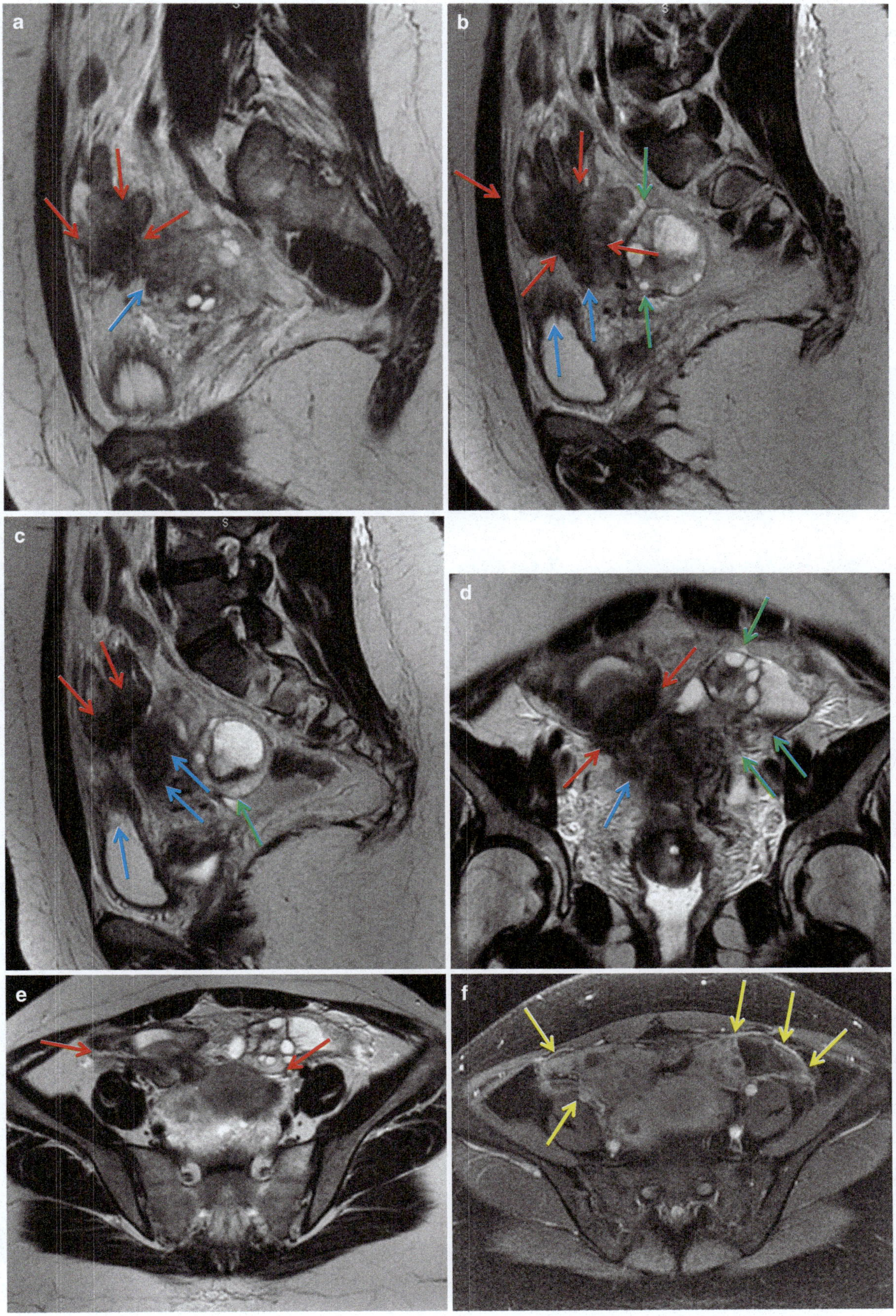

Fig. 4.189 Involvement of the cecum and appendix (red arrows **a–d**) by extension of the lesion in the anterior compartment with bladder and myometrial ligament involvement (blue arrows **a–d**). Note peritoneal endometriosis and multiple adhesions between these structures and adnexas (green arrows **b–d**), in addition to an intense inflammatory reaction with enhancement and peritoneal thickening (yellow arrows in **f**). T2-weighted sequences (**a–e**) and T1 (**f**). (**a**, **c**) Sagittal. (**d**) Coronal. (**e**, **f**) Axial

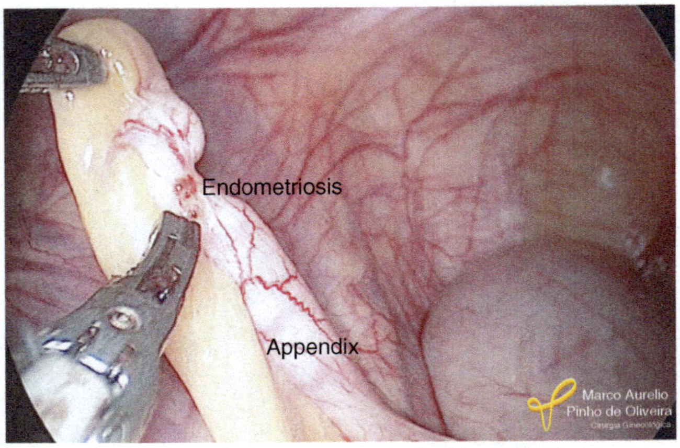

Fig. 4.190 Laparoscopy. Superficial intestinal involvement in the serosa of the appendix, with petechiae and vascular hyperemia

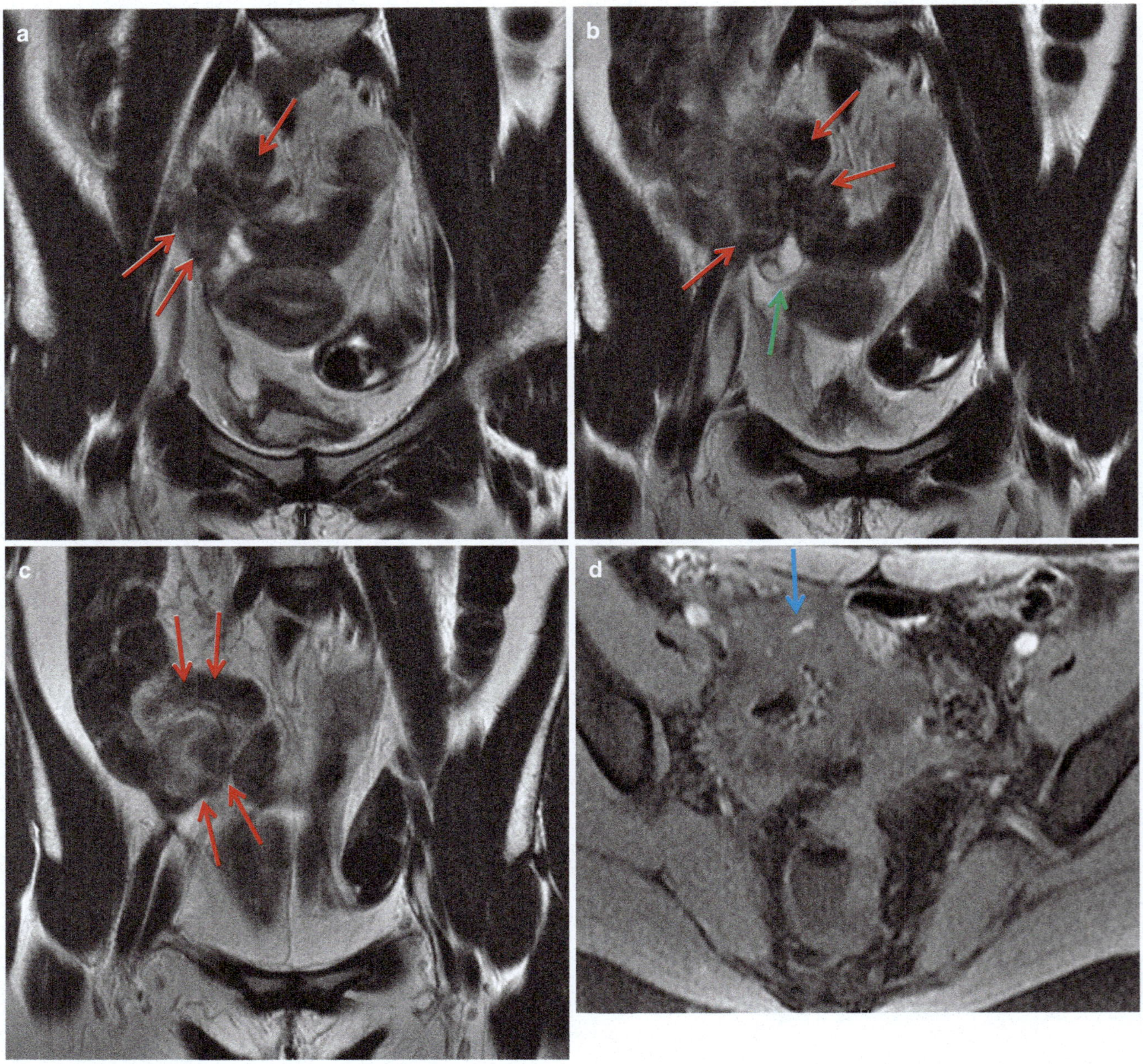

Fig. 4.191 Deep implant in the cecum and ileocecal valve, promoting retraction and deformity (red arrows). Heterogeneous T2-weighted lesion, predominantly hypointense (**a**–**c**), and intermediate signal at T1 (**d**), with discrete bleeding (hyperintense foci—blue arrow in **d**). (**a**, **c**) Coronal. (**d**) Axial. Note distension of appendix by mucocele (green arrow **b**)

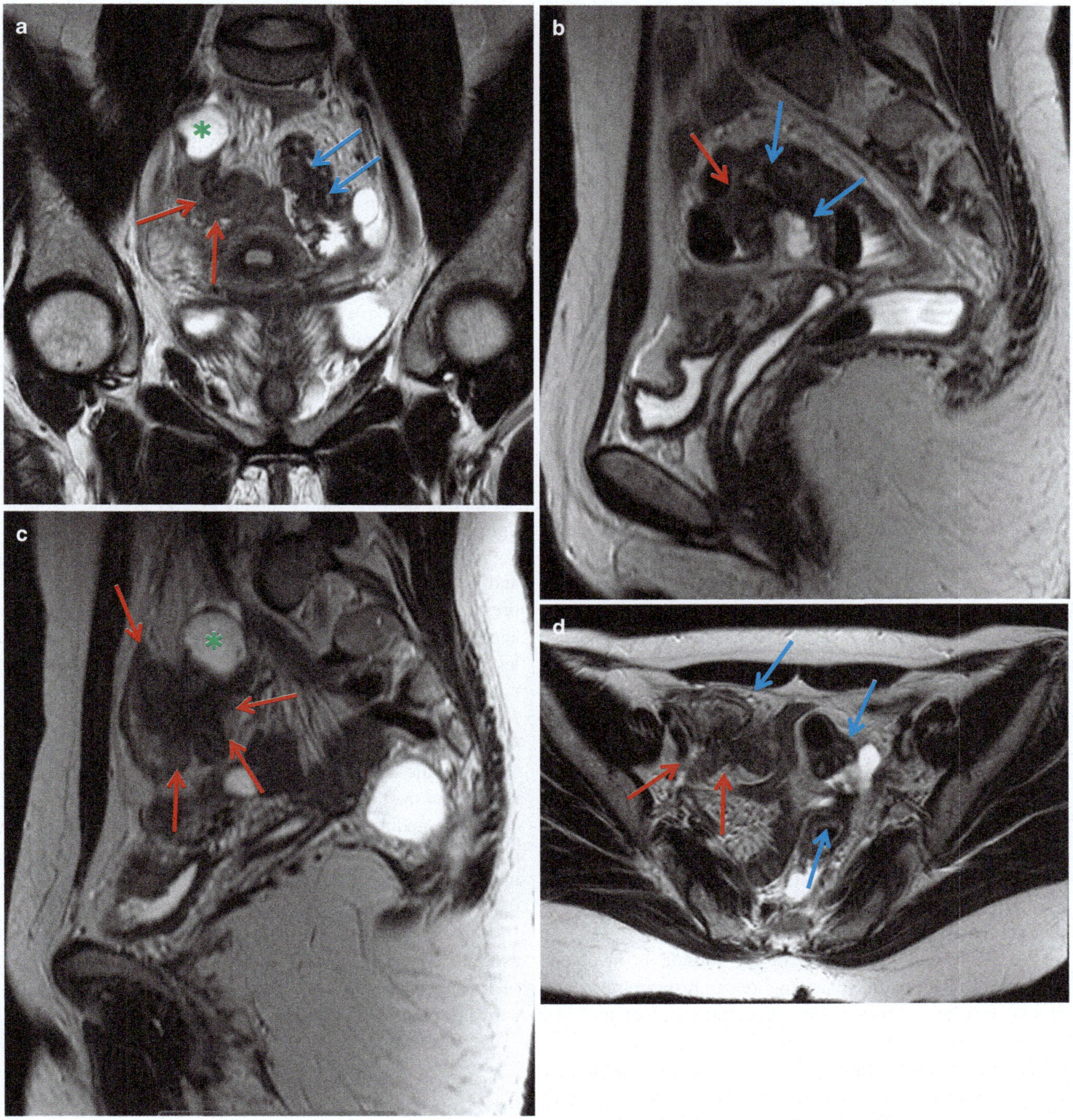

Fig. 4.192 Cecal endometriosis (red arrows), causing parietal thickening, distortion, and retraction (**a**, **d**), in addition to enlargement of the appendix, with formation of pericecal cyst (* in **a**, **c**). Note sigmoid and associated peritoneal endometriosis (blue arrows on **b**, **d**). T2-weighted sequences. (**a**) Coronal. (**b**, **c**) Sagittal. (**d**) Axial

4.5.5 Comments on Treatment

The lesions of the appendix and at the base of the cecum should be routinely removed, because in addition to the association with chronic right flank pain, there is a possibility of the condition worsening (appendicitis).

Moreover, histological evaluation of the appendix is necessary because a carcinoid tumor or even another type of neoplasia may be present.

Terminal ileal lesions and extensive cecal lesions may involve the ileocecal valve and progress to a severe intestinal obstruction. When recognized preoperatively or during surgery, such lesions should be removed.

The appendectomy can be performed with suture threads at the base (with or without invagination of the appendicular stump) or with mechanical suture with linear staplers.

Small lesions at the base of the cecum next to the appendix can also be removed (typhlectomy) using linear endoscopic staplers.

Extensive lesions of the terminal ileum and cecum usually require right hemicolectomy with ileus anastomosis.

4.5.6 Diaphragm

4.5.6.1 Anatomy

The diaphragm is a dome-shaped muscle, which delimits the thoracic cavity from the abdomen.

The peritoneum covers the hepatic face and the parietal pleura the upper face.

4.5.6.2 Common Aspects of Endometriosis

Diaphragmatic endometriosis is rare and often asymptomatic. The symptoms are related to the deep involvement of the muscle [82].

When the entire thickness of the muscle is involved, extension to the pleural space may occur, resulting in pneumonia or a hemothorax. More than 100 cases of thoracic endometriosis have been described [83].

The most plausible theory about this condition is based on retrograde menstruation and subsequent transport of viable cells in the peritoneal fluid of the pelvis to the right diaphragmatic dome [82].

4.5.6.3 Clinical Condition

When symptomatic, diaphragmatic endometriosis is associated with deep lesions involving the full thickness of the diaphragm, with symptoms including pain in the shoulder, epigastrium, chest, or upper right quadrant, probably caused by the irritating effect of the diaphragm implants. The pain can be catamenial [84].

4.5.6.4 MRI and Laparoscopic Findings

Diaphragmatic endometriosis presentation varies at MRI. It may be negative, related to small superficial nodule or holes, observed at laparoscopy. Therefore, a negative exam does not rule out endometriosis.

Lesions identified at MRI exams are usually located at the right posterior subdiaphragmatic area; however, in authors' experience, lesions at the hepatic domus, as well as anteriorly located, may be found. They may present as a micronodule, nodule and a plaque, as well as a hole with a focal liver herniation. Lesions can be unique or may present as a multiple diaphragmatic involvement.

Well-defined elongated hyperintense lesions in the T1- and T2-weighted sequences, especially when using fat suppression, are observed in MRI between the diaphragmatic and hepatic surfaces (Fig. 4.193). Occasionally, hyperintense lesions on T2-weighted sequence do not present hypersignals on the T1-weighted sequence (Fig. 4.194) [85].

4.5.6.5 Comments on Treatment

Small nodules can be removed without the need for resection throughout the thickness of the diaphragm (shaving).

Larger nodules most often reach the pleura, and if the patient is very symptomatic—sometimes having incapacitating pain in the right clavicular region—complete resection of the affected area with opening of the diaphragm is necessary.

In these cases, the surgical treatment is more complex, especially when posterior [83].

In some situations, surgery may be initiated by thoracoscopy after unilateral pneumothorax.

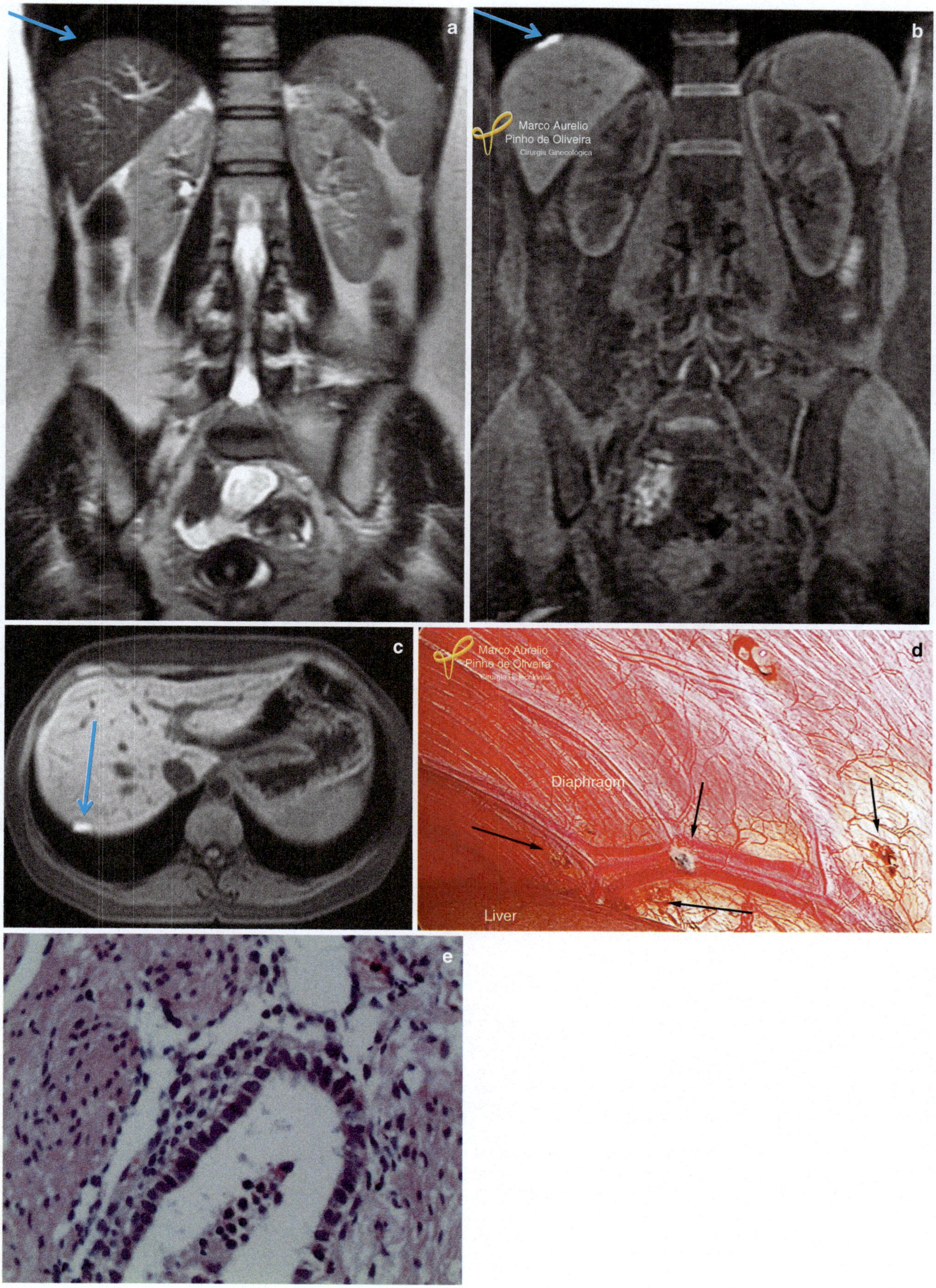

Fig. 4.193 Endometrioses in the right diaphragm (arrows). Elongated lesion, lobulated, well defined, hyperintense in T1-weighted sequences with fat suppression (**b**, **c**) and hypointense on T2 (old bleed in **a**). (**a**, **b**) Coronal. (**c**) Axial. (**d**) Laparoscopy demonstrating implants on the diaphragmatic surface. (**e**) Microscopy (400×) with endometrial gland in the secretory phase surrounded by striated muscle

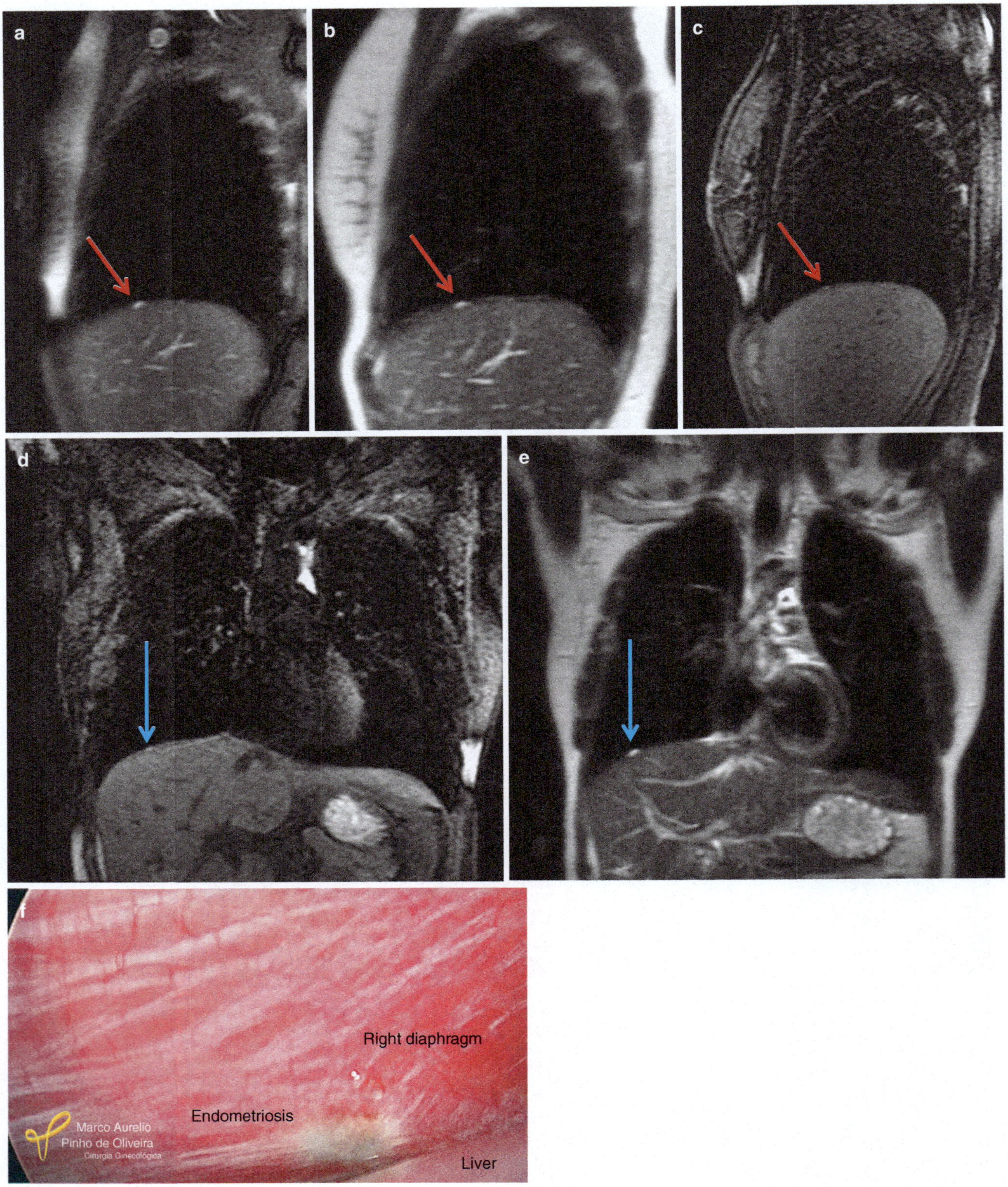

Fig. 4.194 Small lesion in the right of the diaphragm, easily identified on T2-weighted sequence (**e**) and T2 with fat suppression (**a**), hyperintense, with discrete hyperintense signal on T1-weighted sequence (**c**, **d**). (**a**–**c**) Sagittal. (**d**, **e**) Coronal. (**f**) Laparoscopy with lesion penetrating the diaphragm

References

1. Schneider A, Touloupidis S, Papatsoris A, Triantafyllidis A, Kollias A, Schweppe K. Endometriosis of the urinary tract in women of reproductive age. Int J Urol. 2006;13:902–4.
2. Denes FT. Ureteral endometriosis. Int Urol Nephrol. 1980;12:205–9.
3. Chapron C. Deeply infiltrating endometriosis: pathogenetic implications of the anatomical distribution. Hum Reprod. 2006;21:1839–45.
4. Chapron C, Bourret A, Chopin N, Dousset B, Leconte M, Amsellem-Ouazana D, de Ziegler D, Borghese B. Surgery for bladder endometriosis: long-term results and concomitant management of associated posterior deep lesions. Hum Reprod. 2010;25:884–9.
5. Vercellini P, Chapron C, Fedele L, Gattei U, Daguati R, Crosignani P. Review: evidence for asymmetric distribution of lower intestinal tract endometriosis. BJOG. 2004;111:1213–7.
6. Vercellini P, Pisacreta A, Pesole A, Vicentini S, Stellato G, Crosignani P. Is ureteral endometriosis an asymmetric disease? BJOG. 2000;107:559–61.
7. Piketty M, Chopin N, Dousset B, Millischer-Bellaische A, Roseau G, Leconte M, Borghese B, Chapron C. Preoperative work-up for patients with deeply infiltrating endometriosis: transvaginal ultrasonography must definitely be the first-line imaging examination. Hum Reprod. 2008;24:602–7.
8. Bazot M, Darai E, Hourani R, Thomassin I, Cortez A, Uzan S, Buy J. Deep pelvic endometriosis: MR imaging for diagnosis and prediction of extension of disease. Radiology. 2004;232:379–89.
9. Crispi C. Tratado de Videoendoscopia e Cirurgia minimamente invasiva em Ginecologia. 5th ed. Rio de Janeiro: Revinter; 2011.
10. Gabriel B, Nassif J, Trompoukis P, Barata S, Wattiez A. Prevalence and management of urinary tract endometriosis: a clinical case series. Urology. 2011;78:1269–74.
11. Abrão M, Gonçalves M, Dias J Jr, Podgaec S, Chamie L, Blasbalg R. Comparison between clinical examination, transvaginal ultrasonography and magnetic resonance imaging for the diagnosis of pelvic endometriosis. Hum Reprod. 2007;22:3092.
12. Maccagnano C, Pellucchi F, Rocchini L, Ghezzi M, Scattoni V, Montorsi F, Rigatti P, Colombo R. Ureteral endometriosis: proposal for a diagnostic and therapeutic algorithm with a review of the literature. Urol Int. 2013;91:1–9.
13. Takagi H. Novel medical management of primary bladder endometriosis with dienogest: a case report. Clin Exp Obstet Gynecol. 2011;38:184–5.
14. Harada M, Osuga Y, Izumi G, Takamura M, Takemura Y, Hirata T, Yoshino O, Koga K, Yano T, Taketani Y. Dienogest, a new conservative strategy for extragenital endometriosis: a pilot study. Gynecol Endocrinol. 2010;27:717–20.
15. Pérez M, Bazán A, Alonso Dorrego J, Hernández A, de Francisco M, Hernández M, de Santiago J, de la Peña Barthel J. Urinary tract endometriosis: clinical, diagnostic, and therapeutic aspects. Urology. 2009;73:47–51.
16. Fedele L, Bianchi S, Zanconato G, Bergamini V, Berlanda N, Carmignani L. Long-term follow-up after conservative surgery for bladder endometriosis. Fertil Steril. 2005;83:1729–33.
17. Crispi C, de Souza C, Oliveira M, Dibi R, Cardeman L, Sato H, Schor E. Endometriosis of the round ligament of the uterus. J Minim Invasive Gynecol. 2012;19:46–51.
18. Claudon M. The normal ureter. In: Soulie M, Otal P, Joffre F, editors. Radiological imaging of the ureter. Berlin: Springer; 2003. p. 21–36.
19. Kunz G. Adenomyosis in endometriosis—prevalence and impact on fertility. Evidence from magnetic resonance imaging. Hum Reprod. 2005;20:2309–16.
20. Busard M, Mijatovic V, Lüchinger A, Bleeker M, Pieters-van den Bos I, Schats R, van Kuijk C, Hompes P, van Waesberghe J. MR imaging of bladder endometriosis and its relationship with the anterior uterine wall: experience in a tertiary referral centre. Eur J Radiol. 2012;81:2106–11.
21. Bennett G, Slywotzky C, Cantera M, Hecht E. Unusual manifestations and complications of endometriosis—spectrum of imaging findings: pictorial review. Am J Roentgenol. 2010;194:WS34–46.
22. Grasso R, Di Giacomo V, Sedati P, Sizzi O, Florio G, Faiella E, Rossetti A, Del Vescovo R, Beomonte Z. Diagnosis of deep infiltrating endometriosis: accuracy of magnetic resonance imaging and transvaginal 3D ultrasonography. Abdom Imaging. 2009;35: 716–25.
23. Halim A. Human anatomy female pelvis and breast; 2003. 54.
24. Mashfiqul M. Endometriosis of the inguinal canal mimicking a hernia. Singap Med J. 2007;48:157–9.
25. Habiba M, Benagiano G. The incidence and clinical significance of adenomyosis. In: Habiba M, editor. Uterine adenomyosis. New York: Springer; 2016. p. 9–43.
26. Novellas S, Chassang M, Bouaziz J, Delotte J, Toullalan O, Chevallier E. Anterior pelvic endometriosis: MRI features. Abdom Imaging. 2010;35:742–9.
27. Chamié L, Blasbalg R, Pereira R, Warmbrand G, Serafini P. Findings of pelvic endometriosis at transvaginal US, MR imaging, and laparoscopy. Radiographics. 2011;31:E77–E100.
28. Woodward P, Sohaey R, Mezzetti T. Endometriosis: radiologic-pathologic correlation. Radiographics. 2001;21:193–216.
29. Pranay R. Laparoscopic management of moderate: severe endometriosis. J Minim Access Surg. 2014;10:27–33.
30. Luterek K, Barcz E, Bablok L, Wierzbicki Z. Giant recurrent perineal endometriosis in an episiotomy scar—a case report. Polish Gynaecol. 2013;84:726–9.
31. Odobasic A, Pasic A, Iljazovic-Latifagic E, Arnautalic L, Odobasic A, Idrizovic E, Dervisefendic M, Dedić L. Perineal endometriosis: a case report and review of the literature. Tech Coloproctol. 2010;14:25–7.
32. Vimercati A, Achilarre M, Scardapane A, Lorusso F, Ceci O, Mangiatordi G, Angelelli G, Van Herendael B, Selvaggi L, Bettocchi S. Accuracy of transvaginal sonography and contrast-enhanced magnetic resonance-colonography for the presurgical staging of deep infiltrating endometriosis. Ultrasound Obstet Gynecol. 2012;40:592–603.
33. Chapron C, Santulli P, de Ziegler D, Noel J, Anaf V, Streuli I, Foulot H, Souza C, Borghese B. Ovarian endometrioma: severe pelvic pain is associated with deeply infiltrating endometriosis. Hum Reprod. 2012;27:702–11.
34. Clement M. Diseases of the peritoneum. In: Kurman R, editor. Blaustein's pathology of the female genital tract. New York: Springer; 2002. p. 729–89.
35. Brandão A, Ianez P. MR imaging of the pelvic floor: defecography. Magn Reson Imaging Clin N Am. 2013;21:427–45.
36. Thomas E, Cooke I. Impact of gestrinone on the course of asymptomatic endometriosis. BMJ (Clin Res Ed). 1987;294:272–4.
37. Milley P, Nichols D. A correlative investigation of the human rectvaginal septum. Obstet Gynecol Surv. 1969;24:1288–91.
38. Abrão M. Tratamento cirúrgico na endometriose: quando e como fazer. In: Abrão M, editor. Endometriose: uma visão contemporânea. Rio de Janeiro: Revinter; 2000. p. 137–47.
39. Fauconnier A, Chapron C, Dubuisson J, Vieira M, Dousset B, Bréart G. Relation between pain symptoms and the anatomic location of deep infiltrating endometriosis. Fertil Steril. 2002;78:719–26.
40. Fedele L, Bianchi S, Zanconato G, Raffaelli R, Berlanda N. Is rectovaginal endometriosis a progressive disease? Am J Obstet Gynecol. 2004;191:1539–42.
41. Vu D. Surgical anatomy of the uterosacral ligament. Int Urogynecol J. 2010;21:1123–8.
42. Anaf V, Simon P, Nakadi I, Simonart T, Noel J, Buxant F. Impact of surgical resection of rectovafinal pouch of douglas endometriotic

nodules on pelvic pain and some elements of patients' sex life. J Am Assoc Gynecol Laparosc. 2001;8:55–60.
43. Del Frate C, Girometti R, Pittino M, Del Frate G, Bazzocchi M, Zuiani C. Deep retroperitoneal pelvic endometriosis: MR imaging appearance with laparoscopic correlation. Radiographics. 2006;26:1705–18.
44. Bazot M, Gasner A, Ballester M, Darai E. Value of thin-section oblique axial T2-weighted magnetic resonance images to assess uterosacral ligament endometriosis. Hum Reprod. 2010;26:346–53.
45. Kondo W, Ribeiro R, Trippia C, Zomer M. Deep infiltrating endometriosis: anatomical distribution and surgical treatment. Rev Bras Ginecol Obstet. 2012;34:278–84.
46. Fritsch H. Clinical anatomy of the female pelvis. In: Hamm B, Forstner R, editors. MRI and CT of the female pelvis. New York: Springer; 2007. p. 1–24.
47. Schafer A, Langer M. MRI of rectal cancer. In: Schafer AO, editor. Anorectal anatomy. Clinical implications for MR radiologist. New York: Springer; 2010. p. 5–13.
48. Brown G, Kirkham A, Williams G, Bourne M, Radcliffe A, Sayman J, Newell R, Sinnatamby C, Heald R. High-resolution MRI of the anatomy important in total mesorectal excision of the rectum. Am J Roentgenol. 2004;182:431–9.
49. Weed J, Ray J. Endometriosis of the bowel. Obstet Gynecol. 1987;69:727.
50. Remorgida V, Ferrero S, Fulcheri E, Ragni N, Martin D. Bowel endometriosis: presentation, diagnosis, and treatment. Obstet Gynecol Surv. 2007;62:461–70.
51. Pisanu A, Deplano D, Angioni S, Ambu R, Uccheddu A. Rectal perforation from endometriosis in pregnancy: case case report and literature review. World J Gastroenterol. 2010;16:648–51.
52. Remorgida V, Ragni N, Ferrero S, Anserini P, Torelli P, Fulcheri E. The involvement of the interstitial Cajal cells and the enteric nervous system in bowel endometriosis. Hum Reprod. 2004;20:264–71.
53. Ferrero S, Haas S, Remorgida V, Camerini G, Fulcheri E, Ragni N, Straub R, Capellino S. Loss of sympathetic nerve fibers in intestinal endometriosis. Fertil Steril. 2010;94:2817–9.
54. Seracchioli R, Mabrouk M, Guerrini M, Manuzzi L, Savelli L, Frascà C, Venturoli S. Dyschezia and posterior deep infiltrating endometriosis: analysis of 360 cases. J Minim Invasive Gynecol. 2008;15:695–9.
55. Yoon J, Choi D, Jang K, Kim C, Kim H, Lee S, Chun H, Lee W, Yun S. Deep rectosigmoid endometriosis: "mushroom cap" sign on T2-weighted MR imaging. Abdom Imaging. 2010;35:726–31.
56. De Anchorena M. Bowel endometriosis. Prensa Méd Argent. 1999; 86:746–54.
57. Garcia A, Spadoni Neto B, Garcia V, Arruda P, Garcia D. Colonic endometriosis simulating colorectal cancer: report of 2 cases. Revista Brasileira de Coloproctologia. 2006;26:316–20.
58. Guerra G. Endometriose de Reto: Relato de Caso. Revista Brasileira de Coloproctologia. 2004;24:354–7.
59. Oliveira M, Crispi C, Oliveira F, Junior P, Raymundo T, Pereira T. Double circular stapler technique for bowel resection in rectosigmoid endometriosis. J Minim Invasive Gynecol. 2014;21:136–41.
60. Smith J. An atlas of gynecologic oncology; 2003. 82.
61. Ceccaroni M, Clarizia R, Alboni C, Ruffo G, Bruni F, Roviglione G, Scioscia M, Peters I, De Placido G, Minelli L. Laparoscopic nerve-sparing transperitoneal approach for endometriosis infiltrating the pelvic wall and somatic nerves: anatomical considerations and surgical technique. Surg Radiol Anat. 2010;32:601–4.
62. Cottier J. Sciatic endometriosis: MR evaluation. Am J Neuroradiol. 1995;16:1399–401.
63. Manganaro L, Porpora M, Vinci V, et al. Diffusion tensor imaging and tractography to evaluate sacral nerve root abnormalities in endometriosis-related pain: a pilot study. Eur Radiol. 2013;24:95–101.
64. Stoker J, Taylor S, DeLancey J. Imaging pelvic floor disorders, vol. 153. New York: Springer; 2008.
65. Brandão A, Werner H Jr, Daltro P. Ressonância Magnética em obstetrícia e ginecologia. Rio de Janeiro: Revinter; 2003.
66. Shaw R. Atlas of endometriosis; 1993. 25.
67. Hassanin-Negila A. Endometriomas of the abdominal wall: imaging findings. J Radiol. 2006;87:1691–5.
68. Zhao X, Lang J, Leng J, Liu Z, Sun D, Zhu L. Abdominal wall endometriomas. Int J Gynecol Obstet. 2005;90:218–22.
69. Kaunitz A. Needle tract endometriosis: an unusual complication of amniocentesis. Obstet Gynecol. 1979;54:753–5.
70. Oliveira M, de Leon A, Freire E, de Oliveira H. Risk factors for abdominal scar endometriosis after obstetric hysterotomies: a case-control study. Acta Obstet Gynecol Scand. 2007;86:73–80.
71. Horton H, Dezee K, Ahnfeldt E, Wagner M. Abdominal wall endometriosis: a surgeon's perspective and review of 445 cases. Am J Surg. 2008;196:207–12.
72. Hartigan C, Holloway B. MR imaging features of endometriosis at the umbilicus. Br J Radiol. 2005;78:755–7.
73. Yang D. Inguinal endometriosis presenting as a multicystic mass on sonography. JUM. 2007;26:1449–51.
74. Kirkpatrick A, Reed C, Bui-Mansfield L, Russell M, Whitford W. Radiologic-pathologic conference of Brooke Army Medical Center: endometriosis of the canal of Nuck. AJR. 2006;186:56–7.
75. Snell R. Clinical anatomy, 7th ed; 2004. p. 215–7.
76. De Ceglie A. Acute small bowel obstruction caused by endometriosis: a case report and review of the literature. World J Gastroenterol. 2008;14:3430–4.
77. Karaman K, Pala E, Bayol U, Akman O, Olmez M, Unluoglu S, Ozturk S. Endometriosis of the terminal ileum: a diagnostic dilemma. Case Rep Pathol. 2012;2012:1–4.
78. Tsuda M, Yamashita Y, Azuma S, Akamatsu T, Seta T, Urai S, Uenoyama Y, Deguchi Y, Ono K, Chiba T. Mucocele of the appendix due to endometriosis: a rare case report. World J Gastroenterol. 2013;19:5021–4.
79. Kaemmerer E, Westerkamp M, Kasperk R, Niepmann G, Scherer A, Gassler N. Coincidence of active Crohn's disease and florid endometriosis in the terminal ileum: a case report. World J Gastroenterol. 2013;19:4413–7.
80. Ridha J, Cassaro S. Acute small bowel obstruction secondary to ileal endometriosis: report of a case. Surg Today. 2003; 33:944–7.
81. Hapke M, Bigelow B. Mucocele of the appendix secondary to obstruction by endometriosis. Hum Pathol. 1977;8:585–9.
82. Ceccaroni M, Roviglione G, Rosenberg P, et al. Pericardial, pleural and diaphragmatic endometriosis in association with pelvic peritoneal and bowel endometriosis: a and review of the literature. Wideochir Inne Tech Maloinwazyjne. 2012;7:122–31.
83. Jubanyik K, Comite F. Extrapelvic endometriosis. Obstet Gynecol Clin N Am. 1997;24:411–40.
84. Wolthuis A, Aelvoet C, Bosteels J, Vanrijkel J. Diaphragmatic endometriosis: diagnosis and surgical management—a case report. Acta Chir Belg. 2003;103:519–20.
85. Rousset P, Gregory J, Rousset-Jablonski C, Hugon-Rodin J, Regnard JF, Chapron C, Coste J, Golfier F, Revel MP. MR diagnosis of diaphragmatic endometriosis. Eur Radiol. 2016;26(11): 3968–77.

Stratification Risk and Monitoring of Patient by MRI

5

5.1 Patient Risk Stratification

The treatment of deep endometriosis has evolved over the last decade.

Currently, laparoscopy is used only as a therapeutic tool in deep endometriosis and no longer diagnostically, as in the past.

Furthermore, a new therapeutic, medical, and surgical arsenal has emerged, providing increased treatment options for patients.

Thus, the clinical and radiological evaluation of the patient has acquired great value in therapeutic planning.

The current goal of radiology is to provide the gynecological surgeon with the maximum amount of information on the disease in the abdomen and pelvis, allowing the selection of the most appropriate treatment, be it conservative or surgical.

When it has been decided to use surgical therapy, MRI should provide all the details of the lesion, identifying patients with the highest surgical risk and allowing the highest quality and safest procedure.

Thus, it is possible to fulfil the main goal in the treatment of endometriosis: the complete removal of all lesions in a single surgical procedure.

The image in deep endometriosis produced in the most appropriate manner by an experienced radiologist allows the planning of a new therapeutic strategy, personalized through the risk stratification of the patient, separating them into low- and high-risk groups.

For this, the selection of patients by the radiologist should be divided into the steps described below.

1. **Identify the local characteristics**, by organ, of the sites which influence the therapy, that is to say descriptors of the risk lesion for each organ, as already mentioned in the previous section, in Table 4.1.
2. **Check the multifocality of the deep endometriosis**. This means detailing the presence of multiple lesions in the same organ, such as in the intestine, and other organs, such as the bladder and ovaries (Fig. 5.1).
3. **Identify atypical lesion locations**, such as isolated lesions in the pelvic floor, and urethral or bladder involvement due to endometriosis in the anterior abdominal wall. This type of lesion may not be observed at the beginning of laparoscopy; furthermore, the surgical approach may be completely different (Fig. 5.2).
4. **Check associated ovarian and tubal lesions**, which may have implications for the chance of the patients to become pregnant and, in addition, modify the surgery. Ovaries should always be removed from the pelvis during surgery. However, if there is an endometrioma, it must be mobilized and resected [1].
   The tubes must be kept if the surgeon deems that they are still functional. Distended, distorted, or blocked tubes are not functional and may be responsible for chronic pain in the iliac fossa and may further decrease the results of in vitro fertilization (Fig. 5.3).
5. **Note the relationship of the deep lesion to the ureter and urinary obstructive endometriosis**. The ureters are an important anatomical landmark in the pelvis during surgery for deep endometriosis. Thus, it is important to

A. Brandão et al., *Atlas of Deep Endometriosis*, https://doi.org/10.1007/978-3-319-71697-8_5

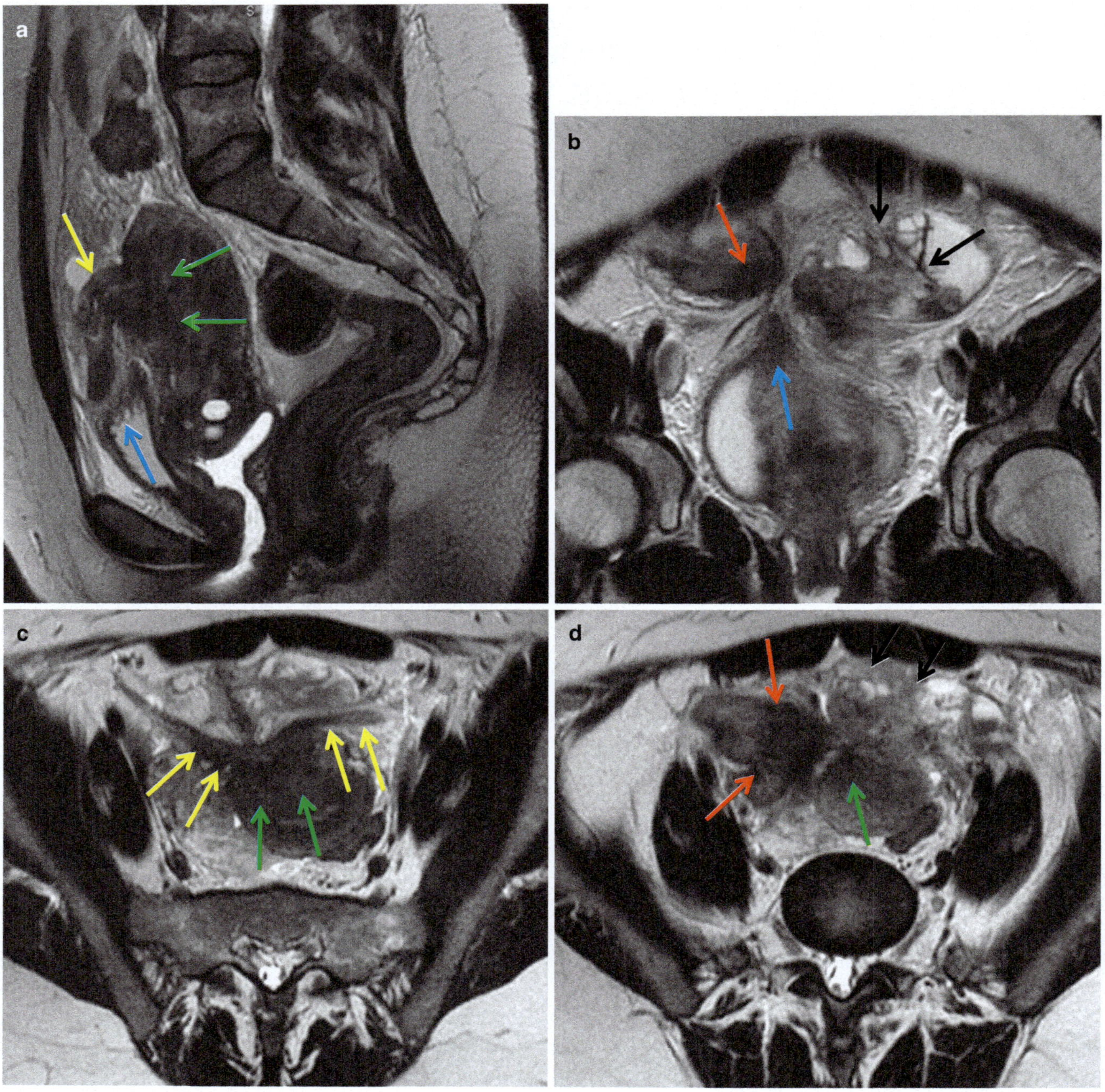

Fig. 5.1 Multifocality of deep endometriosis. Bladder endometriosis (blue arrows), myometrial (green arrows), ligamental (yellow arrows), cecal (red arrows), ovarian (black arrows), and peritoneal, with multiple adhesions. (**a**–**d**) T2-weighted sequences. (**a**) Sagittal. (**b**) Coronal. (**c**, **d**) Axial

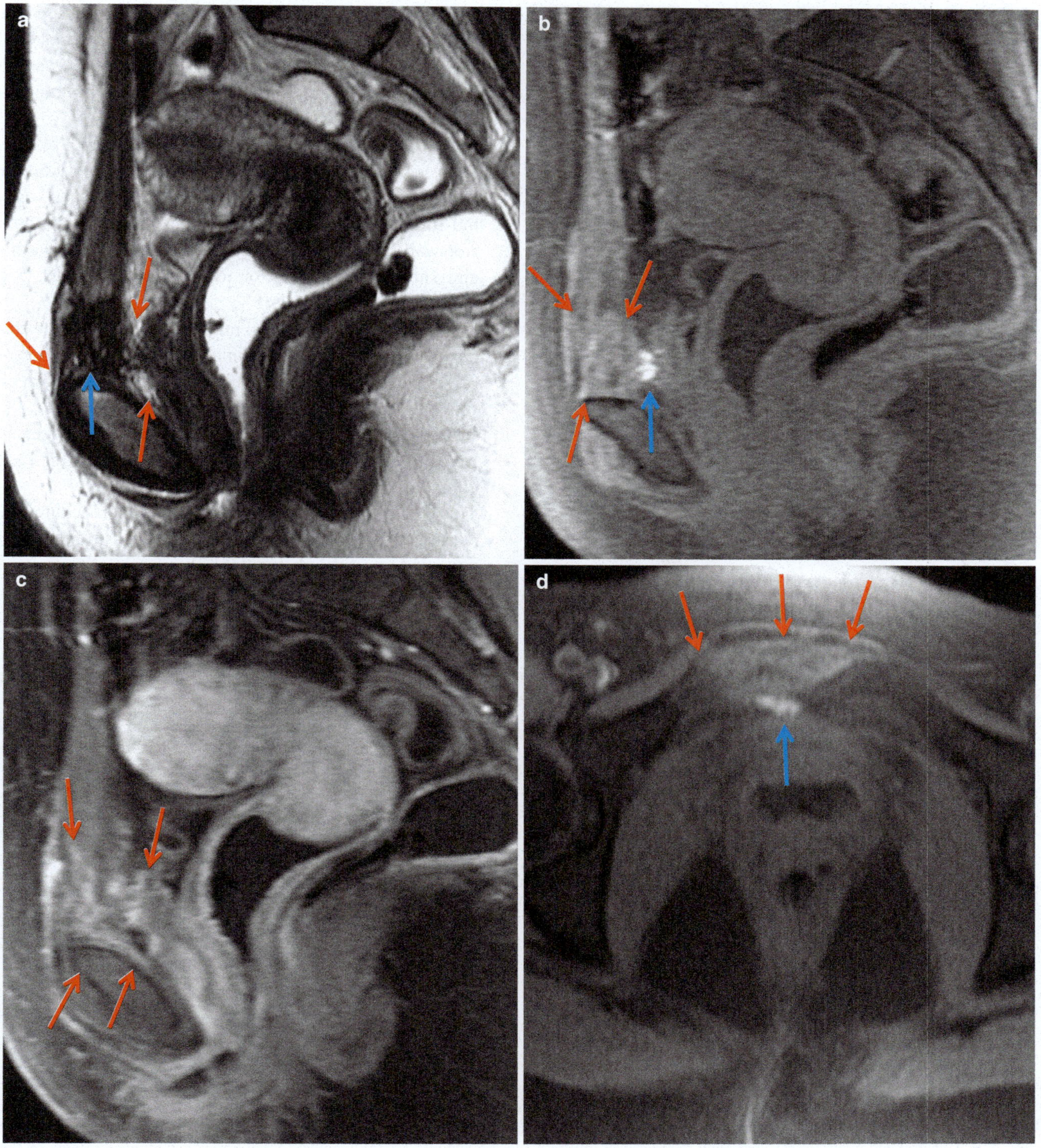

Fig. 5.2 Lesion in an atypical location: abdominal wall insinuated in the extraperitoneal space, compromising the bladder and urethra (red arrows). Lesion in the pubic insertion of the abdominal rectus, with hyposignal in T2 (**a**, **e**) and intermediate signal on T1 (**b**, **d**), and slight enhancement (**c**). Note hyperintense foci in ectopic endometrial tissue on T2 and T1 (blue arrows). (**a**, **e**) T2-weighted sequences. (**b**–**d**) T1-weighted sequences with fat saturation

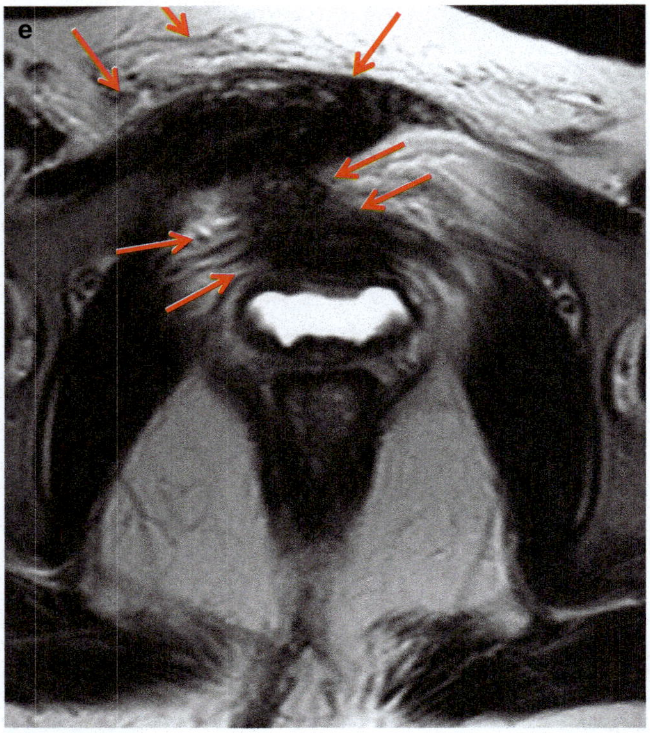

Fig. 5.2 (continued)

describe their distance to the lesion. In addition, when there is a ureteral lesion, its extent and degree of obstruction should be described. Ureteral lesions require partial resection with termino-terminal anastomosis or reimplantation of the ureter (Fig. 5.4) [1].

6. **Quantify the degree of adhesion** promoted by the deep lesion. Adherence can involve several organs in endometriosis. The obliteration of the posterior vaginal fornix is promoted by adhesion between the anterior wall of the rectum and the peritoneum and vagina and should be partially or totally resected (Figs. 5.4 and 5.5).

   The uterosacral ligaments may also be adhere to the adnexa, ureters, nerves, and intestines, resulting in ureterolysis, neurolysis, and identification of pararectal spaces for complete resection of the lesion [1].

   In addition, adhesion may be a consequence of fibrocicatricial tissue from previous surgical procedures, which are common in these patients.

   This type of lesion can hinder new surgical procedures, in addition to causing infertility, dyspareunia, chronic pelvic pain, and intestinal obstruction [2].

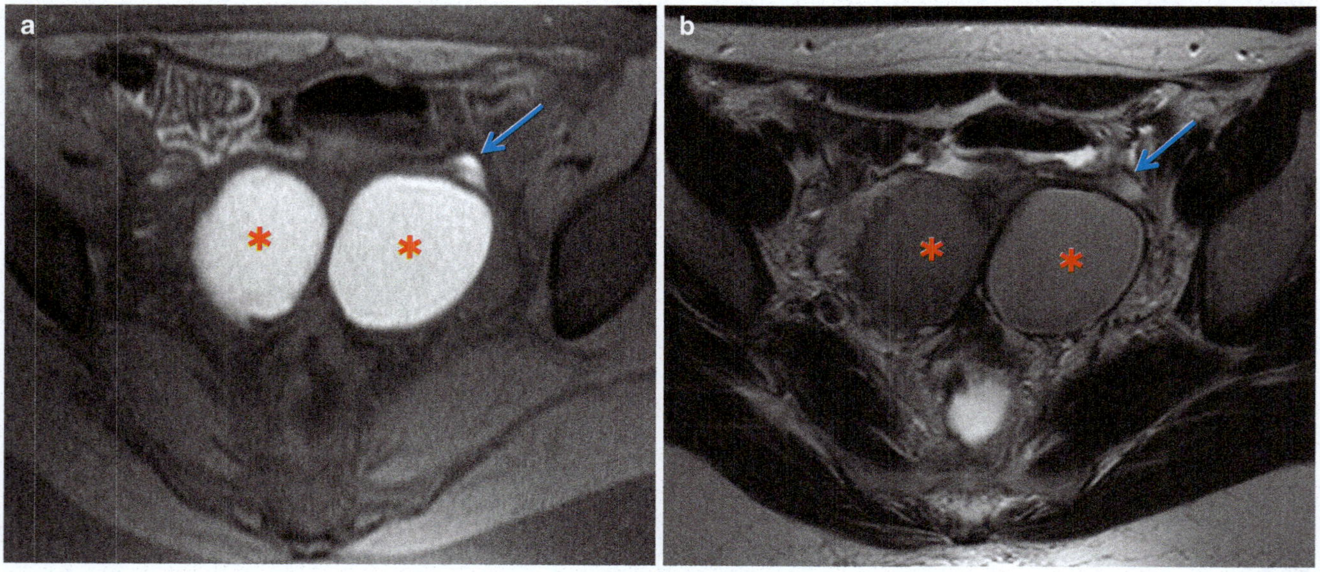

Fig. 5.3 Bilateral endometriomas (* **a–e**) and retrocervical infiltrative lesion and uterosacral ligament (green arrows) and hematosalpinx on the left (blue arrows **a–e**). (**a**, **c**) T1-weighted sequence with fat suppression. (**b**, **d**, **e**) T2-weighted. (**a–d**) Axial. (**e**) Sagittal

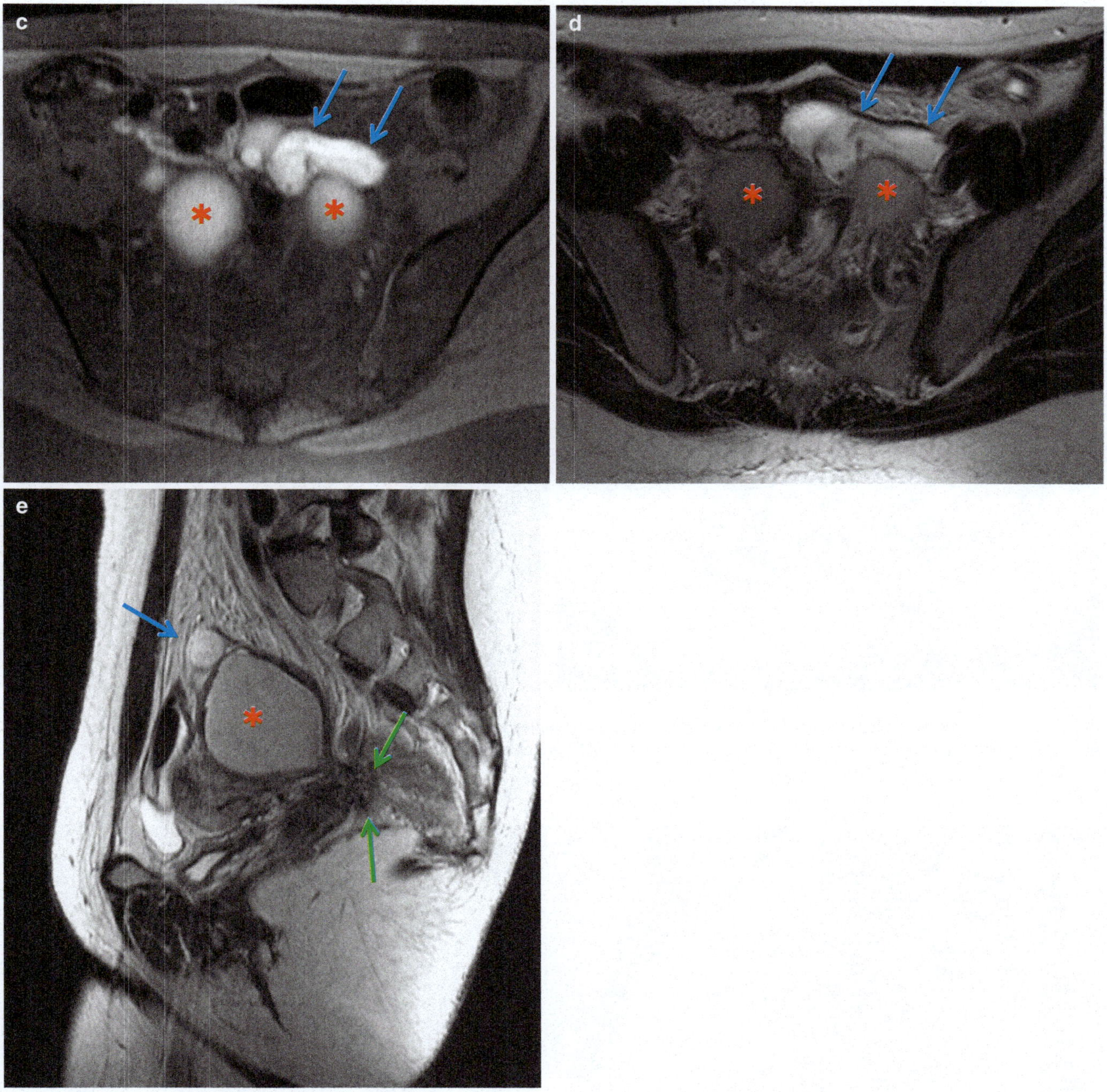

Fig. 5.3 (continued)

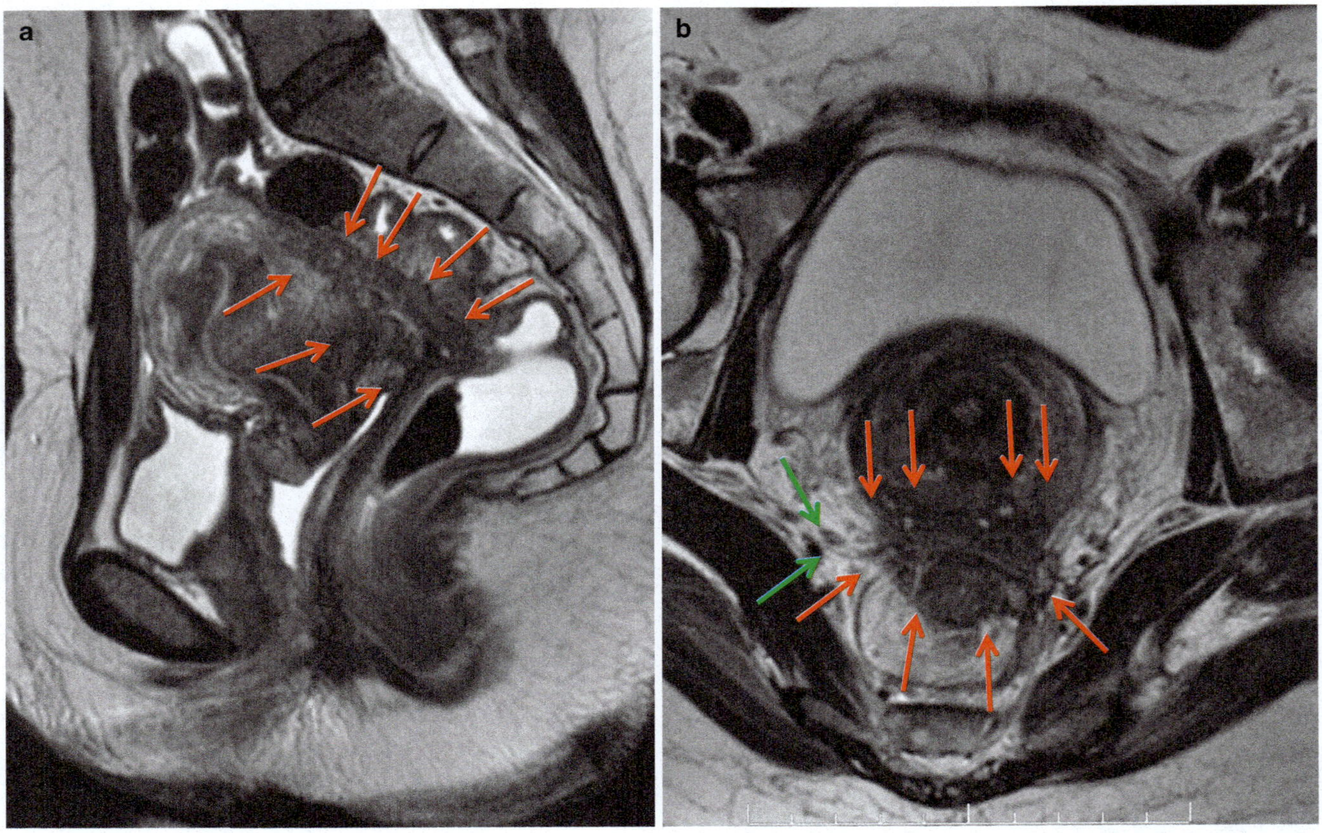

Fig. 5.4 Deep retrocervical lesion with upper plaque-like extension completely obliterating the cul-de-sac and intestinal and parametrial infiltration (red arrows). Relationship with the ureter (green arrow). (**a**, **b**) T2-weighted sequences. (**a**) Sagittal. (**b**) Axial

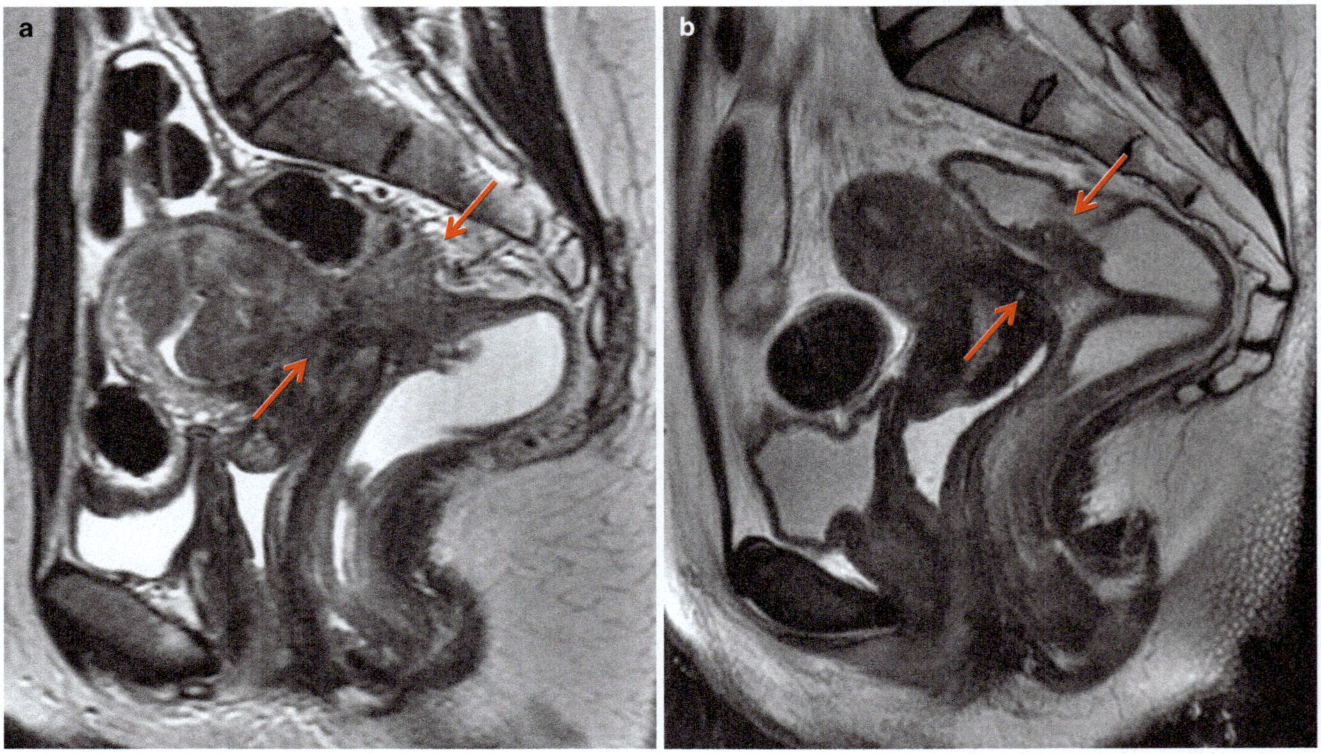

Fig. 5.5 (**a**) Obliteration of the posterior cul-de-sac by retrocervical lesion. Completed by adherence between the rectum, uterus, and vagina, by a retrocervical lesion causing stenosis of the rectum. (**b**) Partial with deep retrocervical and peritoneal lesion with rectal penetration. (**a**, **b**) Sagittal T2-weighted sequences

7. **Characterize the risk of malignancy in the endometriosis**. Endometriosis is a benign pathology with malignant transformation potential.
Genetic alterations (PTEN, p53 mutation of the bcl gene) and a chronic inflammatory state, with cytokine release, modification of mitotic division, and apoptosis similar to the malignant mechanism occur [3].
There is a higher incidence of endometriosis in patients with ovarian neoplasia. On the other hand, the risk of ovarian neoplasia development in these patients is four times greater, and the most common histological types are endometrioid carcinomas and clear-cell carcinomas [3].
However, ovarian endometrioma has a low malignant transformation risk of about 0.7–1.6% in 8 years, with the main risk factors for malignant transformation being advanced patient age and a tumor diameter greater than 9 cm (Fig. 5.6) [1, 4, 5].
The MRI morphological features of suspected malignancy include complex cysts with a solid component, papillary projections, necrosis, thick and irregular septa, bilateral lesions, peritoneal disease, ascites, and lymphadenopathy (Fig. 5.7).
However, these findings are not pathognomonic of malignancy. Multiparametric MRI, with analysis of vascular permeability and diffusion, improves the characterization of

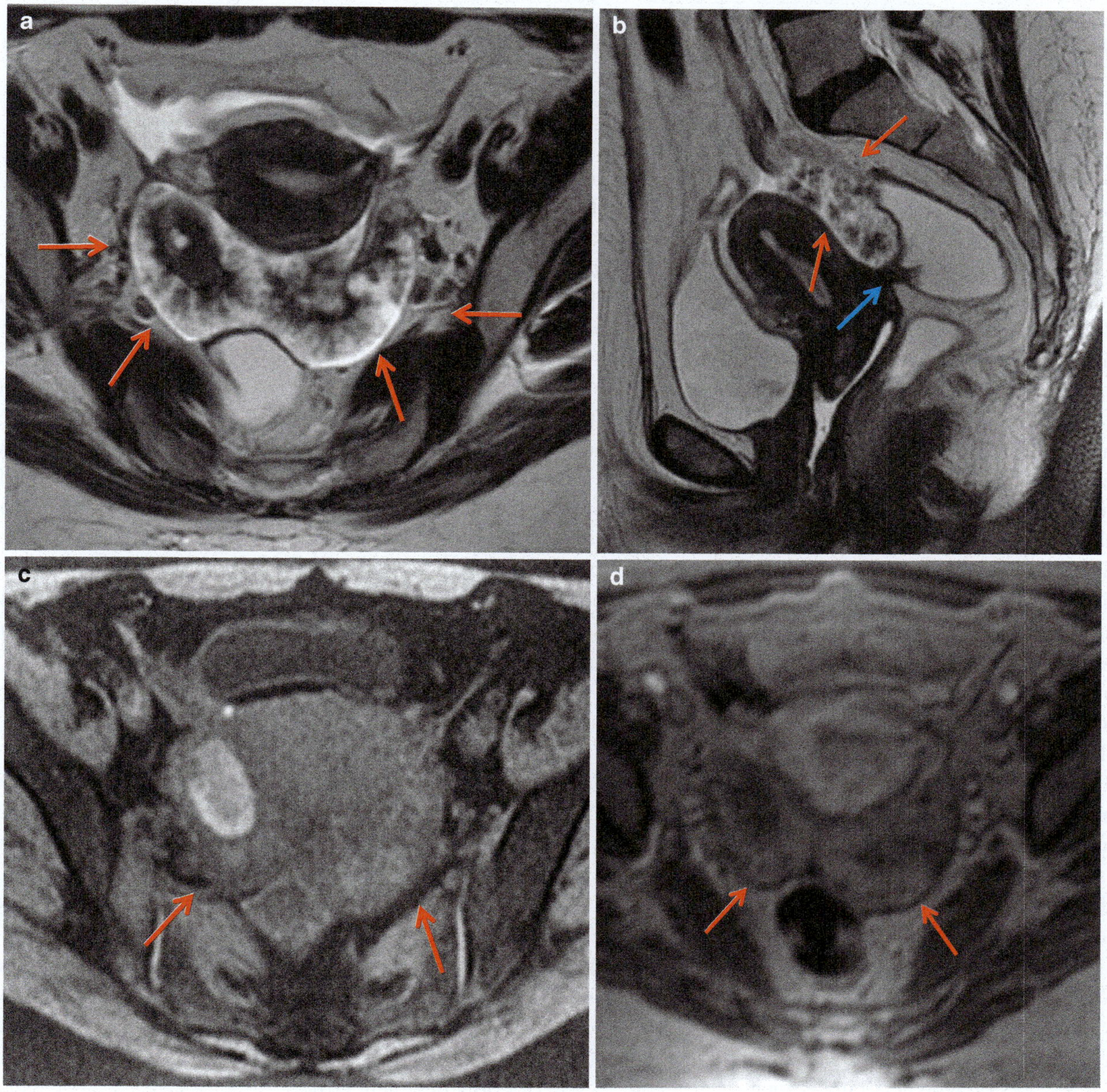

Fig. 5.6 Endometrioid cystadenocarcinoma. Bilateral multiloculated cyst with solid component (red arrows), heterogeneous aspect on T2 (**a**, **b**) with restricted diffusion (hyperintense on **e**), and lower intensity enhancement than the myometrium. Note retrocervical infiltrative lesion (blue arrow **b**). (**a**, **b**) T2-weighted sequences. (**c**) T1-weighted with fat suppression. (**d**) Permeability—DCE. (**e**) Diffusion. (**f**) Laparoscopic aspect of complex cyst

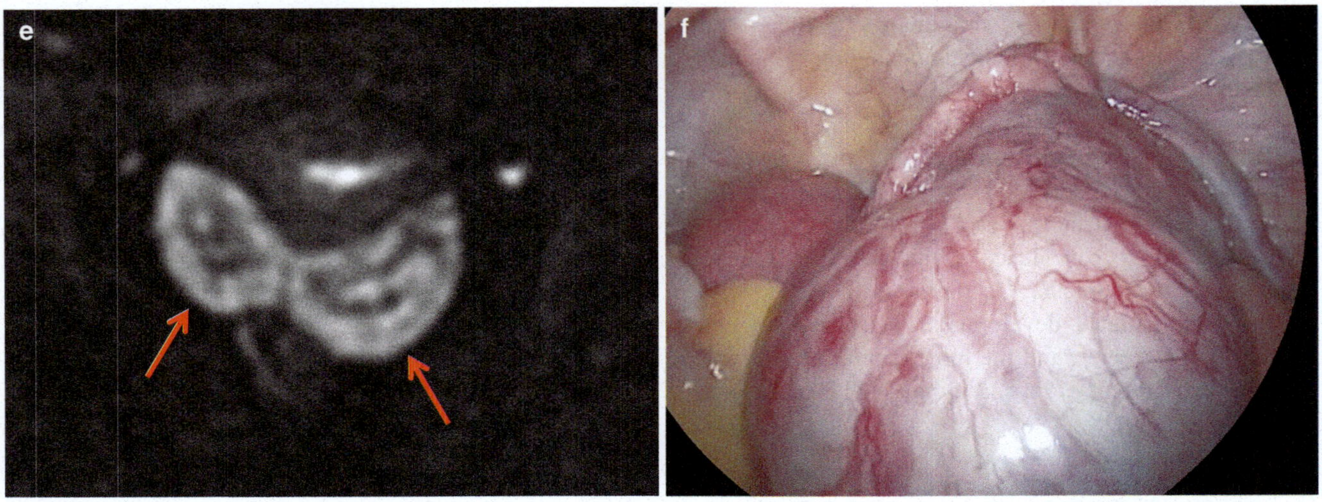

Fig. 5.6 (continued)

ovarian tumors. A solid component with an intermediate signal in the T2-weighted sequence, a high signal in diffusion images, a low signal in the ADC map, and intense and early enhancement with a type 3 curve in the permeability study are signs of malignancy in ovarian lesion (Fig. 5.7) [6]. The literature refers to malignant transformation of endometriosis in extragonadal locations, the most common sites, although rare, being the rectovaginal septum, the colon, the vagina, and the anterior abdominal wall. The histological types mentioned are adenosarcoma and adenocarcinoma [7–9].

8. **Identify other pathologies**, besides endometriosis, of the abdomen and pelvis. The involvement of another condition may have surgical and therapeutic implications, particularly when it affects the uterus. Uterine leiomyoma and adenomyosis can cause chronic pelvic pain, dyspareunia, and infertility and have symptoms similar to endometriosis. Furthermore, the surgical technique can be influenced, adding time and complexity to the procedures (Fig. 5.8).

   The authors considered the highest at risk group of patients to be those who present lesions with the following characteristics:

   (a) Obstructive ureteral lesion
   (b) Obstructive intestinal lesion
   (c) Increased possibility of surgical complications
      - Rectovaginal septum lesion with involvement of the rectum and lower vagina, with greater possibility of rectovaginal fistula
      - Lesion extending to the pelvic floor
      - Lesion with nerve impairment
   (d) Increased possibility of postoperative complications
      - Bilateral parametrial lesion and those with involvement of the sacral roots
   (e) The possibility of malignant transformation

This information enables the surgeon to inform the patient about the possible outcomes, difficulties, and complications of surgical resection.

Moreover, as the appropriate treatment also has the aim of preserving quality of life, staging with MRI allows the surgeon and the patient to choose not to resect all the disease in order to preserve the uterus to still allow the patient to be able to become pregnant and thereby avoid risk of neurological complications.

Endometriosis is a progressive disease. Although it has been described since 1800, the mechanisms responsible for the progression remain unknown despite the progress made in diagnosis and treatment. We still do not know how to discern from an image which patient in the low-risk group will progress to high risk [10].

It is well established that endometriosis grows and regresses in a way dependent on estrogen. The pain may start in a young patient; however, the diagnosis is almost always delayed for several years, affecting the tubo-ovarian structures and compromising fertility.

One of the most important reasons for the progression of the disease is delayed diagnosis [11].

Moreover, the disease can effectively be cured by definitive surgery. However, in young patients with a desire to become pregnant, surgery may be conservative, with follow-up being necessary in most cases, as well as in those who opt for drug treatment [10].

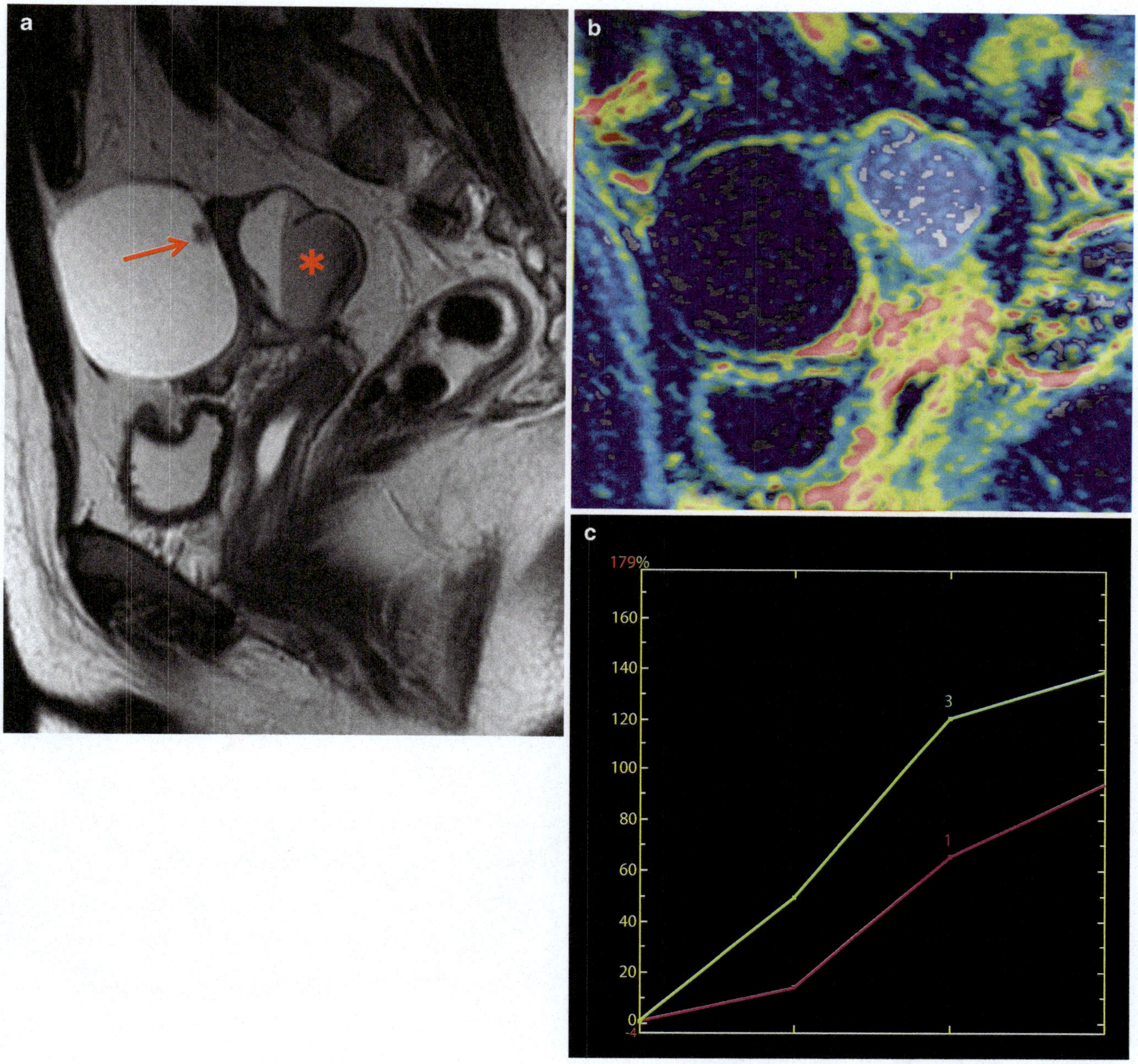

Fig. 5.7 Analysis of vascular permeability improves characterization of ovarian tumors. Solid component with intermediate signal in T2-weighted sequence (arrow) and with a moderate enhancement but smaller in comparison with the myometrium (**b**). ([**b**, **c**] Pink curve in the lesion and green in the myometrium) and type II curve, suggesting borderline lesion. Note endometrioma in the other ovary (*) (**a**)

The progression of endometriosis has been described in the rectovaginal septum in less than 10% of women over a period of 5 years of observation. In addition, an important factor in the severity and progression of endometriosis in adolescents is its association with obstructive anomalies of the Müllerian duct (Fig. 5.9) [11, 12].

Thus, the authors recommend monitoring of asymptomatic patients who opt for nonsurgical treatment. The suggested protocol is for an MRI every 6 months in the first year and then yearly.

Also, we suggest that further examination is carried out if the interval between the MRI and the planned surgery is greater than 6 months (Fig. 5.9).

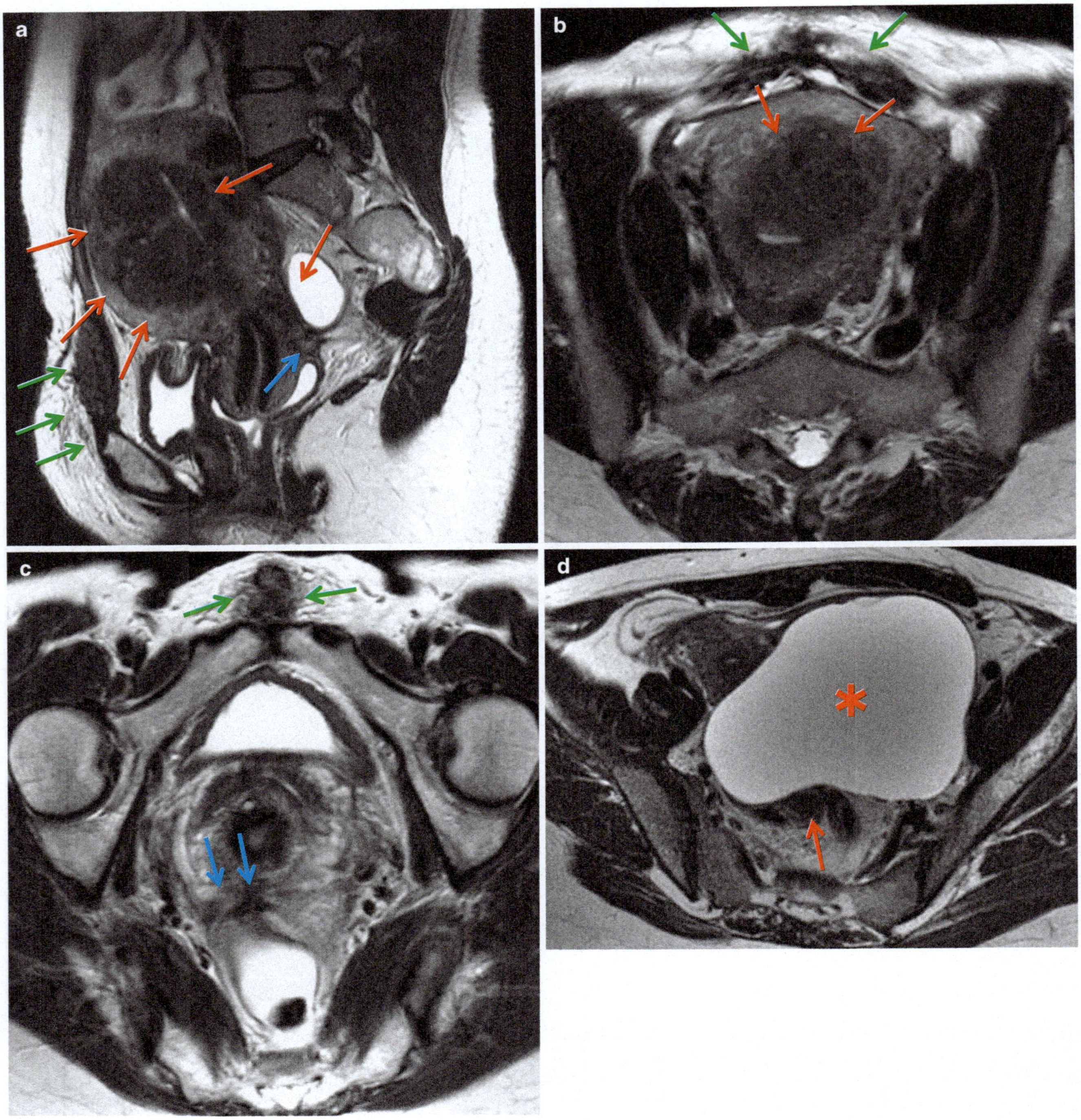

Fig. 5.8 Case 1 (**a–c**): Deep uterine adenomyosis with thickening of the junctional zone and thickening of the anterior wall (red arrows), with symptoms similar to those of endometriosis. Note endometriosis of the anterior wall (green arrow) and discrete retrocervical lesion (blue arrows). Case 2 (**d–f**): sigmoid endometriosis (green arrow), associated with peritoneal pseudocyst (*), as well as a retrorectal cyst (green arrows), multiseptated and heterogeneous (hamartoma). (**a–e**) T2-weighted sequences. (**f**) T1-weighted with fat suppression

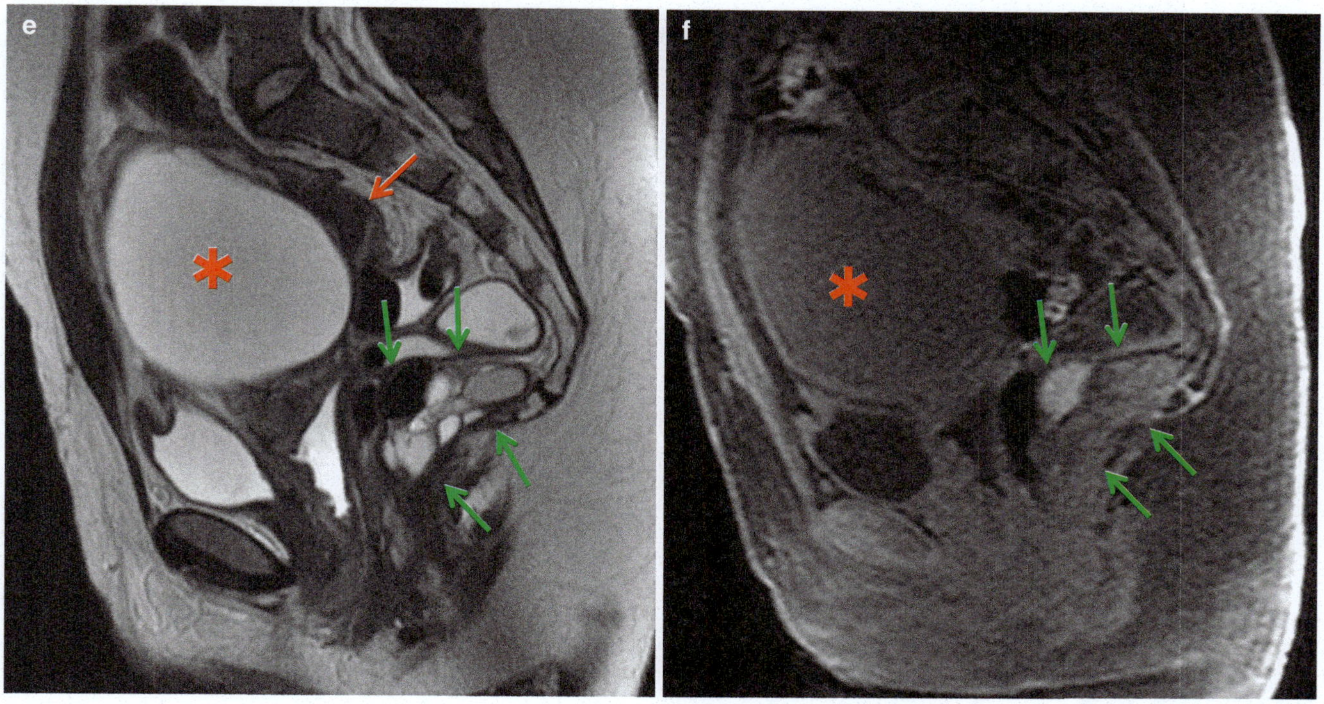

Fig. 5.8 (continued)

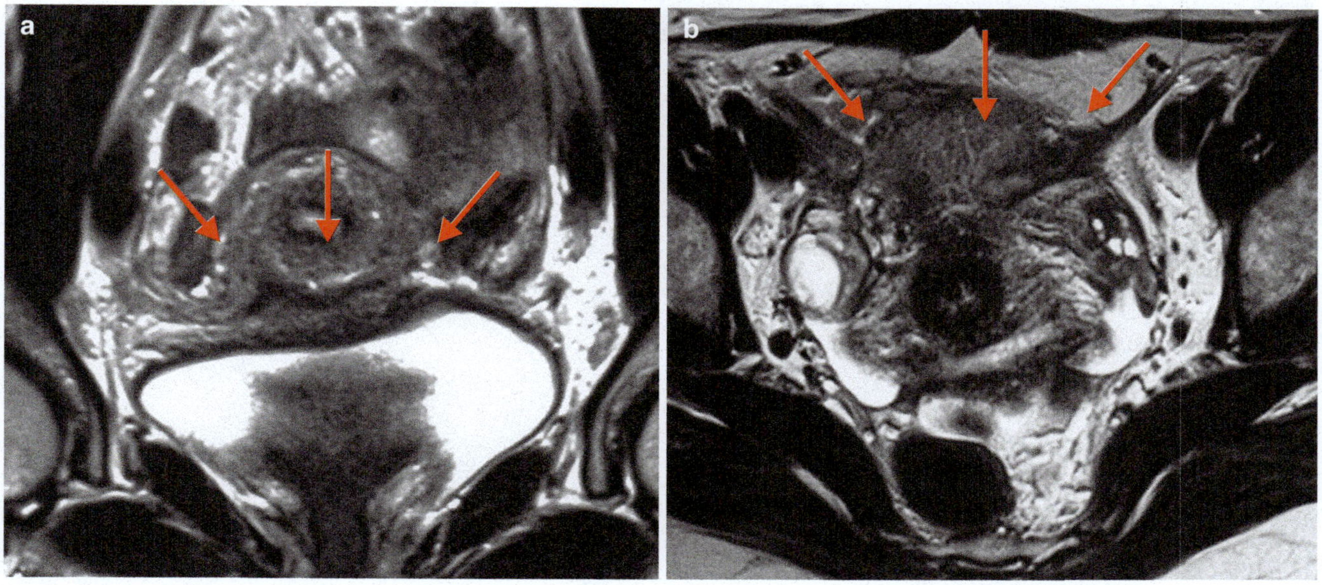

Fig. 5.9 Importance of a new examination before surgery, when the interval between imaging and procedure planning is longer than 6 months. Significant growth of the deep lesion in the anterior compartment from (**a–c**) to (**d–e**), with appearance of myometrial penetration (red line and arrows). (**a–e**) T2-weighted sequences. (**a**, **d**) Coronal. (**c–e**) Axial

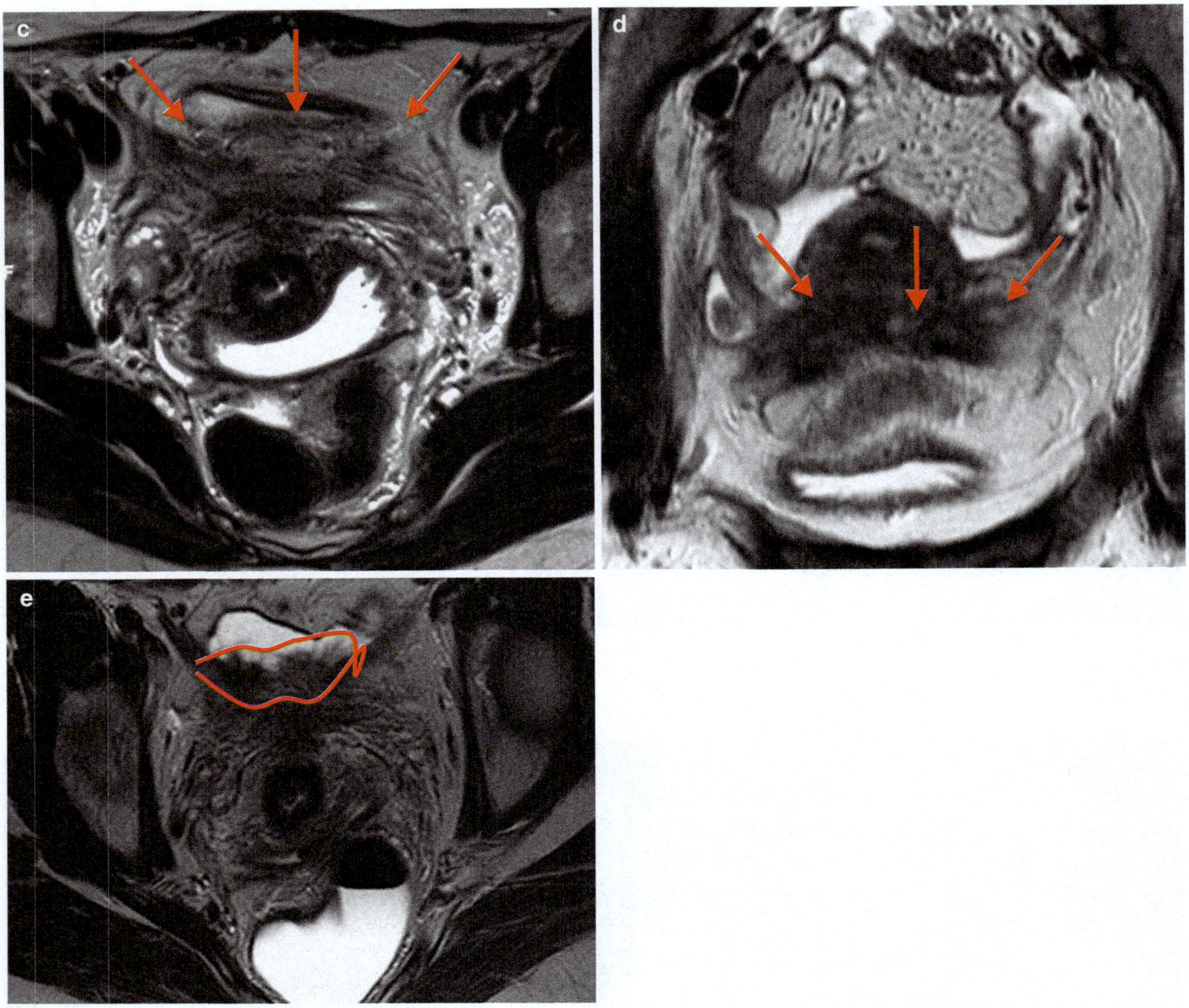

Fig. 5.9 (continued)

References

1. Crispi C. Tratado de videoendoscopia e cirurgia minimamente invasiva em ginecologia. 5th ed. Rio de Janeiro: Revinter; 2011.
2. Somigliana E, Vigano P, Benaglia L, Busnelli A, Vercellini P, Fedele L. Adhesion prevention in endometriosis: a neglected critical challenge. J Minim Invasive Gynecol. 2012;19:415–21.
3. Varma R, Rollason T, Gupta J, Maher E. Endometriosis and the neoplastic process. Reproduction. 2004;127:293–304.
4. Uekuri C, Shigetomi H, Ono S, Sasaki Y, Matsuura M, Kobayashi H. Toward an understanding of the pathophysiology of clear cell carcinoma of the ovary—review. Oncol Lett. 2013;6:1163–73.
5. Kobayashi H, Sumimoto K, Moniwa N. Risk of developing ovarian cancer among women with ovarian endometrioma: 391 a cohort study in Shizuoka, Japan. Int J Gynecol Cancer. 2007;17:37–43.
6. Brandão A, Silva A. Diseases of the female pelvis: advances in imaging evaluation. Magn Reson Imaging Clin N Am. 2013;21:447–69.
7. Fàbregas F, Guimferrer M, Casas F, Caballero S, Xauradó R. Malignant transformation of abdominal wall endometriosis with lymph node metastasis: case report and review of literature. Gynecol Oncol Case Rep. 2014;8:10–3.
8. Ulrich U, Rhiem K, Kaminski M, Wardelmann E, Trog D, Valter M, Richter O. Parametrial and rectovaginal adenocarcinoma arising from endometriosis. Int J Gynecol Cancer. 2005;15:1206–9.
9. Raffaelli R, Piazzola E, Zanconato G, Fedele L. A rare case of extrauterine adenosarcoma arising in endometriosis of the rectovaginal septum. Fertil Steril. 2004;81:1142–4.
10. Kim S, Chae H, Kim C, Kang B. Update on the treatment of endometriosis. Clin Exp Reprod Med. 2013;40:55–9.
11. Brosens I, Gordts S, Benagiano G. Endometriosis in adolescents is a hidden, progressive and severe disease that deserves attention, not just compassion. Hum Reprod. 2013;28:2026–31.
12. Fedele L, Bianchi S, Zanconato G, Raffaelli R, Berlanda N. Is rectovaginal endometriosis a progressive disease? Am J Obstet Gynecol. 2004;191:1539–42.

6 Postsurgical Findings in Deep Endometriosis

6.1 Endometriosis Postsurgical Aspects

The radiologist must be prepared for postoperative analysis of deep endometriosis. Therefore, it is necessary to have knowledge of the pelvic anatomy, the surgical site, and the surgical technique.

Correlation between the surgical report and the pathology helps in understanding the changes seen in MRI. In addition, the MRI findings should be correlated with the images of the previous examination (Fig. 6.1).

Changes can be discreet and difficult to identify, if this routine is not followed.

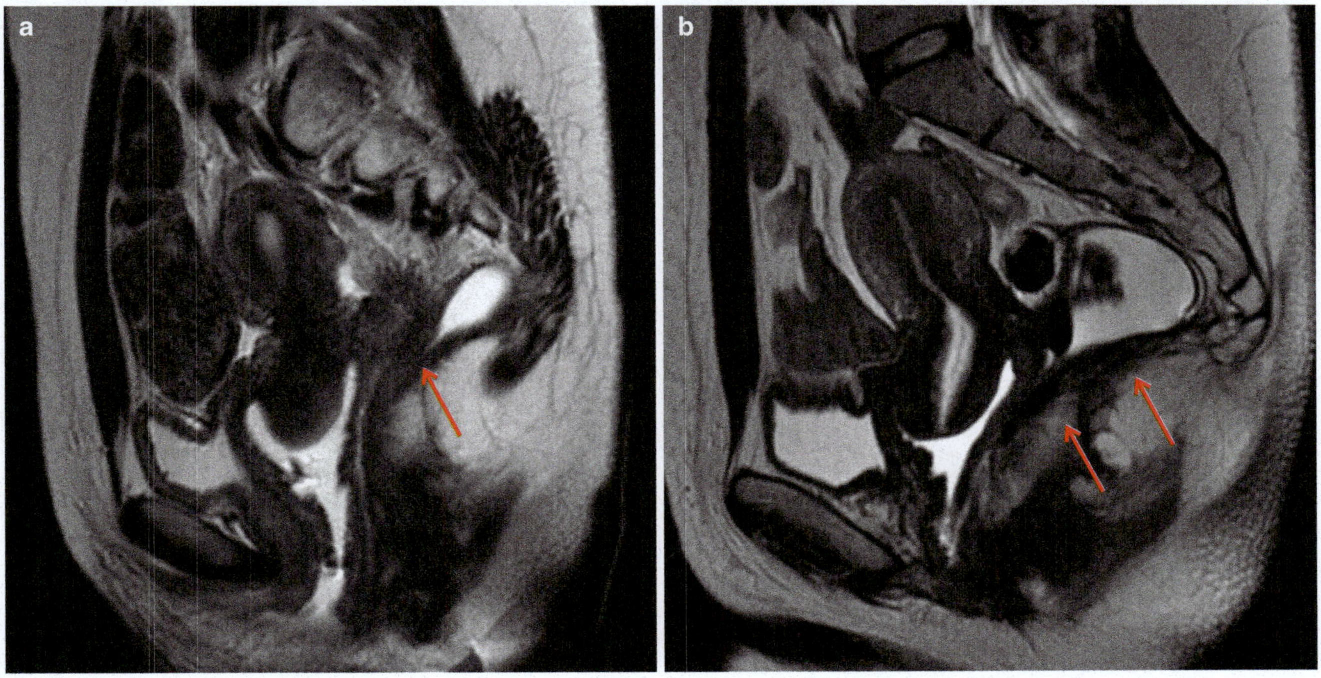

Fig. 6.1 The correlation with the surgical report and the findings of the previous examination aid in the interpretation of the observed changes in the MRI. (Arrows in **a, d**) Right uterosacral ligament endometriosis with extension to the rectum and floor. (Arrows **b, c, e, f**) Fibrous cicatricial tissue on the pelvic floor and on the ligament bed, in addition to signs of colorectal anastomosis. (**a–f**) T2-weighted sequences. (**a–c**) Sagittal. (**d–f**) Axial

A. Brandão et al., *Atlas of Deep Endometriosis*, https://doi.org/10.1007/978-3-319-71697-8_6

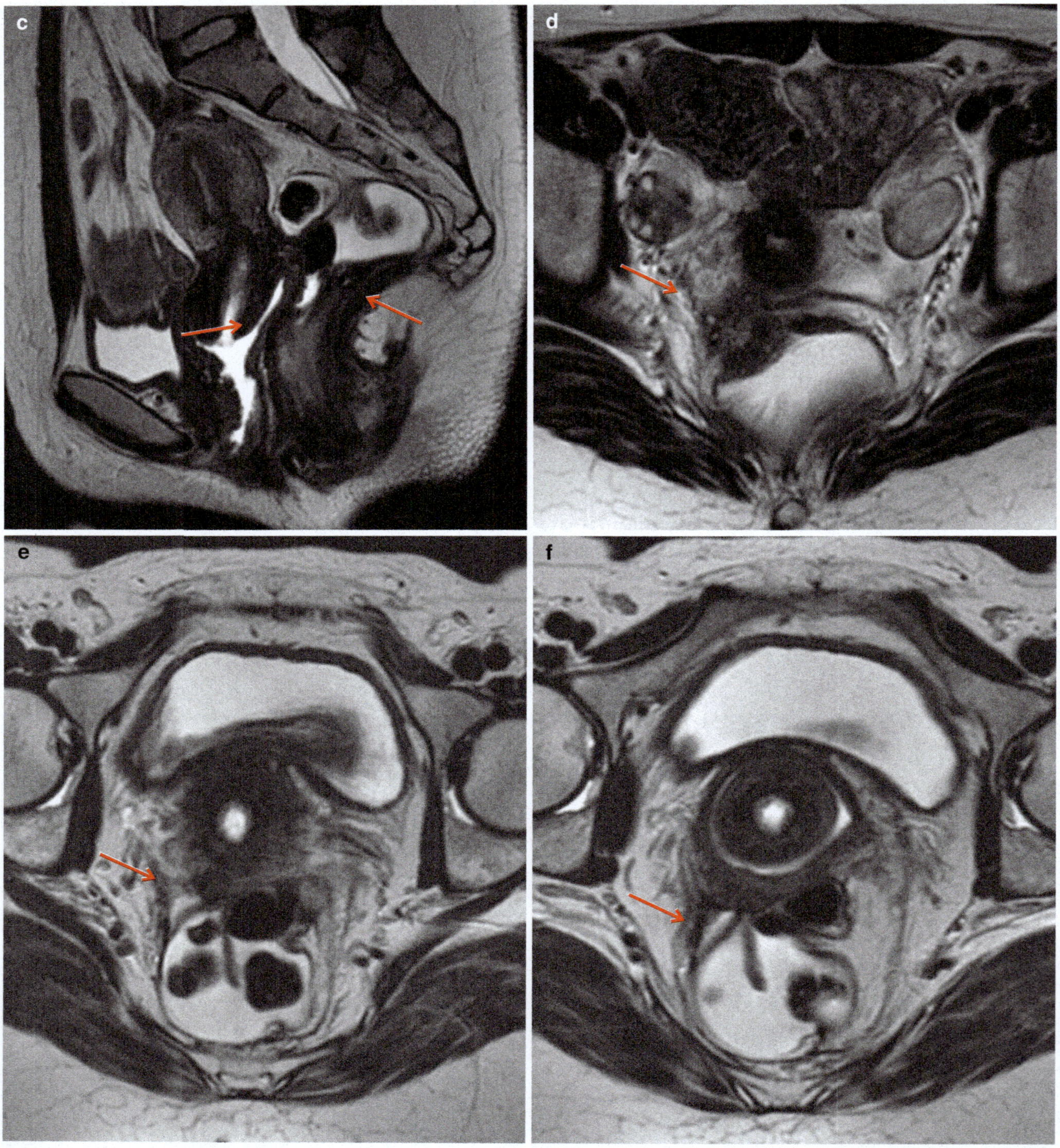

Fig. 6.1 (continued)

Conversely, the findings can be prominent and mimic deep endometriosis.

The most frequently observed changes in the surgical site are fibrocicatricial tissue, magnetic susceptibility artifacts, and signs of resection of the colon, myometrium, and intestine.

6.2 Fibrocicatricial Tissue

Fibrosis is a common consequence of surgery.

In these patients it has a linear aspect, thin and well defined, with a strong hypointense signal in T2-weighted

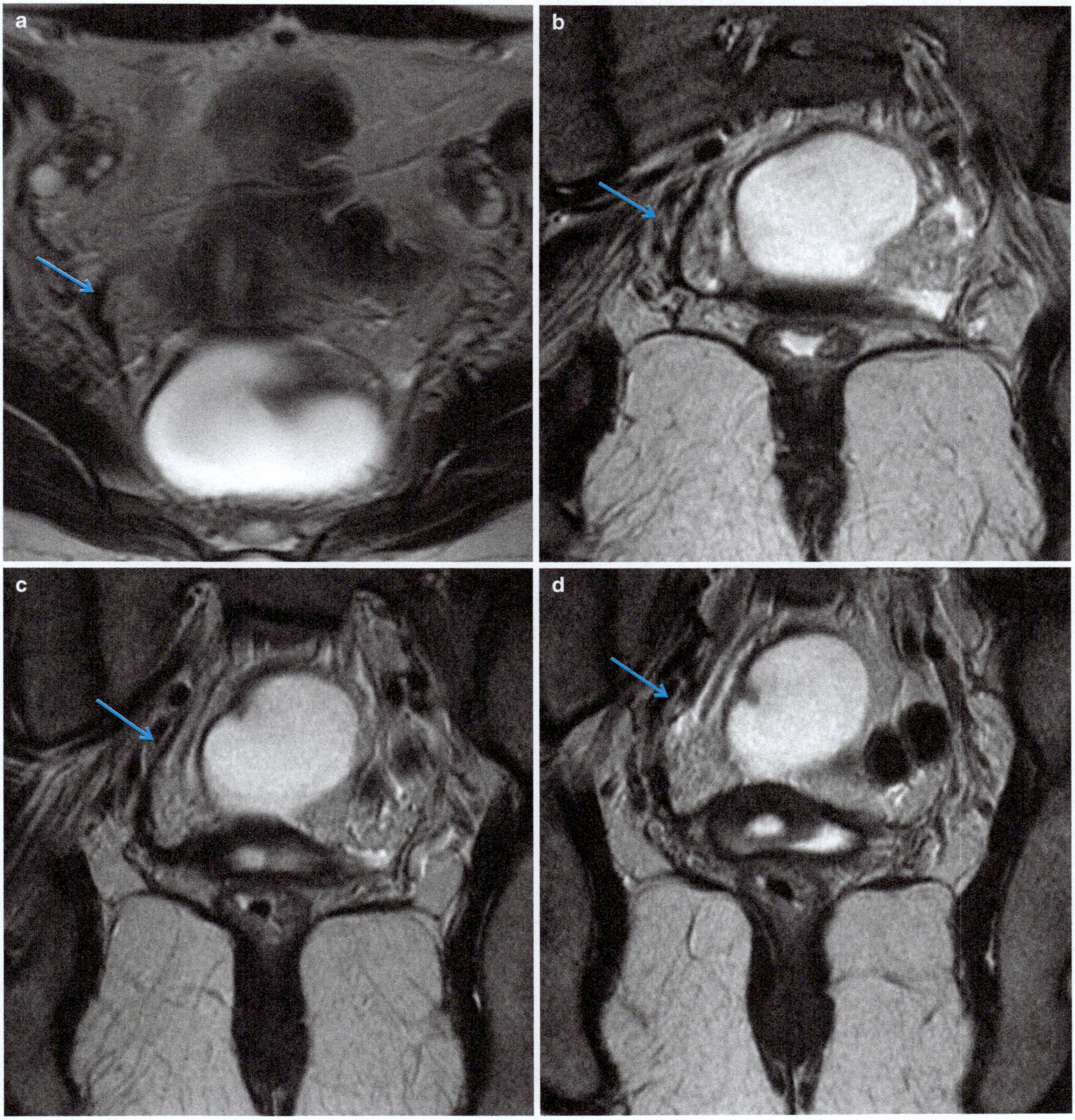

Fig. 6.2 (**a–e**) Fibrosis on the topography of the right uterosacral ligament (arrows **a–e**). Well-defined thin tissue, hypointense on T2-weighted sequence. (**a**) Axial. (**b–e**) Coronal short axis

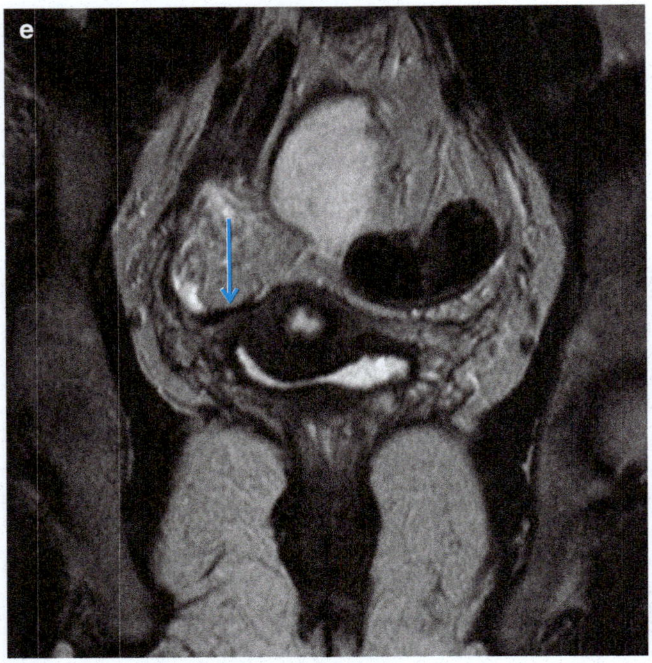

Fig. 6.2 (continued)

sequence without bleeding or gadolinium enhancement (Fig. 6.2).

It is usually identified in the topography of the ligament resection, especially of the uterosacral and parietal peritoneum.

6.3 Foci of Signal Loss in Surgical Site

These represent magnetic susceptibility artifacts related to the surgical procedure and are best evidenced in T1-weighted images obtained in apnea using the gradient-echo technique (Fig. 6.3).

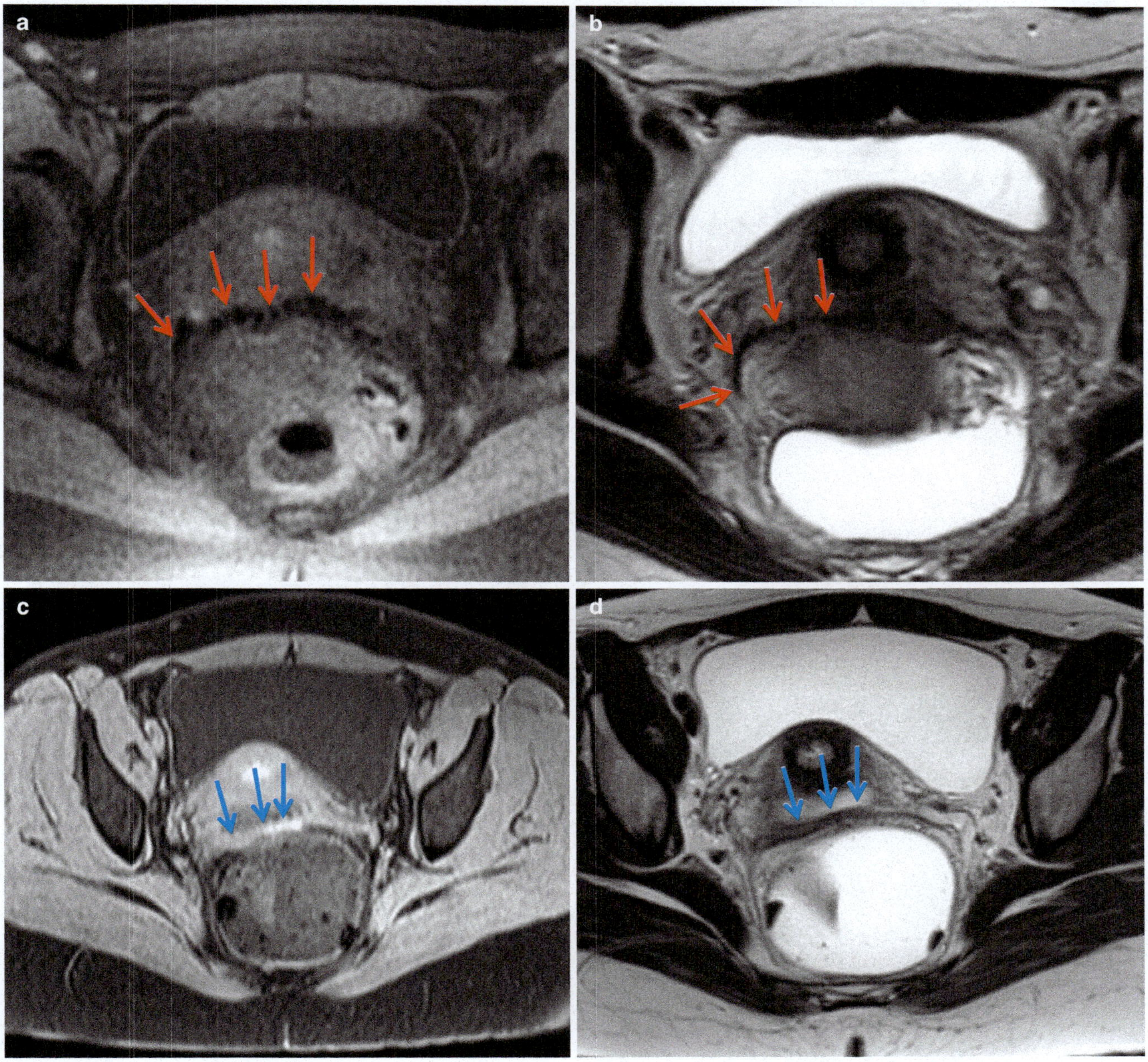

Fig. 6.3 Postoperative retrocervical and uterosacral ligament endometriosis. (**a**, **b**) Magnetic susceptibility artifacts related to the surgical procedure. Note hypointense foci on the T1-weighted images obtained by the gradient-echo technique (**a**) in correlation with fibrous cicatricial tissue identified in the T2-weighted sequence (**b**). (**c**, **d**) Preoperative examination (blue arrows on the lesion)

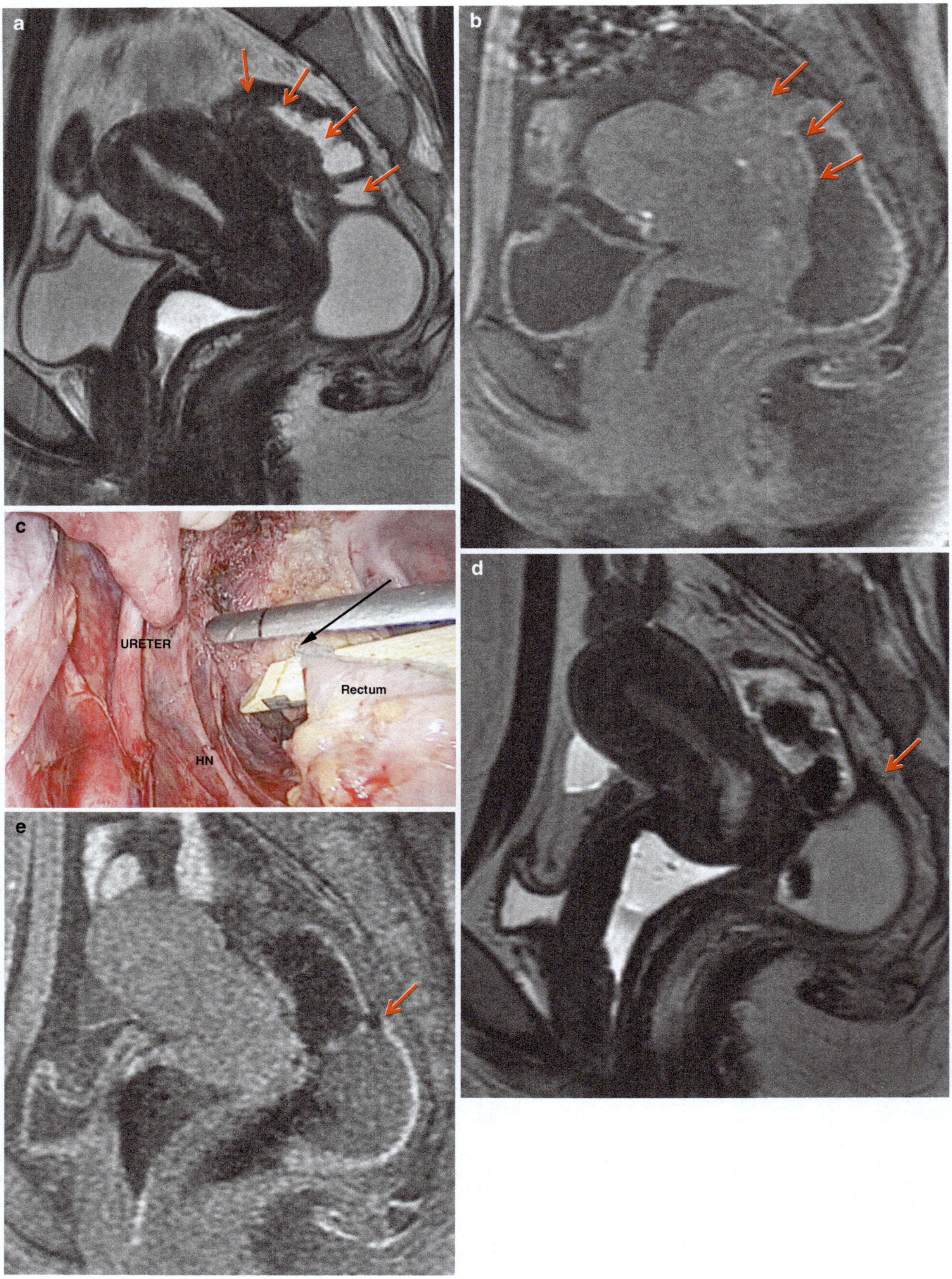

Fig. 6.4 Circular stapling technique. (**a**, **b**) Pre-procedure examination identifying lesion in the sigmoid and upper rectum (arrows). (**c**) Laparoscopy showing resection of the rectum and the staple (arrow). (**d**, **e**) Examination after the procedure. Tissue with hyposignal on T2-weighted sequence and absence of signal on T1, well defined and circular in shape in the plane of the anastomosis (arrows). (**a**, **d**) T2-weighted sequences. (**b**, **e**) T1-weighted with fat suppression

They are accompanied by postsurgical fibrocicatricial tissue and can be observed in intestinal anastomosis and ovarian parenchyma, in addition to the anterior abdominal wall (Fig. 6.4).

6.4 Resection of Posterior Vaginal Fornix and Uterine Cervix

Colpectomy and posterior colpotomy have the effect of reducing the thickness and signal intensity of the vaginal fornix in T2-weighted images with low signal, due to the fibrocicatricial tissue (Fig. 6.5).

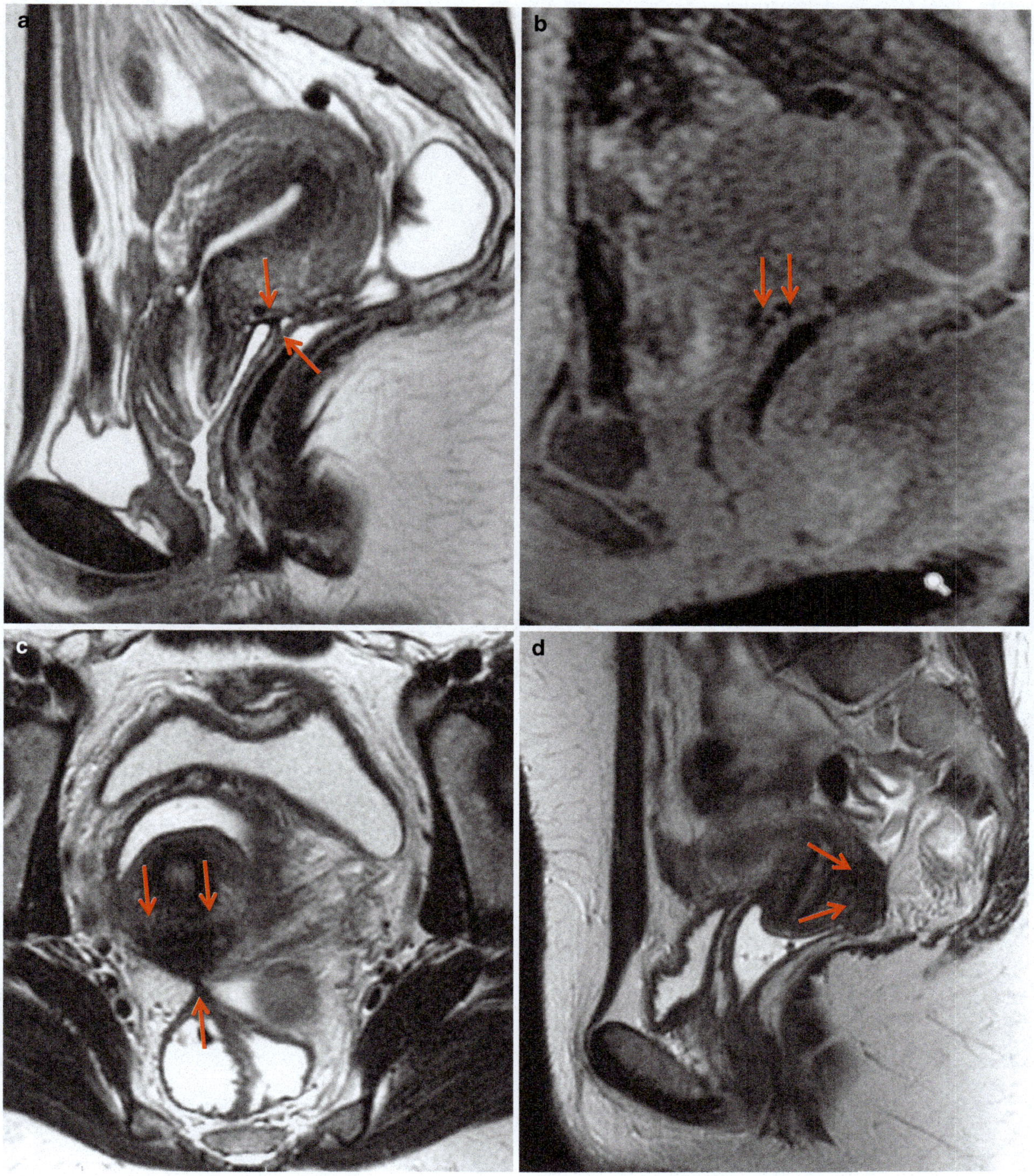

Fig. 6.5 **Case 1**: (**a**, **b**) Postoperative changes of the posterior vaginal fornix. Hypointense on T2 (**a**), due to fibrous scarring tissues. Note hypointense foci on T1 (B). **Case 2**: (**c**, **d**) Preoperative examination with retrocervical endometriosis and superficial involvement of the rectum (arrows). T1- and T2-weighted sequences (**a**, **c**–**f**) with fat suppression (**b**). (**a**, **b**, **d**, **f**) Sagittal. (**c**, **e**) Coronal short axis. (**e**, **f**). Postoperative examination. There is thinning of the vaginal fornix and cervix wall

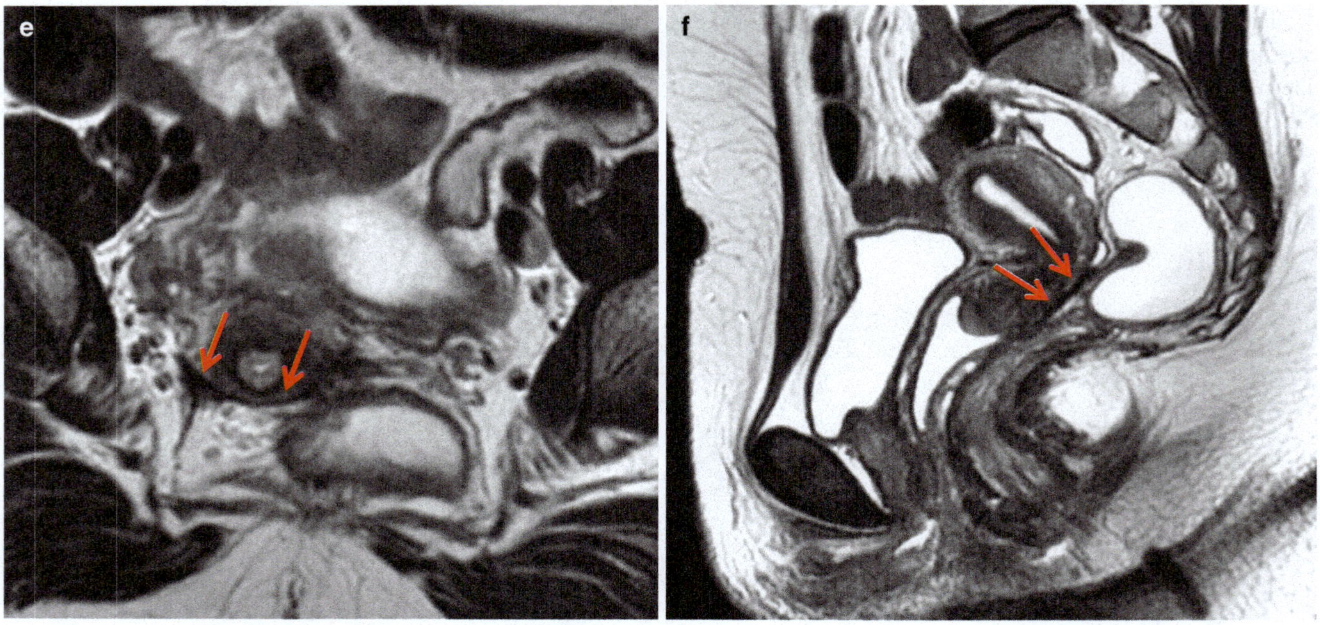

Fig. 6.5 (continued)

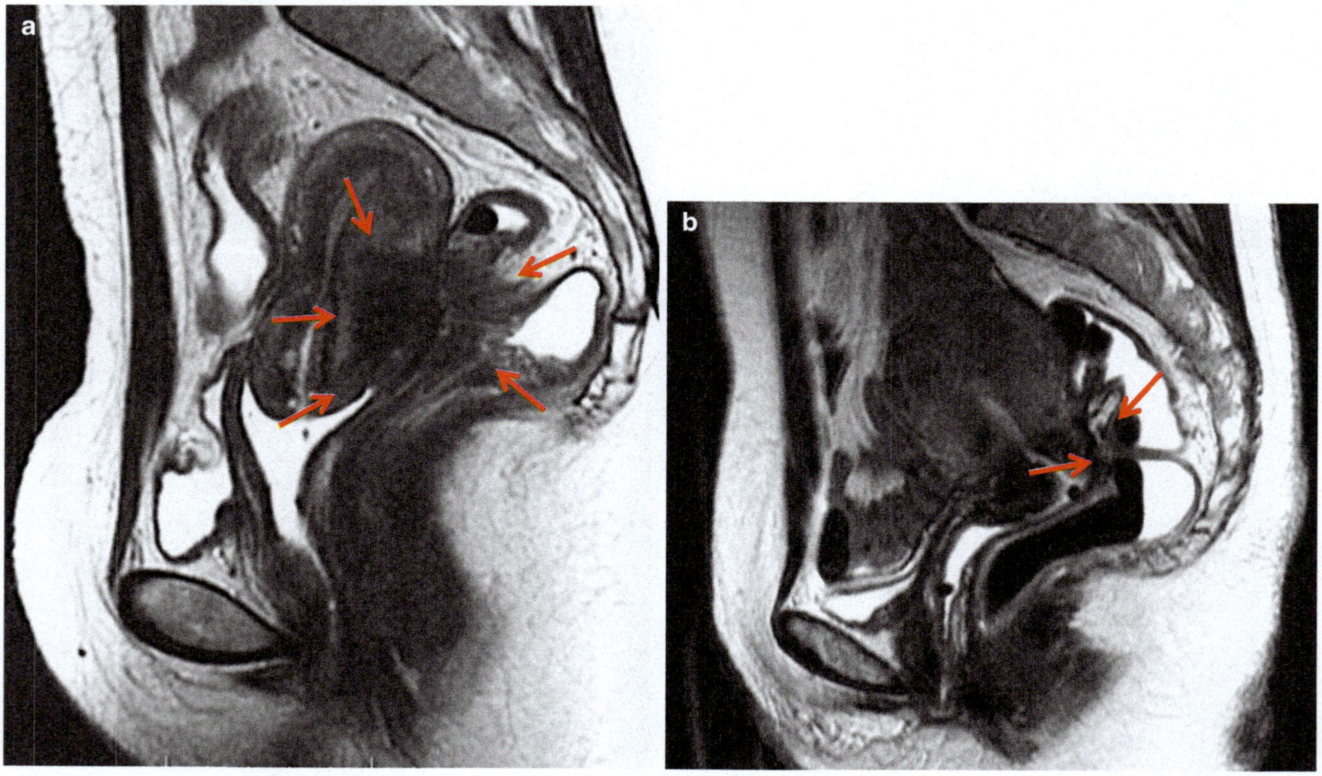

Fig. 6.6 (**a**) Preoperative examination with retrocervical endometriosis and marked myometrial involvement. (**b**) Postoperative examination with findings related to the resection of the myometrial involvement, with irregularity of the contour and focal tapering of the posterior cervical wall, with hypointense signal on T2-weighted without bleeding (**b**). (**a**, **b**) T2-weighted sequences, sagittal

After myometrial resection, irregularities in the contour of the uterus—focal thinning of the uterine wall with a hypointense signal in T2 without bleeding—can be observed (Fig. 6.6).

6.5 Changes in the Parametrium

Changes include ureteral fibrocicatricial tissue caused by manipulation, to ureterolysis, and signs of parametrial resections.

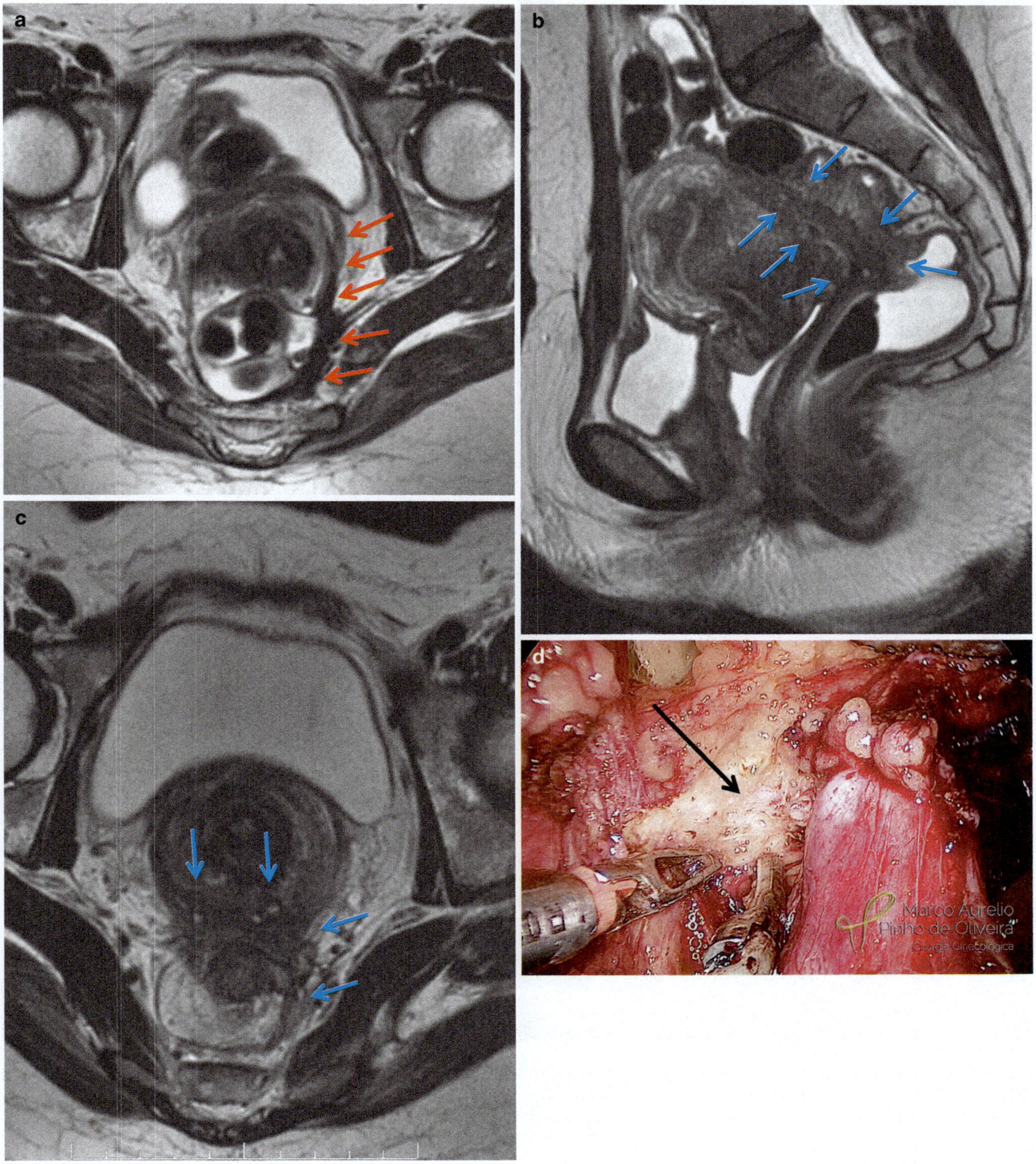

Fig. 6.7 Periureteral and posterior fibrous cicatricial tissue (arrow), well defined, hypointense on the T2-weighted sequence (**a**). (**b**, **c**) Preoperative examination with extensive retrocervical lesion in the rectovaginal septum, completely obliterating the cul-de-sac, vaginal, myometrial, bowel, ligaments, and parametrial ureter impairment. (**a**, **c**) Axial. (**b**) Sagittal. (**d**) Laparoscopy. Resection of right parametrial lesion

After ureterolysis, in some patients, hypointense tissue can be observed in the T2-weighted sequence, periurethral and well defined with no bleeding. Furthermore, there may be slight thickening of the ureter wall and possibly slight dilation (Fig. 6.7).

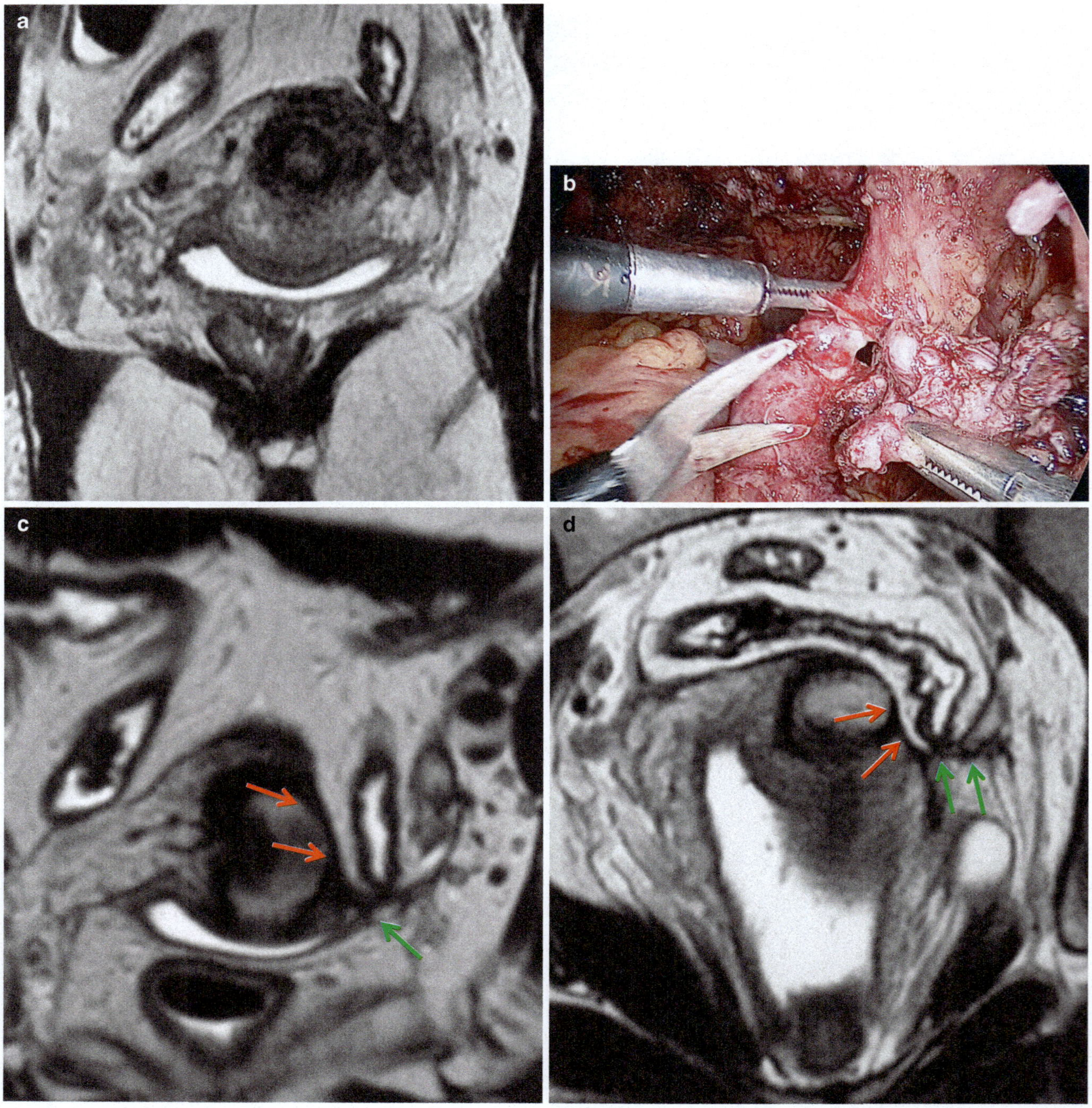

Fig. 6.8 (**a**) Nodule in left parametrium. (**b**) Laparoscopy showing left parametrium infiltration. (**c**, **d**) MRI after the resection of the parametrium. Note asymmetry in relation to the contralateral, reduction of cervical myometrium thickness (red arrows in **d**), and fibrous cicatricial changes in paracolpos (green arrows **c**). T2-weighted sequences

When resection of the lesion includes the parametrium, MRI shows absence of the parametrium, with asymmetry relative to the contralateral side, and may be associated with reduced thickness of the cervical myometrium and fibrocicatricial changes in the paracolpos (Fig. 6.8).

6.6 Colorectal Anastomosis

Resection of bowel lesions promotes a change in the shape of the loop, due to the anastomosis with the colon, and secondary signs in the mesorectum and presacral space.

Circular stapling is well identified by MRI, showing tissue with a hypointense signal in the T2-weighted sequence and no signal in T1, well-defined and with a circular shape in the plane of anastomosis (Fig. 6.4).

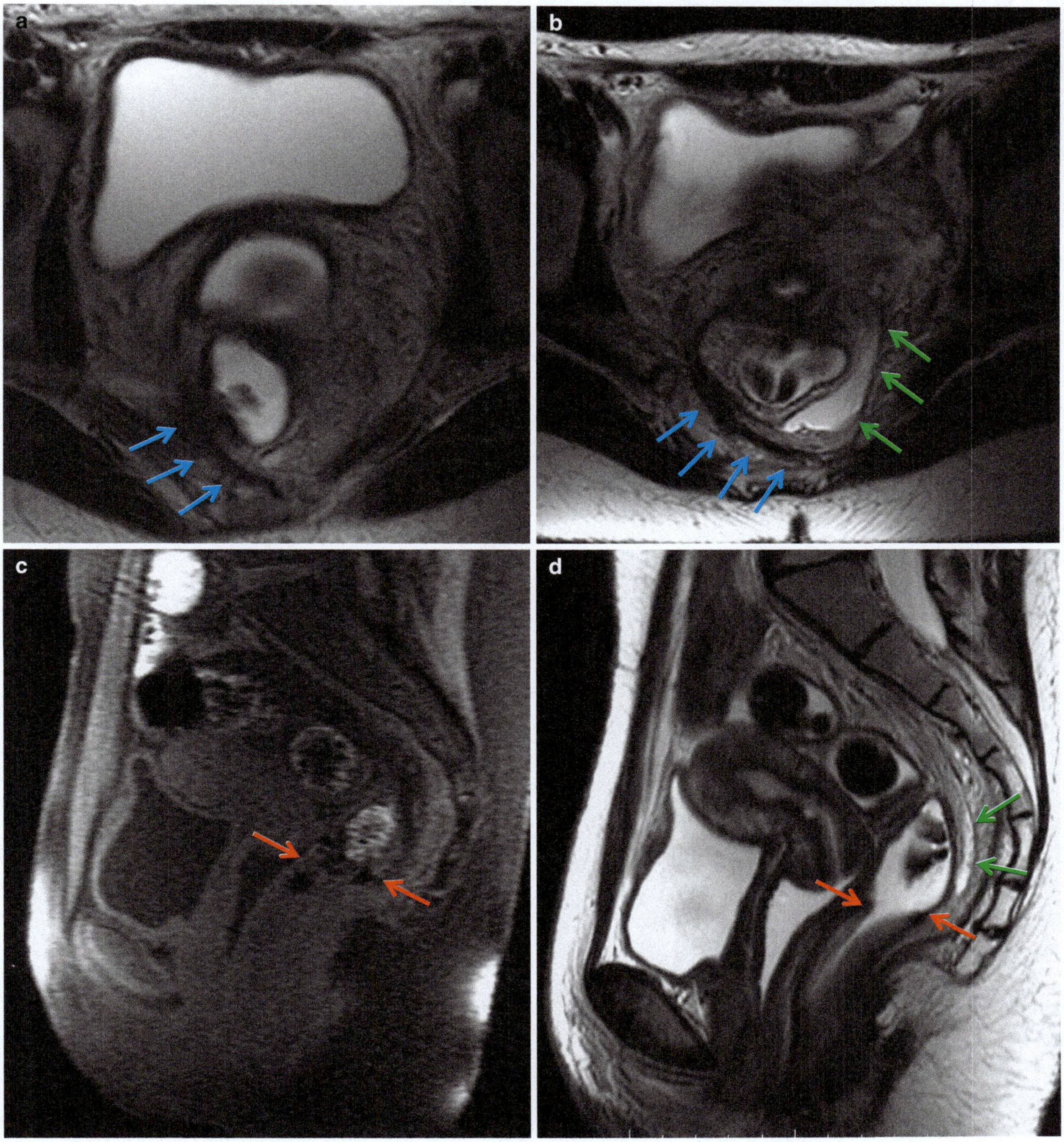

Fig. 6.9 Postoperative findings in the mesorectum with fibrous cicatricial tissue, notably on the right (blue arrows **a**, **b**, **d**, **e**), and fluid accumulation in the pararectal and retrorectal spaces on the left (green arrows in **b**, **d**). Observe artifacts related to stapling (red arrows **c**, **d**). (**a**, **b**, **d**, **e**) T2-weighted sequences. (**c**) T1-weighted with fat suppression. (**a**–**b**) Axial. (**c**–**e**) Sagittal

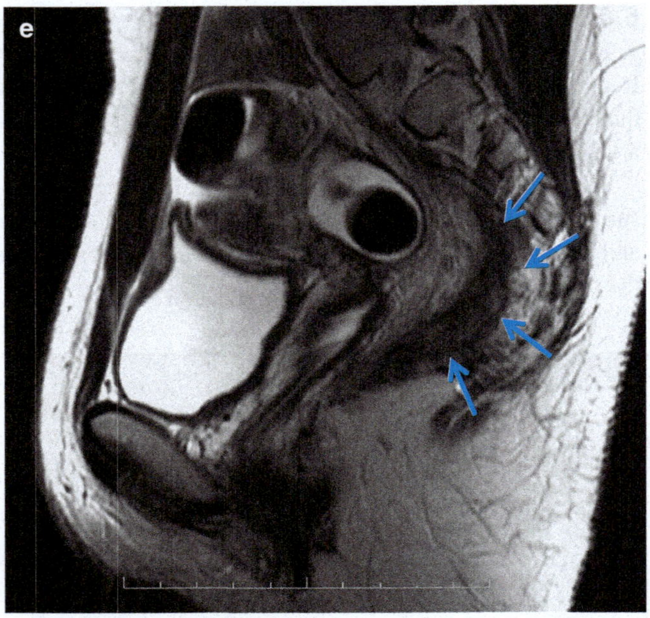

Fig. 6.9 (continued)

In the mesorectum, fibrocicatricial tissue with the same morphological characteristics and intensity can be observed, as well as fluid accumulation in the pararectal and retrorectal spaces. These spaces are virtual but with surgical manipulation are dissected, to achieve either the segmental intestinal or pararectal resection—to isolate the uterosacral ligaments, the nerve plexus, and the posterior vaginal fornix—or the retrorectal to access the levator ani muscle and the presacral roots (Fig. 6.9).

6.7 Complications

Surgical treatment of deep endometriosis is associated with complications such as anastomotic dehiscence, pelvic abscesses, rectovaginal fistulas, and functional urinary and evacuatory disorders, with bladder atony and constipation. The treatment of fistulas often requires further surgery and ileostomia [1, 2].

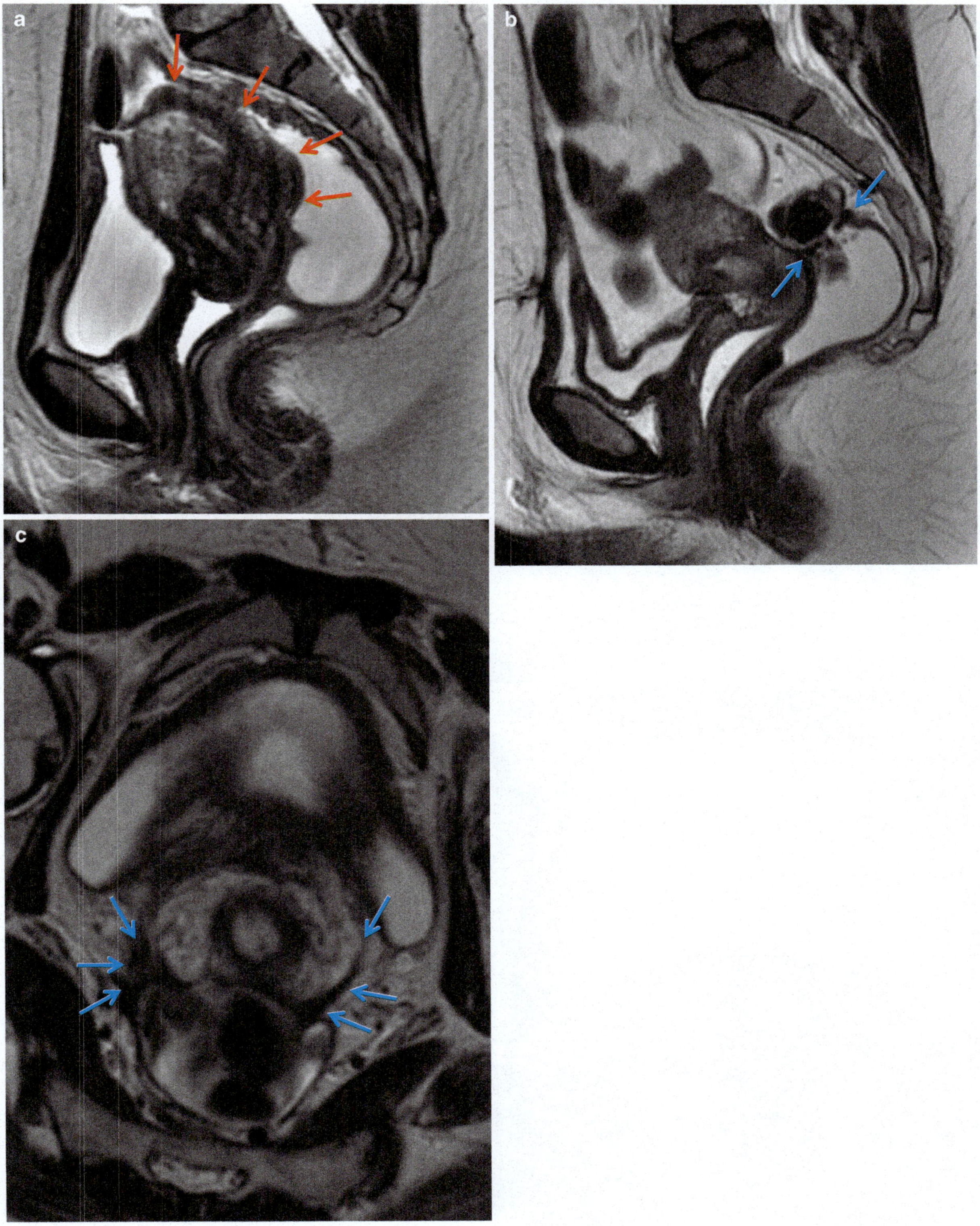

Fig. 6.10 Postoperative of deep endometriosis. Clinical complaints of constipation and significant perianal pain. (**a**) Preoperative examination with retrocervical endometriosis and deep involvement, especially intestinal (arrows). (**b–c**) Postsurgical findings related to stapling and fibrous cicatricial tissue (arrows **b**, **c**) topography of the bilateral hypogastric nerve and inferior hypogastric plexus. (**a**, **c**) T2-weighted sequences. (**a**, **b**) Sagittal. (**c**) Axial

The complications are often related to the level of the intestinal anastomosis; the lower, the greater the rate [1, 3].

However, urinary, sexual, and evacuatory dysfunctions are decreasing with new techniques which affect nerves less.

6.8 Evacuatory Disturbance

Persistent constipation is a frequent complaint of women undergoing colorectal resection for rectal endometriosis, due to stenosis of the colorectal anastomosis and neurological

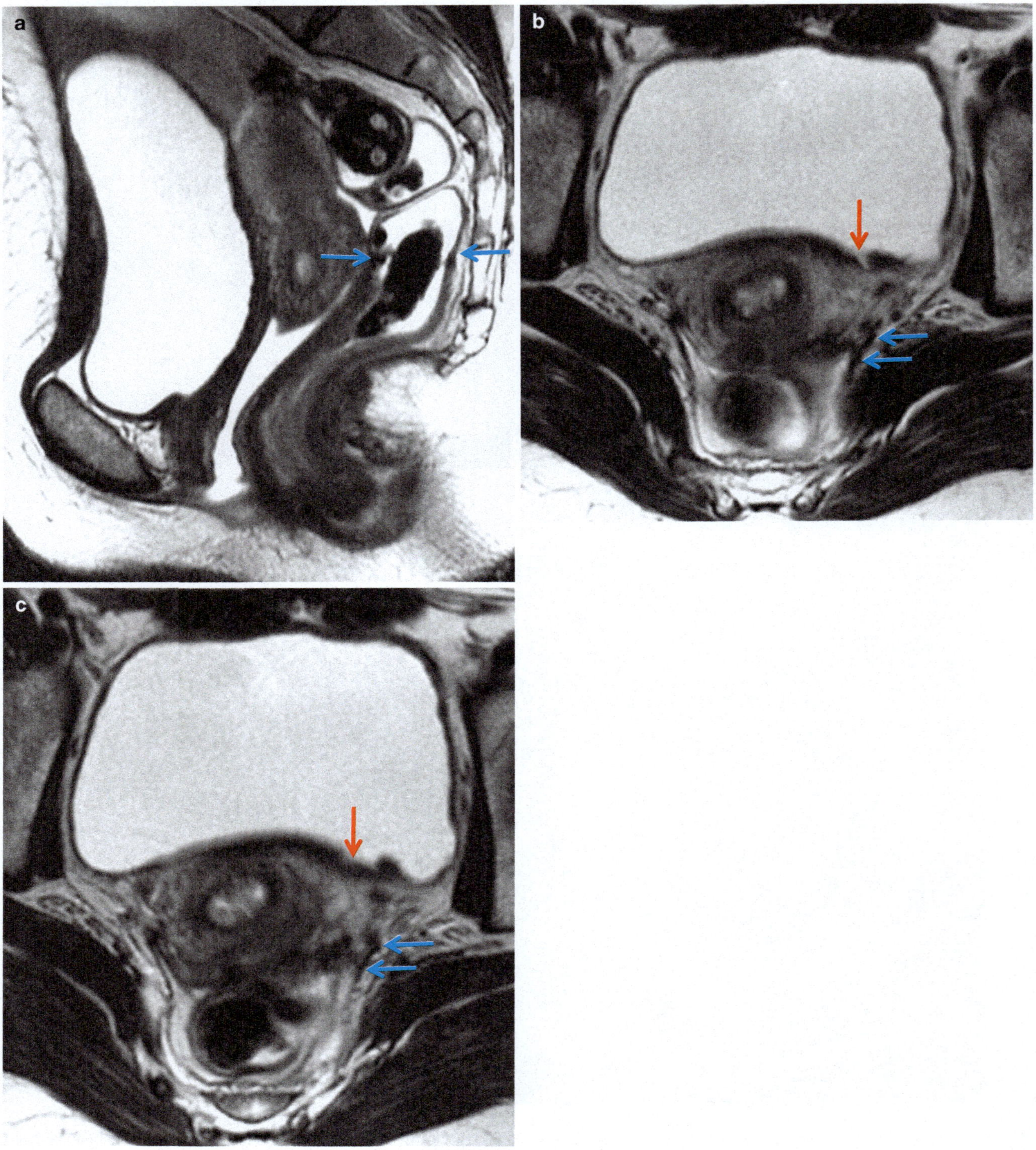

Fig. 6.11 (**a**) Bladder distension due to difficulty in emptying bladder. (**b**, **c**) Observe the thick bladder wall and diverticulum (red arrows), as well as fibrous cicatricial tissue on the left, in the parametrium and intestinal anastomosis (blue arrows)

damage, related to the hypogastric nerve due to extensive dissection around the rectum (Fig. 6.10).

6.9 Bladder Dysfunction

Bladder dysfunction resulting in transient urinary retention or dysuria, usually associated with the injury of the hypogastric nerve or inferior hypogastric plexus branches, often requires extensive resection of the uterosacral liga-

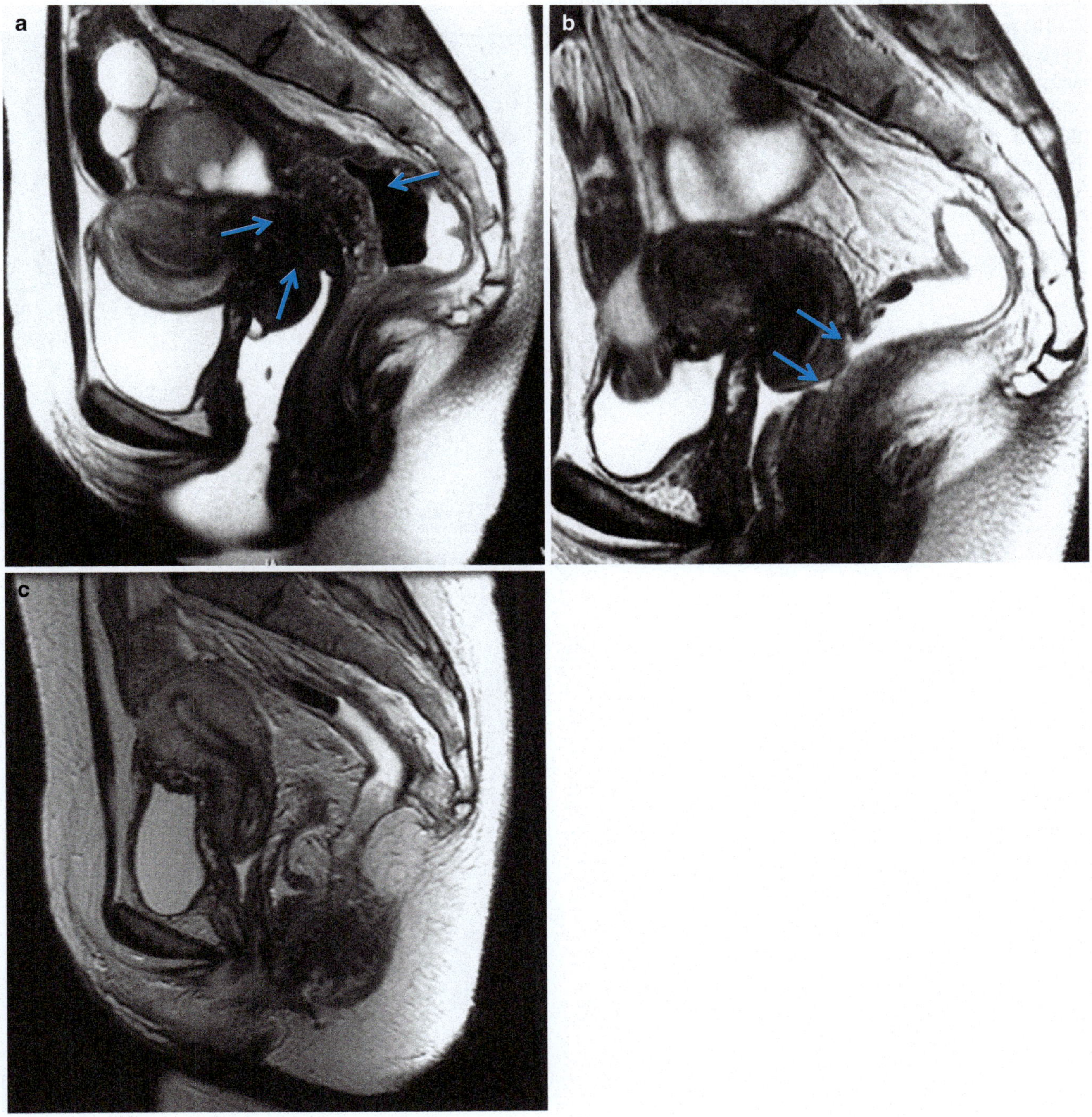

Fig. 6.12 Rectovaginal fistula. Postoperative complication of high-risk endometriotic lesion. (**a**) Preoperative endometriosis involving the lower rectum, retrocervical region, rectovaginal and vaginal fornix (arrows). (**b**) Rectovaginal medial fistula (arrows). (**c**) Postoperative with correction of fistula and restored flow. Note tapering of the posterior wall of the cervix (**a–c**). T2-weighted sequences, sagittal

ment, which may be observed in up to 16% of patients surgically treated for posterior endometriosis [4].

Bladder distention, difficulty voiding, wall thickening, and diverticulum can also be observed (Fig. 6.11).

6.10 Rectovaginal Fistula

A fistula is an abnormal communication between two epithelialized surfaces, in this case between the rectum and vagina.

The incidence is about 2.7%, and the use of the double stapling technique for resecting rectal lesions, especially lower, and partial colpectomy is identified as risk factor (Fig. 6.12) [2].

Fistulas can be low or high, located between the lower third of the rectum and the lower half of the vagina or between the middle third of the rectum and the posterior vaginal fornix.

They are considered small if less 0.5 cm in diameter, average if 0.5–2.5 cm, and large when they exceed 2.5 cm [5].

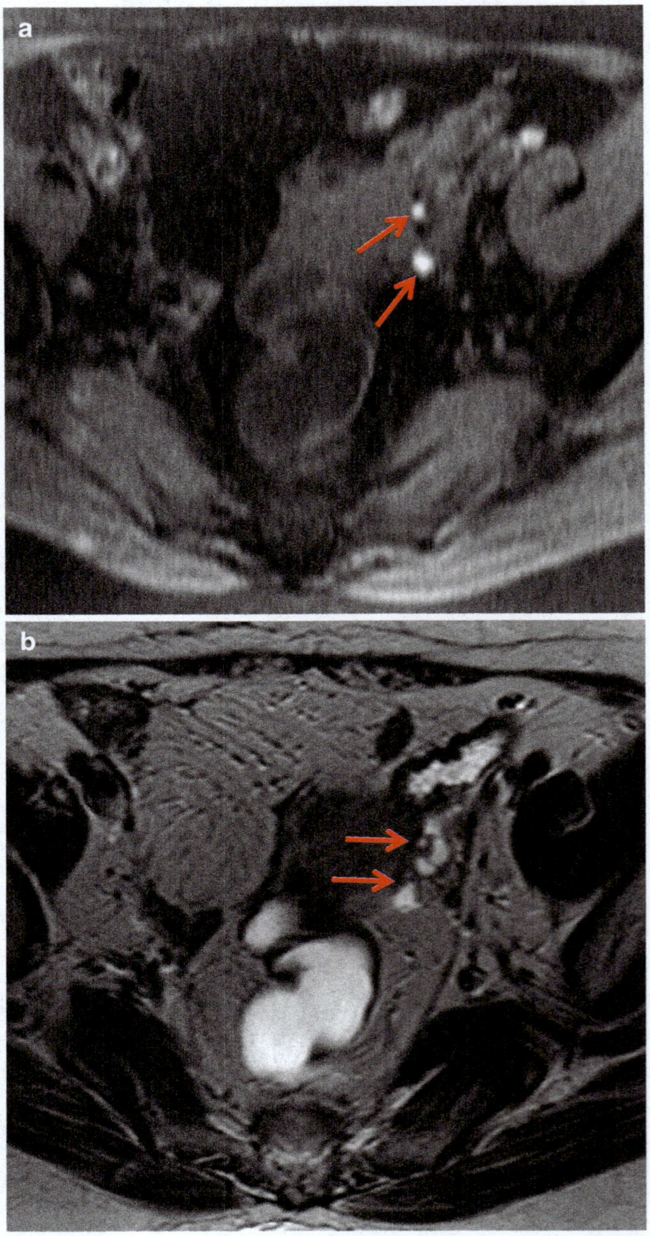

Fig. 6.13 Ovarian endometriosis with small endometriomas (red arrows in **a–c**). Note postsurgical artifacts (hypointense foci) in the parenchyma (blue arrow in **a–c**). (**a–c**) T1-weighted sequences with fat suppression. (**b**) T2-weighted sequence. (**a, b**) Axial. (**c**) Sagittal

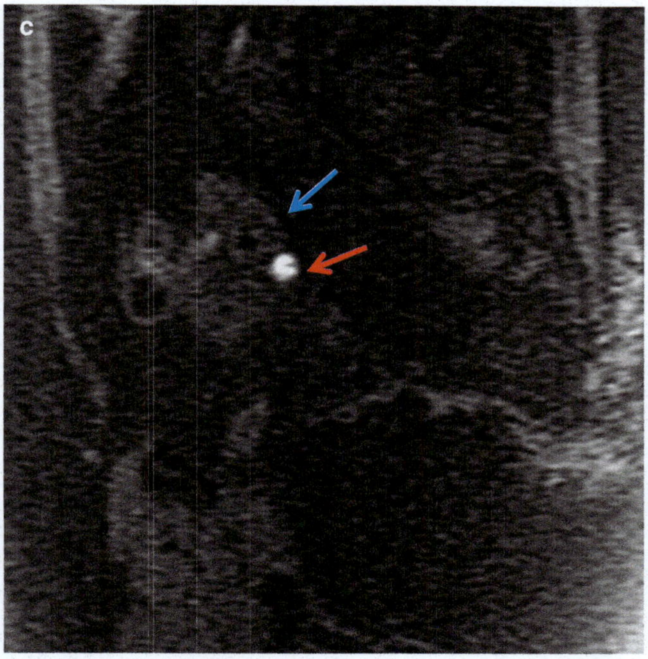

Fig. 6.13 (continued)

6.11 Residual Lesions/Recurrence

The presence of ectopic endometrial tissue in MRI postoperatively may have two explanations, either the surgeon failed to complete the resection or residual disease was intentionally left by choice of the patient and surgeon, such as in the myometrium. Complete myometrium deep endometriosis resection may involve hysterectomy. Thus, if the patient is planning a pregnancy, it may be necessary to leave part of the deep myometrial disease.

Despite advances in surgical techniques, there is a very high variation in the incidence of residual lesions, with an average of 19%, probably related to the definition used for recurrence, type of endometriosis, length of follow-up and surgery, and technical surgical training [6].

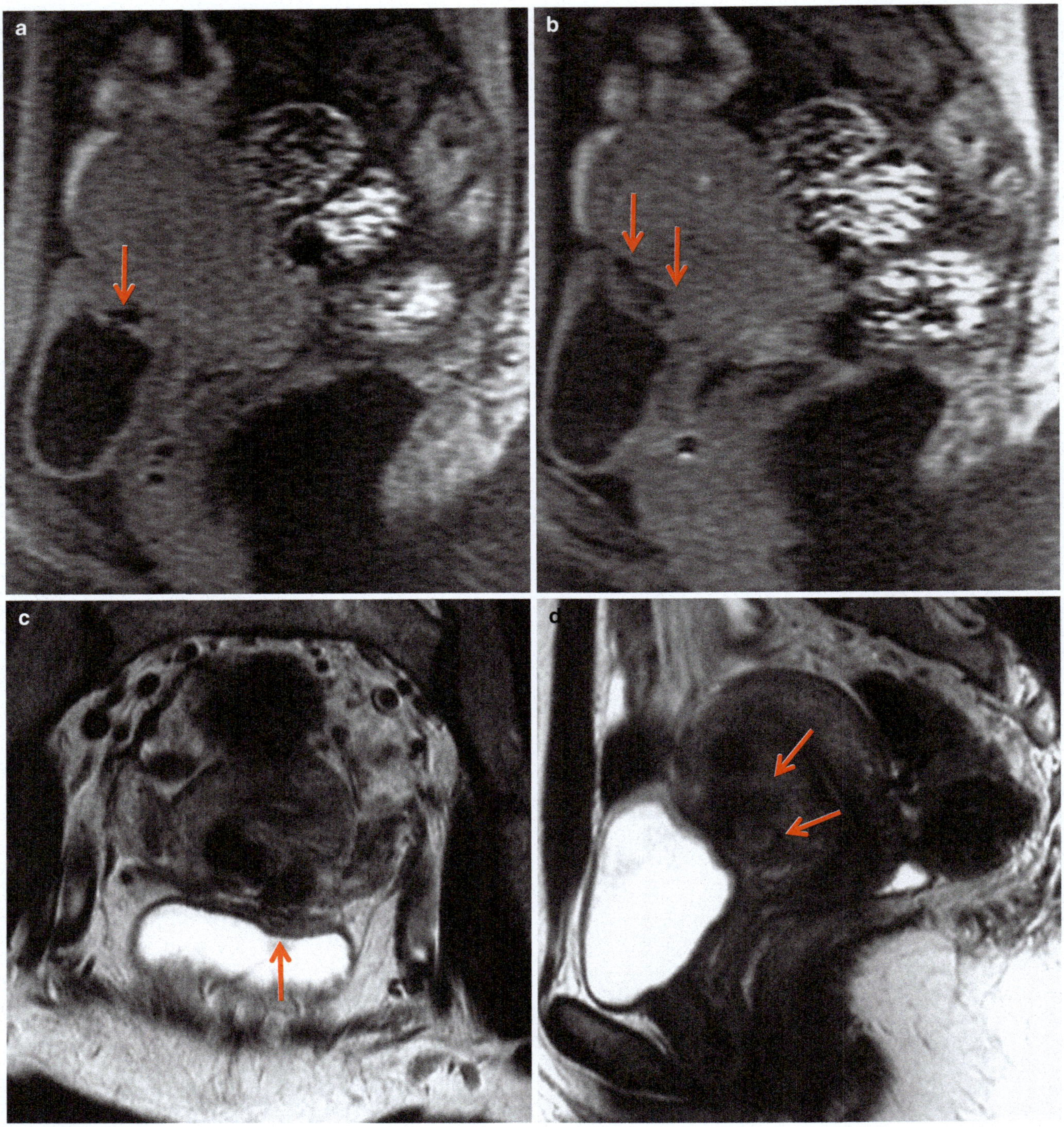

Fig. 6.14 Deep endometriosis after surgery. Progressive increase of the lesion, as well as appearance of ectopic endometrial tissue foci and bleeding. **First exam**: (**a–d**). Asymptomatic. (**a, b**) Fibrous cicatricial tissue with hypointense foci in the anterior compartment (arrows) and discrete hyperintense foci on the superior bladder surface (**c**), as well as myometrial blurring (**c, d**). **Second exam**: (**e–h**) Clinical complaint of occasional pain on urination during the menstrual period. (**e, f**) Infiltrative lesion with mass formation with hyperintense foci in T1- and T2-weighted image (arrows), characterizing ectopic endometrial glands and bleeding, in the fibrous cicatricial tissue. **Third exam**: (**g, h**) Increased lesion with myometrial, bladder, and ligament infiltration (arrows). (**a, b, e**) T1-weighted sequences. (**c, d, f–h**) T2 weighted. (**a, b, d–f**) Sagittal. (**c, g, h**) Coronal short axis

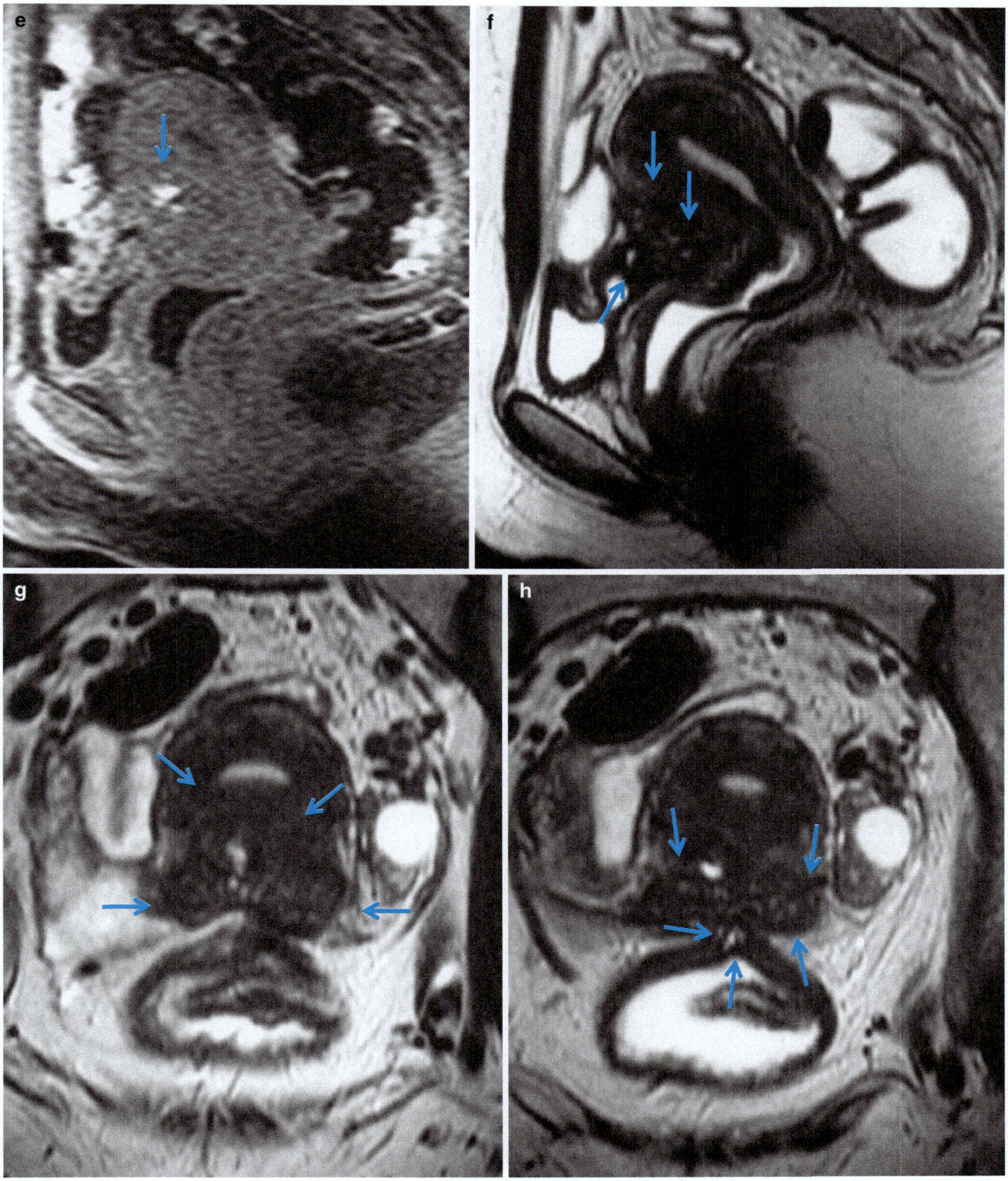

Fig. 6.14 (continued)

Most of the observed residual lesions correlate with the site of the surgical manipulation of the deep endometriosis and ovary.

6.12 Ovary

The ovary is the most common site of recurrence of endometriosis, especially in those who underwent surgical procedure. Incidence rates vary in the literature between 14 and 32% [6].

In most patients there are symptoms (pain or infertility in 75%) [7].

Superficial bleeding spots or endometriomas (Fig. 6.13) can be observed.

6.13 Infiltrative Endometriosis

In infiltrative endometriosis, there is little correlation between pain and clinical recurrence. However, clinical relapse does not always indicate residual disease [7].

Endometriosis should be suspected in these patients when minor bleeding intermingled with fibrosis, an infiltrative lesion with hyperintense foci in T2 is observed, featuring ectopic endometrial tissue, and hyperintense in T1, indicating bleeding (Fig. 6.14).

However, bleeding may be associated with a recent surgical procedure.

In these cases, we suggest always examining the surgical report, talking to the surgeon, and, if in doubt, carrying out a control RMI in 6 months.

References

1. Peixoto Crispi C. Tratado de Videoendoscopia e Cirurgia minimamente invasiva em Ginecologia. 5th ed. Rio de Janeiro: Revinter; 2011.
2. Kondo W. Spontaneous healing of a rectovaginal fistula developing after laparoscopic segmental bowel resection for intestinal deep infiltrating endometriosis. Case Rep Obstet Gynecol. 2013;2013:837–903.
3. Varol N. Rectal surgery for endometriosis: shoud we be aggressive? J Am Assoc Gynecol Laparosc. 2003;10(2):182–9.
4. Roman H. Complications associated with two laparoscopic procedures used in the management of rectal endometriosis. JSLS. 2010;14(2):169–77.
5. Palanivelu C. Laparoscopic management of iatrogenic high rectovaginal fistulas (Type VI). Singap Med J. 2007;48:96–8.
6. Guo SW. Recurrence of endometriosis and its control. Hum Reprod Update. 2009;15(4):441–61.
7. Exacoustos C. Recurrence of endometriomas after laparoscopic removal: sonographic and clinical follow-up and indication for second surgery. J Minim Invasive Gynecol. 2006;13(4):281–8.

Index

A

Abdominal adhesions
- anterior compartment, extensive adherence in, 49, 52
- hyperangulation of loops, 49–51
- kissing ovaries, 48, 49
- pelvic adhesion, signs of, 48
- posterior compartment, lesion in, 49, 53
- posterior deep endometriosis, 55, 56
- redundant sigmoid with uterus, 49, 54, 55

Adenomyosis process, 123
Adnexal lesions, characterization of, 42–44
Anterior abdominal wall
- canal of Nuck
  - endometriosis, 310
  - MRI and surgical finding, 310
  - treatment, 313
- cecum, terminal ileum and appendix, 316–317
  - anatomy, 313
  - clinical condition, 318
  - MRI and laparoscopic finding, 318
  - small bowel endometriosis with discontinuous lesions, 313–315
  - treatment, 322
- diaphragm
  - anatomy, 322
  - clinical conditions, 322
  - endometriosis, 322
  - MRI and laparoscopic finding, 322
  - treatment, 322
- umbilicus
  - anatomy, 300
  - clinical condition, 303
  - endometrioses, 302
  - MRI and surgical findings, 303, 307
  - treatment, 308

Anterior compartment deep endometriosis
- deep bladder lesion with right lateral localization, 68
- empty bladder, 65, 70
- extensive adherence in, 49, 52
- extension pattern, 66
- myometrium
  - anatomy, 122, 206
  - clinical manifestations, 125
  - clinical symptoms, 213
  - endometriosis, 123, 207
  - MRI and laparoscopic findings, 125, 131, 213, 214
  - treatment, 131, 218
- posterior vaginal fornix
  - anatomy, 195, 197–199
  - clinical symptoms, 199
  - MRI and laparoscopic findings, 199
  - treatment, 204
- rectovaginal space
  - anatomy, 161
  - clinical symptoms, 161
  - endometriosis, 161
  - MRI and laparoscopic finding, 165
  - treatment, 172
- rectum and sigmoid
  - anatomy, 219
  - clinical symptoms, 229
  - endometriosis, 221, 224
  - resonance and laparoscopic finding, 229, 231, 232
  - treatment, 232, 234
- retrocervical region
  - anatomy, 137
  - clinical symptoms, 152
  - extension pattern, 141, 142
  - intestinal predominance, 144
  - MRI and laparoscopic finding, 152, 153
  - myometrial penetration, 144
  - treatment, 160
- round ligament
  - anatomy, 107
  - clinical manifestations, 111
  - extraperitoneal portions, 111
  - intraperitoneal portions, 111
  - MRI and laparoscopic finding, 111, 113, 116
  - treatment, 122
- urinary tract
  - bladder anatomy, 71, 74
  - bladder roof, deep lesions in, 75, 77
  - clinical manifestations, 80
  - deep lesions in same patient, 75, 78
  - MRI and laparoscopic finding, 80–87
  - no cleavage plane with right ureteral ostium, 75, 79
  - positive cystoscopy, 75, 76
  - treatment, 87, 88
  - ureter anatomy, 90
  - ureteral endometriosis, 91, 93, 104, 106
- uterosacral ligaments Uterosacral ligaments

B

Bilateral endometriomas, 330
Bilateral ovarian endometriosis with superficial bleeding, 59, 60
Bladder anatomy, 71, 74
Bladder dysfunction, 352
Bleeding cyst, 303
Bowel endometriosis, 25

A. Brandão et al., *Atlas of Deep Endometriosis*, https://doi.org/10.1007/978-3-319-71697-8

C

Canal of Nuck
  endometriosis, 310
  MRI and surgical finding, 310
  treatment, 313
Choriocarcinoma, 44
Colorectal anastomosis, 349

D

Desmoid tumor, 46, 47, 303
Diffusion-weighted sequence (DWI), 42

E

Endometrioid cystadenocarcinoma, 333
Endometrioma, 269, 303
Evacuatory disturbance, 351

F

Fast spin-echo (FSE) pulse sequence, 15
Fibrous stroma, 206

G

Gradient-recalled-echo (GRE) sequences, 14

H

Hourglass-like lesion, 125

I

Infiltrative endometriosis, 197, 355, 356
Infiltrative multifocal intestinal endometriosis, 59, 63
Inflammatory process identification, 45
Inguinal region Canal of Nuck
Intestinal rectal endometriosis, 37
Irregular nodules, 269

K

Kissing ovaries, 48

L

Laparoscopic findings
  bladder deep endometriosis, 80
  cecum, terminal ileum and appendix, 318
  diaphragm, 322
  hypogastric nerve and plexus, 269
  myometrium, 125, 131, 213, 214
  ovarian fossa, 296
  parametrium and paracolpos, 251
  pelvic floor, 284
  posterior vaginal fornix, 199
  rectovaginal space, 165
  retrocervical region, 152, 153
  round ligament, 111, 113, 116
  ureteral endometriosis, 93, 104
  uterosacral ligament, 178, 182, 184
Lateral compartment, 6–7
  hypogastric nerve and plexus
    anatomy, 259
    clinical condition, 269
    endometriosis, 264
    MRI and laparoscopic findings, 269
    treatment, 269
  ovarian fossa Ovarian fossa
  parametrium and paracolpos
    anatomy, 240, 241
    clinical symptoms, 251
    endometriosis, 244
    MRI and laparoscopic findings, 251
    treatment, 259
  pelvic floor Pelvic floor
  ureter, 259
Location of deep endometriosis lesion, 65, 66, 68–70
  anterior compartment
    deep bladder endometriosis, 69
    deep bladder lesion with right lateral localization, 68
    deep lesion, 66
    empty bladder, 70
    extension pattern, 66
  bilateral ovarian endometriosis with superficial bleeding, 59, 60
  infiltrative multifocal intestinal endometriosis, 59, 63
  pelvic location
    abdominal location, 9, 10
    anterior compartment, 2–3
    lateral compartment, 2, 6, 7
    ovarian fossa, 2, 8
    posterior compartment, 2, 4, 5
  posterior lower fornix, 59, 61
  retrocervical lesion, 59, 64
Lower urinary tract endometriosis, 75

M

Magnetic resonance imaging (MRI)
  abdominal wall, endometriosis of, 19, 20
  adnexal lesions, characterization of, 42–44
  canal of Nuck, 310
  deep endometriotic lesions, morphology of, 26
    ligament thickening, 25, 27, 28
    plaque-like, 26, 33, 34
    subperitoneal nodule, 25, 30, 32
  enhancement pattern, 42
  equipment, 13
  inflammatory process identification, 45
  and laparoscopic findings
    bladder deep endometriosis, 80
    cecum, terminal ileum and appendix, 318
    diaphragm, 322
    hypogastric nerve and plexus, 269
    myometrium, 125, 131, 213, 214
    ovarian fossa, 296
    parametrium and paracolpos, 251
    pelvic floor, 284
    posterior vaginal fornix, 199
    rectovaginal space, 165
    retrocervical region, 152, 153
    round ligament, 111, 113, 116
    ureteral endometriosis, 93, 104
    uterosacral ligament, 178, 182, 184
  patient preparation, 21–23
  patient risk stratification, 327
    new examination before surgery, 337
    selection of patients, 327–330, 332–336
  protocol
    pelvic endometriosis protocol, 13, 14
    T1-weighted sequence, 14
    T2-weighted sequence, 15–19

signal intensity
fibrosis and glandular tissue, 36, 38, 39
predominantly fibrous lesions, 35–37
prominent glandular component, lesion with, 36, 40
small non-hemorrhagic abdominal wall deep endometriosis
abdominal adhesion, 46, 48–50, 52–56
gadolinium, 47, 48
umbilicus, 303, 307
Mantle lesion, 34
Mural nodule, 42, 43

O
Ovarian endometriosis, 60, 292, 354
Ovarian fossa
anatomy, 291
clinical condition, 292
endometriosis, 292
MRI and laparoscopic finding, 296
treatment, 300

P
Parametrium changes, 347, 348
Pelvic adhesion, signs of, 48
Pelvic floor
anatomy, 275, 283
clinical presentation, 291
MRI and laparoscopic findings, 284
treatment, 291
Pericervical ring, 175
Peritoneal endometriosis, 134
Peritoneal flow theory, 178
Persistent pelvic pain, 1
Plaque-like lesion, 26, 33, 34
Plaque-like myometrial lesion, 125
Polypoid endometriosis, 36, 42
Posterior compartment, 142, 145–147, 149, 152, 199
extension pattern, 134
lateral extension infiltrating, 134, 135
lesion in, 49, 53
pattern of, 135
peritoneal endometriosis, 134
posterior vaginal fornix, 199
retrocervical region
asymmetric posterior extension, 147
extensive parametrium and bilateral ligament involvement, 146
intestinal predominance, 149
myometrial penetration, 152
superior extension, 145
uterosacral ligaments, lateral extension to, 142
Posterior vaginal fornix
anatomy, 195, 197–199
clinical symptoms, 199
MRI and laparoscopic findings, 199
resection of, 345, 346
treatment, 204
Postsurgical fibrocicatricial tissue, 341
Postsurgical findings
bladder dysfunction, 352
colorectal anastomosis, 349
complications, 350
evacuatory disturbance, 351
foci of signal loss, 343
infiltrative endometriosis, 355, 356
ovary, 354
parametrium changes in, 347, 348
posterior vaginal fornix and uterine cervix, resection of, 345, 346
postsurgical fibrocicatricial tissue, 341
rectovaginal fistula, 353
residual lesions/recurrence, 354
Purely solid mass, 303

R
Rectovaginal fistula, 353
Residual lesions, 354
Retrouterinal lesion, 40

S
Sertoli-Leydig tumor, 44
Spiculated nodules, 269
Subperitoneal nodule, 25, 30, 32

U
Ureteral endometriosis, 91
clinical manifestations, 93
MRI and laparoscopic finding, 93, 104
treatment, 106
Uterine cervix, resection of, 345, 346
Uterosacral ligament
anatomy, 175–177
clinical symptoms, 178
endometriosis, 178
MRI and laparoscopic finding, 178, 182, 184
treatment, 192